NPTI's Fundamentals of Fitness and Personal Training

Tim Henriques, CPT

National Personal Training Institute

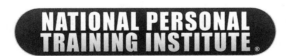

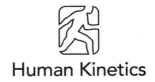

Human Kinetics

Library of Congress Cataloging-in-Publication Data

Henriques, Tim, 1976- author.
  NPTI's fundamentals of fitness and personal training / Tim Henriques.
     p. ; cm.
  National Personal Training Institute's fundamentals of fitness and personal training
  Fundamentals of fitness and personal training
  Includes bibliographical references and index.
     I. National Personal Training Institute, issuing body. II. Title. III. Title: National Personal Training Institute's fundamentals of fitness and personal training. IV. Title: Fundamentals of fitness and personal training.
     [DNLM: 1. Physical Fitness. 2. Physical Exertion--physiology. 3. Physiological Phenomena. 4. Resistance Training--methods. QT 255]
  RC1235
  613.7'11--dc23
                                      2013049300

ISBN: 978-1-4504-2381-6 (print)

Copyright © 2015 by NPTI Educational Resources, Inc.

The web addresses cited in this text were current as of March 2014, unless otherwise noted.

Acquisitions Editors: Michelle Maloney and Roger W. Earle; **Developmental Editor:** Melissa J. Zavala; **Managing Editor:** Rachel Fowler; **Copyeditor:** Bob Replinger; **Indexer:** Nancy Ball; **Permissions Manager:** Dalene Reeder; **Graphic Designer:** Fred Starbird; **Graphic Artist:** Kathleen Boudreau-Fuoss; **Cover Designer:** Keith Blomberg; **Photographs (interior):** © Human Kinetics, unless otherwise noted; **Photo Asset Manager:** Laura Fitch; **Visual Production Assistant:** Joyce Brumfield; **Photo Production Manager:** Jason Allen; **Art Manager:** Kelly Hendren; **Associate Art Manager:** Alan L. Wilborn; **Illustrations:** © Human Kinetics, unless otherwise noted; **Printer:** Sheridan Books

Printed in the United States of America   10   9   8   7   6   5   4   3   2   1

The paper in this book is certified under a sustainable forestry program.

Human Kinetics
Website: www.HumanKinetics.com

United States: Human Kinetics
P.O. Box 5076
Champaign, IL 61825-5076
800-747-4457
e-mail: humank@hkusa.com

Canada: Human Kinetics
475 Devonshire Road Unit 100
Windsor, ON N8Y 2L5
800-465-7301 (in Canada only)
e-mail: info@hkcanada.com

Europe: Human Kinetics
107 Bradford Road
Stanningley
Leeds LS28 6AT, United Kingdom
+44 (0) 113 255 5665
e-mail: hk@hkeurope.com

Australia: Human Kinetics
57A Price Avenue
Lower Mitcham, South Australia 5062
08 8372 0999
e-mail: info@hkaustralia.com

New Zealand: Human Kinetics
P.O. Box 80
Torrens Park, South Australia 5062
0800 222 062
e-mail: info@hknewzealand.com

E5644

Contents

≡16≡ **Practical Application of Nutritional Knowledge** **225**

≡17≡ **Resistance Training Program Design** **245**

≡18≡ **Beginner Workout** **281**

≡27≡ Injury and Rehabilitation 447

Preface

Congratulations! By selecting this book, you have taken a significant step toward becoming a health professional and becoming qualified to work in the fitness field. This book will provide you with in-depth knowledge about the human body—the most amazing, complex, and versatile machine on the planet. In this book we will unlock some of those secrets and learn how the body works and how it responds to exercise. This book will also provide in-depth knowledge about the field of personal training. Personal training is an exciting field that offers many career opportunities. Personal trainers are able to work in a friendly, enjoyable environment where they are not stuck behind a desk all day performing a job that they might not find fulfilling. Many personal trainers enjoy significant autonomy and control over their work schedule. Personal training is an excellent full-time or part-time job that can be financially rewarding. Best of all, personal trainers get to share their knowledge with clients to help them improve their health, fitness, and quality of life. In this field you help others every day that you go to work. A qualified and certified personal trainer assists clients by helping them to achieve goals they never thought possible, by enabling them to improve their fitness levels to enjoy life as fully as possible, and by aiding them in optimizing their health to live as long as possible.

This book was written for personal trainers, although others can read it to learn the secrets that the professionals use to achieve the amazing results that they do. It was specifically written as a text to complement the rigorous curriculum of the National Personal Training Institute (NPTI). NPTI, the leading system of personal training schools in the United States, provides a 500- to 600-hour, 6- to 12-month-long educational program for people who want to become personal trainers.

Surprisingly, schools for personal trainers are relatively rare. Currently, the most common way to become a personal trainer is to purchase study materials (a textbook and perhaps a video), study at home, attend a weekend seminar, and then take a personal training exam. If you pass, you become a "certified" personal trainer, but you are likely not truly qualified. The goal of NPTI is to raise the standards and strengthen the criteria for qualification as a personal trainer. For people who want more from their training, NPTI provides a level of education that goes beyond the textbooks and self-study material to include time in a classroom with an instructor and practical experience and hands-on education in the gym.

The NPTI program includes approximately 100 hours on exercise program design, 100 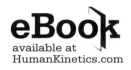 hours on nutrition, 100 hours on anatomy and physiology, and 200 hours of practical experience in the gym with hands-on training. Part of that applied experience is working out every day while you are in the class. You practice personal training on fellow students under the supervision of an instructor and learn all the ins and outs of the equipment in a fitness center. Upon graduation, a successful student receives a diploma in personal training granting that student the title of certified personal trainer (CPT), a certificate in nutrition (the specific title varies by state), and certification in CPR and AED, the latter of which must be renewed on a periodic basis.

This book was written to help address two of the most important questions in fitness: How does the body respond to exercise, and what kind of exercise program should a person follow to achieve specific results? Although this book provides answers to those questions primarily for personal trainers, I believe that anyone with a passion for fitness will benefit from the material contained within the book. Many current fitness books are adequate for the beginner, but they don't provide the complex, in-depth information that many people desire. Textbooks provide that deeper level of knowledge, but those books are tedious to read and include content so esoteric that applying it to a client's workout program is difficult. Worse yet, some textbooks are rooted so deeply in academia that it is obvious that the information provided was not given by authors who have experience in the trenches. Instead, those authors choose to present nice theories without realizing that theory and practical application to real clients are often two different things. My goal with this book is to bridge the gap between those two extremes. I have plucked all the useful information provided in the good textbooks and relate it in the relatively easy-to-read tone that is found is most beginner fitness books. I hope that I have been successful in that venture. In addition, I offer specific exercise programs that my personal-training clients, my students, and I have tried, tested, and proved effective. You can rest assured that the programs presented here will yield results in the gym. I do not just think these programs will work; I know they will work.

A list of key concept references appears at the end of the book. A complete list of all references cited in this book is available at www.HumanKinetics.com/products/all-products/NPTIs-Fundamentals-of-Fitness-and-Personal-Training under the More to Explore section. An instructor guide and presentation package with image bank are available at www.HumanKinetics.com/NPTIs FundamentalsOfFitnessAndPersonalTraining. The instructor guide provides activity ideas for instructors and sample course outlines and syllabi. There are also chapter summaries and suggestions for class projects or student assign-ments for every chapter. The presentation package slides and accompanying image bank include all the art, tables, and photos and can be customized to create presentations. The text in each slide presents the major topics covered in each chapter.

Many people are frustrated with conflicting information, unable to attain and maintain results, and depressed about their bodies and their general state of health. Many people do not like their bodies or even themselves because of this. That is not the way it is supposed to be. Your body is the greatest gift you will ever receive. You should feel exhilarated about what your body is capable of, not ashamed of how it looks or performs. You have the power to change your own body, and with that power comes the ability to help others achieve the same life-changing result. We need strong leaders in the health and fitness industry to show the way, and the best way to lead is by example. It is time to meet that challenge head on and help those around you emerge from the darkness that is poor health and into the light of a healthy and rewarding lifestyle.

I wish you good luck in your venture into the fitness field. A quick look around at the state of health of people today indicates that we are in dire need of your help to improve your clients' physical fitness and health.

Note: This publication is written and published to provide accurate and authoritative information relevant to the subject matter presented. It is published and sold with the understanding that the author and publisher are not engaged in rendering legal, medical, or other professional services by reason of their authorship or publication of this work. If medical or other expert assistance is required, the services of a competent professional person should be sought.

Components of Fitness

Because this book is ultimately for personal trainers, the first task is to define what a personal trainer does. Careers and industries usually have a scope of practice that helps outline what a person's training is and, equally important, what it is not. The scope of practice for a personal trainer is to enhance the components of fitness for the general, healthy population. A personal trainer is educated and trained in ways to improve each of the components of fitness and to apply that information to healthy adults. In this definition the word *general* refers to the age range for clients, referring to people between the ages of 18 and 50. The exact age range can vary depending on a variety of factors, a topic that will be covered in depth in chapter 3. The word *healthy*, in its strictest definition, means absence of disease. For a personal trainer, the primary concern is related to diseases that would affect exercise—metabolic disorders such as diabetes and cardiopulmonary conditions such as hypertension and heart disease. If a client falls outside the general, healthy population, then the client needs to receive medical clearance from another health professional, usually a doctor, before beginning an intense exercise program (3, 93). But exercise of some form or another will benefit almost all people, and most doctors are happy to hear that patients want to begin a fitness regime. The chapter on risk stratification (chapter 3) discusses the types of clients who need to see and receive clearance from a doctor and the limitations that they may have when engaged in personal training.

The second part of the scope of practice references the components of fitness. Traditionally, fitness includes five components— muscular strength, muscular endurance, cardiovascular endurance, flexibility, and body composition—as well as key subcomponents such as speed, power, agility, quickness, and skill (6, 7, 8). Each component covers a specific aspect of a person's overall fitness. Breaking down fitness into separate components helps you, as an aspiring personal trainer, prioritize your efforts with your clients. Each of these components has a corresponding standardized test that you can use to measure your client's starting point and subsequent progress. The following sections explain the five components of fitness and the various ways in which they are tested. The components are presented in no particular order and are not ranked in terms of value. Each is like a spoke in a wheel. One spoke is not necessarily more or less important than another.

MUSCULAR STRENGTH

Muscular strength is the ability of the muscles to contract one time (complete one repetition, or rep) in a specific exercise or movement. This act is called the one-rep maximum, or 1RM. Muscular strength is commonly tested on such exercises as the bench press, squat, deadlift, chest press, and leg press, but a person could perform a 1RM test on any exercise. Safety must be paramount when maxing out (performing one maximum effort), and the proper way to max out is covered in detail in chapter 17. The sports of powerlifting, Olympic weightlifting, and shot put, along with everyday examples such as lifting up the end of a couch, picking up a dog or child, or opening a jar take advantage of muscular strength (66, 85).

MUSCULAR ENDURANCE

Muscular endurance is the ability of the muscles to contract repeatedly (perform multiple reps of an exercise). A muscular endurance test normally involves 20 or more reps. Muscular endurance is commonly tested with the popular exercises of push-ups, sit-ups, and pull-ups, although you can set up almost any kind of muscular endurance test for your clients. Specific exercises or movements test different areas of the body; they do not test the entire body all at once. This aspect of fitness can be referred to as local muscular endurance. The difference between muscular endurance and strength is the number of repetitions completed. For strength, the movement is performed only one time; when your clients perform another rep of the same weight, you have included the element of muscular endurance. The more reps that your client completes, the more important muscular endurance becomes. The fewer reps that your client performs, the more important strength becomes (32).

BODY COMPOSITION

Body composition is the percentage of lean and fat mass in the body, commonly referred to as percent body fat. All mass in the body can be broken down into one of two categories. Body parts that have little fat, such as bone, muscles, and organs, make up a person's lean or fat-free mass. Fat mass is called adipose tissue, or just fat. When clients can "pinch an inch," that part of the body is mostly fat, and when they go on a diet, they are trying to reduce their body fat. If you know your client's percent body fat, you can determine his or her percent body lean. For example, if a client weighs 200 pounds (90.7 kg) and has 20 percent body fat, then the client is 80 percent body lean (4).

Body fat can be measured in many ways, and some methods are more accurate than others. None, however, is perfect, so keep in mind that a calculation of your client's percent body fat is just an estimate. The primary methods of measuring body composition (calipers, bioelectrical impedance, hydrostatic weighing, and DEXA X-ray imaging) are outlined in detail in chapter 3.

FLEXIBILITY

Flexibility is defined as the range of motion (ROM) at a joint. Some joints, such as the shoulder, have a high degree of flexibility; some are fused together, such as the joints in the skull; and some joints offer limited range of motion, such as the bones that make up the spine. The most common flexibility test is the sit and reach, in which you have a client sit on the floor with the legs straight and reach forward for the toes. This test measures the flexibility of the client's hamstrings, gluteals, and lower back. Other tests for flexibility, such as the shoulder elevation test, wall test, and overhead squat test, are outlined in chapter 3.

With flexibility, unlike strength or muscular endurance, more is not always better. Most often, injuries occur in people who are either very inflexible or extremely flexible; people who have a normal, middle-of-the-road level of flexibility experience the fewest injuries (1). When the body is extremely flexible, which is sometimes referred to as hypermobility, the joints are actually loose, which increases the chance of injury, although this condition is relatively rare. If the joints are extremely tight, any exaggerated motion puts extra stress on the joints and on the surrounding muscle, which also contributes to injury (50).

CARDIOVASCULAR ENDURANCE

Cardiovascular endurance is the ability of the heart and lungs to deliver oxygen to the body. *Cardio* means "heart"; *vascular* means "vessels," referring to the arteries and veins that carry blood. Cardiovascular endurance is sometimes referred to as cardiorespiratory endurance; *respiratory* refers to the lungs. It may simply be referenced as aerobic fitness. Someone who can run a marathon or swim a mile has good cardiovascular endurance.

Exercise scientists have developed tests to quantify cardiovascular endurance, and a person's ability on those tests is called $\dot{V}O_2max$. V stands for volume, O_2 is for oxygen, and *max* means "maximal." $\dot{V}O_2max$ is the maximal volume of oxygen that a person can deliver to the body. The units are milliliters of oxygen per kilogram of body weight per minute. That measure is discussed in detail in chapter 3 (2, 22, 105). Maximal tests include the $\dot{V}O_2max$ test and the 1.5-mile (2.4 km) run, and submaximal tests include the Rockport walk test, the fit test, and the step test.

So the five components of fitness are muscular strength, muscular endurance, body composition, flexibility, and cardiovascular endurance. Remember that one of the goals of this book is to help you improve both your own fitness and your clients' fitness. A good philosophy to follow is to realize that you are your first personal-training client. You do not have to look as if you belong on the cover of a magazine, but you should regularly exercise and strive to be fit yourself. You will learn a lot along the way, and you will provide a powerful example to clients if you walk the walk instead of just talk the talk. The message of fitness tends to get lost when it is delivered by people who do not practice what they preach. When in doubt, always try to lead by example.

The scope of practice for a personal trainer is to enhance the components of fitness. Therefore, you need to become an expert in the components of fitness by understanding what they are and knowing the definition and common tests of each component. A focus of this book is to learn how to improve each of those components. With some practice, time, and effort, you will feel comfortable improving these components on yourself and on your clients.

Although the concept of the five components of fitness is generally accepted, it is not meant to be an exhaustive list of all fitness-related abilities. For example, balance, an important ability, is not listed. Speed can be crucial in sport. Skill is important in determining performance in an event, and, of course, a person's nutrition makes a big difference in how his or her body performs. Some include the terms *accuracy* and *coordination* as aspects of fitness, although skill likely accounts for those subcomponents. Nutrition is a factor in body composition. To have a healthy percentage of body fat, a person must be eating at least close to the proper number and right type of calories per day.

Why do you, as an aspiring personal trainer, need to know the five components of fitness? First, knowing the components of fitness will be extremely helpful in setting and achieving fitness goals. Understanding the components of fitness allows you to assess where you are with your own fitness level and where you would like to be; it highlights your strengths and weaknesses. It also highlights your clients' strengths and weaknesses. Whenever possible, try to relate a client's goals to the key components of fitness, because your training and education is in that area.

Second, understanding the five components of fitness helps break down fitness into something more manageable. You are ultimately going to have to decide which components you are going to prioritize for yourself and your clients, and this judgment will guide your training programs. Does your client want to be good at everything, or would that client prefer to specialize? Is the client already proficient at one component of fitness? Does the client need extra work in a particular component of fitness?

Although all components of fitness work together to form an integrated whole, at certain times and during certain events, one component may be vastly more important than the others. In sports that rely primarily on strength or cardiovascular endurance, the components required for success are almost opposites.

A person who wishes to achieve relatively elite levels of performance at a certain activity will have to specialize at some point. One of the benefits of specializing is that doing so focuses the training and allows the athlete to make as much progress as possible with that one ability. The downside, of course, is that you spend less time on the other components. Your client's abilities may not improve in those aspects; in fact, they may even decline (92). In addition, recognize that an average score of fitness would generally be higher for a person who did not specialize than it would be for someone who did, assuming both spent equal time training (see figure 1.1).

As you can see from figure 1.1, one athlete chose to specialize in strength. His cardiovascular endurance, therefore, is relatively low compared with that of aerobic endurance athletes. The second athlete chose to specialize in cardiovascular endurance. His strength, therefore, is low. The third athlete did not specialize in either strength or cardiovascular endurance. As a result, her strength is not as high as that of the strength athlete and her cardiovascular endurance is not as good as that of the aerobic endurance athlete, but the average of her two scores is higher than the average of either the first or the second athlete. She is not a specialist, but she is well rounded. In terms of pure health and not performance, it is probably more beneficial for the body to be well rounded (47).

One thing to keep in mind as we talk about specializing is that you should talk to your clients about specializing only after they have completed the beginner workout, which is described thoroughly in chapter 18. A beginner, someone who has never formally exercised, may come into the gym and say, "I want to bench press a lot, so I am just going to focus on that." But you do not allow that person to jump right into a specialist's program. All good athletes have a solid base of fitness, meaning that they are at least decent at all the components of fitness. Remember to build up the base first and then put the final changes on at the end.

LEGAL ISSUES IN PERSONAL TRAINING

As a practicing personal trainer, you need to be aware of the common legal issues that can affect your business. The good news is that clients rarely sue personal trainers and even more rarely win the case. The bad news is that the general rate of lawsuits is increasing in America, and clients are aware of their ability to sue almost anyone for anything.

If a client sues a personal trainer, the primary claim will be that the personal trainer was negligent. Negligence is defined by *The Free Dictionary* as follows:

Conduct that falls below the standards of behavior established by law for the protection of others against unreasonable risk of harm. A person has acted negligently if he or she has departed from the conduct expected of a reasonably prudent person acting under similar circumstances. In order to establish negligence as a Cause of Action under the law of torts, a plaintiff must prove that the defendant had a duty to the plaintiff, the defendant breached that duty by failing to conform to the required standard of conduct, the defendant's negligent conduct was the cause of the harm to the plaintiff, and the plaintiff was, in fact, harmed or damaged.

In simple terms the definition is saying that the personal trainer was supposed to do something, the personal trainer failed to do that thing, and the client was injured (or worse) because of that action. If the client was not harmed or damaged, the client will not have a strong case. If something happened that a reasonable personal trainer could have not predicted or prevented, the client will not have a strong case. Both aspects need to be clear to find the personal trainer negligent (6).

An examination of lawsuits involving personal trainers and their clients reveals that

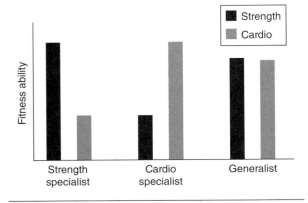

Figure 1.1 Specialization versus generalization.

personal trainers can do several things to safeguard themselves against a lawsuit.

• **Don't make false claims**. If a personal trainer claims to be certified or have special training (for example, claims to be a nutritionist) but is in fact not certified, the personal trainer is setting her- or himself up for trouble. Because the personal trainer is not certified, she or he technically should not be dealing with the client, so anything that happens to the client is much more likely to be the personal trainer's fault (55). Personal trainers should make sure their certifications and specialties are up to date and should avoid claiming that they have education they don't actually have.

• **Have all clients sign a release waiver**. In most legal cases against personal trainers, the waiver is the primary evidence that protects the personal trainer. The waiver should inform the client of the risks associated with exercise including bodily harm and potentially death. The language of the waiver should be clear and explicit. If personal trainers create their own waivers, they should have someone trained in legal matters look over the waiver to make sure that it will hold up in court. The waiver should be a separate form, clearly titled, that the client signs. In one instance of a successful lawsuit against a personal trainer, the waiver was included as part of the financial agreement. It was hard to read, the font was the same as that used in the contract, and the waiver didn't hold up. All clients should sign a waiver regardless of risk stratification or apparent health before they perform any exercise with a personal trainer. A signed waiver is the most important tool in protecting a personal trainer (30).

• **Listen to the client if he or she asks to stop exercising**. If a client asks to stop exercising, the personal trainer needs to listen and respect the wishes of the client. A personal trainer should be able to distinguish between a client's complaint that the exercise is challenging and a client's request to stop the exercise. If a client asks to stop exercising, especially if the request is repeated and done in a serious fashion, and the personal trainer ignores this request and pushes the client on, then the personal trainer may be found negligent because a "reasonable personal trainer" is likely to have listened to the client.

• **Avoid rhabdomyolysis**. Often referred to as *rhabdo* for short, rhabdomyolysis is the breakdown of muscle fibers that leads to the release of muscle fiber contents (myoglobin) into the bloodstream. Myoglobin is harmful to the kidneys and can cause kidney damage. Rhabdo is most commonly caused by a personal trainer's prescription of an exceedingly high number of repetitions with very low weight or calisthenic exercises. For example, having a beginner perform 500 body-weight squats in her or his first session might induce rhabdo (6). Ironically, using an appropriate amount of resistance for beginners (as outlined in chapter 18) will not induce rhabdo because even if the client trains until failure, which is not recommended, the weight would be too heavy for the client to perform the necessary number of reps. The client would simply be unable to keep going. But if the client performs a very large number of reps on an exercise that she or he can do (at least partially), the muscle can become so broken down by the exercise that it will release some of its substances into the bloodstream, some of which can be toxic to the kidneys. Rhabdo can lead to kidney damage, kidney failure, dialysis, and even death. Clients will almost assuredly ask to stop the exercise before this sets in. Reasonable intensity and volume will not produce rhabdo even in untrained, beginning clients.

• **Follow the risk stratification guidelines**. Chapter 3 covers the forms that clients should fill out and the intensity at which they should train when they first work with a personal trainer. Personal trainers who do not follow this standard of conduct run the risk that a client might claim that the personal trainer was negligent and did not properly discover the client's history before exercise. The waiver is still likely to protect a personal trainer in this case, but a qualified personal trainer should seek to learn as much as possible about the client's health history before having the person engage in a workout program. Of course, the personal trainer should follow the recommendations based on the client's risk stratification.

• **Use common sense**. Finally, personal trainers should simply use common sense. Don't modify equipment in the gym for a purpose other than what it was designed for, particularly if the setup appears unsafe. Err on the side of caution with a client—the client is not preparing for the Super Bowl, and everything is not riding on completing that next set or rep. If necessary, reduce the intensity or stop the exercise, do something different, or end the exercise session and allow the client to rest and recover. Pay attention to your clients and ask them how they are feeling. Be cautious when recommending supplementation (particularly if you have no formal training in nutrition), especially supplements that might affect metabolism. Always suggest to clients that they consult with their doctors before taking anything. Stick within your scope of practice and keep the client's well-being at the front of your mind. If clients are lifting heavy weights (for them), be sure that you are in a position to spot them and monitor their safety. Be extra cautious when training an area that has been previously injured, and record all key aspects of the workouts.

Personal trainers should also have liability insurance to help protect them in the event that they are sued. A personal trainer who works for a gym or health club will normally be covered under the umbrella of the club's policy, although the personal trainer should confirm the accuracy of that supposition. A personal trainer who is working independently should carry his or her own liability insurance. Unlike doctors or other health care practitioners who have to set aside a large amount of their income to cover their insurance, personal trainers can usually obtain a million dollars' worth of coverage for $150 or $200 per year. Personal trainers can usually become insured immediately after spending 10 to 15 minutes on a website or on the phone with an insurance company that deals with personal training insurance.

Being sued by a client is unlikely to occur, but it can happen. Personal trainers need to be familiar with what might go wrong so that they can be proactive and work to prevent those issues.

CONCLUSION

The scope of practice for personal trainers is to enhance the components of fitness for the general, healthy population. The classic components of fitness are muscular strength, muscular endurance, body composition, flexibility, and cardiovascular endurance. A personal trainer should know the definitions of those terms and common assessments for each component of fitness.

Luckily, legal cases against personal trainers are reasonably rare, but personal trainers should not rely on the fact that a client is unlikely to sue them. Personal trainers need to avoid being negligent in their duties, and they need to make sure that they are not doing any of the following activities: making false claims, forgetting to have clients sign waivers, ignoring client requests to stop, causing rhabdomyolysis by prescribing excessive exercise, not observing risk stratification guidelines, not having insurance, and not using common sense.

Study Questions

1. What is the scope of practice for certified personal trainers?
   a. to increase the muscularity of all clients
   b. to diagnose and cure clients from all physical ailments
   c. to enhance the components of fitness for the general, healthy population
   d. to adjust the client's musculoskeletal system so that the body functions in perfect harmony

2. Which of the following are three of the five classic components of fitness defined in this chapter?
   a. weight, speed, stamina
   b. power, skill, metabolism
   c. body composition, cardiovascular endurance, muscular endurance
   d. flexibility, power, agility

3. How would a person's body weight generally affect his or her $\dot{V}O_2$max score, assuming that all other variables remained the same?

    a. A lighter body weight would tend to decrease the $\dot{V}O_2$max score.

    b. A lighter body weight would tend to increase the $\dot{V}O_2$max score.

    c. A heavier body weight would tend to increase the $\dot{V}O_2$max score.

    d. $\dot{V}O_2$max is completely independent of body weight; it is not part of the equation.

4. What is rhabdomyolysis?

    a. During hard exercise, the muscles periodically twitch and spasm.

    b. After hard exercise, the muscles immediately grow from the workout.

    c. During hard exercise, myoglobin is released into the bloodstream, which can be harmful.

    d. During hard exercise, muscles eat all the negative bacteria in the system, thus boosting the immune system for 72 hours.

5. Which of the following should a personal trainer do during a personal training session to help minimize the risk of a lawsuit?

    a. Follow risk stratification guidelines and have all clients sign a waiver.

    b. Induce rhabdomyolysis and push new clients past their perceived pain barriers.

    c. Start training before becoming certified and use only high-risk exercises.

    d. Diagnose a client's medical problems and order the client to stop taking all medications prescribed by a doctor.

Principles of Exercise

To have a solid grasp of exercise and the science behind it, you need to understand several principles of fitness. In all fields, core principles and a unifying theory act as a template and provide a foundation for understanding and further study. Darwin's theory of natural selection is that unifying theory for biology. The justification hypothesis is a unifying theory for psychology, and it helps people understand the evolution of language and culture and humankind's unique capacity for self-awareness (15).

Kinesiology—the study of movement—does not yet have a unifying theory. Kinesiology is a young science, and the advanced study of personal training and fitness is relatively new. Thirty years ago personal trainers were rare, and few made that their full-time job. Fifty years ago it was unusual to see someone jogging down the street. Although our field is young, key principles help guide and categorize our knowledge (2, 8).

PROGRESSIVE OVERLOAD

The principle of progressive overload states that to force the body to respond to a stimulus, a person must gradually place a load on the body that it is not accustomed to. The term *overload* simply means a load, often a weight, that is over and above what the body is used to handling. A progressive overload refers to a load that continuously increases as the body adapts. When the body adapts to one load, for example, 50 pounds (22.7 kg), a person must increase the load to 60 pounds (27.2 kg) to continue the response of adaptation.

Normally, this progression is gradual; you don't lift 100 pounds (45.4 kg) and then the next day attempt to lift 200 pounds (90.7 kg). Instead, you might go for 105 pounds (47.6 kg) the next time around. Overload does not have to refer to weight. Increasing reps is another form of overload. And you do not have to increase the load linearly, meaning that you do not have to go up 5 pounds (2.3 kg) or one rep every week, although that kind of increase works well in the beginning stages of training. Rather, the trend over time is for the workouts to become progressively more challenging. Later we will discuss the multiple ways of increasing the load. If your clients begin an exercise program today and train consistently for the next six months, their workout six months from today should be more challenging than their workout today.

A story popular in the fitness world is that of Milo, a wrestler in ancient Greece, who was known for his incredible strength. He reportedly developed that strength by initially picking up a baby calf and carrying it around. He did that every day, and as the calf grew so did his strength. Ultimately, he was able to pick up and carry a fully grown cow. He didn't practice with the baby calf and then try to pick up an adult cow. The same principle applies to lifting weights. We may see people in the gym get used to a certain weight and then try to go up 50 pounds (22.7 kg) because they don't like putting the small weights on the bar. This approach is incredibly foolish. If you go up 5 pounds (2.3 kg) per week in an exercise and continue that for one year, your max will improve by 250 pounds (113.4 kg). Going up by 5 pounds (2.3 kg) per month, progress that many people might snicker at, means an increase of 60 pounds (27.2 kg) per year. Small progress over time adds up to big gains in the long run. As the old proverb goes, the greatest journey is made up of a series of single steps.

SPECIFICITY

The principle of specificity, also known as specific adaptation to imposed demand, or the SAID principle, states that the body will respond specifically to the unique demands placed on it. This rule applies to everything we do. If you run frequently, your body will respond to that activity. The bones in your feet and legs will harden, your leg muscles will build endurance, and your heart and lungs will work more efficiently. But running will have little positive effect on your ability to bench press a heavy weight (10). On the flip side, improving your bench press will likely not help you run 4 miles (6.4 km) in 30 minutes. In simple terms, the principle of specificity says that you become proficient at what you practice. If you want to be a good runner, you need to spend time running. If you want to learn how to shoot foul shots in basketball, you need to practice that activity. If you want to learn to play Ping-Pong, you practice that activity (6, 9, 13). The body will respond to the particular demand placed on it. It will not respond broadly; instead, it will respond specifically.

INDIVIDUAL VARIATION

The principle of individual variation asserts that each person is different and will respond differently to the same stimulus. The variation in response of individuals is not random; rather, a wide array of variables affects how a person responds to exercise. Those variables include but are not limited to genetics, body size, body composition, hormonal levels, sex, training experience, training intensity, stress level, daily sleep, nutritional status, health status, regular use of drugs, and motivation.

Thousands of students have taken the National Personal Training Institute program to become personal trainers. For the first month of that program, those students follow a set workout, similar to the beginner workout described in this book. Although all the students follow the same workout, their results vary. Some make more progress than others do, and some make great gains in certain areas but not as much in other areas. Those results exemplify the principle of individual variation. Individual responses vary.

Although everyone is different, your job as a personal trainer is to assess how the variables are affecting your client's performance. The more control you exert over those variables, the more you will be able to control how the body responds to exercise. If a program isn't working, then you need to ask why and do your best to address the reasons it is not. Did the client really follow the program? What was the client's nutrition plan? How hard did the client work out? Did the client experience zero results, or did the person just not get the results that he or she was looking for? Did you accurately measure the client's abilities before and after to know that he or she didn't really make any progress? What can you change to make sure that the client experiences progress next time? Frustrating though it may be, a period of exercising without making significant progress can be quite educational for the personal trainer in discovering what works and what doesn't. For this reason among others, personal trainers should exercise hard themselves. Finding out what doesn't work on yourself first (and ultimately what does work) is better than having those experiences with a paying client.

FITT PRINCIPLE

The FITT principle refers to the four main variables of any workout program: frequency, intensity, time, and type. Each of these variables must be in proper alignment with the others for maximal fitness gains to occur. You can use these four variables to design a training program and assess the appropriateness of a workout plan for a specific person.

Frequency

Frequency refers both to how often a person works out and to how frequently that person trains each muscle group or body movement. Frequency is normally defined as the number of times in a one-week period. If you train Monday, Wednesday, and Friday, you have a frequency of three times a week. If you complete a total-body workout each time you work out, then your frequency for training each muscle group is also three times per week. But if Monday's workout trains the chest, shoulders, and triceps; Wednesday's workout trains the back, biceps, and abdominal muscles; and Friday's workout trains the legs and lower back (which would be classified as a push–pull and legs workout routine), then your frequency for training each muscle group is one time per week.

Intensity

Intensity refers to how strenuously or vigorously you work out. Intensity is applied to both cardiovascular exercise and resistance training (lifting weights). When training with weights, one way that we measure intensity is as a percentage of the maximum amount of weight you can lift one time, or your one-repetition max, or 1RM. If you can bench 250 pounds (113.4 kg) one time and you are lifting 185 pounds (83.9 kg), you are training with 75 percent of your 1RM. Of course, the closer you are to your 1RM, the more intense the lift is. Additionally, the number of reps that you complete with a given weight is another factor in intensity.

During cardiovascular exercise, intensity is assessed by measuring heart rate, expressed as a percentage of maximum heart rate (MHR). The only way to know your true maximum heart rate is to perform a $\dot{V}O_2$max test, but you can estimate your maximum heart rate. The formula is 220 minus your age. If you are 30 years old, your maximum heart rate is 190 beats per minute; if you are 50, it is projected to be 170 beats per minute. Intensity is the percentage of the max heart rate where you want to train. This value is called your target heart rate (THR), and it normally ranges between 60 and 85 percent of MHR.

You can measure your heart rate with several methods. You can manually take your pulse, you can use the heart rate monitor that is found on most cardiovascular machines, or you can use your own heart rate monitor. For the most reliable and consistent measurement, a heart rate monitor is recommended. A strap that goes around your chest under your shirt transmits your heart rate either to the cardio machine or to a special watch. Training with a heart rate monitor and observing what is happening to your pulse is instructive. You will learn a lot about how you respond to exercise by doing so. You may want to suggest to your clients that they wear a heart rate monitor while training with you, particularly if they are focused on achieving cardiovascular-related goals.

Your heart rate tells you how hard your body is working. Imagine the body as an engine; your heart rate monitor is your tachometer (the gauge that displays an engine's RPMs). The higher you rev that engine, the harder you work and the higher your heart rate goes. And like all engines, the body has a maximum heart rate that it cannot exceed.

Extensive study of aerobic exercise has determined that the range of 60 to 85 percent of MHR is the most productive for most people. If you drop below 60 percent intensity, then the exercise is too easy and your body will not respond optimally to the stimulus. In other words, you won't get all the benefit from the cardio work that you could. Sixty percent intensity is relatively easy; people can often get their heart rate up in this range just by walking (47).

Some form of exercise is always better than nothing. If your clients say to you, "I am exercising at either 50 percent of MHR or not at all," we would prefer that they work at 50 percent rather than not work at all. They will still get some benefit. But you might point out to them that if they are already exercising and spending time to improve their health, they should consider going to at least 60 percent so that they can enjoy more of the benefits of exercise. Working out more intensely doesn't take any longer, and the clients will burn more calories and get into better shape.

The reason that you do not normally go above 85 percent of your max heart rate is not that your heart will explode or be damaged. The justification is much more practical than that. After people go above 85 percent of MHR, the time that they can spend exercising usually drops significantly. Generally, clients should aim for a minimum of 20 minutes of steady-state aerobic exercise to gain health and fitness benefits. If they can't start with that amount, they can do less and work up to 20 minutes. When they have been performing cardiovascular exercise for a while, they will usually want to do it for at least 20 minutes and sometimes up to an hour or more, depending on their goals. In addition, sometimes people do shorter intervals at higher intensity, but the key point is to be aware of the inverse relationship between the intensity of the cardio work and the duration.

As a rule (aerobic endurance athletes will often be an exception), a person can maintain 85 percent of MHR for about 15 minutes. This figure varies between people, and some athletes can maintain it for much longer than 15 minutes, but the average person cannot. Keeping the rule relatively simple, you can last about 15 minutes at 85 percent of MHR, and each percentage point you go up reduces the time that you can sustain it by about a minute. If you exercise at 90 percent of MHR, you can hold that pace for about 10 minutes. At 95 percent you can hold it for about 5 minutes, and if you are at your maximum heart rate you will be able to sustain that pace for 1 minute or less. Again, this general trend is not a rule set in stone. Figure 2.1 highlights the inverse relationship between intensity and duration. As a personal trainer, you need to remember that when training your clients, the harder you make the activity, the shorter it needs to be (41).

Sixty to 85 percent of MHR is a broad range of intensity to work within. If you are 30 years old, then your minimum target heart rate during aerobic exercise should be 114 beats per minute and your maximum target heart rate would be 162 beats per minute. Exercising at 114 beats per minute would feel quite different from exercising at 162 beats per minute; the range can be further broken down to give you some more specific guidelines for yourself and your clients.

The 60 to 70 percent of MHR range is good for beginners. Eliciting some benefit from the exercise is challenging enough; the exercise should not be so difficult that it becomes intimidating and causes the person to dread cardio. The 60 to 70 percent range is also a good range for aerobic exercise that has a long duration, such as 45 minutes or more. If you are going on a 2-hour bike ride, you want to keep your heart rate under 70 percent of MHR so that you have enough energy to finish. This is also a good heart rate if you like to be able to talk during an aerobic exercise session. If you want to talk, read, or watch TV, this intensity will probably suit you best. Finally, if clients simply refuse to exercise at the higher intensity, then this is their only option other than not exercising at all. This range is sometimes referred to as the fat-burning zone because it derives a high percentage of energy from fat, although that subject is a complicated one that is discussed in chapter 22 (31).

The second range is 70 to 85 percent of MHR. This range is commonly called the cardiovascular training zone. A workout in this range is more intense, and with it come several benefits. This range will have the greatest effect on $\dot{V}O_2max$. If you wish to improve your $\dot{V}O_2max$, you need to do most of your training in this zone. If you are an athlete or if you are concerned with your aerobic endurance

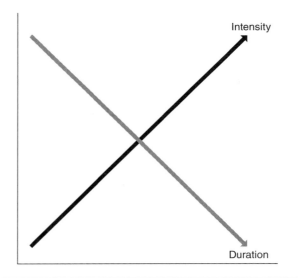

Figure 2.1 The inverse relationship between intensity and duration.

performance—for example, being able to run a certain distance in a certain time—you need to train in this zone. In addition, you will burn more calories minute per minute, which is beneficial to weight loss. Generally, the cardiovascular training zone is more appropriate for intermediate or advanced clients. Exercise in this zone burns more energy from carbohydrate, a topic that is discussed in chapter 22.

Time

Time refers simply to the length of the workout, or its duration. Is the session going to be the typical hour-long workout, is it a two-hour workout, or is it a quick half hour of exercise on the client's lunch break? You need to adapt your clients' workouts to accommodate their time limitations and allot enough time for them to complete the entire workout as planned.

Type

Type refers to the type or classification of exercise, sometimes called mode of exercise. What exactly are your clients doing? Are they performing cardio and, if so, what kind of cardio? Are they running on a track, a treadmill, or a road? Or are they using the rowing machine? If your clients are lifting weights, what exercises are they using? It makes a difference whether they are performing push-ups or bench press, or whether you choose leg presses or squats for them.

The most effective program for your clients will be designed around their goals. This is where you translate the principle of specificity into action. The type of exercises that you choose can make a big difference in the type of gains that they'll achieve. The more specifically your program is tailored to their goals, the more beneficial each workout will be.

The FITT principle is used to design new programs and evaluate existing programs. As a future or current personal trainer, you will likely have friends or clients ask you to look over a program that they have found on the Internet, read in a magazine, or received from a friend. By applying the FITT principle, you can quickly analyze that program. First, you look at the frequency and decide whether the prescribed frequency will produce the desired results. Next, you analyze the intensity, taking into consideration the person's experience, current physical condition, and goals. Does the suggested intensity of the workout match up with the client and his or her goals? You then compare the time that the client is willing to spend on workouts to what is suggested in the program. Finally, what type of exercise is being prescribed? Does it match the client's interests, and will it help the person achieve his or her goals?

SUPERCOMPENSATION

Sometimes called the single-factor model of training, the principle of supercompensation states that after exposure to a stimulus, the body overcompensates, or supercompensates, to that stimulus by storing more of whatever is necessary for future events. The principle of supercompensation is almost like the principle of progressive overload and the principle of specificity combined into one. In broad terms, the principle of supercompensation provides us with an adequate description of how the body responds to exercise by becoming stronger and better prepared for the next exercise session. But when examined closely it does not properly describe how the body responds to exercise, in particular, how the body responds to each individual workout (2).

FITNESS FATIGUE THEORY

Sometimes called the two-factor model of training, the fitness fatigue theory states that a person's physical performance, or physical preparedness, results from a combination of current fitness level and current fatigue level. If you are asked to repeat your workout as soon as you are finished with it, you should perform worse the second time around. This result will occur because of fatigue. If you had to complete it a third time, your performance would decline even more. Although your fitness may have increased from the workout, your fatigue is a negative factor that reduces your overall performance. As you rest, be it for hours or days, your fatigue drops off and your performance improves.

Vladimir Zatsiorsky described the two-factor model of training in *The Science and Practice of Strength Training*. He theorized that the fitness benefit of a workout lasts three times longer than the fatigue deficit (47). If you are sore for three days after your workout, your body will be gaining fitness for up to nine days. The fatigue effect is probably three times stronger than the fitness effect. It has a stronger, immediate effect, but it doesn't last as long. Refer to figure 2.2 for a clearer picture of this concept.

Zatsiorsky developed a formula to predict performance, or what he termed *preparedness*:

$$\text{Preparedness at time t} = \text{initial preparedness} + \text{change in preparedness for one workout} = P(0) + (\text{fitness} - \text{fatigue}) \text{ for one workout}$$

Figure 2.2 illustrates the fitness fatigue theory and its effect on current performance. It also helps answer the question of when the next workout should take place. If you stimulate the body too soon after an intense stimulus (when the performance line is below where it started), overtraining could occur. If you wait too long to work out again after your previous workout, the fitness benefit will diminish and the workouts will not collectively come together to yield better performance.

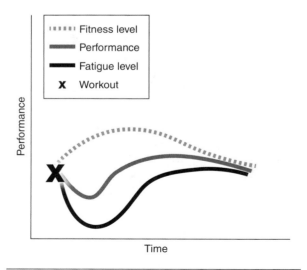

Figure 2.2 Performance is a balance of fitness level and fatigue level.

The fitness fatigue theory is related to a principle that is commonly taught in beginner psychology classes, which is Hans Selye's general adaptation syndrome, sometimes referred to as the GAS model. The GAS model posits that the body goes through a three-phase reaction to stress. The first phase is an alarm phase that occurs while the body is literally encountering the stress or, in this case, a workout. When the stress ends, the body goes into the second phase, the resistance phase. During this phase the stress has been removed and the body is attempting to adapt to the stress in case the stress is encountered again. The third phase of stress is the exhaustion phase, which occurs if the initial stress is too great or if the person is exposed to stress too frequently for the body to adapt to it. In this instance the exhaustion phase is related to the fatigue component of the fitness fatigue theory.

The fitness fatigue theory gives us a better understanding of the how the body responds to a stimulus, such as exercise. It helps us understand what we already know intuitively—that overall ability combined with fatigue results in current performance. But this model, although insightful, can be further developed to add to our understanding of the effects of exercise on the body.

FIVE-FACTOR THEORY OF TRAINING

The five-factor theory of training expands on Zatsiorsky's two-factor model of training. The two-factor model considers fitness level and fatigue level, but in the five-factor model, fitness is separated into two categories: fitness of the physical body (i.e., muscles, bones, tendons, and so on) and fitness of the nervous system, particularly focusing on the brain and nerves. (See chapter 7 for a more detailed discussion about neuromuscular coordination.) The nerves control the muscles and are crucial to performance. Their preparedness can be more important than the preparedness of the muscles themselves, although the two work together as an inseparable unit. The five-factor theory of training has separated the two because the rate of fitness improvement in each system is not the same. For example, as you practice an exercise in the gym, the fitness of your nervous system is improving each minute. Your nervous system is responding to the repetition as you are practicing your technique and learning the skill. Your muscles, however, are being broken down by the training and will need time to heal and recover before their fitness level can increase. One aspect of fitness can improve in minutes; the other aspect will take hours or days to improve (47).

Fatigue is also separated into two categories: physical system fatigue and nervous system fatigue. The physical system and the nervous system also fatigue and recover at different rates. Zatsiorsky posited that fitness benefits last three times longer than any fatigue. This is true for the physical system, but the neuromuscular system can stay fatigued for much longer.

The fifth factor in this model of training is what is termed mind state, or the psychological state of the person while he or she is performing the event. Everyone is familiar with an example of an athlete who performs beyond what was thought possible because of incredible focus and motivation. The opposite also occurs when an athlete who is expected to perform well does not. This result can occur because of nerves or anxiety; the body was ready but the mind state detracted from the athlete's performance.

A formula built upon Zatsiorsky's model can be expressed to help you understand how the five-factor theory of training works in relation to performance.

$$P = (FitNv - FatNv) + (FitPhys - FatPhys) - (100 \text{ percent} - \text{mind state})$$

P = Performance

FitNv = fitness of the nervous system

FatNv = fatigue of the nervous system

FitPhys = fitness of the physical system

FatPhys = fatigue of the physical system

As you can see from this theoretical formula, the goal is to have zero fatigue in both categories so that fatigue will not limit performance. In addition, if a person has optimal mind state, or 100 percent, then 100 percent minus 100 percent equals zero, meaning that optimal mind state does not detract from performance. Suboptimal mind state would detract from performance. If fitness is optimal in both categories, mind state is optimal, and fatigue is at zero, maximal performance will be achieved at that time.

CONCLUSION

Personal trainers must have mastery of seven principles or theories of fitness to ensure that their programs yield results. The principle of specificity dictates that programs will give the user specific adaptations, not general adaptations. The principle of progressive overload makes it clear that over time workouts must increase in difficulty to improve a client's fitness level. The FITT principle expands on the key variables affecting program design including frequency, intensity, time, and type of exercise. The principle of individual variation states that not everyone will respond similarly to the same stimulus. The principle of supercompensation focuses on the idea that at some point after training, the body will supercompensate to adapt to the stimulus. The fitness fatigue theory points out that performance is a balance of a person's fitness and fatigue levels. The five-factor theory of fitness expands on that and suggests the fitness of the muscular system, fatigue of the muscular system, fitness of the nervous system, fatigue of the nervous system, and state of mind can all have a significant effect on performance.

Fitness professionals need to keep the key principles of fitness in mind when creating exercise programs and suggesting routines for others to follow. Ignoring or violating one of these principles will likely yield less than desirable results for clients. New methods and new modes of exercise will always appear, but they must follow and adhere to these principles if they are to have any staying power in the fitness world and any place in your client's training routines.

Study Questions

1. What would be an appropriate use of progressive overload if a client completed a challenging set of 50-pound (22.7 kg) bicep curls for 10 reps the previous week?

   a. 85 pounds (38.6 kg) × 10 reps

   b. 75 pounds (34.0 kg) × 10 reps

   c. 50 pounds (22.7 kg) × 12 reps

   d. 40 pounds (18.1 kg) × 8 reps

2. Considering the principle of specificity, which of the following would be the best supplemental exercise to choose to improve a client's 1RM on the bench press?

   a. barbell incline press

   b. dumbbell decline press

   c. push-ups

   d. chest press machine

3. According to the FITT principle, which of the following changes would most directly increase workout intensity?

   a. increasing treadmill workout time from 20 to 30 minutes at reduced speed

   b. adding a third day of stretching to the workout program

   c. switching from the treadmill to the elliptical machine for the cardio workout

   d. performing cardio at a heart rate of 140 for 30 minutes as opposed to a heart rate of 120 for 30 minutes

4. Which of the following is not one of the five factors in the five-factor theory of fitness?

   a. state of the economy

   b. fitness of the muscular system

   c. fatigue of the nervous system

   d. mind state

5. True or false: The muscular system and the nervous system both improve and show fatigue at the same rate of speed.

   a. true

   b. false

Risk Stratification and Fitness Assessments

One of the most important aspects of your job as a personal trainer is to assess and categorize your client's risk of developing coronary artery disease (CAD). Gone are the days when a personal trainer would high-five a new client and then rush off to the gym to rock out a good workout. The client is putting his or her health in the hands of the personal trainer, and it behooves the personal trainer to discover more about the client's health before setting up an exercise program.

PURPOSES OF STRATIFYING RISK

CAD risk stratification is important for a variety of reasons. First, it pertains to the client's health. You cannot always tell how healthy a person is just by looking at him or her. Our job is to make the client as healthy as possible; we need to learn as much about the client's health as possible before starting an exercise program.

Second, a personal trainer runs the risk of being sued for negligence. To help ensure that all personal trainers are on the same page, the American College of Sports Medicine established guidelines for personal trainers to follow in determining a client's risk level before writing the exercise program. Standard practice is to assess a client in this fashion. If the personal trainer does not do the assessment, he or she is more likely to be held liable for any harm that might come from the client's participation in the exercise program.

Third, knowing the client's risk stratification can help a personal trainer set up a proper program for that client. As will be discussed, some of the risk factors are controllable, and both clients and personal trainers can work hard to reduce a client's risk level.

GOAL OF RISK STRATIFICATION

The overall goal of performing a risk assessment on a client is twofold. The first is simple. We are trying to minimize the risk of an exercise-induced event, which is a health problem brought on by acute exercise. The most significant of these types of events would be a myocardial infarction, or heart attack. Guaranteeing the safety of a client when he or she is exercising is impossible, and it is true that the risk of a heart attack or other event is greater when a person is exercising than when he or she is at rest. The flip side of that equation must be considered as well, and too much time spent at rest without enough exercise will also greatly increase the chance that a health problem will occur. Although health cannot be guaranteed, we can follow certain protocol to minimize the chance that an event will occur. Personal training is a relatively safe activity, and the injury rates for time spent exercising and in the gym are quite low when compared with the rates for almost all other sport or fitness activities.

Following are some guidelines to minimize an exercise-induced event.

- Perform proper risk assessment protocol.
- Medically supervise high-risk clients when they are exercising.
- Have in place a proper and up-to-date emergency action plan (CPR, AED, and first-aid certified).
- Use reasonable exercise intensity and duration.
- Monitor the client as appropriate and at regular intervals.
- Follow standardized warm-up, cool-down, and stretching protocol.
- Minimize competition with beginners and higher risk clients.
- Be aware of the external environment and take the appropriate steps to maintain normal body temperature.

PERSONAL TRAINING FORMS

As a personal trainer, you will have your clients complete a number of relatively standardized forms before they begin training with you. These forms are relatively standardized because the same basic information and content is covered in the form, but the format of the form itself may vary from fitness center to fitness center or from training company to training company. Your particular company may have its own set of forms that it expects you to use (130).

Health History Questionnaire

The primary form used by personal trainers to assess individual clients' level of risk is the health history questionnaire (HHQ). This form covers the eight risk factors and the signs and symptoms of heart disease. Additional information that may be included on this form are an injury history of the client, lifestyle questions about habits such as alcohol use, previous exercise history, information regarding a client's nutrition and weight, information about a client's level of stress, and information about what benefits a client hopes to receive from a personal trainer (increased motivation, learning proper technique, and so on).

Physical Activity Readiness Questionnaire

The physical activity readiness questionnaire (PAR-Q) form is primarily used in a group setting when the HHQ is not practical. The purpose of the PAR-Q is to perform a quick screening of the client to determine whether the client should see a doctor before starting an exercise program (153).

Informed Consent Form

The informed consent form explains both the benefits and risks of the activity discussed, usually either a specific fitness test or the entire training program as a whole. The informed consent should be signed by all clients before activity; it is not limited to those clients who are classified as high or moderate risk. The informed consent, sometimes referred to as a waiver, is extremely important in minimizing a personal trainer's risk in the rare event that a client attempts to sue a personal trainer.

Goal Assessment Form

In this initial phase of questioning, the client should not be bogged down with paperwork. Clients need to be asked in detail about what their goals are and what they hope to accomplish by signing up with a personal trainer. Personal trainers can then delve deeper to understand what the client wants and hopes for. See chapter 4 for more information about goal setting.

Contract

After it has been established that a client will purchase personal training sessions from a personal trainer or fitness company, the client should sign a contract that describes that arrangement in detail. A lawyer should look over or design any contracts that a personal trainer uses to make sure that they will hold up in court (50). Contracts contain (but are not limited to) the following information:

- Client's name and information
- Fitness company name and information
- Original length of term of the contract
- Number of sessions purchased, length of each session, cost of each session, and total cost of the program
- The payment method and system that the client will use to pay for the program (paid in full, monthly, automatic withdrawal, and so on)
- Expiration date for the sessions of the original contract
- Cancellation policy for personal training sessions
- Cancellation policy for the entire contract
- Ability of the fitness company to move the client to another personal trainer if desired
- Automatic renewal procedure of the contract if desired
- Signature of the client
- Signature of the representative of the fitness company

RISK FACTOR ASSESSMENT

A large part of the HHQ is devoted to determining a client's risk stratification. To do this, we need to know where a client stands on eight important risk factors that have been identified to correlate with CAD. The personal trainer simply tallies up the number of yes responses to these simple yes or no questions.

Age

If the client is a male older than 45 years old or a female older than 55 years old, the client has this risk factor. Put simply, the older a person gets, the more likely it is that health problems will affect the person's ability to exercise.

Family History of Heart Disease

If the client has a male first-degree relative (father, brother, or son) who experienced a heart attack or similar issue before age 55 or if the client has a female first-degree relative (mother, sister, or daughter) who experienced a heart attack or similar issue before age 65, the client has this risk factor (103). If the relative had a heart attack or was diagnosed with heart disease, whether or not he or she passed away from the incident, the client checks yes. The client checks yes only once; if the person had a father and two brothers with heart disease, it is a score of one, not three.

Cigarette Smoking

If the client currently smokes cigarettes or has recently quit smoking cigarettes (within six months) but was a regular smoker before that time, the client has this risk factor. Regular smoking is smoking at least one cigarette on a daily basis. This risk factor refers only to the use of tobacco products (42, 64).

Hypertension

Hypertension, or high blood pressure, is defined as a systolic number greater than or equal to 140 mm Hg or a diastolic number greater than or equal to 90 mm Hg. Hypertension is also present if the client is on blood pressure medication, even if the medication is working and the client's blood pressure numbers are now within normal range. Blood pressure can vary; thus, the reading needs to be taken on two separate occasions. If both readings are high, the client has this risk factor. If the elevated readings are new, the client should consult with a doctor; changes in diet and exercise may be enough to lower the reading within normal range. As a personal trainer, remember that you do not make an official diagnosis that the client does indeed have hypertension, but you have information to check yes for the risk assessment. Again, if this is new information to the client, you should suggest a follow-up visit to a doctor for more testing. You can say something like, "I am reading your blood pressure as high; I would suggest that you follow up with your doctor for more clarification" (122–124, 136).

Dyslipidemia

Dyslipidemia refers to cholesterol and lipoproteins in the blood. *Dis* is related to disordered, or out of whack; *lipids* are fat-related compounds; and *emia* refers to the blood, so *dyslipidemia* means that too much fat is in the blood. This risk factor has several values to consider. A personal trainer will not be able to test a client's cholesterol levels; this information comes from a blood test administered by a doctor. If a client has a total greater than or equal to 200 milligrams per deciliter, if the LDL values are greater than or equal to 130 milligrams per deciliter, if the HDL values are less than 40 milligrams per deciliter, or if the client is on cholesterol-lowering medication, the client has this risk factor. If the client met every one of those standards, this is still just one check and counts as a yes for one risk factor (31, 51, 156).

In addition, a client may have a negative risk factor associated with cholesterol. This risk factor is the only one that has a negative risk factor. If the HDL values are greater than or equal to 60 milligrams per deciliter, then one of the risk factors can be erased. HDL is part of total cholesterol, and as such a client might have a total over 200 but an HDL of 70. That would erase this risk factor (one positive factor for the 200; one negative factor for the 70; 1 − 1 = 0). If the client did not have high total cholesterol, this negative risk factor can be used to erase any other single risk factor. They are all equally weighted; thus, any risk factor can be negated.

Impaired Fasting Glucose Levels

Fasting glucose levels indicate a client's ability to handle and process glucose. If the body is unable to maintain normal glucose levels and the blood sugar rises, insulin is not working properly and the person may be more likely to develop diabetes. This condition does not indicate that the client has diabetes (and personal trainers do not make a diagnosis anyway), but it does indicate that the client may be prediabetic. Fasting glucose levels are often tested twice to ensure accurate results. Personal trainers do not administer this test to their clients; clients get their results from their doctor. An impaired fasting glucose score of greater than 100 is a risk factor for CAD.

Obesity

A high amount of body weight and body fat has been shown to correlate with a large number of health problems, including heart disease, stroke, and diabetes (88). Not enough information is available to provide exact guidelines for body-fat levels associated with disease; instead, body mass index (BMI) and waist circumference are used to determine obesity. These values work relatively well for large groups but can be inaccurate for individuals. Therefore, personal trainers can use their best judgment when classifying a client as obese or not. In general, a truly obese person (not just a heavy, muscular individual) exceeds the BMI standard, the waist circumference standard, and the unhealthy body-fat standard (greater than 22 percent body fat for males and greater than 35 percent body fat for females) at the same time (52).

To be classified as obese, a client needs a BMI of greater than 30, calculated by dividing the person's weight in kilograms by his or her height in meters squared, or a waist circumference of greater than 102 centimeters for males (40 inches) or greater than 88 centimeters (35 inches) for females. The waist circumference indicated here is the thinnest part of the waist between the xiphoid process and the belly button.

Sedentary Lifestyle

If the client does not participate in 30 minutes or more of moderate intensity physical activity on at least three days a week for at least three months, the client has this risk factor.

After the personal trainer has received the necessary information on all these values, he or she simply sums the total number of risk factors. Possible sums range from minus one to eight risk factors. The personal trainer records this number on the HHQ because it will be used shortly to assist with risk classification.

Current Diseased Condition

The personal trainer should directly ask clients if they have been officially diagnosed with a disease that might affect their ability to exercise and overall health. These diseases are typically metabolic, cardiovascular, or pulmonary in nature. Common examples include heart disease, diabetes, cancer, HIV, and AIDS. If the client has been diagnosed with a disease, skip the next section and proceed to the risk classification section. If the client has not been diagnosed with a disease, then proceed to the following section about signs and symptoms of diseases.

Signs and Symptoms of Disease

Besides analyzing the eight risk factors, the personal trainer needs to go over a second section of questions with the client. The purpose of evaluating the risk factors is to assess the client's potential for developing a disease, but the client may already have a disease that might affect exercise. Diseases of this type are generally cardiovascular, pulmonary, or metabolic diseases, and their presence will be expressed through specific signs or symptoms. When a personal trainer asks a client about his or her experience with the signs or symptoms of disease, the personal trainer generally asks, "Are you now or do you regularly experience . . . ," and the client responds with a yes or no to each sign or symptom question. The following list covers the key signs or symptoms to ask clients about and includes a brief description of those signs and symptoms.

Chest Pain, Discomfort, or Angina Equivalent

A feeling of pressure, heaviness, constricting, or squeezing in the chest, neck, or jaw area can indicate the existence of CAD.

Shortness of Breath (SOB) at Rest or Mild Exercise

Dyspnea is abnormal uncomfortable awareness of breathing that occurs in unexpected situations such as rest or mild exertion. This mindfulness is common with intense exercise or even brief but vigorous exercise involving large muscle groups (for example, climbing the steps while carrying a load of laundry might invoke this briefly), but people should not have trouble breathing while at rest or with gentle movement. This is a key symptom for cardiac or pulmonary disease.

Syncope or Dizziness

Syncope is a loss of consciousness. Syncope or dizziness that occurs during exercise can indicate a problem with the cardiovascular system and needs to be checked by a doctor. This condition is more common after exercise, but it should not be ignored.

Orthopnea or Paroxysmal Nocturnal Dyspnea

Orthopnea is trouble breathing when in a supine position that is relieved by sitting upright. Paroxysmal nocturnal dyspnea is trouble breathing while sleeping at night when lying down. This symptom can indicate problems with the function of the heart.

Ankle Edema

If the client experiences bilateral ankle edema at night, it can indicate a problem with the blood flow in the body.

Palpitations or Tachycardia

Palpitations are an unpleasant awareness of a fast heartbeat; tachycardia is an abnormally high resting pulse (greater than 100 beats per minute). These symptoms can be caused by an improperly functioning heart or other issues such as anxiety or fever.

Intermittent Claudication

Intermittent claudication refers to pain that occurs in a muscle that is stressed by exercise, and it tends to indicate a lack of blood flow to the muscle. This pain is reproducible with activity, does not come on at random, and usually disappears after the activity ceases. This symptom can indicate the presence of CAD or diabetes.

Heart Murmurs

Heart murmurs are not necessarily problematic, but they should be looked at by a doctor, because some types of heart murmurs can contribute to exercise-induced events. If a client has a heart murmur but has been told by a doctor that the condition is not an issue, then the client does not have this symptom. But if the client has a heart murmur but does not know what its effects are, then the client has this symptom.

Unusual Fatigue or SOB During Usual Activities

If a client is exceedingly tired, fatigued, or low on energy during activities that he or she usually performs with ease, the symptoms can indicate the prevalence of a disease and should be looked at by a doctor.

RISK CLASSIFICATION

After the personal trainer has the answers to the previous sets of questions (number of risk factors, disease status, and signs and symptoms of disease), he or she is then able to classify the client based on that information. All clients will be placed into one of three categories: low, moderate, or high risk. The risk classification then determines whether the client can proceed without the approval or clearance from a doctor, and it will provide the personal trainer with guidelines about what exercise intensity is appropriate for the specific client.

Low Risk

Clients who have minus one, zero, or one risk factor are classified as low risk. They do not have any signs or symptoms of a disease, nor do they have an actual disease. Clients who are low risk are considered within the scope of practice for the personal trainer, and these clients can exercise at both moderate and vigorous intensity. Clients who are low risk do not

need to be cleared by a doctor before beginning an exercise program, although it is appropriate to suggest that all clients receive clearance to be extra safe (1).

Moderate Risk

Clients who are classified as moderate risk have two or more risk factors (two through eight risk factors). They do not have any signs or symptoms of a disease, nor do they have an actual disease. Clients who are classified as moderate risk are considered outside the scope of practice for the personal trainer if they perform vigorous exercise. Clients who are classified as moderate risk are able to work with a personal trainer and perform moderate exercise without medical clearance. If the personal trainer wishes the client to perform vigorous exercise, the client should be cleared by a doctor to do so (1).

High Risk

Clients who are classified as high risk have one or more signs or symptoms of a disease or have an actual disease. Clients who are classified as high risk are considered outside the scope of practice for the personal trainer. Clients who are classified as high risk must be given medical clearance before beginning any physical activity with a personal trainer. The doctor then places the client inside the personal trainer's scope of practice either with limitations as to exercise type and intensity or with no limitations. The only way for a client to be classified as high risk is for the client to have a sign, symptom, or actual disease; the risk factors are not used for this placement (1).

The exercise permitted for clients in the CAD risk categories is classified as moderate exercise or vigorous exercise. To follow the preceding guidelines, those terms must be operationally defined.

Moderate Exercise

Moderate exercise is defined as intensity between 40 and 60 percent of $\dot{V}O_2$max or heart rate reserve (HRR), intensity between three and six metabolic equivalents of task (METs), or intensity within the person's capacity that he or she can comfortably sustain for a prolonged period (at least 45 minutes).

Vigorous Exercise

Vigorous exercise is defined as intensity greater than 60 percent of $\dot{V}O_2$max or HRR, intensity greater than six METs, or exercise intense enough to represent a substantial cardiorespiratory challenge. Note that what many personal trainers would define as vigorous differs from this textbook definition. Almost all traditional activity thought of as true exercise will be vigorous in nature. This definition is more conservative; 60 percent of $\dot{V}O_2$max usually corresponds to just above 70 percent of MHR. Any exercise intense enough to fail the talk test will likely be classified as vigorous.

After a client has been assessed and ultimately classified, the personal trainer is then armed with appropriate exercise guidelines. A client classified as low risk should not proceed immediately to advanced programs if he or she is a beginner. A classification of low risk simply means that the client is able to perform exercise of an intense nature at the personal trainer's discretion; it does not mean the client must perform only vigorous exercise. If a client is classified as moderate risk and does not have medical clearance, the personal trainer can train the client only at moderate intensity. You can remember that moderate risk equals moderate intensity. The personal trainer should strongly suggest that the client receive medical clearance in a prompt fashion, because the client will likely be fully cleared and placed back in the scope of practice. The personal trainer will then be able to implement more intense exercise, and the client will reach his or her goals faster.

If a client is classified as high risk, the personal trainer is not able to train that client. Essentially, that classification is stating that the client may likely, or already does, have a disease and that exercise might cause an exercise-induced event. Thus, exercise must be avoided until further information is available. If the client has arrived for an hour-long session or has signed up for an initial consulta-tion, the personal trainer does not have to wrap up the session after five minutes and dismiss the client. The personal trainer can use that time to discuss in detail the client's goals and exercise history. The personal trainer might go over certain aspects of nutrition. This is a good time to teach a client how to read a food label and calculate calories if he or she doesn't know how to do that already. The personal trainer can demonstrate how to use certain pieces of equipment in the gym, although the client cannot perform any activity until cleared by a doctor. Clients are not usually turned off by this mandate to see a doctor before beginning exercise; instead, they are often pleased and impressed that the personal trainer cared enough about their health to make this a requirement.

FITNESS ASSESSMENTS

After performing risk stratification and classification, the personal trainer can perform certain fitness assessments on the client. These assessments can be part of an initial consultation, they might take place early in a client's contract to establish a baseline, or they might occur at regular intervals during the training to measure results (144). Many fitness assessments are available. Fitness assessments should not be considered mandatory; they should be viewed as tools that will help the personal trainer assess and measure the client. Those tools will ultimately help the personal trainer design a proper exercise program for the client. Personal trainers need to choose assessments that are specific to each client. The assessments used to measure Grandma's ability will likely be different from the assessments used to measure a college athlete's ability. All assessments can be broken down into resting or active assessments (table 3.1). Resting assessments are performed before active assessments so that they are not affected by the performance of the active test.

Sex

Most forms have the words *male* and *female* to circle or boxes to checkmark.

Table 3.1 Resting and Active Fitness Assessments

Resting fitness assessments	Active fitness assessments
Sex	Sport-specific tests
Age	Muscular strength
Height	Muscular endurance
Weight	Cardiovascular endurance
Body mass index	Flexibility
Resting pulse	
Heart rate reserve	
Blood pressure	
Body composition	
Body circumferences	
Waist–hip ratio	

Age

Because age can be a risk factor, asking a client's age is important. Another term used to describe age is chronological age.

Height

In the United States, height is traditionally measured in feet and inches. The metric system can be used if preferred; the conversion is 1 inch equals 2.54 centimeters. The average height for American adult males is 5 feet, 9.5 inches plus or minus 3 inches (176.5 cm plus or minus 7.6 cm). For females, it is 5 feet, 4 inches plus or minus 2 inches (162.5 cm plus or minus 5 cm).

Weight

In the United States, body weight is usually measured in pounds. The metric system can be used if preferred; 1 kilogram equals 2.2 pounds. The average weight for American adult males is 191 pounds (86.6 kg) (notably up from 166 pounds [75.3 kg] in 1960). For females, it is 160 pounds (72.6 kg) (up from 140 pounds [63.5 kg] in 1960).

Body Mass Index

Body mass index (BMI) is a ratio that compares two variables: height and weight. The formula for BMI is

$$BMI = \text{weight in pounds} \div (\text{height in inches})^2 \times 703$$

or (metric version)

$$BMI = \text{weight in kilograms} \div (\text{height in meters})^2$$

Example 1: 135-pound female who is 5 feet, 5 inches tall

$$135 \div (65 \times 65) = 135 \div 4{,}225 =$$
$$0.0319526 \times 703 =$$
$$22.46 \text{ BMI, healthy category}$$

Example 2: 176-pound male who is 5 feet, 8 inches tall

$$176 \div (68 \times 68) = 176 \div 4{,}624 =$$
$$0.038062 \times 703 =$$
$$26.75 \text{ BMI, overweight category}$$

Example 3: 235-pound male who is 6 feet, 2 inches tall

$$235 \div (74 \times 74) =$$
$$235 \div 5{,}476 =$$
$$0.042914 \times 703$$
$$= 30.17 \text{ BMI, obese category}$$

Use table 3.2 to categorize a client based on BMI.

The average BMI for Americans, both males and females, is 27.5. Keep in mind that BMI factors in only height and weight; it does not calculate body-fat percentage. A male who is 5 feet, 10 inches (177.8 cm) and weighs 215 pounds (97.5 kg) at 5 percent body fat will have the same BMI as a male of the same height and weight at 30 percent body fat. Both clients are classified as obese according to table 3.2. BMI is useful when looking at large groups of

Table 3.2 BMI Categories

BMI	Category
<18.5	Underweight
18.5–24.9	Healthy
25.0–29.9	Overweight
30.0–34.9	Obese (level I or mild obesity)
35.0–39.9	Obese (level II or moderate obesity)
≥40.0	Obese (level III or morbid obesity)

Reprinted from National Institutes of Health and National Heart, Lung, and Blood Institute 1998.

people, but it is of limited value when looking at individuals, particularly in the fitness world.

Resting Pulse

The number of times that the heart beats in one minute at rest is the resting pulse or resting heart rate (RHR). Personal trainers should take a client's pulse by finding it at the radial artery, recording it for 15 seconds, and multiplying that number by four. Figure 3.1 indicates the location of the radial artery on the forearm near the wrist.

Heart Rate Reserve

The difference between the number of heartbeats in one minute at rest and the client's maximal heart rate is heart rate reserve (HRR). This value is part of the Karvonen heart rate formula and is calculated by subtracting the resting heart rate from the estimated maximal heart rate. The goal is to have a high heart rate reserve.

$$MHR - RHR = HRR$$

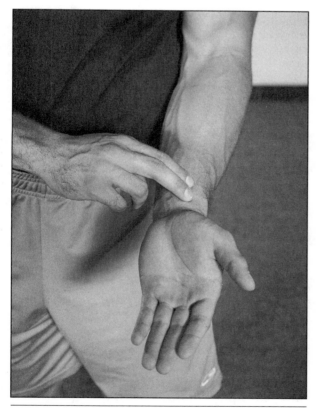

Figure 3.1 Location of the radial artery.

Blood Pressure

The pressure that the blood exerts against the arterial walls is blood pressure. It is expressed as one number over another number. The top number is the systolic blood pressure, and the bottom number is diastolic blood pressure. Normal blood pressure is around 120/80. Hypertension is defined as a blood pressure number greater than or equal to 140/90 (122). The diastolic number is the most important in classifying blood pressure, and it is used in table 3.3.

Body Composition

Several methods are available to estimate percent body fat; some are reasonably inexpensive and easy to do, and others require more time, money, or special equipment. Consult table 3.4 for the classifications and typical percent body-fat levels of people who excel in a variety of sports. Also, appendix G describes how to calculate lean body mass (LBM) and fat weight after a body composition test is performed.

Hydrostatic Weighing

The principle behind this method, also known as underwater weighing, is that fat floats and lean mass (muscle, bone) sinks. Think about what happens when you throw a chicken breast in water. It sinks, right? Well, so do muscles. The name for this law is Archimedes' principle, which states that for an equal weight, lower-density objects have a larger surface area and displace more water than higher-density objects do.

This test is performed in a giant aquarium or small pool (see figure 3.2). In the pool a plastic chair is suspended from an overhead scale. The client sits in the chair, tips his or her head forward to be under the water line, blows all the

Table 3.3 Diastolic Blood Pressure Classifications

Diastolic BP	Classification
90–104	Mild hypertension
105–119	Moderate hypertension
≥120	Severe hypertension

Table 3.4 Percent Body Fat Descriptive Data for Athletes in Various Sports

Classification and typical percent body fat of athletes playing the sport		Sport
Extremely lean		
Males	<7%	Gymnastics
Females	<15%	Bodybuilding (at contest)
		Wrestling (at contest)
		Cross-country
Very lean		
Males	8-10%	Men's basketball
Females	16-18%	Racquetball
		Rowing
		Soccer
		Track and field decathlon (men)
		Track and field heptathlon (women)
Leaner than average		
Males	11-13%	Men's baseball
Females	19-20%	Canoeing
		Downhill skiing
		Speed skating
		Olympic-style weightlifting
Average		
Males	14-17%	Women's basketball
Females	21-25%	American football quarterbacks, kickers, linebackers
		Hockey
		Horse racing (jockey)
		Tennis
		Discus throw
		Volleyball
		Women's softball
		Powerlifting
Fatter than average		
Males	18-22%	American football (linemen)
Females	26-30%	Shot put

Reprinted, by permission, from NSCA, 2008, Administration, scoring, and interpretation of selected tests, by E. Harman and J. Garhammer. In *Essentials of strength training and conditioning*, 3rd ed., edited by T. Baechle and R.W. Earle (Champaign, IL: Human Kinetics), 290; data from D.C. Nieman, 1995, *Fitness and sports medicine*, 3rd ed. (Palo Alto, CA: Bull).

air out of the lungs, and remains motionless for 10 seconds (long enough to measure his or her weight underwater). From that information and other data, the client's body density is calculated (see appendix H) and entered into a formula to determine an estimate of the client's percent body fat.

The drawbacks of hydrostatic weighing stem mainly from the need for specialized equipment and an experienced tester. Most fitness centers do not perform hydrostatic weighing. The test takes about 10 to 15 minutes per person, so it is not feasible for large groups of people. Finally, not everyone is comfortable being in the water, particularly because the person has to exhale with the head underwater, which is an unusual sensation. But some colleges and athletics settings do offer hydrostatic weighing, and it's an option worth considering. The standard error for hydrostatic weighing is 2.7 percent.

Skinfold Calipers

The primary method that personal trainers use to determine a client's body fat is skinfold calipers. The personal trainer records measurements from the right side of the client's body whenever possible. The caliper simply provides

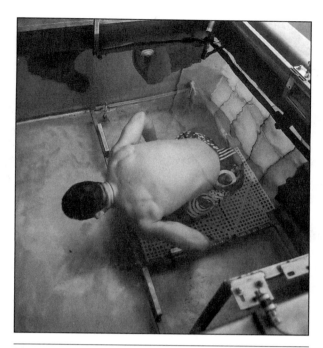

Figure 3.2 Hydrostatic weighing.

a millimeter measurement of the thickness of a pinch. That number is then entered into a formula to calculate the subject's body-fat percentage. Several formulas are used, and each relies on measurements from various sites on the body. Generally, the greater the number of sites that are used, the more accurate the test.

The main benefit of the calipers is that they are inexpensive and easy to use. This method of measuring body fat is offered free or for a minimal fee at most gyms, and it can be performed in a few minutes. But the calipers are not perfect. They assume that all people store fat in the same places, even though vast differences appear (you have probably seen a person with a lean upper body and a fat lower body), and certain formulas are more or less accurate with certain populations and ethnicities. The generalized formulas often do not account for race, although there is some evidence that races have different body densities and body composition. Also, not everyone's skin is the same tightness, and getting a caliper reading on a person with very tight skin can be difficult. Tester error can be large, meaning that if the person doesn't know how to measure the body fat correctly at the various sites, the numbers will be off. Finally, the sample size

from which the body-fat information is drawn is relatively small and may not generalize well to the entire population. The standard error for body-fat calipers is approximately 3.5 percent (146).

To get the most valid results, the same person should measure the subject's body fat each time. This approach can be a benefit to the personal trainer. For a client to see consistent results, the same person should take the client's body-fat measurement. Body fat should not be measured after a workout because the skin might be too tight because of a pump and it may be more slippery (75). The tester records the actual numbers obtained at each site (instead of just the end body-fat percentage). The personal trainer should not be too concerned with a client's exact percentage of body fat according to a chart; instead he or she should look for a general trend of decreasing body fat.

Recommendations regarding the technique for using a caliper include the following:

- Hold the caliper in the right hand and pinch the client with the left hand.
- Pinch the skinfold with the first two fingers and the thumb; for most measurements, the pinching fingers face down and the posterior side of the hand faces away from the client.
- Pinch the appropriate site and pull the skin and fat away from the muscle and bone to create the skinfold.
- Measure the thickness of the skinfold with the caliper by placing the tongs of the caliper directly below the thumb and forefingers up against the client's body. Allow the caliper to compress the skinfold briefly and settle before reading the measurement to the nearest half millimeter. Then open up the caliper tongs, remove it from the skinfold, and release the pinch. The pinching hand is the first hand on and the last hand off.

Skinfold Sites There are 10 common sites to measure a client's body fat with calipers, although no current formula uses all the sites at one time. Table 3.5 lists the common body-fat sites and guidelines about the specific location on the body.

Figure 3.3 shows the location of the various skinfold measurement sites on the body.

Skinfold Formulas Four formulas are commonly used to estimate body fat. Each formula uses different sites and has different positives and negatives. None of the formulas is more

Table 3.5   Skinfold Caliper Measurement Sites and Guidelines

Anatomical sites	Right side of the body for all measurements
Biceps	Vertical fold, halfway between the shoulder and elbow, directly on the biceps
Triceps	Vertical fold, midway between the elbow and shoulder
Chest	Diagonal fold, midway between the upper armpit and nipple
Midaxillary	Horizontal fold, directly below the armpit
Lower back	Horizontal fold, directly over the kidneys and 2 inches (5 cm) to the right of the spine
Inferior angle of the scapula (subscapular)	Diagonal fold, directly below and slightly medial to the bottom of the shoulder blade
Iliac crest (suprailiac)	Diagonal fold, at height of the iliac crest, 3 to 4 inches (7.6 to 10 cm) from the navel where the abs and the obliques meet
Abdomen	Vertical fold, 1 inch (2.5 cm) to the right of the navel
Quadriceps (front of thigh)	Vertical fold, midway between the kneecap and top of the thigh
Calf	Vertical fold, inside of the leg on the largest part of the calf

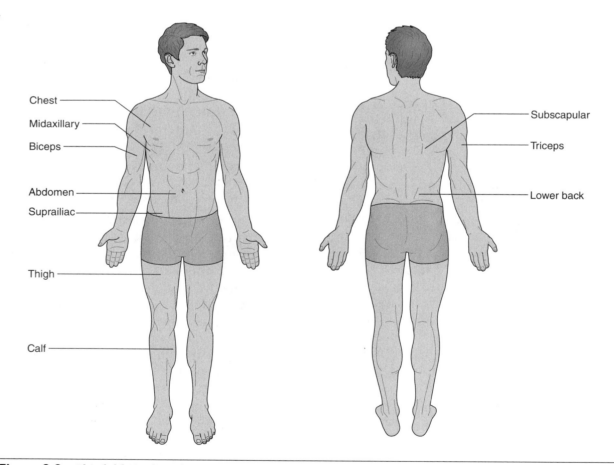

Figure 3.3   Skinfold site locations.

accurate than plus or minus 3 percent, even when administered by a skilled tester. Refer to table 3.6 for a summary of common formulas to estimate percent body fat from skinfold testing; note that some, but not all, of the formulas described in this section are included in the table. Appendix H provides additional formulas.

- The Durnin–Womersley formula is the most popular method for taking body fat and is found in most fitness centers,

although a better practice is to use several or all the formulas to establish a more accurate assessment of the client. This formula uses four sites that are the same for men and women: biceps, triceps, subscapula, and suprailiac.

Pros: Uses four sites instead of three; clients do not need to wear special clothing because the sites are usually easily accessible; it is the most common formula; detailed tables exist to determine body fat easily.

Table 3.6 Equations for Calculating Estimated Body Density From Skinfold Measurements Among Various Populations

SKF sites[a]	Population subgroups	Sex	Age	Equation	Reference
S7SKF (chest + abdomen + triceps + subscapular + suprailiac + midaxillary + thigh)	Black or Hispanic	Women	18-55 years	Db (g/cc)[b] = 1.0970 − 0.00046971 (S7SKF) + 0.00000056 (S7SKF)^2 − 0.00012828 (Age)	Jackson et al.
S7SKF (chest + abdomen + triceps + subscapular + suprailiac + midaxillary + thigh)	Black or athletes	Men	18-61 years	Db (g/cc)[b] = 1.1120 − 0.00043499 (S7SKF) + 0.00000055 (S7SKF)^2 − 0.00028826 (Age)	Jackson and Pollock
S4SKF (triceps + anterior suprailiac + abdomen + thigh)	Athletes	Women	18-29 years	Db (g/cc)[b] = 1.096095 − 0.0006952 (S4SKF) − 0.0000011 (S4SKF)^2 − 0.0000714 (Age)	Jackson et al.
S3SKF (triceps + suprailiac + thigh)	White or anorexic	Women	18-55 years	Db (g/cc)[b] = 1.0994921 − 0.0009929 (S3SKF) + 0.0000023 (S3SKF)^2 − 0.0001392 (Age)	Jackson et al.
S3SKF (chest + abdomen + thigh)	White	Men	18-61 years	Db (g/cc)[b] = 1.109380 − 0.0008267 (S3SKF) + 0.0000016 (S3SKF)^2 − 0.0002574 (Age)	Jackson and Pollock
S2SKF (triceps + calf)	Black or white	Boys	6-17 years	% BF = 0.735 (S2SKF) + 1.0	Slaughter et al.
S2SKF (triceps + calf)	Black or white	Girls	6-17 years	% BF = 0.610 (S2SKF) + 5.1	Slaughter et al.
Suprailiac, triceps	Athletes	Women	High school and college age	Db (g/cc)[b] = 1.0764 − (0.00081 3 suprailiac) − (0.00088 3 triceps)	Sloan and Weir
Thigh, subscapular	Athletes	Men	High school and college age	Db (g/cc)[b] = 1.1043 − (0.00133 3 thigh) − (0.00131 3 subscapular)	Sloan and Weir

[a]SKF = sum of skinfolds (mm); Db = body density.

[b]Use population-specific conversion formulas to calculate %BF from Db.

Reprinted, by permission, from NSCA, 2008, Administration, scoring, and interpretation of selected tests, by E. Harman and J. Garhammer. In *Essentials of strength training and conditioning*, 3rd ed., edited by T. Baechle and R.W. Earle (Champaign, IL: Human Kinetics), 288; adapted, by permission, from V.H. Heyward, 2014, *Advanced fitness assessment and exercise prescription*, 7th ed. (Champaign, IL: Human Kinetics), 238.

Cons: Usually gives the highest body-fat percentage for the client compared with the other formulas; it measures only the upper body; seems to produce the largest error with lean men.

- The Jackson–Pollock seven-site formula involves taking body fat at seven sites: chest, midaxillary, triceps, abdomen, suprailiac, thigh, and subscapula. These sites are the same for men and women.

 Pros: Uses seven sites, which often results in lower body-fat percentages than those produced by the Durnin–Womersley formula.

 Cons: Uses more invasive sites (chest, thigh, midaxillary); tables to determine body fat quickly are not as common.

- The Jackson–Pollock three-site formula uses only three sites, and the sites differ for men and women. For men the sites are chest, abdominal area, and thigh. For women the sites are triceps, suprailiac, and thigh.

 Pros: The use of three sites is the quickest test; it involves a specific formula for men and for women; it may be more accurate.

 Cons: Use of only three sites collects less data; the personal trainer has to remember the correct sites for the two sexes.

- The Parillo nine-site formula uses the most sites. This formula was developed by John Parillo as a method of assessing bodybuilders because he believed that the other formulas were not accurate enough to differentiate very low levels of body fat.

 Pros: Was developed for a practical, real-life application; uses more sites than any other method; good for showing change with lean people; easiest formula to memorize and calculate.

 Cons: Method was developed without calculating body density, which is a standard part of body-fat calculations; sample size of subjects is unknown; may not be as accurate for populations with a high percentage of body fat.

Bioelectrical Impedance

Bioelectrical impedance uses a small device (see figure 3.4) that sends an electrical signal through the body to detect what type of tissue is present. Some tissue conducts electricity well, but other tissue does not. A bioelectrical impedance test is actually measuring total body water, and from there the amount of lean mass and ultimately fat mass can be estimated. Normally, these machines cost between $50 and $200, but clinical ones can cost thousands. The more expensive bioelectrical impedance machines report a standard error of 2.8 percent when compared with hydrostatic weighing; the cheaper models are likely less accurate. A person's body water can fluctuate a fair amount, and that will alter how the machine assesses the percentage of body fat. Food and waste can also affect the reading. These devices are generally more accurate for those in the middle of the spectrum; very lean and obese people are often misread on the bioelectrical impedance test. Personal trainers like this method because tester error and variance does not exist, and the test is quick, inexpensive, and noninvasive. The big negative is simply that this method is not that accurate and does not show change as well as body-fat calipers do. Bioelectrical impedance devices often give the person his or her BMI calculation at the same time (which has nothing to do with the body fat scanned; the machine simply has the BMI formula in it and uses the input height and weight to calculate it).

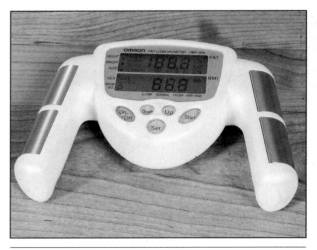

Figure 3.4 Bioelectrical impedance device.

Bod Pod

The Bod Pod is a machine that uses air displacement plethysmography to determine percent body fat. The subject sits in an oval-shaped machine, much like a giant egg (see figure 3.5). Each test takes about five minutes to complete. The machine finds the subject's weight and volume and from there estimates his or her body composition. The principle is the same as that used in hydrostatic weighing, but this test is quicker and more convenient because the person does not have to get wet or put his or her head under water. The Bod Pod is reported to have a standard error of 3 percent.

DEXA Imaging

This procedure measures body fat using dual-energy X-ray absorptiometry (DEXA or DXA) imaging of the body. A computer scans the body and takes pictures of the inside of the body, similar to an MRI. It then puts all the pictures together and estimates how much body fat the subject has. This procedure can be relatively expensive, and it obviously requires a specialized machine. Because this method involves using an actual picture of the body instead of formulas to estimate how the specific body acts, it is the new gold standard for taking body fat. DEXA imaging is believed to be the most accurate of the methods currently available. The subject

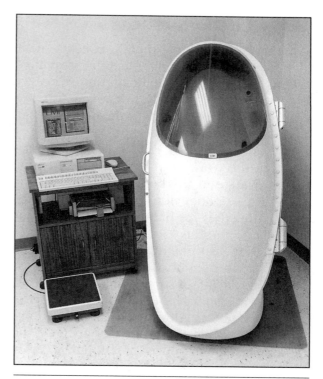

Figure 3.5 Bod Pod machine.

can usually learn his or her bone density at the same time with this test. The biggest negative with this method is that it involves some radiation; performing this test regularly would likely not be ideal for health (4). An example of a DEXA machine is seen in figure 3.6.

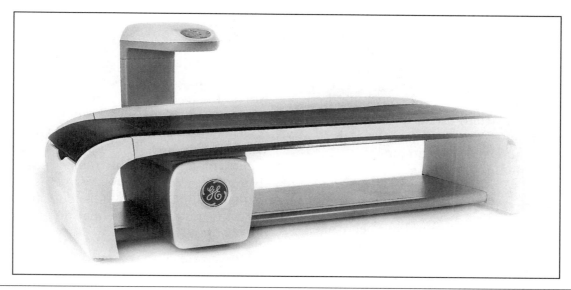

Figure 3.6 DEXA machine.

Body Circumferences

Another common and generally effective mode that personal trainers can use to assess their clients is to calculate body circumferences at different areas of the body. In simple terms, this method involves taking tape measurements of various sites. The tape measure is an excellent tool for showing change. As a client progresses through the workout program, documenting actual change in the body is useful. But the tape measure does not do a good job of discriminating the type of tissue that it is measuring. If a client adds 2 inches (5 cm) to his or her thigh measurement, we are unable to tell from that information alone if the increase was all muscle, all fat, or some combination. Thus, the tape measure alone does not allow us to calculate body fat. Although some institutions, such as the military, use it for that purpose, the tape measure does not give us enough accurate information to make a body-fat calculation in the fitness world (11).

When calculating body measurements, two measurements can be recorded. The most common method is to have the client stand relaxed in anatomical position and record the various sites. The client can flex or contract the muscles in an area, which can affect the measurement. This most commonly occurs with arm measurements, but it can be used in most sites. Some clients are interested in this number purely for ego, which is fine, but recording a flexed measurement does have value to a personal trainer because it helps monitor change quicker than a relaxed measurement.

Listed in table 3.7 are the common circumference measurement sites and guidelines about how to obtain an accurate assessment of that region of the body. See figure 3.7 for an illustration of the body circumference measurement sites.

Waist–Hip Ratio

After the tape measurements have been taken, a personal trainer can figure out the client's waist–hip ratio. This assessment of body fat and health helps put the BMI into perspective. Larger but leaner clients usually retain a relatively narrow waist. Clients who have significant body fat usually have a wider waist. The waist–hip ratio is found by simply dividing the waist measurement (at the smallest part) by the hip measurement.

Waist measurement ÷ hip measurement = waist–hip ratio

The ratios listed in table 3.8 are age and sex specific. The thicker the waist is, the more likely it is that the person is storing a significant amount of fat around the organs. The excess fat is linked to health problems. The ratios should be considered in the light of all the information available. For example, if a female had a waist of 23 inches (58.4 cm) and hips of 26 inches (66 cm), she would have a waist–hip ratio of .88 and be deemed unhealthy. Further examination, however, shows that a 23-inch (58.4 cm) waist is very thin, as are 26-inch (66 cm) hips. This woman is not overfat. She will likely have a low BMI (certainly below 30 and likely closer to 20 or below) and a low body-fat reading (certainly below 35 percent). Therefore, logic dictates that she not be labeled unhealthy even though she meets one criterion. Instead, she is simply not as "hippy" as a normal female, but that would not indicate a high probability of poor health. Use of the waist–hip ratio in conjunction with other measures of health such as body-fat percentage, BMI, and the waist measurement itself gives a more accurate picture.

ACTIVE ASSESSMENTS

After performing the resting assessments, the personal trainer can take active assessments. Not all the assessments listed here need to be used on each client. Clients can have one training session devoted to testing, in which the whole session is spent conducting these assessments, or the personal trainer may choose to perform one or two assessments during a regular training session. If the personal trainer conducts multiple assessments in one day, the order of tests matters.

Testing Order

There is no universal agreement about the proper order of exercise tests, but several stan-

Table 3.7 Body Circumference Measurement Sites and Guidelines

Body site	How to measure	Notes
Neck	Anatomical position, around the base of the neck	Same area that a man's tie would cover.
Shoulders	Anatomical position, at widest part of the shoulder girdle Flexed: shoulders puffed up, standing tall	Around the middle deltoids and across the chest and back; tape measure should meet on the back.
Chest	Anatomical position across the nipples and upper back Flexed: chest puffed up, standing tall	Client lifts arms up to get tape measure around the body; arms must return to the side; tape measure should meet on the back.
Waist 1	Anatomical position, at thinnest part of the waist Flexed: waist sucked in (made small) as much as possible	Usually a bit above the belly button.
Waist 2	Anatomical position, around the belly button Flexed: waist sucked in as much as possible	
Upper arm	Anatomical position, around thickest part of the right upper arm Flexed: upper arm raised out to the side, elbow flexed, palm supinated, and upper arm musculature contracted, at thickest part	Just below the deltoids; tape measure should meet on the outside of the arm.
Forearm	Anatomical position, at thickest part of the forearm Flexed: elbow flexed approximately 90 degrees, palm pronated, wrist flexed, forearm musculature contracted, at thickest part	Just below the elbow joint.
Wrist	Anatomical position, around the wrist	Just before the hand, right after the distal portion of the radius and ulna; often used for frame size assessment.
Hips	Anatomical position, widest part of the hip girdle	Around the middle part of the gluteal muscles and greater trochanter; tape measure should meet on the side.
Thigh 1	Anatomical position, legs staggered slightly, at thickest part of the right thigh Flexed: thigh musculature contracted	Close to the groin; include the adductors; tape measure should meet on the outside of the leg.
Thigh 2	Anatomical position, legs staggered slightly, midpoint on the right thigh between the anterior superior iliac spine (ASIS) and the patella Flexed: thigh musculature contracted	Halfway down; does not include the adductors; tape measure should meet on the outside of the leg.
Calf	Anatomical position, thickest part of the right calf Flexed: foot plantar flexed and calf musculature contracted	Slightly below the knee on the thickest part.

dards should be followed. The completion of one test can affect, either positively or more likely negatively, the performance of a subsequent test, so the personal trainer needs to be aware of the interaction between tests. Here are the common standards:

- Resting assessments occur before active assessments.
- Sport-specific assessments occur before other active assessments.
- Muscular strength tests occur before muscular endurance tests.
- Flexibility tests are performed last.

Most of the disagreement occurs over where to place cardiovascular endurance tests in the assessment. No single answer is perfect; cardiovascular endurance tests should be placed in the testing order based on their importance to the client and the personal trainer. For a strength athlete, cardiovascular endurance is less

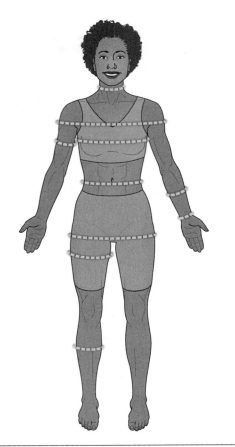

Figure 3.7 Body circumference measurement site locations.

Table 3.8 Waist–Hip Ratio Classifications

Sex	Unhealthy waist–hip ratio	
	<60 years old	≥60 years old
Males	>0.95	>1.03
Females	>0.86	>0.90

important than strength, so the strength tests should be performed first. For a cardiovascular endurance athlete, the reverse is true. For the regular client, strength tests will generally have less negative effect on cardiovascular endurance tests than vice versa, but ultimately the personal trainer will choose where to place those tests (54).

Sport-Specific Tests

Three common tests related to sport performance may be appropriate for clients, depending on their goals.

40-Yard (37 m) Dash

- Protocol
  - Warm up and perform two practice runs on a flat, straight surface.
  - Sprint the distance at maximal speed.
  - Perform the test twice, allow sufficient rest between the trials, and record the average to the nearest .1 second.
- Normative data (table 3.9)

T-Test

- Protocol
  - Set up the testing area as shown in figure 3.8.
  - Warm up and perform a practice run.
  - Sprint forward from cone A to cone B and touch the base of the cone with the right hand.
  - Shuffle to the left to cone B and touch the base of the cone with the left hand.
  - Shuffle to the right to cone C and touch the base of the cone with the right hand.
  - Shuffle to the left to cone B and touch the base of the cone with the left hand.
  - Run backward from cone B to pass by cone A (there is no need to touch cone A).
  - Stop the stopwatch as cone A is passed by.
  - Perform the test twice, allow sufficient rest between the trials, and record the best score to the nearest .1 second.
- Normative data (table 3.9)

Vertical Jump

- Protocol
  - Rub chalk on the fingertips of the dominant hand.
  - Stand with the dominant shoulder next to the wall and reach as high as possible with the dominant hand.

Table 3.9 Vertical Jump, T-Test, 40-Yard (37 m) Sprint, Hexagon Test, and 300-Yard (274 m) Shuttle Descriptive Data* for Various Groups

Group, sport, or position	Vertical jump inches	Vertical jump cm	T-test seconds	40-yard (37 m) sprint seconds	Hexagon test seconds	300-yard (274 m) shuttle seconds
NCAA Division I college American football split ends, strong safeties, offensive and defensive backs	31.5	80		4.6-4.7		<59
NCAA Division I college American football wide receivers and outside linebackers	31	79		4.6-4.7		<59
NCAA Division I college American football linebackers, tight ends, safeties	29.5	75		4.8-4.9		<61
College basketball players (men)	27-29	69-74	8.9			
NCAA Division I college American football quarterbacks	28.5	72		4.8-4.9		
NCAA Division I college American football defensive tackles	28	71		4.9-5.1		<65
NCAA Division I college basketball players (men)	28	71				
NCAA Division I college American football offensive guards	27	69		5.1		<65
Competitive college athletes (men)	25-25.5	64-65	10.0	5.0	12.3	
NCAA Division I college American football offensive tackles	25-26	64-66		5.4		<65
Recreational college athletes (men)	24	61	10.5	5.0	12.3	
High school American football backs and receivers	24	61		5.2		
College baseball players (men)	23	58	9.2			
College tennis players (men)	23	58	9.4			
High school American football linebackers and tight ends	22	56		5.4		
College American football players	21	53		5.35		
College basketball players (women)	21	53	9.9			
17-year-old boys	20	51				
High school American football linemen	20	51		4.9-5.6		
NCAA Division II college basketball guards (women)	19	48				
NCAA Division II college basketball forwards (women)	18	46				
NCAA Division II college basketball centers (women)	17.5	44				
Sedentary college students (men)	16-20.5	41-52	11.1	5.0	14.2	
18- to 34-year-old men	16	41				
Competitive college athletes (women)	16-18.5	41-47	10.8	5.5-5.96	12.9	
College tennis players (women)	15	38	11.1			
Recreational college athletes (women)	15-15.5	38-39	12.5	5.8	13.2	
Sedentary college students (women)	8-14	20-36	13.5	6.4	14.3	
17-year-old girls	13	33				
18- to 34-year-old women	8	20				

*The values listed are either means or 50th percentiles (medians). There was considerable variation in sample size among the groups tested. Thus, the data should be regarded as only descriptive, not normative.

Reprinted, by permission, from NSCA, 2008, Administration, scoring, and interpretation of selected tests, by E. Harman and J. Garhammer. In *Essentials of strength training and conditioning*, 3rd ed., edited by T. Baechle and R.W. Earle (Champaign, IL: Human Kinetics), 278; data from G.M. Adams, 1998, *Exercise physiology lab manual*, 3rd ed. (Dubuque, IA: McGraw-Hill).

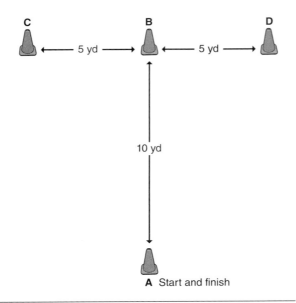

Figure 3.8 T-test diagram.

- With the fingertips, mark the highest standing reach point on the wall.
- Squat down slightly and then quickly jump up with the dominant hand. Touch the wall at the highest jump reach point.
- Measure the difference between the highest standing reach point and the highest jump reach point.
- Perform the test three times, allow sufficient rest between the trials, and record the best score to the nearest .5 inch or 1 cm.
- Normative data (table 3.9)

Muscular Strength Tests

Maximum strength can be assessed by determining a client's one-repetition maximum (1RM) in major resistance training exercises such as the bench press, shoulder press, squat, deadlift, power snatch, power clean, chest press, machine leg press, or hip sled. Use caution in having clients lift maximal weight; some clients should not perform 1RM testing until they have an initial strength base. The personal trainer should make the decision to administer 1RM testing to a client in a certain exercise based on the client's capabilities. Refer to the section "1RM Testing" in chapter 17 for a detailed description of the proper protocol and to tables 3.10 through 3.17 for the normative data for commonly tested exercises.

Definitions of the Strength Classifications

Tables 3.12 through 3.17 provide five labels, or classifications, that correspond to a client's score from a 1RM test based on his or her body weight:

Untrained

- An expected level of strength in a healthy person who has not trained on the exercise before but can perform it correctly
- The minimum level of strength required to maintain a reasonable quality of life in a sedentary person

Novice

- A person training regularly for a period of three to nine months
- A strength level that supports the demands of vigorous recreational activities

Intermediate

- A person who has engaged in regular training for up to two years
- A degree of specialization in the exercises and a high level of performance at the recreational level

Advanced

- A person with multiyear training experience who has definite goals in the higher levels of competitive athletics

Elite

- Athletes who are competing in strength sports
- Attained by approximately 2 percent of those who weight train

Table 3.10 Relative Strength Norms for 1RM Bench Press

Percentile rankings* for men	Age						
	20-29	30-39	40-49	50-59	60+		
90	1.48	1.24	1.10	0.97	0.89		
80	1.32	1.12	1.00	0.90	0.82		
70	1.22	1.04	0.93	0.84	0.77		
60	1.14	0.98	0.88	0.79	0.72		
50	1.06	0.93	0.84	0.75	0.68		
40	0.99	0.88	0.80	0.71	0.66		
30	0.93	0.83	0.76	0.68	0.63		
20	0.88	0.78	0.72	0.63	0.57		
10	0.80	0.71	0.65	0.57	0.53		

Percentile rankings* for women	Age					
	20-29	30-39	40-49	50-59	60-69	70+
90	0.54	0.49	0.46	0.40	0.41	0.44
80	0.49	0.45	0.40	0.37	0.38	0.39
70	0.42	0.42	0.38	0.35	0.36	0.33
60	0.41	0.41	0.37	0.33	0.32	0.31
50	0.40	0.38	0.34	0.31	0.30	0.27
40	0.37	0.37	0.32	0.28	0.29	0.25
30	0.35	0.34	0.30	0.26	0.28	0.24
20	0.33	0.32	0.27	0.23	0.26	0.21
10	0.30	0.27	0.23	0.19	0.25	0.20

Norms were established using a Universal bench press machine.

*Descriptors for percentile rankings: 90 = well above average; 70 = above average; 50 = average; 30 = below average; 10 = well below average.

Data for women provided by the Women's Exercise Research Center, The George Washington University Medical Center, Washington, D.C., 1998.

Data for men provided by The Cooper Institute for Aerobics Research, *The Physical Fitness Specialist Manual*, The Cooper Institute, Dallas, TX, 2005.

Reprinted, by permission, from V.H. Heyward, 2014, *Advanced fitness assessment and exercise prescription*, 7th ed. (Champaign, IL: Human Kinetics), 162.

Table 3.11 Relative Strength Norms for 1RM Leg Press

Percentile rankings* for men	Age					
	20-29	30-39	40-49	50-59	60+	
90	2.27	2.07	1.92	1.80	1.73	
80	2.13	1.93	1.82	1.71	1.62	
70	2.05	1.85	1.74	1.64	1.56	
60	1.97	1.77	1.68	1.58	1.49	
50	1.91	1.71	1.62	1.52	1.43	
40	1.83	1.65	1.57	1.46	1.38	
30	1.74	1.59	1.51	1.39	1.30	
20	1.63	1.52	1.44	1.32	1.25	
10	1.51	1.43	1.35	1.22	1.16	
Percentile rankings* for women	**Age**					
	20-29	30-39	40-49	50-59	60-69	70+
90	2.05	1.73	1.63	1.51	1.40	1.27
80	1.66	1.50	1.46	1.30	1.25	1.12
70	1.42	1.47	1.35	1.24	1.18	1.10
60	1.36	1.32	1.26	1.18	1.15	0.95
50	1.32	1.26	1.19	1.09	1.08	0.89
40	1.25	1.21	1.12	1.03	1.04	0.83
30	1.23	1.16	1.03	0.95	0.98	0.82
20	1.13	1.09	0.94	0.86	0.94	0.79
10	1.02	0.94	0.76	0.75	0.84	0.75

Norms were established using a Universal leg press machine.

*Descriptors for percentile rankings: 70 = above average; 50 = average; 30 = below average; 10 = well below average.

Data for women provided by the Women's Exercise Research Center, The George Washington University Medical Center, Washington, D.C., 1998.

Data for men provided by The Cooper Institute for Aerobics Research, *The Physical Fitness Specialist Manual*, The Cooper Institute, Dallas, TX, 2005.

Reprinted, by permission, from V.H. Heyward, 2014, *Advanced fitness assessment and exercise prescription*, 7th ed. (Champaign, IL: Human Kinetics), 163.

Table 3.12 Bench Press Standards for Adults

Pounds (kg) Body weight	Adult men				
	Untrained	Novice	Intermediate	Advanced	Elite
114 (51.7)	85 (38.6)	110 (49.9)	130 (59.0)	180 (81.6)	220 (99.8)
123 (55.8)	90 (40.8)	115 (52.2)	140 (63.5)	195 (88.5)	240 (108.9)
132 (59.9)	100 (45.4)	125 (56.7)	155 (70.3)	210 (95.3)	260 (117.9)
148 (67.1)	110 (49.9)	140 (63.5)	170 (77.1)	235 (106.6)	290 (131.5)
165 (74.8)	120 (54.4)	150 (68.0)	185 (83.9)	255 (115.7)	320 (145.1)
181 (82.1)	130 (59.0)	165 (74.8)	200 (90.7)	275 (124.7)	345 (156.5)
198 (89.8)	135 (61.2)	175 (79.4)	215 (97.5)	290 (131.5)	360 (163.3)
220 (99.8)	140 (63.5)	185 (83.9)	225 (102.1)	305 (138.3)	380 (172.4)
242 (109.8)	145 (65.8)	190 (86.2)	230 (104.3)	315 (142.9)	395 (179.2)
275 (124.7)	150 (68.0)	195 (88.5)	240 (108.9)	325 (147.4)	405 (183.7)
319 (144.7)	155 (70 .3)	200 (90.7)	245 (111.1)	335 (152.0)	415 (188.2)
≥320 (145.1)	160 (72.6)	205 (93.0)	250 (113.4)	340 (154.2)	425 (192.8)

Pounds (kg) Body weight	Adult women				
	Untrained	Novice	Intermediate	Advanced	Elite
97 (44.0)	50 (22.7)	65 (29.5)	75 (34.0)	95 (43.1)	115 (52.2)
105 (47.6)	55 (24.9)	70 (31.8)	80 (36.3)	100 (45.4)	125 (56.7)
114 (51.7)	60 (27.2)	75 (34.0)	85 (38.6)	110 (49.9)	135 (61.2)
123 (55.8)	65 (29.5)	80 (36.3)	90 (40.8)	115 (52.2)	140 (63.5)
132 (59.9)	70 (31.8)	85 (38.6)	95 (43.1)	125 (56.7)	150 (68.0)
148 (67.1)	75 (34.0)	90 (40.8)	105 (47.6)	135 (61.2)	165 (74.8)
165 (74.8)	80 (36.3)	95 (43.1)	115 (52.2)	145 (65.8)	185 (83.9)
181 (82.1)	85 (38.6)	110 (49.9)	120 (54.4)	160 (72.6)	195 (88.5)
198 (89.8)	90 (40.8)	115 (52.2)	130 (59.0)	165 (74.8)	205 (93.0)
≥199 (90.3)	95 (43.1)	120 (54.4)	140 (63.5)	175 (79.4)	220 (99.8)

Note: If the bar does not make contact with the chest above the bottom of the sternum with a momentary pause, these standards do not apply.

© Killustrated & Lon Kilgore, PhD. Updated strength performance standards are available at http://lonkilgore.com/freebies/freebies.html.

Table 3.13 Shoulder Press Standards for Adults

Pounds (kg)	Adult men				
Body weight	Untrained	Novice	Intermediate	Advanced	Elite
114 (51.7)	55 (24.9)	75 (34.0)	90 (40.8)	110 (49.9)	130 (59.0)
123 (55.8)	60 (27.2)	80 (36.3)	100 (45.4)	115 (52.2)	140 (63.5)
132 (59.9)	65 (29.5)	85 (38.6)	105 (47.6)	125 (56.7)	150 (68.0)
148 (67.1)	70 (31.8)	95 (43.1)	120 (54.4)	140 (63.5)	170 (77.1)
165 (74.8)	75 (34.0)	100 (45.4)	130 (59.0)	155 (70.3)	190 (86.2)
181 (82.1)	80 (36.3)	110 (49.9)	140 (63.5)	165 (74.8)	220 (99.8)
198 (89.8)	85 (38.6)	115 (52.2)	145 (65.8)	175 (79.4)	235 (106.6)
220 (99.8)	90 (40.8)	120 (54.4)	155 (70.3)	185 (83.9)	255 (115.7)
242 (109.8)	95 (43.1)	125 (56.7)	160 (72.6)	190 (86.2)	265 (120.2)
275 (124.7)	95 (43.1)	130 (59.0)	165 (74.8)	195 (88.5)	275 (124.7)
319 (144.7)	100 (45.4)	135 (61.2)	170 (77.1)	200 (90.7)	280 (127.0)
≥320 (145.1)	100 (45.4)	140 (63.5)	175 (79.4)	205 (93.0)	285 (129.3)
Pounds (kg)	Adult women				
Body weight	Untrained	Novice	Intermediate	Advanced	Elite
97 (44.0)	30 (13.6)	40 (18.1)	50 (22.7)	65 (29.5)	85 (38.6)
105 (47.6)	35 (15.9)	45 (20.4)	55 (24.9)	70 (31.8)	90 (40.8)
114 (51.7)	35 (15.9)	50 (22.7)	60 (27.2)	75 (34.0)	100 (45.4)
123 (55.8)	40 (18.1)	50 (22.7)	60 (27.2)	80 (36.3)	105 (47.6)
132 (59.9)	40 (18.1)	55 (24.9)	65 (29.5)	85 (38.6)	110 (49.9)
148 (67.1)	45 (20.4)	60 (27.2)	70 (31.8)	95 (43.1)	120 (54.4)
165 (74.8)	50 (22.7)	65 (29.5)	75 (34.0)	105 (47.6)	135 (61.2)
181 (82.1)	50 (22.7)	70 (31.8)	80 (36.3)	110 (49.9)	140 (63.5)
198 (89.8)	55 (24.9)	75 (34.0)	85 (38.6)	115 (52.2)	150 (68.0)
≥199 (90.3)	60 (27.2)	80 (36.3)	95 (43.1)	125 (56.7)	160 (72.6)

Note: If the subject bends the knees, leans back with the shoulders behind the hips, or does not completely extend the elbows, these standards do not apply.

Table 3.14 Squat Standards for Adults

Pounds (kg) Body weight	Adult men				
	Untrained	Novice	Intermediate	Advanced	Elite
114 (51.7)	80 (36.3)	145 (65.8)	175 (79.4)	240 (108.9)	320 (145.1)
123 (55.8)	85 (38.6)	155 (70.3)	190 (86.2)	260 (117.9)	345 (156.5)
132 (59.9)	90 (40.8)	170 (77.1)	205 (93.0)	280 (127.0)	370 (167.8)
148 (67.1)	100 (45.4)	190 (86.2)	230 (104.3)	315 (142.9)	410 (186.0)
165 (74.8)	110 (49.9)	205 (93.0)	250 (113.4)	340 (154.2)	445 (201.8)
181 (82.1)	120 (54.4)	220 (99.8)	270 (122.5)	370 (167.8)	480 (217.7)
198 (89.8)	125 (56.7)	230 (104.3)	285 (129.3)	390 (176.9)	505 (229.1)
220 (99.8)	130 (59.0)	245 (111.1)	300 (136.1)	410 (186.0)	530 (240.4)
242 (109.8)	135 (61.2)	255 (115.7)	310 (140.6)	425 (192.8)	550 (249.5)
275 (124.7)	140 (63.5)	260 (117.9)	320 (145.1)	435 (197.3)	570 (258.5)
319 (144.7)	145 (65.8)	270 (122.5)	325 (147.4)	445 (201.8)	580 (263.1)
≥320 (145.1)	150 (68.0)	275 (124.7)	330 (149.7)	455 (206.4)	595 (269.9)
Pounds (kg) Body weight	Adult women				
	Untrained	Novice	Intermediate	Advanced	Elite
97 (44.0)	45 (20.4)	85 (38.6)	100 (45.4)	130 (59.0)	165 (74.8)
105 (47.6)	50 (22.7)	90 (40.8)	105 (47.6)	140 (63.5)	175 (79.4)
114 (51.7)	55 (24.9)	100 (45.4)	115 (52.2)	150 (68.0)	190 (86.2)
123 (55.8)	55 (24.9)	105 (47.6)	120 (54.4)	160 (72.6)	200 (90.7)
132 (59.9)	60 (27.2)	110 (49.9)	130 (59.0)	170 (77.1)	210 (95.3)
148 (67.1)	65 (29.5)	120 (54.4)	140 (63.5)	185 (83.9)	230 (104.3)
165 (74.8)	70 (31.8)	130 (59.0)	150 (68.0)	200 (90.7)	255 (115.7)
181 (82.1)	75 (34.0)	140 (63.5)	165 (74.8)	215 (97.5)	270 (122.5)
198 (89.8)	80 (36.3)	150 (68.0)	175 (79.4)	230 (104.3)	290 (131.5)
≥199 (90.3)	85 (38.6)	160 (72.6)	185 (83.9)	240 (108.9)	305 (138.3)

Note: If the squat is not performed below parallel, these standards do not apply.

© Killustrated & Lon Kilgore, PhD. Updated strength performance standards are available at http://lonkilgore.com/freebies/freebies.html.

Table 3.15   Deadlift Standards for Adults

Pounds (kg)	Adult men				
Body weight	Untrained	Novice	Intermediate	Advanced	Elite
114 (51.7)	95 (43.1)	180 (81.6)	205 (93.0)	300 (136.1)	385 (174.6)
123 (55.8)	105 (47.6)	195 (88.5)	220 (99.8)	320 (145.1)	415 (188.2)
132 (59.9)	115 (52.2)	210 (95.3)	240 (108.9)	340 (154.2)	440 (199.6)
148 (67.1)	125 (56.7)	235 (106.6)	270 (122.5)	380 (172.4)	480 (217.7)
165 (74.8)	135 (61.2)	255 (115.7)	295 (133.8)	410 (186.0)	520 (235.9)
181 (82.1)	150 (68.0)	275 (124.7)	315 (142.9)	440 (199.6)	550 (249.5)
198 (89.8)	155 (70.3)	290 (131.5)	335 (152.0)	460 (208.7)	565 (256.3)
220 (99.8)	165 (74.8)	305 (138.3)	350 (158.8)	480 (217.7)	585 (265.4)
242 (109.8)	170 (77.1)	320 (145.1)	365 (165.6)	490 (222.3)	595 (269.9)
275 (124.7)	175 (79.4)	325 (147.4)	375 (170.1)	500 (226.8)	600 (272.2)
319 (144.7)	180 (81.6)	335 (152.0)	380 (172.4)	505 (229.1)	610 (276.7)
≥320 (145.1)	185 (83.9)	340 (154.2)	390 (176.9)	510 (231.3)	615 (279.0)
Pounds (kg)	Adult women				
Body weight	Untrained	Novice	Intermediate	Advanced	Elite
97 (44.0)	55 (24.9)	105 (47.6)	120 (54.4)	175 (79.4)	230 (104.3)
105 (47.6)	60 (27.2)	115 (52.2)	130 (59.0)	190 (86.2)	240 (108.9)
114 (51.7)	65 (29.5)	120 (54.4)	140 (63.5)	200 (90.7)	255 (115.7)
123 (55.8)	70 (31.8)	130 (59.0)	150 (68.0)	210 (95.3)	265 (120.2)
132 (59.9)	75 (34.0)	135 (61.2)	160 (72.6)	220 (99.8)	275 (124.7)
148 (67.1)	80 (36.3)	150 (68.0)	175 (79.4)	240 (108.9)	295 (133.8)
165 (74.8)	90 (40.8)	160 (72.6)	190 (86.2)	260 (117.9)	320 (145.1)
181 (82.1)	95 (43.1)	175 (79.4)	205 (93.0)	275 (124.7)	330 (149.7)
198 (89.8)	100 (45.4)	185 (83.9)	215 (97.5)	285 (129.3)	350 (158.8)
≥199 (90.3)	110 (49.9)	195 (88.5)	230 (104.3)	300 (136.1)	365 (165.6)

Note: If the knees, hips, and upper back are not completely extended, these standards do not apply.

© Killustrated & Lon Kilgore, PhD. Updated strength performance standards are available at http://lonkilgore.com/freebies/freebies.html.

Table 3.16 Power Clean Standards for Adults

Pounds (kg)	Adult men				
Body weight	Untrained	Novice	Intermediate	Advanced	Elite
114 (51.7)	55 (24.9)	105 (47.6)	125 (56.7)	175 (79.4)	205 (93.0)
123 (55.8)	60 (27.2)	110 (49.9)	135 (61.2)	185 (83.9)	225 (102.1)
132 (59.9)	65 (29.5)	120 (54.4)	150 (68.0)	200 (90.7)	240 (108.9)
148 (67.1)	75 (34.0)	135 (61.2)	165 (74.8)	225 (102.1)	265 (120.2)
165 (74.8)	80 (36.3)	145 (65.8)	180 (81.6)	245 (111.1)	290 (131.5)
181 (82.1)	85 (38.6)	160 (72.6)	195 (88.5)	265 (120.2)	310 (140.6)
198 (89.8)	90 (40.8)	165 (74.8)	205 (93.0)	280 (127.0)	325 (147.4)
220 (99.8)	95 (43.1)	175 (79.4)	215 (97.5)	295 (133.8)	345 (156.5)
242 (109.8)	100 (45.4)	185 (83.9)	225 (102.1)	305 (138.3)	355 (161.0)
275 (124.7)	105 (47.6)	190 (86.2)	230 (104.3)	315 (142.9)	365 (165.6)
319 (144.7)	110 (49.9)	195 (88.5)	235 (106.6)	320 (145.1)	375 (170.1)
≥320 (145.1)	115 (52.2)	200 (90.7)	240 (108.9)	330 (149.7)	385 (174.6)
Pounds (kg)	Adult women				
Body weight	Untrained	Novice	Intermediate	Advanced	Elite
97 (44.0)	30 (13.6)	60 (27.2)	70 (31.8)	95 (43.1)	115 (52.2)
105 (47.6)	35 (15.9)	65 (29.5)	75 (34.0)	100 (45.4)	125 (56.7)
114 (51.7)	40 (18.1)	70 (31.8)	80 (36.3)	110 (49.9)	135 (61.2)
123 (55.8)	40 (18.1)	75 (34.0)	85 (38.6)	115 (52.2)	145 (65.8)
132 (59.9)	45 (20.4)	80 (36.3)	90 (40.8)	120 (54.4)	150 (68.0)
148 (67.1)	50 (22.7)	90 (40.8)	100 (45.4)	135 (61.2)	165 (74.8)
165 (74.8)	50 (22.7)	95 (43.1)	110 (49.9)	145 (65.8)	185 (83.9)
181 (82.1)	55 (24.9)	100 (45.4)	120 (54.4)	155 (70.3)	195 (88.5)
198 (89.8)	60 (27.2)	110 (49.9)	125 (56.7)	165 (74.8)	205 (93.0)
≥199 (90.3)	65 (29.5)	115 (52.2)	135 (61.2)	175 (79.4)	220 (99.8)

Note: If the bar is caught below a 90-degree knee angle or is caught and ridden down below parallel, the applicability of these standards is voided.

© Killustrated & Lon Kilgore, PhD. Updated strength performance standards are available at http://lonkilgore.com/freebies/freebies.html.

Table 3.17 Power Snatch Standards for Adults

Pounds (kg)	Adult men				
Body weight	Untrained	Novice	Intermediate	Advanced	Elite
114 (51.7)	45 (20.4)	80 (36.3)	95 (43.1)	135 (61.2)	160 (72.6)
123 (55.8)	50 (22.7)	85 (38.6)	105 (47.6)	145 (65.8)	175 (79.4)
132 (59.9)	55 (24.9)	95 (43.1)	115 (52.2)	155 (70.3)	185 (83.9)
148 (67.1)	60 (27.2)	105 (47.6)	130 (59.0)	175 (79.4)	205 (93.0)
165 (74.8)	65 (29.5)	115 (52.2)	140 (63.5)	190 (86.2)	225 (102.1)
181 (82.1)	70 (31.8)	125 (56.7)	150 (68.0)	205 (93.0)	240 (108.9)
198 (89.8)	75 (34.0)	130 (59.0)	160 (72.6)	220 (99.8)	250 (113.4)
220 (99.8)	80 (36.3)	135 (61.2)	170 (77.1)	230 (104.3)	265 (120.2)
242 (109.8)	85 (38.6)	140 (63.5)	175 (79.4)	235 (106.6)	275 (124.7)
275 (124.7)	90 (40.8)	145 (65.8)	180 (81.6)	245 (111.1)	285 (129.3)
319 (144.7)	95 (43.1)	150 (68.0)	185 (83.9)	250 (113.4)	290 (131.5)
≥320 (145.1)	100 (45.4)	155 (70.3)	190 (86.2)	260 (117.9)	300 (136.1)
Pounds (kg)	Adult women				
Body weight	Untrained	Novice	Intermediate	Advanced	Elite
97 (44.0)	25 (11.3)	50 (22.7)	55 (24.9)	75 (34.0)	95 (43.1)
105 (47.6)	30 (13.6)	55 (24.9)	60 (27.2)	80 (36.3)	100 (45.4)
114 (51.7)	35 (15.9)	55 (24.9)	65 (29.5)	85 (38.6)	110 (49.9)
123 (55.8)	35 (15.9)	60 (27.2)	70 (31.8)	90 (40.8)	115 (52.2)
132 (59.9)	35 (15.9)	65 (29.5)	75 (34.0)	95 (43.1)	120 (54.4)
148 (67.1)	40 (18.1)	70 (31.8)	80 (36.3)	110 (49.9)	135 (61.2)
165 (74.8)	40 (18.1)	75 (34.0)	90 (40.8)	115 (52.2)	150 (68.0)
181 (82.1)	45 (20.4)	80 (36.3)	95 (43.1)	125 (56.7)	155 (70.3)
198 (89.8)	50 (22.7)	90 (40.8)	100 (45.4)	135 (61.2)	165 (74.8)
≥199 (90.3)	55 (24.9)	95 (43.1)	110 (49.9)	140 (63.5)	175 (79.4)

Note: If the bar is caught below a 90-degree knee angle or is caught and lowered below parallel, these standards do not apply. Also, no press-out is allowed.

© Killustrated & Lon Kilgore, PhD. Updated strength performance standards are available at http://lonkilgore.com/freebies/freebies.html.

Table 3.18 provides three classifications of a client's score from a maximal test.

Decent

- Another way of saying "not bad for someone who trains"
- Most likely associated with a client who had to work out to achieve that level of strength
- Describes clients who are strong enough that their everyday life is not limited by their strength level
- Likely requires 6 to 12 months of consistent training

- A good milestone for a beginner client to work toward
- Failure to lift 50 percent of this level defined as weak

Good

- Difficult to achieve this level without hard training
- Classified as strong by most people
- Achievable for most people with three to five years of hard training
- A good milestone for an intermediate client to work toward

Table 3.18 Strength Standards for Males and Females

Exercise	Male			Female		
	Decent	Good	Great	Decent	Good	Great
Squat	315 lb 142.9 kg) or 1.5 × BWT	405 lb (183.7 kg) or 2 × BWT	455 lb (206.4 kg) or 2.5 × BWT	95 lb (43.1 kg) or 0.75 × BWT	155 lb (70.3 kg) or 1.25 × BWT	205 lb (93.0 kg) or 2 × BWT
Bench press	225 lb 102.1 kg) or 1.25 × BWT	315 lb (142.9 kg) or 1.5 × BWT	365 lb (165.6 kg) or 2 × BWT	65 lb (29.5 kg) or 0.5 × BWT	105 lb (47.6 kg) or 0.75 × BWT	135 lb (61.2 kg) or 1 × BWT
Deadlift	315 lb (142.9 kg) or 1.5 × BWT	405 lb (183.7 kg) or 2 × BWT	495 lb (224.5 kg) or 2.75 × BWT	115 lb (52.2 kg) or 1 × BWT	185 lb (83.9 kg) or 1.5 × BWT	225 lb (102.1 kg) or 2 × BWT
Standing military press	105 lb (47.6 kg)	165 lb (74.8 kg)	225 lb (102.1 kg)	45 lb (20.4 kg)	65 lb (29.5 kg)	95 lb (43.1 kg)
Leg press	410 lb (186.0 kg)	720 lb (326.6 kg)	1,000 lb (453.6 kg)	180 lb (81.6 kg)	360 lb (163.3 kg)	450 lb (204.1 kg)
45-degree bent-over row	225 lb (102.1 kg)	275 lb (124.7 kg)	315 lb (142.9 kg)	65 lb (29.5 kg)	105 lb (47.6 kg)	135 lb (61.2 kg)
Push-up (military style for females)	30	60	90	5	25	50
Dip	20	40	60	1	15	30
Pull-up	10	20	30	1	5	12
E-Z bicep curl	80 lb (36.3 kg)	135 lb (61.2 kg)	180 lb (81.6 kg)	40 lb (18.1 kg)	60 lb (27.2 kg)	80 lb (36.3 kg)
Skull crusher	70 lb (31.8 kg)	115 lb (52.2 kg)	150 lb (68.0 kg)	35 lb (15.9 kg)	55 lb (24.9 kg)	75 lb (34.0 kg)
Elbow plank	1:30	3:00	5:00	1:30	3:00	5:00

Note: All exercises are performed with free weights, good form, no supportive gear other than a belt, and drug free. All are for a 1RM unless otherwise noted, and the weight of the bar is included in all the exercises when applicable. If both a weight and a body-weight level are given, the lifter may use whichever number is lighter.

Great

- Likely the 99th percentile or higher of the normal population
- But does not mean great for an athlete
- May not be achievable for all people; rarely achieved without long-term hard training (compare to state, national, and world records for a score significantly higher than this level)

Muscular Endurance Tests

Muscular endurance can be evaluated by tests that involve a client performing many repetitions with a submaximal effort or statically holding a certain body position for a maximum amount of time. In addition to the tests described in this section, the plank, pull-up, and dip exercises and the static flexed arm hang can be selected to assess a client's muscular endurance.

Push-Up

- Protocol
  - Men assume the standard push-up starting position with the hands shoulder-width apart and the elbows and body straight. Women start similarly except that the knees rather than the feet contact the ground. The knees are flexed at 90 degrees, and the ankles are crossed.
  - Lower the body until the chest makes contact with a tester's fist (men) or the torso makes contact with a foam roller (women).

- Press the body up until the elbows are fully extended.
- Perform as many repetitions as possible.
- Normative data (table 3.19)

Partial Curl-Up (Crunch)

- Protocol
  - Assume a supine position on a mat with the knees at a 90-degree angle and the arms at the sides resting on the floor. The fingers are touching a 4-inch-long (10 cm) piece of tape placed at the ends of the fingers. A second piece of tape is placed 4 inches (10 cm) away from the first piece of tape.
  - Set a metronome to 50 beats per minute and perform a curl-up to lift the shoulder blades off the mat in cadence with the metronome.
  - During the curl-up, slide the arms and fingers on the floor to meet the second piece of tape.
  - In cadence with the metronome, uncurl back to the starting position.
  - Perform as many repetitions as possible, without a pause, up to a maximum of 25.
- Normative data (table 3.20)

YMCA Bench Press

- Protocol
  - Set the metronome to 60 beats per minute (to time the performance of 30 repetitions per minute, spending one second to lower the bar and one second to raise the bar).
  - Get into the proper body position to perform the bench press exercise; men use an 80-pound (36 kg) bar and women use a 35-pound (16 kg) bar.
  - Lift the bar off the upright rack and listen to the cadence of the metronome.
  - Lower the bar down to touch the chest lightly in cadence with the metronome.
  - Push the bar up to full elbow extension in cadence with the metronome.
  - Perform as many repetitions as possible, without a pause.
- Normative data (table 3.21)

Cardiovascular Endurance Tests

A key component of fitness, especially as it relates to general health, is cardiovascular endurance. As discussed in chapter 1, car-

Table 3.19 Fitness Categories by Age Groups and Sex for Push-Ups

Category	Age and sex									
	20-29		30-39		40-49		50-59		60-69	
	M	F	M	F	M	F	M	F	M	F
Excellent	36	30	30	27	25	24	21	21	18	17
Very good	35	29	29	26	24	23	20	20	17	16
	29	21	22	20	17	15	13	11	11	12
Good	28	20	21	19	16	14	12	10	10	11
	22	15	17	13	13	11	10	7	8	5
Fair	21	14	16	12	12	10	9	6	7	4
	17	10	12	8	10	5	7	2	5	2
Needs improvement	16	9	11	7	9	4	6	1	4	1

Source: *Canadian Physical Activity, Fitness & Lifestyle Approach: CSEP-Health & Fitness Program's Appraisal and Counselling Strategy*, 3rd edition, ©2003. Reprinted with permission from the Canadian Society for Exercise Physiology.

Table 3.20 Percentiles by Age Groups and Gender for Partial Curl-Up

Rating	Age (years)					
	15-19	20-29	30-39	40-49	50-59	60-69
Men						
Excellent	25	25	25	25	25	25
Very good	23-24	21-24	18-24	18-24	17-24	16-24
Good	21-22	16-20	15-17	13-17	11-16	11-15
Fair	16-20	11-15	11-14	6-12	8-10	6-10
Needs improvement	≤15	≤10	≤10	≤5	≤7	≤5
Women						
Excellent	25	25	25	25	25	25
Very good	22-24	18-24	19-24	19-24	19-24	17-24
Good	17-21	14-17	10-18	11-18	10-18	8-16
Fair	12-16	5-13	6-9	4-10	6-9	3-7
Needs improvement	≤11	≤4	≤5	≤3	≤5	≤2

Source: *Canadian Physical Activity, Fitness & Lifestyle Approach: CSEP-Health & Fitness Program's Appraisal and Counselling Strategy*, 3rd edition, ©2003. Reprinted with permission from the Canadian Society for Exercise Physiology.

Table 3.21   YMCA Bench Press Norms

Percentile	Age and sex											
	18-25		26-35		36-45		46-55		56-65		>65	
	M	F	M	F	M	F	M	F	M	F	M	F
90	44	42	41	40	36	33	28	29	24	24	20	18
80	37	34	33	32	29	28	22	22	20	20	14	14
70	33	28	29	28	25	24	20	18	14	14	10	10
60	29	25	26	24	22	21	16	14	12	12	10	8
50	26	21	22	21	20	17	13	12	10	9	8	6
40	22	18	20	17	17	14	11	9	8	6	6	4
30	20	16	17	14	14	12	9	7	5	5	4	3
20	16	12	13	12	10	8	6	5	3	3	2	1
10	10	6	9	6	6	4	2	1	1	1	1	0

Score is number of repetitions completed in 1 minute using an 80-pound (36 kg) barbell for men and a 35-pound (16 kg) barbell for women.

Reprinted, by permission, from NSCA, 2008, Administration, scoring, and interpretation of selected tests, by E. Harman and J. Garhammer. In *Essentials of strength training and conditioning*, 3rd ed., edited by T. Baehle and R.W. Earle (Champaign, IL: Human Kinetics), 282; adapted from YMCA, 2000.

diovascular endurance can be quantified by calculating a client's $\dot{V}O_2max$, or the number of milliliters of oxygen the body can provide per kilogram per minute. The most important thing to note about that equation is that body weight is a component of aerobic fitness. Having both a high $\dot{V}O_2max$ and a high body weight is extremely difficult. As a person's body weight goes up, the heart and lungs increase in size, but those organs will not increase in size at the same rate as the rest of the body does. A 400-pound (181.8 kg) person cannot have a heart that is proportionally the same size as the heart of a 150-pound (68.2 kg) person who is in good shape. This truism means two things to you as a personal trainer. First, a person who really wants to excel at cardiovascular events needs to be at a relatively low body weight (and relatively lean at the same time). Second, when your clients start to lose body weight, they will often find that their "energy" levels go up. What has really happened is that their $\dot{V}O_2$max has improved, thus reducing the energy they need to get through their daily life. They therefore have more energy reserves and feel better. Even a 5- or 10-pound (4.5 to 9.1 kg) weight change can be quite noticeable.

Males generally have a higher $\dot{V}O_2$max than females, about 5 or 6 points higher, because males tend to have larger hearts and lungs than females do, even at the same body weight (104, 110).

Your client's $\dot{V}O_2$max can be determined in two ways—either by measuring it during a maximal exercise test or by estimating it from a submaximal test.

Measuring $\dot{V}O_2$max

A client's $\dot{V}O_2$max can be directly measured with a truly maximal test. This test is usually performed by having the client exercise on a treadmill wearing a mask that covers the nose and mouth, similar to a scuba mask, with tubes that connect to a computer. The computer monitors the amount of oxygen that the client inhales and exhales and calculates the difference. This difference is the amount of oxygen that the body is using. The client begins the test at a slow walk on a level treadmill. The technician gradually increases the speed or the incline of the treadmill until the client is running as hard as he or she can go. The client will likely reach his or maximum speed in 8 to 12 minutes (110). That point is your client's $\dot{V}O_2$max, when he or she is delivering the maximal amount of oxygen to the muscles (104). In the end, you will get a two-digit score representing your client's $\dot{V}O_2$max. The scores generally range from about 20 milliliters per kilogram per minute to 80 milliliters per kilogram per minute; the higher the score, the better. A person with a score of 20 milliliters per kilogram per minute would have a poor $\dot{V}O_2$max and might even get winded going up one flight of stairs, whereas a person with a $\dot{V}O_2$max of 80 milliliters per

kilogram per minute would probably be an Olympic-level athlete.

Estimating $\dot{V}O_2$max

Performing a measured $\dot{V}O_2$max test is useful for athletes, particularly those involved in aerobic endurance events, but it is not feasible or appropriate for all people. Beginners and people with heart issues will probably not do a max test, and some people just don't have access to the equipment. If this is the case, you can estimate your client's $\dot{V}O_2$max by performing a submax test, a test in which the client does not work as hard as possible. *Submax* means "submaximal," so by having your client work at just a moderate level of intensity, you can get information about how his or her body is responding to exercise, and from that you can estimate the true $\dot{V}O_2$max. Of course, this method has more error, but it is easier to do.

Rockport Walk Test

- Protocol
    - Use a stopwatch to measure the time needed to cover 1 mile (1.6 km) as quickly as possible by fast walking (walking only; no jogging or running).
- Normative data (table 3.22). Note: This test is for clients 18 to 69 years old.

Step Test

- Protocol
    - Place a 12-inch (30 cm) box or step on a flat surface.
    - Set the metronome to 96 beats per minute (to time the performance of 24 steps per minute using one second for each part of the stepping movement: right foot up, left foot up, right foot down, left foot down).
    - Listen to the cadence of the metronome and then complete three minutes of stepping.
    - After the last step, sit down and (within five seconds) measure the recovery heart rate for one minute.
- Normative data (table 3.23)

Table 3.22 Norms for the Rockport Walk Test

	Clients aged 30-69 years (min:s)	
Rating	Males	Females
Excellent	<10:12	<11:40
Good	10:13-11:42	11:41-13:08
High average	11:43-13:13	13:09-14:36
Low average	13:14-14:44	14:37-16:04
Fair	14:45-16:23	16:05-17:31
Poor	>16:24	>17:32
	Clients aged 18-30 years (min:s)	
Percentile	Males	Females
90	11:08	11:45
75	11:42	12:49
50	12:38	13:15
25	13:38	14:12
10	14:37	15:03

Reprinted, by permission, from J. Morrow, A. Jackson, J. Disch, and D. Mood, 2011, *Measurement and evaluation in human performance*, 4th ed. (Champaign, IL: Human Kinetics), 201.

Table 3.23 Male and Female Norms for Recovery Heart Rate Following the 3-Minute Step Test (beats/min)

	Age (years)					
Rating	18-25	26-35	36-45	46-55	56-65	66+
	Male					
Excellent	70-78	73-79	72-81	78-84	72-82	72-86
Good	82-88	83-88	86-94	89-96	89-97	89-95
Above average	91-97	91-97	98-102	99-103	98-101	97-102
Average	101-104	101-106	105-111	109-115	105-111	104-113
Below average	107-114	109-116	113-118	118-121	113-118	114-119
Poor	118-126	119-126	120-128	124-130	122-128	122-128
Very poor	131-164	130-164	132-168	135-158	131-150	133-152
	Female					
Excellent	72-83	72-86	74-87	76-93	74-92	73-86
Good	88-97	91-97	93-101	96-102	97-103	93-100
Above average	100-106	103-110	104-109	106-113	106-111	104-114
Average	110-116	112-118	111-117	117-120	113-117	117-121
Below average	118-124	121-127	120-127	121-126	119-127	123-127
Poor	128-137	129-135	130-138	127-133	129-136	129-134
Very poor	142-155	141-154	143-152	138-152	142-151	135-151

Reprinted, by permission, from J. Morrow, A. Jackson, J. Disch, and D. Mood, 2011, *Measurement and evaluation in human performance*, 4th ed. (Champaign, IL: Human Kinetics), 200.

1-Mile (1.6 km) Run

- Protocol
    - Use a stopwatch to measure the time it takes to cover 1 mile (1.6 km) as fast as possible by running, jogging, or fast walking.
- Normative data (table 3.24). Note: This test is for clients 6 to 17 years old.

1.5-Mile (2.4 km) Run

- Protocol
    - Use a stopwatch to measure the time needed to cover 1.5 miles (2.4 km) as fast as possible by running, jogging, or fast walking.
    - Convert the seconds portion of the finishing time to minutes by dividing it by 60. For example, 9:15 (9 minutes and 15 seconds) converts to 9.25 minutes (15 ÷ 60 seconds = 0.25 minute).
    - Calculate an estimate of $\dot{V}O_2max$ (in ml/kg/min) using this equation:

$$\dot{V}O_2max = 483 \div \text{time in minutes} + 3.5$$

- Normative data (tables 3.25 and 3.26)

Flexibility Tests

Tests for flexibility are joint specific, just as muscular strength tests are specific to the muscles involved in the exercises used for testing. Common tests include the overhead squat, shoulder elevation, wall glide, and the test described in this section, the sit and reach.

Sit and Reach

- Protocol
    - Warm up, remove shoes, and sit on the floor with the knees straight and the heels pressed against the front of the sit-and-reach box.
    - Slowly reach forward as far as possible with both hands placed evenly over each other to push the sliding guide bracket along the top of the sit-and-reach box; keep the knees straight and the heels pressed against the front of the box. Pause momentarily at the most forward-flexed position.
    - Repeat the test twice and record the best score.

Table 3.24 Norms for 1-Mile Run (min:s)

	Percentile					
	Boys			Girls		
Age	85	50	15	85	50	15
6	10:15	12:36	16:30	11:20	13:12	16:45
7	9:22	11:40	15:00	10:36	12:56	16:00
8	8:48	11:05	14:10	10:02	12:30	15:19
9	8:31	10:30	12:59	9:30	11:52	14:57
10	7:57	9:48	13:07	9:19	11:22	14:00
11	7:32	9:20	12:29	9:02	11:17	14:16
12	7:11	8:40	11:30	8:23	11:05	14:12
13	6:50	8:06	10:39	8:13	10:23	14:10
14	6:26	7:44	10:18	7:59	10:06	12:56
15	6:20	7:30	9:34	8:08	9:58	13:33
16	6:08	7:10	9:22	8:23	10:31	14:16
17	6:06	7:04	8:56	8:15	10:22	13:03

Table 3.25 Percentile Values for Maximal Aerobic Power ($\dot{V}O_2$max; ml · kg⁻¹ · min⁻¹)

Percentage	Age (years) 20-29	30-39	40-49	50-59	60-69	Percentage	Age (years) 20-29	30-39	40-49	50-59	60-69
	Males						Females				
90	54.0	52.5	51.1	46.8	43.2	90	47.5	44.7	42.4	38.1	34.6
80	51.1	47.5	46.8	43.3	39.5	80	44.0	41.0	38.9	35.2	32.3
70	48.2	46.8	44.2	41.0	36.7	70	41.1	38.8	36.7	32.9	30.2
60	45.7	44.4	42.4	38.3	35.0	60	39.5	36.7	35.1	31.4	29.1
50	43.9	42.4	40.4	36.7	33.1	50	37.4	35.2	33.3	30.2	27.5
40	42.2	42.2	38.4	35.2	31.4	40	35.5	33.8	31.6	28.7	26.6
30	40.3	38.5	36.7	33.2	29.4	30	33.8	32.3	29.7	27.3	24.9
20	38.1	36.7	34.6	31.1	27.4	20	31.6	29.9	28.0	25.5	23.7
10	35.2	33.8	31.8	28.4	24.1	10	29.4	27.4	25.6	23.7	21.7

Reprinted, by permission, from NSCA, 2012, Fitness testing protocols and norms, by E.D. Ryan and J.T. Cramer. In *NSCA's essentials of personal training*, 2nd ed., edited by J.W. Coburn and M.H. Malek (Champaign, IL: Human Kinetics), 239; data from American College of Sports Medicine, 2010, *ACSM's guidelines for exercise testing and prescription*, 8th ed. (Philadelphia: Lippincott Williams & Wilkins).

Table 3.26 $\dot{V}O_2$max Descriptive Data for Athletes in Various Sports

Classification and typical $\dot{V}O_2$max of athletes playing the sport (ml · kg⁻¹ · min⁻¹)		Sport
Extremely high		
Males	70+	Cross-country skiing
Females	60+	Middle-distance running
		Long-distance running
Very high		
Males	63-69	Bicycling
Females	54-59	Rowing
		Racewalking
High		
Males	57-62	Soccer
Females	49-53	Middle-distance swimming
		Canoe racing
		Handball
		Racquetball
		Speed skating
		Figure skating
		Downhill skiing
		Wrestling
Above average		
Males	52-56	Basketball
Females	44-48	Ballet dancing
		American football (offensive, defensive backs)
		Gymnastics
		Hockey
		Horse racing (jockey)
		Sprint swimming
		Tennis
		Sprint running
		Jumping

(continued)

Table 3.26 *(continued)*

Classification and typical V̇O₂max of athletes playing the sport (ml · kg⁻¹ · min⁻¹)		Sport
Average		
Males	44-51	Baseball, softball
Females	35-43	American football (linemen, quarterbacks)
		Shot put
		Discus throw
		Olympic-style weightlifting
		Bodybuilding

Reprinted, by permission, from NSCA, 2008, Administration, scoring, and interpretation of selected tests, by E. Harman and J. Garhammer. In *Essentials of strength training and conditioning*, 3rd ed., edited by T. Baehle and R.W. Earle (Champaign, IL: Human Kinetics), 282; data from D.C. Nieman, 1995, *Fitness and sports medicine*, 3rd ed. (Palo Alto, CA: Bull).

- Normative data (table 3.27); note that the norms are based on a zero point—the point at which the tips of the fingers reach the toes—of 26 cm (to convert inches to centimeters, multiply by 2.54).

USING THE RESULTS OF A FITNESS ASSESSMENT

Performing the tests provides some valuable information to the personal trainer. First, it serves as a baseline assessment to let the personal trainer know where the client is on certain components of fitness. As the client progresses through the training program, the client can be retested and change can be

shown. Beginners will make progress more rapidly than intermediates or advanced clients will, so they should probably be tested more frequently. To chart progress, beginners should be tested every one to three months, intermediates every two to four months, and advanced clients every three to six months.

Testing clients on standardized tests presented in this text is useful because the personal trainer can then compare the client with others. That knowledge can help clarify the client's strengths and weaknesses. For example, if a female client could perform 45 push-ups but needed 25 minutes to complete the 1.5-mile (2.4 km) run, she clearly performed well on a muscular endurance test but poorly on a cardiovascular test. That client may prefer

Table 3.27 Fitness Categories by Age Groups for Trunk Forward Flexion Using a Sit-and-Reach Box (cm)

Category*	Age									
	20-29		30-39		40-49		50-59		60-69	
	M	F	M	F	M	F	M	F	M	F
Excellent	40	41	38	41	35	38	35	39	33	35
Very good	39	40	37	40	34	37	34	38	32	34
	34	37	33	36	29	34	28	33	25	31
Good	33	36	32	35	28	33	27	32	24	30
	30	33	28	32	24	30	24	30	20	27
Fair	29	32	27	31	23	29	23	29	19	26
	25	28	23	27	18	25	16	25	15	23
Needs improvement	24	27	22	26	17	24	15	24	14	22

These norms are based on a sit-and-reach box in which the zero point is set at 26 cm. When using a box in which the zero point is set at 23 cm, subtract 3 cm from each value in this table.

Source: *Canadian Physical Activity, Fitness & Lifestyle Approach: CSEP-Health & Fitness Program's Appraisal and Counselling Strategy*, 3rd edition, ©2003. Reprinted with permission from the Canadian Society for Exercise Physiology.

to train muscular endurance in the gym, but improving her $\dot{V}O_2$max will likely yield the greatest improvement to her health. If a client is an athlete, comparisons can be made to other athletes in the same sport to identify strengths and weaknesses. For example, if a male soccer player had a $\dot{V}O_2$max of 75 milliliters per kilogram per minute and a bench press 1RM of 85 pounds (38.6 kg), he does not need to work on his $\dot{V}O_2$max because it is already significantly higher than that of other soccer players. But his bench press 1RM is quite low, so he needs to do more work in the weight room, which will translate to better performance on the field. Of course, at high levels, mastery of the sport-specific skills (such as dribbling and shooting in soccer) will have the greatest effect on sport performance (78).

Personal trainers can use the tests to help plan the workout program. If a client simply says, "I want to get fit," that information is likely not enough for a personal trainer to construct a detailed workout. If the client completes a battery of tests and as a result says, "I want to get fit so that I can perform more pull-ups, hold a plank longer, have a higher vertical jump, and have bigger arms," the personal trainer can use that information to develop an exercise program specific to that person. The personal trainer can then take the client through a routine, retest the client two months later, discover the effectiveness of the program, and make modifications to keep the client moving toward his or her goals.

Finally, effective tests can highlight areas or issues that clients may not be aware of. For example, a client may be focused on losing weight, but if the client performs an overhead squat flexibility test and scores poorly, the personal trainer can educate the client about the importance of flexibility and other components of fitness to help the client become healthier overall.

CONCLUSION

Personal trainers need to classify each client based on the risk stratification scale and the assessments that are appropriate to use with that client. Personal trainers should be familiar with the various forms that clients will fill out; the risk factors for coronary artery disease; the signs and symptoms of coronary artery disease; and the indicators that classify clients as low, moderate, or high risk.

Also, personal trainers can use a battery of various assessments for their clients to gain better understanding of their fitness levels. Assessments are broken down into resting and active categories. Personal trainers should understand that assessments should be performed in a specified order to minimize the fatigue effect of previous assessments. All assessments are simply tools available to the personal trainer; no assessments are mandatory for all clients.

Study Questions

Use the following information to answer study questions 1 and 2.

A 40-year-old male wishes to begin a personal training program. He is 5 feet, 10 inches (177.8 cm) tall and weighs 187 pounds (84.8 kg), and his waist is 36 inches (91.4 cm). He walks twice a week for an hour and plays racquetball twice a week. His dad passed away at 78 from heart disease; his other relatives are still alive. He does not smoke, and his blood pressure is 130/85, for which he is on medication. His total cholesterol is 215. His LDL is 145, and his HDL is 48. He has a fasting glucose of 89. He has no signs or symptoms of a disease, and he does not have a disease that would affect his metabolism.

1. What is this client's risk stratification?
   a. low risk
   b. moderate risk
   c. high risk

2. What types of activity are you able to do with this client without a medical clearance?
   a. This client can engage in both moderate and vigorous exercise.
   b. This client can engage in only moderate exercise; he needs a clearance for vigorous exercise.

c. This client can engage only in resistance training at any intensity; he needs a clearance for any cardiovascular work.

d. This client cannot engage in physical activity until he is cleared by a doctor.

3. Put the following tests in the order in which you would perform them, assuming that all tests were performed on the same day:

Push-up test

1RM bench press test

Resting pulse

Body fat

a. resting pulse, body fat, 1RM bench press test, push-up test

b. body fat, resting pulse, 1RM bench press test, push-up test

c. resting pulse, push-up test, 1RM bench press test, body fat

d. push-up test, 1RM bench press test, body fat, resting pulse

4. Which of the following is a sign or symptom of coronary artery disease?

a. fasting glucose level of 105

b. muscular strength ranked in the bottom 25 percent

c. being on blood pressure or cholesterol medication

d. tachycardia, shortness of breath, and unusual fatigue

5. What waist–hip ratio is considered the maximum healthy value for a female?

a. 1.11

b. .95

c. .85

d. .67

Setting Goals

Helping your clients set proper goals will help ensure that they see the results they want. In addition, their success will increase your client retention rate. You need to understand what clients really mean when they share their fitness goals. Clients will not use "personal trainer speak"; they will not ask you to help them increase their $\dot{V}O_2max$, for example. Instead they will offer vague ideas about looking good, feeling better, and getting stronger. Occasionally, they may even say something that they don't mean. Consider the two following scenarios:

> A male client walks up to a personal trainer and expresses interest in personal training. The client says that he would like to "get better at push-ups." The personal trainer asks the client why he wants to get better at push-ups, and the client responds, "To have a bigger chest and arms." The personal trainer clarifies, "So what you are really looking for is a program to increase the size of your chest and arms?" The client retorts, "Yeah, that's what I said."

> A female client walks up to a personal trainer and expresses interest in personal training. The client says that she wants stronger legs. The personal trainer asks the client why she wants stronger legs, and the client responds, "So I can run a half marathon faster." The personal trainer clarifies, "So what you are really looking for is a program to reduce your half marathon time?" to which the client responds, "Yes, that's what I said."

In both scenarios, the client started by leading the personal trainer down the wrong road. In the first scenario the client indicated that he wanted to improve his push-up ability, which a knowledgeable personal trainer will generally associate with muscular endurance. In the second scenario the client indicated that she wanted stronger legs. A personal trainer would logically think of squats and the component of muscular strength. But in reality those clients wanted something else, and only by exploring their goals did the personal trainer realize what they actually wanted. If the personal trainer had not done that, he might have helped the male client complete 20 more push-ups after three months only to be fired because he didn't make his client's chest and arms bigger. The personal trainer needs to understand the client's goals. The job of the personal trainer is not to judge clients for their goals. If the personal trainer in the second scenario told the client that running half marathons was stupid and that she would be better off lifting weights, he would very likely lose the client. A wise personal trainer also needs to be aware that clients often worry that the personal trainer will decide what they need to do without even asking them what their goals are. They worry that a personal trainer will take one look at them and then decide how they should proceed, often with the fear that they might become a mini version of the personal trainer. Sometimes clients do want to emulate their personal trainers, but not all of them do. Indeed, the more impressive a personal trainer's physique is or the more elite his or her athletic ability is, the more worried a client may be about becoming a clone. The personal trainer needs to reassure the client that the personal trainer will use his or her knowledge to help the client reach personal goals, not force the client to become a look-alike of the personal trainer (21).

GOAL-SETTING GUIDELINES

When asking clients to go over their goals, as a personal trainer, you should initially sit back and just let them talk. You should practice reflective listening and essentially repeat back to them what they are saying. Do not put words in their mouths, do not cut them off and finish their sentences for them, don't assume you know what their goals are, and do not judge their goals. Initially, just listen. After the client has spoken, then you can try to understand and further refine the client's goals. A useful acronym to help that process is *SMART*:

- S—specific
- M—measurable
- A—attainable
- R—realistic
- T—time based or timeline

Some people prefer the acronym *SMARTER*, in which the *E* refers to *exciting* and the last *R* refers to *recorded*, which simply means that your goals are written down (9, 17).

Specific

Goals should be specific; this means that clients clearly define what it is they are trying to do. They should not just say, "I want to look better." Instead, they should say, "I am currently at 25 percent body fat, and I want to get down to 20 percent body fat," or "My arms are currently 14 inches (35.5 cm), and I want them to be 15 inches (38 cm)."

Objective

Goals should be objective and measurable; this means that if you were to ask another personal trainer whether your client achieved the goal, the answer would be obvious and backed up by a measurable change. The opposite of objective is subjective, which is what most goals are but is what you want to guide the client away from. Clients often have vague, subjective goals such as feeling better or feeling younger. Those goals are too vague and need to be more clearly defined to be better understood. Try to make most goals performance based. Athletes commonly set such goals, but the general clientele doesn't focus on this. Performance-based goals are helpful for all clients because they are automatically specific and objective. Such goals guide the subsequent training program and serve as motivation during training. In addition, a performance-based goal is more empowering because the client has more control over the goal and can see specific and concrete progress.

Realistic

Goals should be realistic; this is another way of saying that goals should be attainable. The point of this goal is not to doubt someone's capacity or downplay his or her ability. But focusing on a huge, long-term goal can be frustrating, especially if your clients are currently far from that goal. The best thing to do is to break down that goal into smaller segments. If a person wants to lose a significant amount of weight, 200 pounds (90.7 kg), for example, the task can seem overwhelming, and the client can easily become discouraged. But a goal to lose 50 pounds (22.7 kg), or 20 pounds (9.1 kg), or even 10 pounds (4.5 kg) will seem more doable. Focus your client's energy on just the first 20 pounds, make that the goal, and allow the person to feel successful after attaining it. After the client succeeds, you do the same thing again with the next 20 pounds, but the client should go into that next phase feeling encouraged by his or her initial success. If the client can do that 10 times, he or she has lost 200 pounds.

Time Based

Good goals are time based, which means that they have a timeline or a date by which they will be achieved. The client should say, "I want to lose 12 pounds (5.4 kg) in the next three months," and as that time ticks by, he or she needs to lose that weight. A client who wants to lift a certain amount of weight or run a certain time should have a goal date for accomplishing that task.

Having a timeline serves two purposes. First, it causes people to act. Seeing the date on the calendar and seeing it get closer helps start them moving. Second, the date can be motivating. When a competition nears for athletes, they tend to crank up their energy and activity. They know that the competition is near and that if they don't train hard now, they will never have a chance to do so.

Control

People should have control over their goals. One way to do this is to set a process goal. A process goal is a goal that you (or your client) are directly in control of. A person who is just beginning to work out could set a goal to go to the gym 12 times this month. The person is in control of that goal, and nothing or nobody can stop him or her from doing that. Process goals are empowering because people know that it is up to them to accomplish the goal. Some people focus on outcome goals. Our society emphasizes the outcome of an event, but the problem is that we can't control outcome goals. Instead, people should focus on things that they have control over (2). If people focus on everything in their control, concentrate on their execution, and execute as well as possible, the desired outcome often occurs.

Components of Fitness

When setting goals, a good approach is to formulate them in relation to the five components of fitness—strength, muscular endurance, cardiorespiratory endurance, flexibility, and body composition. These components are objective and measurable. If your clients say that they want to look better, that goal can be vague and difficult to define. But if your clients say that they want to reduce their body fat, you can help them with that goal. A personal trainer's scope of practice is to enhance the components of fitness for the general, healthy population and relate all goals to the components of fit-

ness and their subcategories. See table 4.1 for examples of common general or subjective fitness goals and the more specific goals related to components of fitness.

Translating a client's goals can also mean revising them so they are more detailed, objective, time based, and measurable. Here are some more examples of goals that personal trainers will commonly hear. The initial goal is the client's original statement; the revised goal is that statement fleshed out by the personal trainer with more details from the client.

Initial goal: "I want to lose weight."

Revised goal: "I want to lose 15 pounds (6.8 kg) of body fat in three months."

Initial goal: "I want to gain weight."

Revised goal: "I want to gain 10 pounds (4.5 kg) of weight and at least 7 pounds (3.2 kg) of muscle in three months."

Initial goal: "I want to increase my energy."

Revised goal: "I want to improve my $\dot{V}O_2$max from a 29 to a 35 in three months."

Table 4.1 Translating Common Goals to Specific Goals

Common goal	Specific goal
Look better	Decrease body fat Increase muscle size
Feel better	Decrease body fat and weight Increase $\dot{V}O_2$max Increase strength Increase flexibility
Have more energy	Increase $\dot{V}O_2$max Decrease body fat and weight
Tone up	Decrease body fat Increase muscle size
Get stronger	Increase muscle strength Increase muscle size Increase muscle endurance
Feel younger	Increase $\dot{V}O_2$max Increase strength Increase flexibility Decrease body fat
Get bigger	Increase muscle size Increase muscle strength
Lose weight	Decrease body fat Decrease body weight

Initial goal: "I want to improve my flexibility."

Revised goal: "I want to improve the flexibility of my hamstrings, lower back, and shoulders, and I want to score a 20 on the sit and reach in two months and perform an easy wall glide."

Initial goal: "I want to get bigger."

Revised goal: "I want to gain 3 inches (7.6 cm) on my chest, 1.5 inches (3.75 cm) on my arms, and 2 inches (5 cm) on my thighs in six months."

Initial: "I want to get stronger."

Revised: "I want to bench press 315 pounds (142.9 kg) for one rep in six months."

Initial: "I want more endurance."

Revised: "I want to perform 30 push-ups, 10 pull-ups (each in one minute), and a three-minute plank on my next muscular endurance test, which is two months away."

Initial: "I want to tone up."

Revised: "I want to decrease my body fat by 5 percent and increase my muscles (as shown by an increase in muscular strength and endurance tests) in two months."

TYPES OF GOALS

Goals can be classified into four types, differentiated by how long it will take to achieve the goal.

Ultimate Goals

Ultimate goals are goals that people dream about achieving at some point during their life. Honestly, most ultimate goals are never achieved, but with the knowledge gained from this book, you may be able to help your clients achieve one or more of their ultimate goals. A person may be 5, 10, or even 20 years away from achieving a goal that he or she has always wanted to reach.

Ideally, these ultimate goals are process goals, but that is not always the case. Ultimate goals can be especially motivating because they truly represent a person's dream, but they can also be defeating. Sometimes, particularly when a person starts out, the goal is so far away that attaining it may seem impossible. This circumstance presents an interesting catch-22; if the goal is too easy, it isn't really an ultimate goal and achieving it will not be that rewarding. On the other hand, if the goal is too difficult, the person may never achieve it, which can be frustrating and discouraging. Unattainable goals can cause people to give up on their efforts altogether. Even if a person fails at one ultimate goal, he or she should not give up. When the ultimate goal seems far away, the wise approach is to break that larger goal down into more achievable levels and manageable periods and then work toward those somewhat smaller goals.

Long-Term Goals

Long-term goals normally take about six months to a year to achieve, although in some instances it might take as long as four or five years. If the time frame is much longer than that, the goal is an ultimate goal. Long-term goals are difficult to achieve but can be accomplished with consistent effort. The person needs to design a game plan and follow it. Examples of long-term goals are the following: lose 50 pounds (22.7 kg), increase bench press by 75 pounds (34.0 kg), add 4 to 6 inches (10 to 15 cm) to chest measurement, decrease running pace by 1 minute per mile (by 37 seconds per km), run a marathon, walk 50 miles (80.5 km) in one day, reduce 40-yard (37 m) dash speed by .3 second, and so forth. An average person (one not already elite) could complete most of the preceding goals in about a year. Remember, when a person is just starting, he or she makes progress quickly, and after someone has been training for a long time, progress comes more slowly.

Short-Term Goals

Short-term goals are interim goals designed to help people achieve their long-term goals.

They are normally one to four months in duration; two to three months is the most common period. Usually, several short-term goals strung together will lead to the accomplishment of the long-term goal. People should feel confident that they can achieve short-term goals with some hard work. The goals should not be daunting; they should be realistic and motivating. If a person is doubtful about his or her ability to achieve a short-term goal, then it is too difficult and it should be scaled back. Examples of common short-term goals are the following: run 3 miles (4.8 km) without stopping, increase bench press by 20 pounds (9.1 kg), take 2 inches (5 cm) off waist measurement, lose 10 pounds (4.5 kg), increase push-up and sit-up scores, and consistently eat four or five meals per day for two months (26).

Daily Goals

Goals that people have for themselves every day are daily goals. Because people have many daily goals and because they aren't that hard to achieve, they are sometimes perceived as the least significant goals. In fact, the opposite is true. Daily goals are the most important goals that people can have. Without them, people have no chance to achieve short-term, long-term, or ultimate goals. Generally, our brains work backward. We set a goal that is far away and then backtrack our way to that goal. Real life, however, works by going forward. We have to take baby steps every day, and if we do that, natural progress will lead us to our larger goals. In fact, when the time comes to hit those long-term and even ultimate goals, they just become the daily goal for that day. The fact that daily goals are the most important and the easiest to achieve should be motivating. People have within themselves the power to achieve almost anything they want, as long as they are willing to put the effort into it. If people can just take care of today, each and every day, they will be successful (36).

Common daily goals include going to the gym, eating the meals planned for the day, finishing all scheduled sets, completing the scheduled time for a cardio workout, accomplishing other daily tasks to allow time to work out, getting a reasonable night's sleep, being prepared for each workout, getting out of bed on time, and maintaining academic grades to be eligible to compete.

TIMELINE FOR GOALS

Clients often ask personal trainers what they can realistically expect the body to do in a certain time frame. For example, they might want to lose weight, but they are not sure how long it will take to do so in a healthy fashion. Fad diets and supplement marketing insist that progress will be nearly instantaneous, when often that is not the case.

Generalizing about what kind of progress a client will make is difficult. Remember the principle of individual variation: People respond differently to the same stimulus. In addition, remember that if clients are new to exercise or new to a particular type of activity, their starting level will be low but they will likely make rapid progress in that area. If clients have been performing an activity for a while and are used to exercise, their starting level should be higher but they will make progress more slowly.

Although it is challenging to predict exactly how the body will respond to an exercise program, it can be beneficial to have a general idea of the progress that a person might make, assuming that he or she is working out hard, training consistently, and following a good diet. Remember, if your clients want to change how they look or how much they weigh, nutrition is more important than their workout plan. That statement might sound bizarre, but it is true. This point doesn't mean that working out isn't important; rather, it highlights the real importance of nutrition (19).

Outlined in table 4.2 is a list of common client goals, the rate of progress that they can expect in striving toward that goal, and the results that they often achieve in a three-month period.

Three months is a good timeline because it is long enough for your clients to see some definite results. If they have been working hard and haven't seen any changes in three months, it is time to alter the program. Some personal

Table 4.2 Realistic Rates of Change for a Typical Personal-Training Client

Goal	Realistic progress	Change in three months
Body composition changes		
Lose weight	Lose 1–2 lb (.5–1 kg) of fat per week or 1% of body weight	Lose 5–25 lb (2.3–11.4 kg)
Gain weight	Gain .5–1 lb (.2–.5 kg) of muscle per week	Gain 5–10 lb (2.3–4.5 kg)
Lose body fat	Lose up to 1% a week max	Lose 4–8%
Increase measurements		
Large area*		Add 1–2 in. (2.5–5 cm)
Small area**		Add .5–1 in. (1.3–2.5 cm)
Decrease measurements		
Large area*		Lose 1–3 in. (2.5–7.6 cm)
Small area**		Lose .5–1 in. (1.3–2.5 cm)
Performance changes		
Increase $\dot{V}O_2$max		Increase about 5 ml/kg/min
Increase bench press		Increase 5–20 lb (2.3–9.1 kg) or 5–10%
Increase squat		Increase 10–40 lb (4.5–18.2 kg) or 5–10%
Increase deadlift		Increase 10–40 lb (4.5–18.2 kg) or 5–10%
Increase sit and reach		Increase 1–3 in. (2.5–7.6 cm)
Increase sit-ups in 1 minute		Increase 5–10
Increase push-ups in 1 minute		Increase 5–10
Increase pull-ups or chin-ups		Increase 1–5
Decrease 1.5-mile (2.4 km) run time		Decrease 0:30–2:00

Note: Advanced athletes will progress much more slowly; beginners may improve more rapidly.

*Large measurements include shoulders, hips, chest, and waist.

**Small measurements include thigh, upper arm, calves, neck, and forearms.

training businesses experience significant success by selling contracts that are at minimum three months long. Selling a client four or eight sessions is fine, but all that can do is get the ball rolling; three months is enough time to feel and see some real results.

In general, a few weeks of training is needed for people to start to feel the effects. After two to three weeks of regular exercise, people often comment that they have more energy and feel better about themselves. After one to two months beginners should notice significant change in their performance. They should be able to lift more weight or perform more reps (or both) on most exercises. Two months, or three at the most, is needed to begin to see some changes in the body. Muscles become

firmer and more noticeable, the waist becomes slimmer, and more lines appear on the body. In this length of time, performance (as measured by the five components of fitness) improves significantly.

Setting proper goals is a huge step in the right direction because doing so serves to guide actions. Proper goals help personal trainers make sure that the programs are the most suited to their specific clients. Measuring the results serves as a useful benchmark and learning stick as a personal trainer learns and refines over time what works best. Of course, goals are just one step. Anyone can write down a goal on a piece of paper; the second step is to hit the gym and apply some real effort to that program to get the most out of it.

CONCLUSION

Personal trainers should encourage clients to set SMART goals, and they should be aware of the difference between process goals and outcome goals. Whenever possible, the personal trainer should relate the client's goals to the components of fitness. Goals can be classified according to their time frame into daily, short-term, long-term, and ultimate goals. Personal trainers should be familiar with realistic rates of progress for the various components of fitness so that they can help their clients set goals for themselves.

Study Questions

1. Which of the following is a process goal?

    a. I will bench press 315 pounds (142.9 kg).

    b. I will win today's game.

    c. I will score three touchdowns in tonight's game.

    d. I will cook my food in advance and eat 1,500 calories today.

2. Which type of goal is considered under the client's control?

    a. outcome goal

    b. process goal

3. A client can bench press 155 pounds (70.3 kg) after three months of training. He or she hopes one day to be able to bench press 300 pounds (136.1 kg). That goal would be an example of a

    a. long-term goal

    b. short-term goal

    c. daily goal

    d. process goal

4. A client weighs 150 pounds (68.0 kg) and wishes to lose weight. What is the maximum realistic fat loss per week a personal trainer should seek to achieve with this client?

    a. 2 pounds (1.1 kg) of fat a week

    b. 1.5 pounds (.7 kg) of fat a week

    c. 1 pound (.45 kg) of fat a week

    d. .5 pounds (.23 kg) of fat a week

5. True or false: The more advanced a client is, the faster he or she will make progress in a program.

    a. true

    b. false

Conducting a Personal Training Session

The heart of personal training lies in the one-on-one (or group) sessions that a client has with a personal trainer. Thus, being a good personal trainer requires the ability to conduct positive and beneficial personal training sessions. The point of this chapter is to cover the information necessary to be able to do that.

GUIDELINES FOR THE PERSONAL TRAINER

The personal trainer has a significant responsibility to the client, not only because he or she has a contractual obligation to the client but also because the client is depending on the personal trainer to reach the goals that were set in the beginning of the program.

The Personal Trainer Is in Charge

With each personal training session at least two people will be involved: the client, who is the one receiving the training, and the personal trainer, the person who is conducting the session. As the personal trainer, you are in charge. You decide when the session starts and ends, what exercises will be performed and in what order, and how much weight and how many reps will be completed. You are in charge of everything from A to Z about the personal training session.

The power dynamic in a personal training session can be complex. On one hand, the client is ultimately in power because he or she has hired you and can fire you anytime. On the other hand, you are the health professional, and the client has hired you to tell him or her how to get in shape and improve health and fitness.

A personal trainer who is confident, knowledgeable, and self-assured will usually not have much problem setting the tone for the session. But if a personal trainer is timid, seems confused, appears weak, or lacks confidence, the client may fill the void and assume the leadership position. This should not happen, and if it does, problems and complications will occur down the road. Personal trainers should avoid saying things such as, "What do you want to work on today?" or "What do you feel like doing?" or "Well, I was thinking we might try to squat today, if that's OK with you." Be confident, have a plan for the day, and follow it (67).

Be Prepared and Start on Time

A personal trainer can help set the tone by being on time for each session, or even a few minutes early. If a session begins at 8:00 a.m., do your best to be ready at 8:00 a.m. sharp. Being ready means being in your uniform, at the appointed meeting place, with the workout created and prepared for that day's session. Ready does not mean walking into the gym at 8:03 a.m., going to the bathroom, getting dressed, combing your hair, slapping together a quick workout on a Post-It note, and emerging at 8:14 a.m. finally prepared for the session.

Remember, the client is paying you for a set time, most commonly an hour, at a going rate of usually $60 per hour or more, so the client is in essence paying you a dollar a minute for your services. Showing up 5 or 10 minutes late is unacceptable.

A prepared personal trainer will have the workout designed and written down. You will have referred back to previous workouts and drafted a session that is current, is relevant, and follows the principles of specificity and progressive overload. If the workout requires a stopwatch, cones, foam roller, or anything else, you should ensure that all that equipment is available and ready for use.

Shake Hands to Start and End the Session

To signify the start of a personal training session, approach and greet the client and shake his or her hand. This action indicates that you are in charge of the session, and it signals formally that the training session has begun. A client might be ready 5 or 10 minutes early, but you might need that time for whatever reason, and that is OK. The session doesn't begin when the client is ready; it begins when the personal trainer is ready, which should be exactly on time. Not shaking the client's hand immediately upon arrival lets the client know that you need that time and that the session will begin shortly.

In addition, shaking hands at the end of the session is appropriate. Sometimes it is not clear exactly when the session will end. You do not want your client to finish that last set of crunches just to have you mumble goodbye and walk away. Nor does the session automatically end when the 60 minutes is up; you don't want to abandon your client when he or she is in the middle of a set. Instead, you formally end the session. You might say something like, "That wraps up our workout for today. Great job!" or, "That was the last exercise for today. I'll see you next Monday at 7," and then shake hands to finish the session. This is also a good time to confirm when the next scheduled meeting is and to see whether your client has any questions about the fitness program. Even

with long-standing clients, shaking hands at the start and end of each session is a good habit.

Stay Near the Client at All Times

After you are officially on the clock with the client, the client should receive your undivided attention. Part of that attention is simply physically staying near the client nearly all the time, with just a few exceptions. Going to get a towel for the client or setting up the next machine is acceptable, but any time spent away from the client should be short and for a specific purpose. You are responsible for the client's safety at all times during the session, and you can't fulfill that responsibility if you are far away from your client. The gym is a potentially dangerous environment—weights can roll, bars can move, medicine balls can fly, and other members don't always pay attention to what they are doing. If a client is squatting, you should be in spotting position at all times. Even if the weight is easy for the client to lift, a problem could occur if another member accidentally bumps the bar or a dumbbell rolls into the platform (49, 104).

This rule applies to the warm-up as well. The personal trainer should not officially start the session and then send the client off by him- or herself to warm up on the treadmill for five minutes. You should accompany the client to the treadmill, set it up the way you wish, and then use that time to talk to the client. This is a good time to find out how the client is really feeling. Is the client sore from the previous workout? How has the client's nutrition plan been going? Small talk and catching up are OK as well. You want the client to bond with you, and small talk helps create that bond.

Control the Cardio Machine

The personal trainer should set up the cardiovascular machines and be the one who pushes the buttons to set the level, speed, and incline to whatever is appropriate. The only exception to this is if you can't reach or can't access the appropriate the buttons. In this case, you can tell the client what to do.

You want to establish this protocol for two primary reasons. First, if you program the machine, it will always be set at the level you want. If the client sets the treadmill and you then override the plan, negative feelings could develop. Second, you establish that the client does not touch the controls on the machine; therefore, he or she will not alter the intensity in the middle of the workout. Allowing clients to program the machine in the beginning often gives them the idea that they can modify the intensity of the exercise during the routine. In addition, asking clients to program the machine is unrealistic and unfair. Part of what they are paying for is your expertise in setting up anything related to exercise.

Adjust the Equipment Settings

You should lead the client to whatever machine or apparatus is to be used, literally walking in front of the client because the client may not know where you are headed next. In addition, you should properly adjust the equipment for each client. During an equipment orientation, you can explain how and why the machine is set up the way it is, but in a regular personal training session you should just set it up. The client should not be expected to know how to adjust the machine or whether it is properly aligned.

From reviewing previous workouts, which you will have done as part of your preparation, you will know the proper settings and need not waste time recalibrating the alignment for each machine. If the client is new or performing a new exercise, making an adjustment after you see the client perform the movement is OK. Getting it right is paramount, no matter how many tries it takes. After the setting is correct, do yourself a favor and record it for future reference. A good personal trainer should know how to adjust all the equipment in the gym, whether or not he or she regularly uses each piece of equipment (33).

Record the Workout in the Log

The personal trainer should record the workout in its entirety either during or shortly after the session. If you allow too much time to pass after the completion of the session before you record it, you will not remember some of the details of the workout. You want to include everything pertinent in the workout log, from the first minute to the last. The workout log serves several important functions:

- It keeps an accurate record of what happened during the session.
- It allows the personal trainer to track the client's progress.
- It serves as a learning tool by giving the personal trainer an idea of what works and what does not.
- It serves as a time diary for the workout.
- It makes creation of future workouts significantly easier.
- It serves as a legal record of what happened during the workout in the rare instance that the personal trainer is sued.
- It serves as a resource for billing so that personal trainers and fitness companies know how many personal training sessions were completed each day, week, or month. For that reason among others, clients usually initial or sign their workout log after a session is completed.

The personal trainer does not need to give the workout log to the client, but a client's request for a copy of a specific workout can certainly be accommodated. In addition, in case of a legal dispute, a personal trainer should not give the workout log to a lawyer without first consulting his or her own lawyer.

Choose the Sets, Weight, Rest, and Reps for Each Exercise

Remember that the personal trainer is in charge and dictates how the session proceeds. The personal trainer chooses the appropriate number of warm-up and work sets, the amount of weight, the number of reps, and the duration of rest for each exercise.

After a client completes a set, you should ask yourself how many reps you want the client to perform on the next set. Should the number of reps be the same, higher, or lower than the previous set? Then you should decide how long the client will rest before the next set begins. Shorter rest, of course, means less complete recovery. Then you should ask yourself how hard the previous set was. Only after calculating all that information should you decide what weight is appropriate for the client. In general, use the following guidelines, assuming that the first set was quite challenging.

- If you want more reps and rest time will be adequate, then usually the weight is lowered. A decrease of 5 to 20 percent is standard, and a 10 percent decrease in weight is the norm. If rest time is very short, then a 20 percent or greater drop is called for (34).

- If you want an equal number of reps to the previous set and the rest time is adequate, the weight can stay the same. If the rest time is short, the weight is usually dropped by 5 to 10 percent (34).

- If you want a lower number of reps and the rest time is adequate, the weight should be increased. An increase of 2.5 to 10 percent is standard. If you want a lower number of reps and the rest time is short, the weight generally remains unchanged (34).

Load and Remove the Weights

The personal trainer is responsible for loading the weight on a machine or barbell, both sides if necessary. Think of it as valet personal training; you, as the personal trainer, are there to take care of your client. Most clients will not assist you in loading or unloading the weight, usually because they don't know what you are doing or how to calculate the correct weight. Some clients, especially those more experienced and seasoned in fitness, will assist you, and that is fine if they wish to do so. You should take light dumbbells to the client and then replace them when the client finishes. If you are not working in your own private studio, you are responsible for replacing all weights and unloading all bars as soon as the client is finished working with them. In general, personal trainers should follow the guidelines given to the regular members of

the club. If the weight is too heavy for you to move or lift, then you can ask the client to set up and remove that weight.

You are also responsible for making sure that the weight is loaded correctly and evenly, if necessary. Even if the client chooses to help you, it is ultimately your responsibility to set up everything correctly. Miscommunications can occur. If a personal trainer says, "Let's go to 225," does that mean to go to a total weight of 225 pounds or to put two 25-pound plates on each side of the bar? It is a good idea to get in the habit of visually checking and actually feeling the bar before each set to make sure that it is evenly loaded and that the collars are in place.

Do Not Work Out Together Unless Preapproved

Generally, a personal trainer and a client should not work out together. When a personal trainer is working out, his or her focus will likely be directed inward instead of at the client, where it should be. But some personal trainers do enjoy working out with their clients. Being paid to work out is nice, and some clients find exercising with their personal trainers and seeing them in action—walking the walk—to be highly motivating. If you wish to work out alongside your client, first make sure that doing so is an accepted policy with your employer. Second, ask the client in explicit terms whether he or she would like to use a personal training session as a workout session with you. Before the workout has begun, you need to establish clearly whether the client is paying for the session. The client might think that the mutual workout session is free. Even if a client agrees to pay for the session, do not assume in the future that the understanding will always be in place. Each time that you wish to work out with the client, you should clarify that the client will be paying for the session. In addition, for safety reasons the client should lift while you are resting between sets so that you are always able to spot the client and keep him or her safe. When a personal trainer and a client are performing bench presses side by side at the same time, the activity can hardly be called safe and supervised.

Be Professional and Respectful of the Client at All Times

The personal trainer should remain professional and respectful of the client at all times. A friendship may develop, and the environment in the fitness center may create a relaxed atmosphere, but the personal trainer should always remember that the person is a client first and foremost. Even when a particular client might be comfortable with a less professional relationship, keeping things professional and respectful at all times is the best approach.

Becoming too friendly with a client can interfere with normal business operations. For example, if your client who is also a friend cancels on you with little notice, will you feel comfortable charging him or her? Another possibility is that a client might develop feelings for a personal trainer, and a personal trainer who is behaving in a relaxed or unprofessional way might incidentally encourage those feelings to develop. If you do sense that a client is developing an emotional attachment to you, you can try being extremely professional and courteous with the client without opening yourself up to him or her at all. If that does not work or if the client makes unwanted advances toward you, it is usually best to have a direct, sit-down talk with the client and perhaps a supervisor to reestablish the boundaries of the relationship. If you still are unable to resolve the issue, you might think about trading or switching the client to another personal trainer who would be a better fit (82).

Make the Client First Priority

In a busy fitness center, a gym member may ask a personal trainer for help while a personal trainer is conducting a session. This request does not observe proper etiquette, but not all gym goers follow proper etiquette all the time. You can handle each situation case by case, but in general you can respectfully decline to help the gym member because the client is your first priority and is paying for your services. You might handle the situation by saying something like, "I am sorry I can't assist you at the moment, I am working with a client right now. As soon as our session is over, I would be happy to help you out in any way I can." If the request is for a small thing, such as a spot, and you know someone else in the gym—another personal trainer who is free, a gym employee, or perhaps another friendly and qualified gym member—you might suggest that the gym member contact that person. People can sometimes be a little pushy, and allowing someone other than your client to have five minutes of your time during the session is not appropriate. The client is not paying you to help someone else; he or she is paying you for personal attention. In the case of a true emergency that might require a CPR-certified responder or something of a similar nature, those guidelines can be suspended.

Be Timely

A good personal training session is usually managed down to the minute. If you are stopping a session short of the full time, the client is not receiving his or her money's worth and you are not doing everything you can to improve the person's health and fitness. You can always perform another set, complete another minute of cardio, stretch a little bit longer, work on a weak point, improve mobility, perform some conditioning, or any number of other things to fill the time. As you become more established in your profession, you will have back-to-back sessions lined up, so one session will start at 8:00 and end at 8:59, and the next will start at 9:00. Busy personal trainers may literally find themselves shaking the hand of one client to signal the end of a session and then turning around and shaking the hand of another client to signal the beginning of that one.

If you wish to run over the prescribed time with a client, you should do so only if you do not have a client waiting for you and the client is able to exceed the allotted time. Not all clients will be able to run late because they may have scheduled meetings or appointments to make after their usual ending time. If both the personal trainer and the client are able to run late, then the personal trainer can do that. Both parties should understand that the additional time results in no additional fees to the client unless explicitly stated otherwise. Clients often appreciate a few extra minutes of a personal trainer's time because it indicates the personal trainer is genuinely interested in improving the client's health and fitness as opposed to looking to clock out as soon as possible.

A more common scenario is that the client is late. If a client has hired a personal trainer for 60 minutes, the personal trainer is obligated to the client for that time, no more and no less. If a client arrives for a session 15 minutes late, then 15 of the 60 minutes have been used up, and the client has 45 minutes remaining with the personal trainer. If you have another client following that particular session, then the session must end at the regularly scheduled time. If the client is able to extend the workout and you are able and willing to do so, then allowing the session to run long is a possibility. You should be aware that extending the personal training session rewards the client for being late. You should clearly indicate that extending the session might be possible in a particular instance but that it will not always be the case, so the client should arrive on time.

If the client is continually late, you can initiate a conversation about this tardiness and determine whether another arrangement might be better for both the client and you. You should not feel obligated to extend a session or feel guilty about ending a session at the designated time, and you should not inconvenience other clients to accommodate a client who was late.

If you have waited for a long time for a late client, you can assume that the person isn't going to show and that the session is, in effect, canceled. But you should establish a predetermined wait time and have clients agree to it at the signing of the contract. For example, if your policy is that after a client is 20 minutes late to a 60-minute session, the session is canceled, you need to make all clients aware of this policy. An uncomfortable scenario will occur if the client shows up 30 minutes late, flustered but ready to exercise, discovers that you have left the building, and learns then that he or she will still be charged for the session. Industry standard is that the personal trainer will wait half as long as the scheduled session for the client, without notice, before the session is considered canceled and charged to the client.

Accept That Adjustments Can Be Made on the Fly

Earlier in this chapter the importance of being prepared and ready for a personal training session was stressed; being prepared is the mark of a good personal trainer. But no matter how prepared you might try to be, confounding variables will at times conspire against you. The gym might be particularly crowded, a machine might be broken, or the client might show up limping from a pick-up basketball game the night before. Now you need to modify the workout. That is OK. Use the knowledge gained from this text and other resources, make a quick but logical decision, and come up with a substitute plan. Something is always better than nothing. You might change just one little thing, or you might have to change the whole workout. Do what is necessary for your client. The more experienced you become, the easier this will be. But that is not an excuse for an experienced personal trainer to show up for training sessions with no preparation. Just because you can create a good workout in your head in two minutes does not mean that you should. Designing a thoughtful, long-term plan that emphasizes specificity and overload is important to the client's overall progress, and you cannot do this on the fly.

Make the Call

As stated earlier, the personal trainer needs to have an idea of the goal weight, sets, reps, and rest for each exercise. For every set that a client performs, you should have an idea about how many reps the client will complete, but having an idea is not a guarantee that it will happen. Perhaps the client is feeling particularly strong and is able to get two additional reps on a set. Perhaps the client is unusually tired and can't perform the prescribed reps. In all instances, you make the call. So at some point in the middle of the set, usually about halfway or a bit beyond, you will instruct the client on how many reps to perform (36).

For example, let's say that a female client is preparing to bench press 75 pounds (34 kg). You should know beforehand that this female's best set at 75 pounds (34 kg) is 10 reps. You might say something like, "OK, we are ready for the next set. You have lifted for this for 10 reps before. Let's see if we can beat that. Give it your best shot." You are not sure whether the client will be able to perform 8, 10, 11, 12, or 14 reps with the weight. Giving clients a range is useful so that they have some idea of what is expected of them and how they should approach the set. A tough set of 20 reps is quite different mentally and physically from a tough set of 3 reps, and the client should know what to expect.

In our example, you watch the client begin the set of bench presses, cueing her and encouraging her. Around rep 4 to 6, based on how the set looks so far, you determine how many reps the client should attempt. If the client gets to 5 reps but begins to shake and become wobbly in her form, you may tell her to go for only 2 or 3 more reps and then finish the set. If the client is looking good at 6 reps, you can tell the client to aim for 5 or 6 more reps to set a new record and to follow progressive overload. If the client looks super strong and her form is perfect, you might just tell the client, "Keep going, looking great," at rep 6. Then at rep 10 you can make the call, maybe having the client shoot for 13 or 14 reps, if the set is awesome. After a set like that, you should tell the client how well she performed to enhance the feelings of intrinsic motivation that come from accomplishing something positive.

One last note: Asking a client to "do one more rep" is appropriate to say only two or three times. Clients know that they need to work hard to achieve results, but they can become frustrated if a personal trainer or coach always moves the target and pulls that carrot out of reach. In addition, if a personal trainer is always finding that clients can complete additional reps, then he or she is not doing a good job of predicting what they are capable of in the first place.

Learn How to Read Clients

In personal training, you must learn how to understand your clients' actions and words.

Sometimes clients will be direct and will say exactly what they have on their mind, but more often they will give little hints or use body language to indicate how they are feeling. The ultimate measure of a personal trainer is his or her retention rate. Clients who stay with and re-sign with a personal trainer are pleased and believe that they are getting their money's worth. If a client moves off to another personal trainer or stops training with the personal trainer, then something happened. It is not always within a client's control to stay with a personal trainer, but more often than not it is (67, 74).

The number one reason that people do anything is because it is fun. Fun beats results or health or aesthetics; people continually perform activities that are fun. The job of the personal trainer is to make the training session fun at some level. That doesn't mean that every minute is fun and that the personal trainer just tells jokes and nothing gets done; it means that the client must rank the session overall as fun or enjoyable at least in part. The goal is not to make clients hate exercise; it is to make them love exercise so that they continue it for the rest of their lives (1).

A big part of conducting a successful personal training session is setting up the appropriate intensity for the client. Some clients like extremely intense workouts that leave them gasping for breath, but others do not. Some personal trainers like to train people in an intense fashion; others do not. Generally, the goal is to work clients just a little bit harder than they would work themselves.

To assess intensity, the rating of perceived exertion (RPE) chart is useful. For resistance training and exercise in general, the 1 to 10 scale RPE chart is highly effective (96). At the end of important work sets, ask the client on a scale of 1 to 10 how hard that set was, with 1 being super easy and 10 being extremely hard. You should predict in your own mind what the client will say before he or she says it. If you are within 1 point, then you are most likely reading the client correctly. If you are far off, however, by 3 or more points, you are not reading the client correctly and you are not accurately assessing how challenging the workout is to him or her. Perceived exertion is often more important than actual exertion. After you ask that question, a good follow-up question is to ask the client on a scale of 1 to 10 where he or she expects to be; don't assume that all clients expect to be at the same number. This tool is valuable because the client is telling you whether the set was either too hard or too easy. If a client tells you that the previous set was a 6 on the RPE chart and then says that he or she expects to be at an 8, you need to make the set harder, plain and simple. If the client says that the set was a 9 but expects to be at a 7, he or she is asking you to make it easier; you are pushing the client too hard. One set like that in a workout is no problem, but if you continually ignore the client and keep pushing too hard, you might alienate him or her.

At the end of the workout, repeat this series of questions but now ask, "On a scale of 1 to 10, how hard was that workout?" Have the client focus on the difficulty of the entire workout as opposed to just a single set. Again, predict what the client will say and see whether you are making an accurate read. Whether you agree with your client's numerical assessment does not matter; more important is that you are empathizing with the client and seeing what he or she is going through. Follow up by asking the client where he or she expects to be when ranking the entire workout. This information will tell you directly whether the workout was too hard, too easy, or just right. If you are more than 2 points off on a regular basis, you will likely have problems down the road. Clients may become increasingly dissatisfied that your expectations are not in line with their own.

Be Receptive to Feedback

If you feel comfortable doing so, ask for feedback on how the session went and how it could be improved. When you ask for feedback, you must be open to receiving it. If you get defensive at the client's first suggestion, the client will be unlikely to provide any additional feedback. If the client is giving you feedback and you are having a hard time making sense of it, you might ask him or her to suggest a solution. For example, if a client comments that you did not spot him or her very well on the

bench press but doesn't elaborate, you might ask how you can perform the spot next time to avoid that problem. Constructive criticism will contain a solution (37).

GUIDELINES FOR THE CLIENT

In a perfect world, personal trainers could pick their clients, but it doesn't always work that way. You can lay out some guidelines and expectations for your clients, just as guidelines and expectations apply to you, the personal trainer.

Do Not Whine

There is no crying in baseball, and there is no whining in weightlifting. You can joke about this rule with your clients, but you need to enforce it. A simple strategy to handle whining is to make things harder when the client whines. If the client complains that the 15-pound (6.8 kg) dumbbells are quite heavy, he or she will find the 20-pound (9.1 kg) dumbbells even heavier. You must be sure that the heavier weight is safe for the particular client before using this technique. If it is, this approach tends to solve the problem rapidly.

Do Not Allow Negative Self-Talk

If you catch clients using negative self-talk, downplaying themselves, or saying that they can't do it, point it out, tell them that negative self-talk is not allowed, and ask them to correct their language. What the mind believes will happen often does happen, and we as personal trainers want to use that power to our advantage, not to our disadvantage. For some people this approach is quite a change, but they will find it a welcome change after years of negativity (27).

Recognize That the Personal Trainer Is in Charge

Remind clients of this point occasionally if they try to run the session or dictate the plan.

Remind them why they hired you. You are an expert in the field, and you are using your knowledge to help them.

Have an Open Mind

Often many effective methods can be used to accomplish the same goal. Humans have been fit for hundreds of years, and they did not all train the same way or use a specific modality. Hard work, sweat, perhaps a bit of blood, commitment, and consistency can accomplish a lot.

VALUE OF A PERSONAL TRAINER

Occasionally a potential client will question the value of a personal trainer. He or she might comment that personal trainers are overpaid and not worth the money, that training and working out is easy and that anyone can do it, and so on. Personal trainers need to understand the real value that clients gain by having a personal trainer. They can use this knowledge to combat the previous arguments and feel more comfortable in recommending their own services. People expect that you, the personal trainer, will be regularly working out and striving to achieve your own fitness goals. You may or may not choose to hire a personal trainer, but you should at least find a good workout partner with whom you are compatible (6).

Good personal trainers are first and foremost reliable and dependable. They show up on time for every workout. Clients should be able to expect that of you. Personal trainers should have a positive attitude and increase the energy of the environment rather than deplete it. Personal trainers are fun to be around, but they are serious about fitness. They should know what the client's goals are and they should work to help the client achieve those goals. They should be honest with the client, even if what they say is not always what the client wants to hear. The bottom line is that personal trainers should help make a client's workouts more productive and more enjoyable. If they do that, chances are that they are good personal trainers. Personal trainers offer the following additional benefits:

- A client is less likely to skip a workout if he or she is meeting somebody. Even a highly self-motivated client won't want to work out on some days. Knowing that he or she is meeting somebody and will be letting the personal trainer down by failing to show increases the likelihood that the client will go (66).

- When clients are training hard, a personal trainer can be there to spot them and keep them safe. No one feels comfortable having to wander around the gym and either ask the same person for a spot repeatedly or ask people who may not know how to spot.

- A personal trainer will push clients to work harder than they would by themselves. A personal trainer can encourage a client to perform 12 reps when the client would have stopped at 10, or motivate the client to lift an extra 10 pounds (4.5 kg). Hard work equals good results; harder work equals better results.

- A personal trainer can make the workout more fun. That doesn't mean that everything is always pleasurable, but the client should enjoy the overall experience. Working out with someone usually adds to the fun, and the number one reason why people do anything is that the activity is fun. If you make working out fun for your clients, they are more likely to continue with it long term. That is good for them and good for you (90).

- Workouts are more social when they are shared with another person. Human beings are social by nature, so we generally tend to enjoy being around other people, at least people whom we like. In addition, people bond through activity. The more intense the activity is, the more people bond. In few other relationships do clients spend two or three hours every week with just one other person. The relationship can develop into one that both parties come to enjoy and look forward to.

• Working with a personal trainer might cause a better hormonal release in the client. One hypothesis asserts that when people are in a physical competition or are being judged on their performance (which a personal trainer will do to some extent), the body releases more testosterone than it does when they do the same activity alone (65).

WORKOUT LOG

Another key to success for long-term training is keeping a training log or workout journal, and personal trainers need to do this for their clients. Amazingly, many relatively serious people work out hard but do not keep a journal. Their general lack of progress, however, is not surprising. Keeping a workout log is essential if you want your clients to make consistent progress. A log will tell you what is working and, equally important, what is not working. It will keep an accurate record of what you did; memory is not nearly as reliable, particularly when dealing with 10, 20, or 30 clients on a regular basis. If you have a client follow a workout program for three months and his or her 1RM bench press goes up 30 pounds (13.6 kg), you have a blueprint of a plan that increases the 1RM in the bench press. If you need to tweak the plan, so be it, but if the person hits a plateau or is stuck in a rut, you have a detailed plan of what you did to make the bench go up 30 pounds. Repeating that plan will likely increase the bench again. There is also some logic in applying that effective plan to another client with the same goals. The principle of individual variation states that the second client is not guaranteed to experience the same progress, but the plan has a good chance of being effective for that client as well and is certainly a good starting point from which to make further modifications (49).

One of the first things to do with new clients is to set up a workout log for them. It doesn't need to be anything fancy; a notebook large enough to record the information often works well. The notebook should be sturdy enough to withstand some abuse in the gym and the passage of time, so don't get the cheapest one you can find. Gyms and fitness companies often provide training sheets for personal trainers to record their clients' workouts. Those can be effective, and they might be convenient for submitting, although the single sheets tend to become lost or misplaced over time.

When you are writing down your clients' workouts, you want to record everything that is important to how they performed and what you did with them. Of course, you record the name of the exercise, the weight, the number of reps, and the number of sets that the client performed. You should make a note of the rest time, either for that specific exercise or just by recording the total workout time, which allows you to figure out how long you were letting the client rest on average. In addition, record warm-ups, cardio, and stretching.

You might want to ask clients what their body weight is each day, although that can be a little invasive. If clients are interested in changing their weight, a better approach is to educate them about the process. You can suggest that the client weigh in each day and record it somewhere. Some people are turned off by the idea of weighing themselves each day, but doing so is a good idea. The research is clear that people who weigh themselves regularly lose more weight and keep the weight off for longer than those who do not.

When people weigh themselves every day, they learn how the body fluctuates and what foods and activities make them gain and lose weight. They can learn whether they are achieving any weight-gain or weight-loss goals that they have set for themselves. Body weight can fluctuate 2 to 3 pounds (.9 to 1.4 kg) in either direction, so if people weigh themselves only once a week, a month can pass before they see whether any real change has occurred. You must ultimately do what works best for your clients at that particular time. You do not need to force clients to weigh in or have public weigh-ins or anything like that, which can make the problem worse. Over time, as clients become more comfortable with you as their personal trainer and begin to see results in the gym, they will start to trust your opinion more, even if it differs from their own.

When recording the workouts, a suggestion is to write down one workout per page. Generally, one workout will take a whole page. If it doesn't, you may be inclined to want to save paper, but cramming several workouts onto one page makes it hard to refer back to and find specific bits of information. In addition, recording the day and the date will make your log an easy-to-use reference book. Most people perform similar exercises on certain days. For example, those who resistance train at least three times a week train the chest muscles on Mondays. If you want to see what your client did for his or her chest routine three weeks ago, you may not remember the exact date, but if you just look at Mondays and go back three weeks, you should find the information rapidly.

Other things to include are how easy or hard a set was. If a set was unusually tough, note that so you know not to increase the intensity too much next time. Conversely, if a set was very easy, you can make a bigger jump the next time around. If something bothered the client—for instance, a military press bothered his or her shoulder—make note of that. If the client later tells you that he or she was exceptionally sore after a workout, you can go back and try to figure out the cause. If the client's nutrition has been poor or he or she was sick or didn't get enough sleep, write all that down. Record the settings on the machines so that you can set up quickly each time. Your goal is to record all the information that will enable you to duplicate the workout later when you have forgotten the details.

Another important thing to record is whether you spotted the client on an exercise and how many reps you spotted him or her on. Providing a client with a spot offers several benefits. Of course, the number one purpose of a spot is to keep the client safe, which is your first priority. Having a spot allows the client to push that extra bit without worrying about what will happen if he or she fails; the spot removes fear from the lifter. The spotter can help the client perform forced reps, if that is desired. Any reps that a client receives a spot on should be distinguished from those reps that do not receive help. An effective way of

recording reps that received help is to designate them with a "+" sign. For example, a written record of "200 × 8 + 2" indicates that the client lifted 200 pounds (90.7 kg) for 8 reps and then performed 2 additional reps while receiving assistance from the spotter. This performance on the set is important to differentiate from 200 × 10. As soon as your hands touch the bar, the handle, or the implement, you are providing a spot. Just the act of someone else stabilizing the bar with his or her fingers can make the exercise much easier.

The spotter provides valuable cues and feedback to the client, letting him or her know about form and technique. The spotter should also motivate the client. That motivation should match what the client is looking for (a yell, gentle words of encouragement, and so on) and match the intensity of the set; a warm-up set needs little encouragement, but a lifetime best for an experienced exerciser likely needs a lot of encouragement. The spotter can also provide a lift off or help the client start in the proper position. Finally, the spotter should be counting the reps so that the client knows where he or she is in the set and how many more reps remain to do.

Table 5.1 shows a sample page from a workout log. The total time is at the top, in this case 1:15, which is how long the workout took to complete, so this workout was 1 hour and 15 minutes long from start to finish. The day and date are on the upper-left section of the page, and the body weight is in the upper-right section of the page. Then the workout is listed. You read it as you would a book, so go left to right all the way across, down a line, and then start over. The name of the exercise is listed first, followed by the weight lifted and the number of reps performed. In this example, the bench press was the first resistance training exercise performed. The client completed three warm-up sets first—the bar by itself at 45 pounds (20.4 kg), 135 pounds (61.2 kg), and then 185 pounds (83.9 kg). He then began the true training sets. He lifted 225 pounds (102.1 kg) for 12 reps, rested, lifted 245 pounds (111.1 kg) for 10 reps, rested, and then lifted 265 pounds (120.2) for 8 reps, which was hard for him.

Table 5.1 Sample Workout Log

Monday, 12/12/14	1:15	210 pounds
Treadmill	5-minute warm-up at 4.0 mph at 2% grade	–
Bench press	45 × 12 185 × 8 245 × 10	135 × 8 225 × 12 265 × 8 Tough!
Incline press	135 × 10 205 × 10	185 × 12 225 × 6 + 2
Pec (short rest of 0:30) (seat at 4)	180 × 12 130 × 12	150 × 12
Straight-bar tricep push-down	60 × 15 100 × 12	90 × 15 110 × 10 Form so-so
Rope push-down	40 × 15 60 × 12	50 × 12
Tricep extension machine (seat 2, pad 5)	100 × 12 140 × 12 + 2	120 v 12
Bike	5-minute cool-down at level 7 at 80 RPMs	–
Stretch pecs, shoulders, and triceps for 5 minutes		

This log does not specify exactly how long the client rested between sets, but we can estimate it from the length of the workout. The workout was 1 hour and 15 minutes long. From that, subtract a 5-minute warm-up, a 5-minute cool down, and 5 minutes for stretching. That leaves 1 hour, during which 23 total sets were completed. By dividing 23 sets into 60 minutes, we calculate that each set took about three minutes. One set takes approximately 1 minute for the actual lift, which means that the client rested about 2 minutes between sets. Certainly, on some exercises, resting a little longer is natural, and on others, the rest is shorter, so we can estimate that this client was resting 2 to 3 minutes after each set of the bench press.

A workout log is a vital tool for a client or anyone interested in understanding and improving performance. You want to find out what worked and what didn't. All good scientists take notes on their research, and you should as well. Put simply, people who aren't keeping a workout log aren't serious about working out.

A workout log is also an extremely valuable tool for a personal trainer. First, it records the workout. A full-time personal trainer likely has 15 to 25 clients training an average of twice a week. That amount of information is far too much to store in your head, week in and week out.

The workout log also serves as a record for what happened from a liability point of view. Imagine that a client got hurt or worse and you were sued. Did you warm up the client? Did you use any method of assessing how the client was feeling? Were you evaluating intensity, pulse, rating of perceived exertion, and so forth? Was your progression logical? If the client had already completed 100 pounds (45.4 kg) for 10 reps, trying 105 pounds (47.6 kg) for 8 reps is logical, but trying 350 pounds (158.8 kg) for 6 reps is not.

Finally, the workout log serves as an accurate record for billing purposes. Clients often buy 8, 12, or 24 sessions in a package. What happens if a dispute arises over the number of sessions that have been completed? You can easily solve that issue by showing the client the workout log. A good idea is to have the client initial the log after each session. Personal trainers often have to turn in their completed, signed workouts before being paid, so if you turn in 60 completed sessions for that pay period (usually two weeks), you know that you will be paid for 60 sessions. In summary, record those workouts. Everyone will be the better for it.

CONCLUSION

The personal trainer must conduct and be in control of the personal training session. The job includes setting up and adjusting everything for the client and planning the workout with an appropriate intensity and duration. Personal trainers need to develop the ability to read clients so that they can provide better customer service. They also have to provide guidelines to their clients regarding behavior and attitude to help increase the effectiveness of the training sessions.

Personal trainers should record a client's workout in a workout log, including the date, day of the week, exercises performed, weight, reps, sets, rest time, cardio work, stretches completed, and so on. A good workout log allows the trainer to duplicate the session again later. Workout logs are important for legal protection, billing summaries, and record keeping, and the information contained within can assist the personal trainer in programming future workouts.

Study Questions

1. The ideal time for a personal trainer to start the personal training session is
   a. five minutes before the session is scheduled to begin
   b. five minutes after the session is scheduled to begin
   c. at the exact time the session is scheduled to begin
   d. when the client indicates that he or she is ready to work out

2. Why are workout logs useful as a billing tool?
   a. Workout logs record the number of sessions conducted.
   b. Workout logs record the rate of progress that the client is achieving.
   c. Workout logs allow the personal trainer to record the client's settings on the equipment.
   d. Workout logs allow the personal trainer to keep an accurate record of exactly what occurred during the training session.

3. Which of the following is not a benefit to suggesting to clients that they weigh themselves on a regular basis?
   a. Clients will learn what their natural weight fluctuation is per day.
   b. Clients will catch any change in weight early on rather than after a significant change has occurred.
   c. The emotional stress of regularly weighing in will burn more calories per day.
   d. Studies show that people who regularly weigh in keep lost weight off longer.

4. When should a personal trainer make the call and tell the client how many reps to perform during a challenging work set?
   a. after the first rep is complete
   b. at or just after reaching the approximate halfway point of the goal number of reps
   c. after the client makes a face or shows other external signs of exertion
   d. after the client reaches failure

5. If a client does not help the personal trainer load the weights, what should the personal trainer do?
   a. Explain what weight goes on the bar so that the client knows how to load it properly.
   b. Leave one side of the bar unloaded so that the client gets the hint for the next set.
   c. Tell the client that loading the weight provides a better workout and instruct the client to load both sides of the bar from now on.
   d. Do not expect the client to help load the weights; that is the personal trainer's job.

Basic Anatomy

Knowledge of anatomy is a foundation for understanding the rest of this book. To understand how exercise programs should be designed and why certain exercises are more or less effective than others, you must be familiar with anatomy. Our focus will be on the musculoskeletal system, which means that we will focus on the muscles and bones.

People are often intimidated by anatomy, but studying muscles can be fun. If you want to be a personal trainer, you need to understand how the muscles and bones work in the body. Once you understand anatomy, you can look at any exercise, even an exercise that you have never seen before, and figure out what muscles are working. In addition, you can watch an athlete move and figure out what muscles are involved in that movement and what needs to be trained to improve performance. The bottom line is that you can't be a good personal trainer without at least a basic (and preferably a deep) understanding of anatomy.

BONES

To get started, we are going to look at the bones in the body. Muscles attach to the bones, and the bones are the anchors for the muscles, as well as the frame that gives the body its shape. Most people are at least a little familiar with bones because they have seen skeletons before, either models or on TV. Bones remain long after the rest of the body is gone—they are the hardest and most durable part of the anatomy—but do not think of bones as just dead tissue inside the body. Bones are not like steel rods that do nothing. They are made up of living tissue and are constantly changing.

Weight-bearing exercise can increase bone density, whereas aging, some diseases, and poor nutrition can make bones thin, brittle, and weak. Bone tissue produces cells, and it requires nutrients to function properly. The body contains over 200 bones in (206 in the normal adult human body), but we are going to focus on the major ones.

All bones in the body can be broken down into two categories: the axial skeleton and the appendicular skeleton. The axial skeleton consists of the bones that make up the core, or axis. Other than the spine, these bones are not significantly involved in movement (2, 41). The axial skeleton comprises four key components:

- Skull and face—many fused bones
- Ribs—12 pairs, for both men and women
- Vertebral column—the spine, or backbone
- Sternum—the breastbone

The appendicular skeleton consists of all the bones in the limbs, the appendages, and their girdles (figure 6.1). A girdle is the place where the limb attaches to the axial skeleton. We have two main girdles: the shoulder and the hip. The bones of the appendicular skeleton are extremely important in locomotion (movement).

When we talk about the anatomy of bones and muscles, we normally refer to the body as being in anatomical position (47). In this position a person is standing up, feet slightly apart, palms forward, thumbs out.

The appendicular skeleton starts with a description of the bones of the upper body.

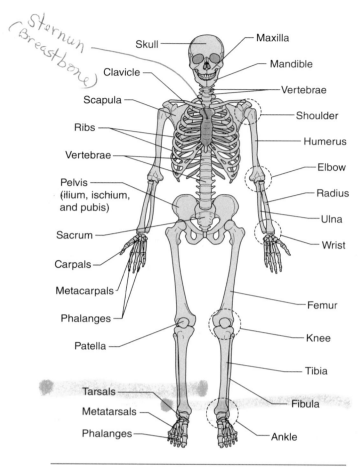

Sternun
(Breastbone)

Figure 6.1 The human skeleton.

Bones
in Avg Adult
body 206

- The shoulder girdle is composed of two bones.
    - Clavicle—commonly called the collarbone. If you go to the top of the sternum and then work your way out to your shoulder, you can follow along the ridge of your clavicle.
    - Scapula—commonly called the shoulder blade. Many muscles surround this area, but if you reach across your body as if you were trying to scratch your upper back, you can feel a ridge of bone that belongs to your scapula. This ridge extends to the bony flat part on top of your shoulder.
- The arm itself has three main bones in it, not including the wrist and hand.
    - Humerus—the bone in the upper arm that runs between the elbow and the shoulder. When your bang your elbow against something, you

might exclaim that you hit your funny bone. Actually, you have hit your ulnar nerve, which runs behind your humerus bone, but through a pun on the word *humerus* (how humorous), it has come to be called the funny bone.

- Radius—the bone in the lower arm on the thumb side. In anatomical position, this bone is on the outside or lateral part of the forearm. From your thumb, work your way up your forearm to about where a watch would be and press down to locate your radius. This is where you should take the pulse; the radial artery is so named because it sits on the radius. As you get closer to your elbow, your radius is covered by muscles and is harder to feel.
- Ulna—the bone in the lower arm on the pinky (little finger) side. In anatomical position (remember, palms are forward) the ulna is on the inside, or medial, part of the forearm. From your pinky, work your way up your forearm above your wrist to find your ulna. You can follow your ulna all the way up your forearm to your elbow. The point of your elbow is part of your ulna. Your humerus ends a couple of inches before that point.
- The wrist and hand have many small bones in them.
    - Carpals—eight small bones in the wrist. These unusually shaped bones look somewhat like small pebbles. Your wrist goes from the end of the radius and ulna to the beginning of your hand, an area about 1 inch (2.5 cm) long. To remember that the bones in the wrist are called carpals, recall that carpal tunnel syndrome is a problem with the wrist.
    - Metacarpals—five bones in the hand, one per finger including the thumb. If you feel the back of your hand, you can normally feel where each bone is. These bones are long and thin, about the size of a chicken-wing bone.

- Phalanges—the set of bones that make up your fingers. The fingers are called digits, and the phalanges are the bones in the digits. You have 14 phalanges in each hand, three in each finger and two in the thumb.

The appendicular skeleton in the lower body is structurally similar to that in the upper body, with a few small differences.

- The hip girdle (remember that the girdles are part of the appendicular skeleton) consists of three bones instead of two, which in adulthood are fused together and called the pelvis or pelvic girdle (46).
  - Ilium—a relatively large, flat, fan-shaped bone. The ilium makes up the top of the hip girdle. From your waistline on your side, go up about 1 to 2 inches (2.5 to 5 cm) and then push in and down to touch the top of your ilium. It runs toward the front of your body and toward your back to your vertebral column. It is the highest (most superior) bone in the hip girdle.
  - Pubis—sometimes called the pubic bone. This bone is in the front (anterior) of the body. It is well below the belly button and just above the genitals. It is shaped like half a donut (the front half).
  - Ischium—the lowest bone (most inferior) in the hip girdle. The ischium is also shaped like half a donut, and when it is put together with the pubic bone, it makes a full donut or circle (44). This bone is not to be confused with the ilium. *Ischium* has an *s* in it, and you can remember it as your "sit" bone, because when you are sitting upright you are sitting on this bone. If you slouch when you are sitting, you are sitting on your tailbone, or *coccyx*, the bottom portion of the vertebral column.
- Each leg has three main bones (and one secondary bone), not including the ankles or feet (45).

- Femur—the thigh bone. The largest and longest bone in the body, the femur goes from the hip down to the knee.
- Tibia—the shinbone. From your kneecap, if you move your fingers about 2 inches (5 cm) down, you should run into a hard bump, which is your tibia. It runs all the way down to your ankle and makes up part of the upper medial (inside) aspect of your ankle. It is the largest bone in the lower leg because it supports the weight of the body and is medially positioned.
- Fibula—the smaller bone in the lower leg. If you go back to that bump under your kneecap (tibia) and then move your fingers about 3 to 4 inches (7.6 to 10 cm) around the outside of your knee, you should come to another bump on the upper outside of your calf. This is where your fibula begins. It runs all the way down your leg and makes up the upper outside (lateral) part of your ankle. When you reach down and touch the outside of your ankle just above your shoe, you are touching your fibula. This bone is broken more often than the tibia is. When football players are tackled from the outside, this bone might break. People often mispronounce or misspell this bone; it is not the "fibia." You can remember that *fibula* has an *l* in it, which stands for "little" or "lateral." The word *tibia* does not have an *l* in it.
- Patella—the kneecap. One difference between the arm and leg bones is the existence of the patella. The elbow does not have an elbow cap, but the knee does, and the kneecap is called the patella. This bone floats, meaning that it is not directly attached to another bone. With your leg straight and relaxed, you can probably move this bone around a bit. The patella helps increase the biomechanical advantage of the quadriceps muscles.

- Like the bones of the wrist and hand, the bones of the ankles and feet are small and unusually shaped.
  - Tarsals—seven bones in the ankle. These bones are similar to the carpals in the wrist. It is believed that as we evolved, what would have been the patella in the elbow moved down to the join the wrist to make the eighth carpal, which would explain why there are eight carpals and seven tarsals. You can remember that the tarsals are located in the foot because *t* is for both "toes" and "tarsals." The tarsals extend farther into the foot than the carpals do in the wrist. The tarsals go about halfway down the foot. The largest tarsal is the heel bone, or the calcaneus.
  - Metatarsals—five bones in the foot. Again, there is one metatarsal for each toe. The metatarsals are located in the distal half of the foot.
  - Phalanges—the set of bones that make up the toes. The toes, just like the fingers, are called digits, and the bones in the digits are called phalanges. Again, each foot has 14 phalanges, 3 in each toe except the big, or great, toe, which has 2. You have 56 phalanges in your body; more than a quarter of the bones in your body are located in the fingers and toes.

The body contains more bones than those listed, notably those in the skull and vertebral column. But the ones listed make up the appendicular skeleton, which serves as a common attachment site for muscles.

MUSCLES

Muscles are the second part of the musculoskeletal system that we will be studying. The body has more muscles than it does bones. Approximately 650 named muscles and many smaller, unnamed muscles are found in the body. This book focuses on the major muscles used during exercise, the muscles that people actively attempt to improve (36).

Muscle Naming

To design and follow an exercise program and to understand why certain exercises are effective, you need a basic understanding of the muscles of the body—where they are and what they do. Remember that muscle tissue can contract. Muscles usually start (originate) on a bone, cross a joint (where two bones meet), and then end (insert) on another bone. The main purpose of the skeletal muscles is to move bones, thereby initiating movement such as walking or throwing.

As you gain a deeper knowledge of anatomy, you will benefit by beginning to change your vocabulary. Right now, we are going to learn the more scientific names for each of the major muscles. After you learn the name, try to use it when you are thinking or talking about that muscle. Table 6.1 provides a list of the common names for muscles and the more scientific "gym" name for that particular muscle group, which is the name that personal trainers usually use when referring to a muscle. In chapters 11, 12, and 13 you will learn the full scientific names of the muscles that make up each group, along with their placement on the skeleton and function in the body (16).

If you are wondering where the abductors are, they are not part of the outer thigh; that is still the quads. Instead, they are the outer part of your butt, close to where your hip pocket would be. Think *b* for *butt*, so the abductors are part of your butt, or glutes.

Obviously, you need to know which muscles are working to assess the effectiveness of a certain exercise. When you see exercises listed in this book, the muscles involved will usually be referred to with the gym names. For example, a push-up works the muscles of the pecs, delts, and triceps, to name a few. As you will learn, the names often encompass multiple muscles. For example, there are three gluteal muscles, three hamstrings, five adductors, and so on, but going from step 1 of knowing the common name to step 2, which is knowing the more accurate and scientific name, is a good start. Having a basic understanding of the composition of muscles and muscle tissue is important. Figure 6.2 shows the location and provides the

Table 6.1 Muscle Name Vocabulary

Upper body	
Common name	**Gym name**
Chest	Pecs
Middle and upper back	Lats
Shoulders	Delts
Front arm	Biceps
Back arm	Triceps
Neck region (between neck and shoulders)	Traps
Lower back	Erectors
Stomach	Abs
Sides	Obliques
Front forearm	Forearm flexors
Back forearm	Forearm extensors
Lower body	
Common name	**Gym name**
Butt	Glutes
Thigh	Quads
Back of thigh	Hamstrings
Inside of thigh	Adductors
Calves	Two main muscles—gastrocnemius, soleus
Front shin	Tibialis anterior

gym names of many of the superficial muscles of the human body.

Types of Muscle Tissue

Muscle tissue is unique in the body in that it is the only tissue (along with its surrounding fascia) that is able to contract. Some tissues can stretch and then rebound (such as your skin), but no other tissue can actively contract. The body contains three primary types of muscle tissue.

Smooth Muscle

Smooth muscle is found in the stomach and intestines. Its action is involuntary, meaning that it contracts without conscious thought. When you eat food, after you have swallowed, your body works to digest it whether you think about it or not.

Cardiac Muscle

This specialized muscle tissue is found in the heart. The action of cardiac muscle, like that of smooth muscle, is involuntary. As you read

this book your heart is beating without any conscious effort or intention. Some people can exert some control over their heartbeat, increasing or decreasing it with a thought, but in general the heart beats without any conscious control (39).

Skeletal Muscle

Sometimes called striated muscle because of its striped appearance under a microscope, skeletal muscle is the kind of muscle tissue found in the external muscles, the muscles that move the body (37). Skeletal muscle is so named because it attaches to and moves the bones or the skeleton. It makes up the chest, legs, arms, and so forth. Its movement is considered voluntary because you can control your skeletal muscle. You can choose to raise your arm above your head or not. Occasionally, your skeletal muscle malfunctions and contracts on its own (a cramp), but in general you are in control of these muscles. In this book we focus on this type of muscle tissue (10).

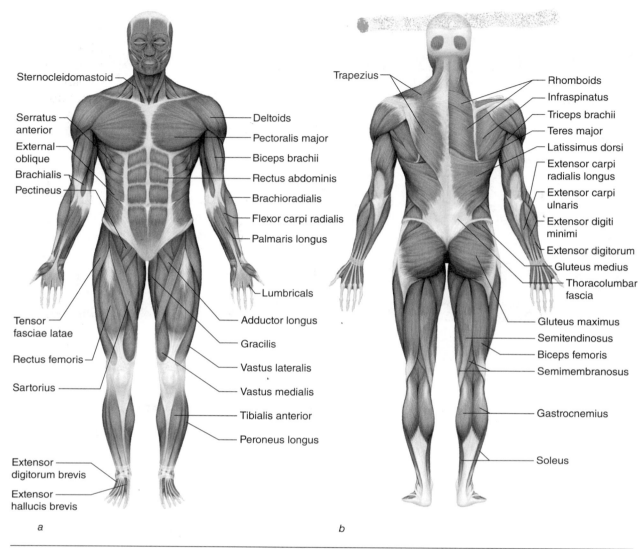

Figure 6.2 Superficial muscles of the human body: *(a)* front view; *(b)* rear view.

Skeletal muscle is composed of muscle fibers. A muscle fiber is the same thing as a muscle cell; it is just a specialized cell. One cell equals one fiber. A muscle fiber is long and thin but bigger than most cells. You could see a muscle fiber with your naked eye. It is about the size of a human hair. Most muscle fibers are a few centimeters long, although the length differs among the various muscles.

Muscle Fiber Structure

Some very small muscles have just a few muscle fibers in them, such as the small muscles that control the movements of your eyes. Most of the major skeletal muscles, such as your pectorals and biceps, have thousands of muscle fibers in each muscle. Imagine that you were putting someone's hair into a ponytail. If you wrapped up the ponytail tightly, it would not be that big, but it would be made up of many individual hairs. You can imagine your muscles in the same way. Your biceps is probably about as big around as that ponytail (or ideally a little bigger). Imagine how many muscle fibers are in your biceps (most humans have 170,000 to 480,000 muscle fibers in their biceps brachii) (17).

Microscopic muscular anatomy is complex, and research into it is ongoing. Presented here is an overview of this anatomy. The goal is to help you develop a basic understanding of the molecular structure of a muscle and its application to personal training. This synopsis is not complete or comprehensive. For more detail, refer to an anatomy or physiology textbook or consult *Supertraining* by Yurki Verkhoshansky and Mel Siff (51).

If you were to examine one muscle fiber, you would discover that it is made up of a bundle of miniature fibers (see figure 6.3). These minifibers are called myofibrils and are too tiny to see with your eyes. The myofibrils, meaning "little muscle fibers," are arranged in a bundle. Imagine a tractor-trailer hauling a bunch of hollow steel pipes. The steel pipes would be arranged in a bundle and tied together so that they don't fall apart. The overall configuration of those steel pipes is similar to a muscle fiber; each individual steel pipe is like a myofibril. Each single skeletal muscle fiber contains an average of 1,000 myofibrils (15).

Now examine one individual myofibril as seen in figure 6.4. If you looked at it closely you would see that it is made up of sections lined up end to end. Each of those sections is a sarcomere. Sarcomeres are extremely small; there are about 4,500 sarcomeres in one centimeter. The sarcomere is important because it is the smallest contractile unit in a muscle. You can visualize sarcomeres as looking a bit like oil drums lying on their sides.

If you were to examine one sarcomere magnified and bisected so that you could see inside it, you would see that it contains two kinds of myofilaments. These two myofilaments are called actin and myosin. Actin is a thin filament, whereas myosin is thick. Each sarcomere contains more actin filaments than myosin filaments.

Myosin filaments have something called cross bridges on them. These cross bridges connect the myosin to the actin filaments. The actin filaments are connected to the ends of each sarcomere. When a muscle contracts, the actin filaments are pulled toward each other by the myosin filaments. As they draw near each other, they pull the edge of the sarcomere together. This process repeats itself thousands of times within each sarcomere in the muscle as the muscle contracts (19).

Each muscle fiber is made up of a bundle of myofibrils. All cells have walls to keep certain contents inside the cell and certain contents outside the cell. The cell wall of the muscle fiber is called the sarcolemma. The cell wall acts as a protective barrier for the cell. Surrounding

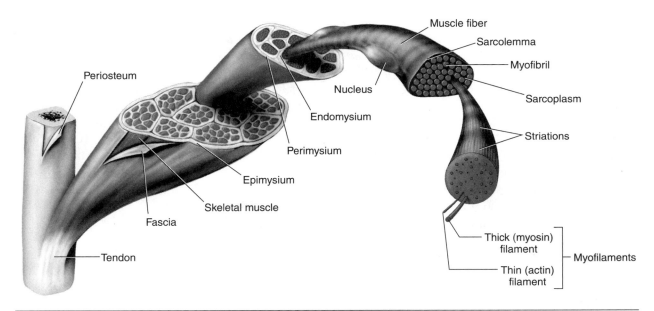

Figure 6.3 Varying levels of complexity in muscle tissue.

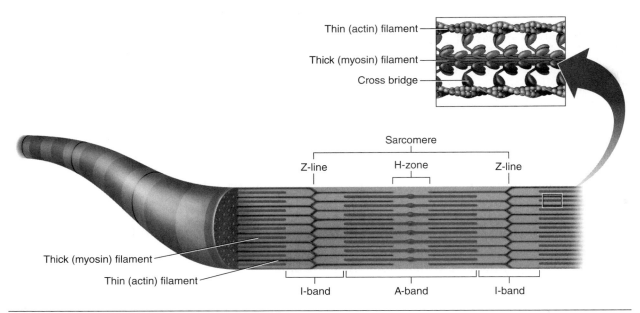

Figure 6.4 Makeup of a single skeletal muscle fiber cell.

the cell wall is a membrane of connective tissue called endomysium, a wrapping that surrounds and is continuous with the muscle fiber.

Inside a muscle, muscle fibers are arranged together in bundles, similar to the way that the myofibrils are arranged. But there are more myofibrils than there are muscle fibers per bundle. A bundle of muscle fibers is called the fasciculi (plural form) or sometimes a fasciculus (singular form). A fasciculus is a group of muscle fibers tied together; most fasciculi have 10 to 100 muscle fibers in them. Go back to the ponytail example. Imagine that you have the hair pulled back and are ready to put it in a ponytail. Well, perhaps you want to braid the hair, so you separate out different sections that will all ultimately make up that one ponytail. Each section of hair is a bundle of hair follicles that will be tied off. A bundle of muscle fibers is a fasciculus, and that fasciculus is surrounded by connective tissue called perimysium. The perimysium covers and wraps up fasciculi, just as the endomysium covers and wraps up a muscle fiber.

Let's return to the ponytail example. You have several different sections of hair, each tied off, that you are going to put in one ponytail. The ponytail itself is a bunch of hair that has been sectioned off. A muscle itself (such as a biceps or quadriceps) is a bundle of fasciculi wrapped together. And a muscle is covered by connective tissue called epimysium. This tissue surrounds the muscle and is continuous with the tendon to which it attaches. To remember that epimysium is the outermost covering of muscle, think about epidermis, which is our skin, the outermost covering of our body. Both words have the same prefix (4).

Attempting to understand muscle structure can be daunting. Start from the largest structure (a muscle) and then go to the smallest structure (a myofilament); next time, reverse that order. Developing an understanding of the structure of muscle will help you understand how a muscle responds to training. Outlined here is a condensed list of the important terms to help you focus your efforts. This list goes from large to small.

- Epimysium—tissue that surrounds a muscle and attaches to the tendon
- Muscle—a bundle of fasciculi
- Perimysium—tissue that surrounds fasciculi
- Fasciculi—a bundle of muscle fibers
- Endomysium—tissue that surrounds a muscle fiber

- Sarcolemma—the membrane of a muscle fiber
- Muscle fiber—a muscle cell made up of a bundle of myofibrils
- Myofibril—microscopic muscle fiber made up of a row of sarcomeres
- Sarcomere—the smallest contractile unit in a muscle; contains myofilaments
- Myofilaments—two small filaments (actin and myosin) crucial in muscular contraction
- Actin—the thin myofilament that slides along the myosin pulling the sarcomere ends closer together, resulting in contraction
- Myosin—the thick myofilament that doesn't appear to move; has many cross bridges
- Cross bridges—globular heads that attach the myosin to the actin

Muscle Fiber Types

Skeletal muscles are further understood to contain two types of fibers: slow twitch and fast twitch (27). Slow-twitch, or Type I, muscle fibers are relatively small, and they tend not to grow very large, even when trained. They have a good blood supply and are resistant to fatigue, so they are able to contract repeatedly without getting too tired. But slow-twitch muscle fibers are relatively weak. They can't generate high levels of power (20). You would use primarily slow-twitch muscle fibers when performing anything that requires many reps, such as jogging, walking, cycling, and rowing (25). Slow-twitch muscle fibers are sometimes called red muscle fibers because of their color; they are the dark meat in animals, such as a chicken thigh.

The second kind of muscle fiber is the fast-twitch, or Type II, muscle fiber. Fast-twitch muscle fibers are larger than slow-twitch fibers, and they increase in size after training. Fast-twitch muscle fibers become fatigued easily, but they are able to generate a large amount of force. They are used primarily in sprinting, jumping, throwing, and lifting weights.

Anytime you are trying as hard as you can, you are using your fast-twitch muscle fibers. Type II muscle fibers are sometimes called white muscle fibers because of their appearance. They are the white meat in animals, such as a chicken breast. Keeping things simple for now, you can think of fast-twitch and slow-twitch muscle fibers as having characteristics opposite of each other. We will learn more about these types of fibers in chapter 7.

CONCLUSION

Within a personal trainer's scope of practice is understanding basic anatomy, including the major bones of the body and the part of the skeleton that they belong to, the large muscles groups and their scientific names, the microscopic structures within a muscle, and the two main types of skeletal muscle. Personal trainers need to understand anatomy if they wish to be at the top of their field.

Study Questions

1. Which of the following bones are in the axial skeleton?
   a. skull, clavicle, humerus, ribs
   b. vertebral column, pelvic girdle, femur, tibia
   c. skull, vertebral column, ribs, sternum
   d. ribs, sternum, humerus, shoulder girdle
2. What two bones make up the shoulder girdle?
   a. ilium, ischium
   b. scapula, radius
   c. clavicle, ilium
   d. scapula, clavicle
3. What is the smallest contractile unit in a muscle?
   a. sarcomere
   b. fasciculi
   c. muscle fiber
   d. epimysium

4. What covers a muscle fiber?

a. sarcomere

b. endomysium

c. perimysium

d. epimysium

5. What is the big muscle on the posterior of the upper body?

a. pecs

b. delts

c. lats

d. quads

Nervous System

Movement of the body is usually initiated in the brain. The brain controls the muscles and tells them what to do. Remember that skeletal muscles are voluntary, meaning that they are under our control. Movement is created by nerves and muscles working together, which is called neuromuscular coordination. Neuromuscular coordination is the ability of the nerves and muscles to work together efficiently to produce coordinated movement, sometimes called skill. Don't think of someone as being coordinated or uncoordinated; instead, think of someone as being highly skilled or unskilled in a certain activity. That skill may or may not translate to other activities.

As mentioned, neuromuscular coordination is the ability of the nerves and the muscles to work together. One section of that definition has already been studied in chapter 6, the muscles, and we will now examine the nerves. The purpose of nerves is to relay messages to and from the brain. Think of nerves as wires much like those in a computer or TV. Nerves are visible to the naked eye. People often assume that they are microscopic, but they are similar in size to arteries and veins. We can imagine that nerves look like flattened pieces of spaghetti in both size and shape. Like most transporters in the body, they are larger at their origin near the spinal cord and become smaller in the distal part of the limbs.

TYPES OF NERVES

Two types of nerves are found in the body. Sensory nerves (also called afferent nerves) send messages about the outside world to the brain. When you touch a hot stove, the nerves in your fingers send a signal up to the brain that the stove is hot. When you look at something, nerves in your eye send the signal to your brain. Sensory nerves send information from receptors in the body to the brain.

Motor nerves (or efferent nerves) send signals from the brain out to the body, namely the muscles. When you touch the hot stove, a signal travels along the sensory nerves from your hand to your brain. Your brain computes the signal and then sends another signal down your motor nerves to the muscles in your arm to move your hand. These signals have the potential to travel very fast, as in the situation when your hand is burning. Your hand moves or all muscles seem to move almost immediately, but in that split-second your brain both received and sent signals: "The stove is hot!" and then "Move the hand!"

Motor nerves hold the most interest for personal trainers, because those nerves control the muscles. The impulse starts in the brain, travels down the spinal cord, exits the spinal cord, and travels down to the specific muscles necessary to produce the movement. The nerve then branches off and hits specific muscle fibers in that one muscle (or group of muscles) to initiate movement.

MUSCLE CONTRACTION PROCESS

The muscle contraction process is a complex process that can be explained in several simple steps. You need to become familiar with some specific terms before learning about how a nerve controls the muscle.

- Action potential (AP)—nervous impulse from the brain, analogous to electricity traveling down a wire
- Neurotransmitters—chemical messengers used by neurons to signal other cells
- Acetylcholine (Ach)—the neurotransmitter involved in muscular contraction
- Neuromuscular junction—the space (synapse) between the nerve endings and the muscle fibers (1, 9–11, 14)
- Motor unit—one motor nerve and all the muscle fibers that it innervates
- Sarcoplasmic reticulum (SR)—tiny tubes surrounding a myofibril that hold calcium

The process begins with the brain initiating a conscious movement. For example, if you want to bring your arm up over your head to ask a question in class, your brain sends an action potential down the spinal cord. Just above the base of your neck, the nerves that control your shoulder (deltoids) exit from the vertebral column. This action potential travels down the nerve all the way until the nerve ends. The nerve innervates (connects to) multiple muscle fibers, in this case muscle fibers of the deltoid. The action potential travels all the way to the end of the nerve right near those muscle fibers.

At the end of each motor nerve and its branches are small sacs. These sacs hold a neurotransmitter called acetylcholine (Ach). The purpose of the action potential is to travel down the nerve and hit the sacs. This causes the sacs to open up. Ach falls out and permeates the muscle fiber.

Ach is so small that it is able to go through the membrane and cell wall of a muscle fiber (the endomysium and sarcolemma) and right into the myofibrils. A bunch of tubes called the sarcoplasmic reticulum (SR) surround the myofibrils. Ach interacts with the sarcoplasmic reticulum. When Ach hits the SR, it tells the SR to open up and release calcium ions, which are stored inside the SR.

The SR releases calcium ions into the myofibril. These calcium ions are small enough to penetrate the sarcomere, which houses the actin and myosin myofilaments. When calcium enters the sarcomere, it signals the cross bridges on the myosin to connect to the actin. After these cross bridges are firmly connected, the myosin heads swivel, much like a screw or a gear, and that action pulls the actin filaments toward each other. The actin filaments are connected to the ends of each sarcomere (Z-line). As the actin come toward each other, the sarcomere shortens or contracts. This shortening of the sarcomere, done throughout the muscle fibers and the muscle itself, causes the muscle to contract on the scale that we are used to. Thus, your deltoid contracts to help raise your arm above your head (17, 22).

Muscle will stop contracting when the brain stops sending an action potential to the nerve. This would stop Ach from being released, which would stop the SR from releasing the calcium. As the calcium levels diminish in the sarcomere, the myosin cross bridges would swivel in reverse and actin would pull apart, resulting in a relaxed muscle. At times you may want your muscle to contract, but it will not, such as when you want to keep performing an exercise but you are too tired to continue. You may be out of Ach for the moment, your muscle may be out of fuel (see chapter 8), your muscle may have by-products in it that are causing the fatigue, or other elements may be contributing to the situation (23, 24). Here is a summary of the simple steps that your body goes through when a muscle contracts.

1. Brain sends an action potential down nerve.
2. AP travels to end of nerve and hits neuromuscular junction.
3. AP causes acetylcholine to be released at end of nerve.
4. Ach diffuses into muscle cells.
5. Ach interacts with sarcoplasmic reticulum.
6. SR releases calcium into the sarcomere.
7. Calcium causes myosin cross bridges to swivel and connect with actin.
8. Myosin pulls actin filaments toward each other, shortening the sarcomere.
9. Muscle contracts.

Muscular contraction is complex, and we are still learning about the sequence of events and the relevance of certain biochemicals. The purpose of this book is not to provide a definitive and exhaustive explanation of how muscles work but instead to give you, the personal trainer, a deeper level of knowledge and a greater understanding of the actions taking place in the body, which in turn should allow you to understand how exercise affects the body at a more systemic level. The images presented in figure 7.1 through 7.4 help illustrate the key points of the muscle contraction process.

MOTOR UNIT

A motor unit is one motor nerve and all the muscle fibers that it innervates (4). As the fundamental working unit in a muscle, the motor unit is important to understand. Think of a motor unit as a light switch. You have the switch, and then you have all the lights that the switch controls. In your body, most muscles have many muscle fibers per motor unit (one switch that controls a bunch of lights). Earlier, slow-twitch muscle fibers were differentiated from fast-twitch muscle fibers. Likewise, we can label the motor units; thus, there are slow-twitch motor units and fast-twitch motor units.

Slow-twitch motor units have fewer fibers per motor unit (with an average of close to 200). Fast-twitch motor units have more fibers per motor unit (with an average of 1,000 to 2,000).

The motor units operate on the all-or-none principle, which states that either all the muscle fibers in one single motor unit contract or none of them contract. If one motor unit has 200 muscle fibers, either all 200 of those fibers contract and follow the previously described procedure or none of them do. You can't get 100 out of the 200 fibers to contract; the body is not wired to do that (43).

Again, consider the light switch example. When you turn on a light, it is either all on or all off; there is no in between. You can't move the switch up slightly and have the light come on just a little bit (motor units don't have rheostats). Another example is a gun. When you pull the trigger of a gun hard enough, it fires, and you cannot control how fast the bullet flies out. It doesn't just plop out if you pull the trigger lightly. Conversely, if you squeeze the trigger hard, the bullet doesn't fly out extra fast. Either you shoot the gun or you don't.

This concept also negates the idea that a muscle fiber contraction can be strong or weak. At the motor unit level, either all the muscle fibers contract or none does; you can't have a weak or partial contraction when you are fresh.

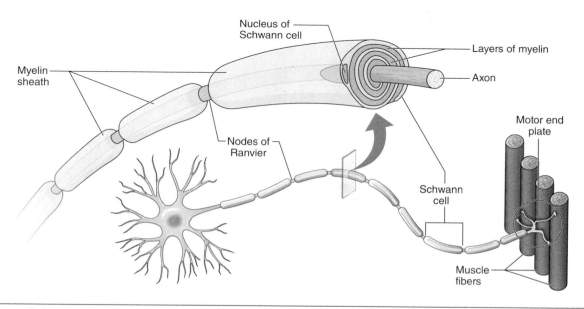

Figure 7.1 Action potential traveling down a motor nerve.

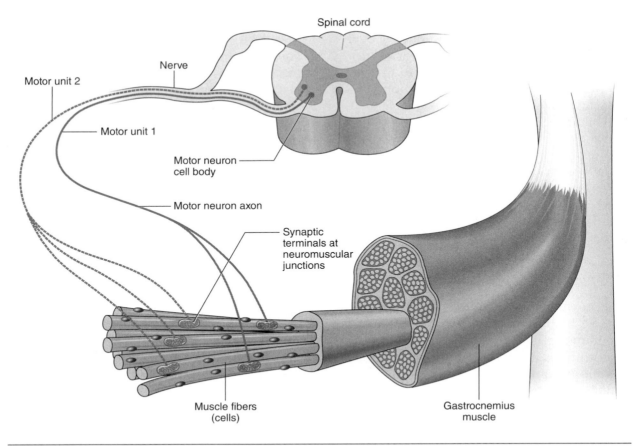

Figure 7.2   One motor nerve connecting to muscle fibers.

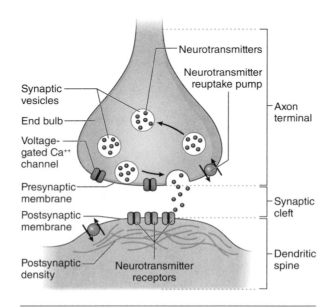

Figure 7.3   Neuromuscular junction.

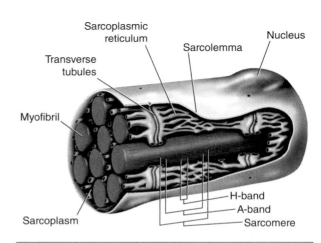

Figure 7.4   Sarcoplasmic reticulum surrounding the myofibril.

FACTORS AFFECTING FORCE PRODUCTION

The all-or-none principle can seem counterintuitive. Obviously, we can control how much force our muscles generate. The concepts of motor unit recruitment and frequency of activation explain how both statements can be true. These factors, combined with others, determine overall force production.

Motor Unit Recruitment

One motor unit has multiple muscle fibers, and they all work together under the all-or-none principle. Each individual muscle, however, has many motor units in it. We can control (somewhat) how many motor units we use, or recruit, to accomplish a certain task. Imagine that your biceps has 50 motor units in it and that each motor unit is capable of generating about 1 pound (.45 kg) of force. To pick up a glass of water, which weighs about 1 pound, you will use two or slightly more motor units; the rest will stay inactive. To pick up a book bag that weighs 10 pounds (4.5 kg), you will recruit 11 or more motor units. To curl a 40-pound (18.1 kg) dumbbell, you will need at least 41 motor units; you will probably feel as if you are using all your motor units. And to curl a 75-pound (34.0 kg) dumbbell, you will need to get stronger or get some help. Right now, you can generate only 50 pounds (22.7 kg) of force, so you can't successfully lift the 75-pound (34.0 kg) dumbbell without cheating. Motor unit recruitment refers to your ability to control and use your motor units—in other words, how much of your muscle you are currently using and how much you are able to use.

Studies have shown that beginners and people who are performing exercises that they are unfamiliar with have relatively poor motor unit recruitment, often around 50 percent of the total number of motor units in the muscle. Using the previous example, you might have the ultimate potential to curl 50 pounds (22.7 kg), but if the exercise is new to you, you might be able to lift only 25 pounds (11.3 kg). The additional weight will be too hard to control. This problem is particularly noticeable in exercises that require a higher level of skill, such as a bench press. To perform a bench press successfully, you have to lie down and then balance a long (7 feet, or 2.1 m), relatively heavy (45 pounds, or 20.4 kg) bar. People who have never done this before may have the strength to do it but lack the coordination needed. The bar wobbles and doesn't move evenly, and the reps don't mimic each other. After a few weeks of practice, the same person may be able to bench press the bar with ease, not because he or she is stronger from a physiological perspective, but because the person has become more skilled in the exercise (12).

As your skill in certain exercises increases, your motor unit recruitment increases. You are able to use more of the motor units that you have. But people rarely use 100 percent of their motor units, even when they try to do so. Generally, experienced lifters recruit about 80 percent or more of their motor units, depending on the person and the situation. In extreme situations, people can possibly recruit more motor units than they can in normal situations. Generally, in weight training the goal is to use a significant number of motor units because only the motor units stimulated by exercise will change and respond to exercise. If a client lifts 15 pounds (6.8 kg) but is strong enough to lift 100 pounds (45.4 kg), that lift is so easy that the client will use only a few of his or her motor units and thus will experience limited results. If the client is pushed harder, he or she will recruit more motor units and experience better results. Again, the principle of specificity comes into play; only the specific parts of the muscle worked will respond and adapt to that exercise.

Frequency of Activation

Frequency of activation is the second way that we can control how much force a muscle generates. To review, a muscle contracts because an action potential (electrical impulse) travels down the nerve and causes the muscle to contract. But your brain doesn't normally send just one action potential; instead, it sends many action potentials that follow one another. Frequency of activation refers to the frequency of those action potentials—how fast and how many of them your brain sends out. When you are trying to generate high levels of force, your brain sends out action potentials frequently and rapidly. Lower amounts of force call for fewer and less frequent action potentials.

Remember that we have introduced the concept of two major kinds of motor units—a slow-twitch motor unit and a fast-twitch motor unit. They are so named because of the kind of twitch that they can accept from the nerve. A twitch is the name for each minicontraction that an action potential initiates. Slow-twitch motor units can accept twitches only at a relatively slow rate, and if they receive twitches faster than they can process them, the extra twitches are ignored. This situation is like yelling at a slow person to run faster. Assuming that the person is trying as hard as possible, asking him or her to go faster won't have any effect. Because these slow-twitch fibers can't receive impulses as quickly and because they can process only a certain number in a given span of time, their force is limited. For those reasons, they produce relatively weak contractions. But because these muscle fibers contract less frequently, they are better able to recover between contractions. They are thus more resistant to fatigue and have better endurance.

Fast-twitch motor units can receive more impulses in a given period than slow-twitch motor units can. They can therefore generate more force and cause a stronger contraction. But these motor units fatigue much sooner than the slow-twitch units do.

Note that all muscle contractions (twitches) occur fast in relation to our general sense of time. The difference between slow and fast twitches is a matter of milliseconds, but that difference is enough to cause the different characteristics in the muscle fibers. When dealing with electricity, milliseconds are significant. If the concept of slow- and fast-twitch motor units is confusing, there is a simpler way to look at it. When people move quickly or try really hard, they use primarily fast-twitch motor units. If people move slowly or barely try, they use primarily slow-twitch motor units.

The purpose of learning about frequency of activation and motor unit recruitment is to understand how muscles contract and how we can regulate the force of that contraction. Let's use one more example. Imagine that you had 10 guns lined up pointing at a target and each gun held 10 bullets. If you wanted to cause minimal damage to that target, you could fire one gun one time. If you wanted to inflict more damage, you could fire each gun one time, so that 10 bullets strike the target. Think of the number of guns fired as the number of your motor units recruited. You have many in each muscle, and you can control how many you use. If you wanted to cause maximum damage to the target, you could fire all 10 guns 10 times. This would send 100 bullets streaking toward the target. How frequently you pull the trigger of each gun is frequency of activation. You can pull the trigger either many times or a few times, and your action has a great effect on what happens. But you cannot control how hard each bullet strikes the target. The all-or-none principle comes into play. Either the bullet fires from the gun or it does not. Either all of the muscle fibers in a motor unit contract or none of them do.

✳Neuromuscular Coordination

The ability to control your motor unit recruitment and your frequency of activation is collectively called neuromuscular coordination. This chapter started by stating the definition of neuromuscular coordination as the ability of nerves and muscles to work together; that ability is changeable, meaning that over time it can improve, remain stable, or deteriorate. Neuromuscular coordination is specific to a certain activity; you might have good coordination in a bench press and poor coordination in a squat, or good coordination in pitching a baseball but poor coordination in shooting a basketball. Neuromuscular coordination is not just one broad ability that can be ranked for all people; instead, it is a series of specific skill sets that can vary greatly, both between individuals and even within a single individual.

Muscle Size

The size of a muscle can have an effect on how much force it produces. Most people know this intuitively; larger people tend to be stronger than smaller people. Athletes in heavier weight classes lift more than athletes in lighter weight classes do. The cross-sectional area of a muscle, its girth, correlates with strength. The length of a muscle is not as well correlated with strength. Muscle size is changeable over time. Together, neuromuscular coordination and muscle size are the two most important factors in determining strength, and they are somewhat controllable (20).

Preloading

The concept of preloading involves placing a load on a muscle before asking it to contract concentrically. Here is a simple example to illustrate. Place one hand on your heart and lift just your pointer finger up. Then hit your chest as hard as you can with your finger. Try it a few times and note the force developed by your finger. Now, repeat the process, but this time when your finger is up, use the thumb on your other hand like a trigger and let your finger press against it before you let it go. Hit your chest again. What happened? If you did the experiment right, you should notice a significant difference between the first hit to your chest and the second hit. The second time involved preloading; you loaded up the muscles that contract your finger before they actually moved the finger. If you ever perform an eccentric movement before a concentric movement, the muscle is preloaded. When you preload a muscle, the strength of that muscle improves significantly.

Preloading can be used in the gym. Free-weight exercises are usually preloaded. If you complete a bench press, first you hold the weight in your hands above your chest, bring it down, and then push it back up. Holding the weight involves preloading the muscles involved. Some machines, however, do not use preloading. Most machines for your chest require you to sit down, grasp the handles at the bottom of the range of motion, and then push forward to lift the weight up. You go from no load to full load right away; no preloading occurs with those machines.

Preloading is a useful technique, and in general you want to use exercises that involve preloading. This technique increases both the safety and the benefit of the exercise. If you are using machines or exercises that don't involve preloading, try to perform them in a way that includes preloading. Clients who work with a personal trainer gain the benefit of always having a partner in the gym. For example, you can help the client complete the first rep on a chest press machine so that he or she starts with the arms straight. Don't count the first rep (because the client didn't do it alone) and then begin the exercise. Some exercise machines have foot pedals or other methods of helping the person begin the exercise. Take advantage of these when they are available.

Prestretching

Prestretching is stretching a muscle immediately before that muscle contracts. Prestretching does not mean stretching out for five minutes and then beginning a workout; it means that the muscle involved must stretch (elongate) right before it contracts (shortens). Pretend that you have a ball in your hand and are going to throw it across the room. Put your hand up as if you are going to throw the ball. Now, as you go to throw, what is the first movement your body makes? Most people draw the hand back farther before throwing. Think of swinging a baseball bat. First you cock the bat back and then you swing it. If you kick a soccer ball, first you pull your leg back and then you kick. Prestretching occurs in almost every sporting event that involves strength, power, and speed.

Prestretching works because in some ways muscles are like rubber bands. They are elastic, meaning that after they stretch out they want to rebound back to their original shape. The more they stretch out, the more they want to rebound. In addition, components in your muscles called muscle spindles cause a protective contraction when your muscles are stretched. We will talk more about this later, but in general, muscle spindles detect a stretch on a muscle and then cause a corresponding contraction. This is called the stretch reflex. The faster and greater the stretch is, the stronger the resulting contraction is.

If a muscle is prestretched, but a delay occurs between the stretch and the contraction, the stretch reflex will dissipate and the contraction will be weaker. For example, in a power lifting competition in which you perform a bench press, you must lower the bar to your chest, pause it on your chest, and wait for the judge to tell you to press. Then, after the command is given, you can push the bar back up. This purpose of the pause in competition is to prevent people from gaining momentum by slamming the bar on the chest and to make the lift easier to judge. The pause makes the bench press harder because it lessens the effect of the stretch reflex. In a bench press, the muscle stretches as the bar is lowered and then contracts as the bar is pushed back up. The longer the pause is, the harder the lift is.

Prestretching and preloading sometimes work together. For example, the first rep on some weight machines involves neither a prestretch nor a preload. If you are performing a chest press on a machine, the first rep starts at your chest, so there is no prestretch and no preload, as mentioned earlier. Have you ever noticed that on some machines the first rep is extra tough, the next three or four reps aren't that hard, and then the reps get harder again as you get tired? That fluctuation in effort occurs because that first rep doesn't involve either a prestretch or a preload. Providing a client with a liftoff ensures that the initial rep includes both a prestretch and a preload. During resistance training, if a muscle is prestretched it is automatically preloaded, but the reverse of that scenario is not always true (a preload does not guarantee a prestretch).

Angle of Pennation

A muscle's angle of pennation describes how its muscle fibers are arranged in relation to the tendon that runs through the muscle. Muscle fibers are arranged in three main ways. In some muscles, the fibers run parallel to the tendon. The biceps is a good example of a fusiform arrangement. The muscle fibers run straight up and down, just as the tendon does. In other muscles, called unipennate muscles, the fibers run off at an angle from one side of the tendon. The muscle looks almost like a feather; the feathers are the muscle fibers, and the hard center spine that the feathers are anchored in is the tendon. Examples include the small muscles in your lower leg and your glutes. This arrangement of fibers is stronger than the parallel arrangement (35). Another arrangement of fibers is called bipennate. Bipennate muscles have a tendon running through the center of the muscle and muscle fibers coming off at an angle to either side of the tendon. An example of this type of arrangement is the main muscle in the quadriceps, the rectus femoris. Bipennate muscles are the strongest type of muscle. Figure 7.5 illustrates the various angles of pennation found in muscle tissue.

Changing the angle of pennation is difficult, although some studies have shown that when large amounts of hypertrophy occur a slight change can result. In addition, not everyone has the same angle of pennation for each muscle. Therefore, some muscles in the body are stronger than others, even if they are the same size.

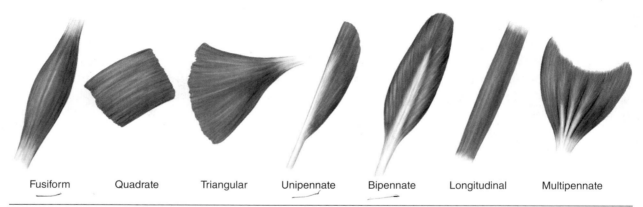

| Fusiform | Quadrate | Triangular | Unipennate | Bipennate | Longitudinal | Multipennate |

Figure 7.5 Various angles of pennation of muscle tissue.

Joint Stability

Some joints are more stable than others, allowing greater strength to be developed around them. For example, the hips are much more stable than the shoulders, which helps to explain why the legs are far stronger than the arms. Also, everyone's joints are not created equal. Some people's joints are genetically stronger than the joints of others. Elite arm wrestlers' shoulder joints are more stable than a normal person's shoulder joint and can therefore handle greater force. An injury to muscle, tendon, ligament, or other connective tissue will likely compromise joint stability and significantly limit strength. The specific shape of a person's bones, the placement and thickness of tendons and ligaments, and the way that the bones fit together all combine to affect joint stability. Adding muscle (or even fat) around a joint or using an artificial wrap like a knee or wrist wrap increases its stability. In that way, a joint's stability improves, but training cannot overcome all genetic factors.

Muscle Position

The position that your muscle is in when contracting makes a big difference in how much strength it can generate. Most muscles are able to generate maximum force when starting from a position that is slightly reduced from anatomical position. For example, your biceps generate the most force when you begin with your arms in a slightly bent position and then contract them fully. This occurs because of the way that the actin and myosin filaments overlap. When a muscle is being stretched, the actin and myosin filaments overlap very slightly, which makes for a poor connection that does not allow maximum strength to be generated. Think of sitting in a chair and having someone stretch your arms out to the side and behind your back. In that position you will be vulnerable and weak. When the actin and myosin filaments overlap more, the muscle contraction is much more powerful.

At the other extreme, if you fully contract a muscle, that muscle is in a strong position to resist being moved, but its available range of motion is too short to generate much force.

When the elbow is almost fully bent, the biceps cannot generate a lot of extra force. If you bend your elbow and then try to smack your other hand, the muscle will not generate much force because it can only move another inch or two (a few centimeters) before it is fully contracted. The last inch or two of a tricep push-down or leg extension is always tough because the muscle is almost fully contracted and getting that extra inch of contraction against a challenging resistance is difficult.

The practical application of this concept is evident in exercises that use a large range of motion. You will have weak points and strong points along that range of motion. In addition, in exercises that use a very short range of motion, maximum force will be limited. Generally, training through a relatively full range of motion is best on most exercises. The benefits and drawbacks of partials will be discussed in a later section (44).

Muscle Fibers and Motor Units

The number of muscle fibers that a person has can affect his or her maximum strength. A person with a greater number of muscle fibers can ultimately increase his or her strength more than a person with fewer muscle fibers can. Currently, the research is not clear on whether an adult body can grow new muscle fibers with resistance training (this is called hyperplasia) (53).

As previously stated, within each muscle the muscle fibers are controlled by a nerve, and this combination forms a motor unit. A motor unit is either a slow-twitch motor unit or a fast-twitch motor unit (controlling slow- or fast-twitch muscle fibers). Different people and different muscles have a differing percentage of slow- and fast-twitch motor units. Muscles that are postural and designed for continuous work, such as the soleus in the calf, tend to be dominated by slow-twitch motor units. Other muscles that are more for power and striking, such as the gastrocnemius, have fast-twitch motor units. Not all people have the same percentage, even in the same muscle. One client might have 80 percent fast-twitch motor units in the pecs, another might have 50 percent, and someone else might only have 35 percent. The majority of muscles on most people seem to follow a rough 50-50 split. Whether we have the ability to change those motor units and their muscle fibers through training is an area of debate, although recent research and anecdotal evidence are suggesting that through proper, long-term training, we can alter those percentages somewhat.

Muscle Age

The age of the muscle, or more simply the age of the person, has an effect on how much force can be produced. Very young muscle (i.e., the muscle of a child) tends to be relatively weak because the muscle is small and neuromuscular coordination is not well developed. Muscle also weakens as a person ages, and this deterioration becomes pronounced in older adults. Common sense tells us that a 70-year-old man is not normally as strong as a 30-year-old man (although some 70-year-old men are very strong; the highest deadlift on record for those over 60 years old is an amazing 705 pounds [319.8 kg]).

Muscle undergoes sarcopenia, a reduction in size and strength, as it ages. Unfortunately, as we age we also tend to become less active, which compounds the sarcopenia and creates a negative snowball effect on fitness and health. The fast-twitch motor units degrade more with age than the slow-twitch motor units do, and that finding should make intuitive sense.

When it comes to aging, there is good news and bad news. Generally, the body begins to age at about 30 years old. That age might seem young, but that is when most bodily processes begin to decline. The good news is that maximum performance in both muscle strength and cardiovascular endurance is normally reached in the 30s, often the late 30s. Some athletes are still peaking in their early 40s. Compare that outcome with sports in which athletes peak at 16 and are considered old at 20, such as gymnastics and figure skating. A tremendous amount of training and a long time is needed for the body to adapt before elite levels can be reached in sports that require muscle strength or cardiovascular endurance. In addition, the body is able to respond to both cardiovascular exercise and resistance training at any age. You can be 80 years old when you begin an exercise program and become more fit at 81 than you were at 80 (or even 70 for that matter).

Muscle Damage

Muscle damage can affect how much force a muscle can produce. Of course, a serious injury will severely limit the strength that a muscle can produce. This protective defense mechanism prevents further harm. But a less serious injury, or perhaps even an "injury" that many people experience every day, delayed-onset muscle soreness (DOMS), can affect the force produced by a muscle. This last condition is called delayed onset because soreness doesn't usually kick in until about one to two days after the intense workout, and it can then last anywhere from just one day up to a week or possibly even more. Although DOMS is common, the exact mechanism for causing it has not been determined. What is clear is that a sore muscle is weaker than a fresh one, and the sorer that muscle is, the weaker it is.

Mind State

Mind state, or mental readiness, can affect how much force a person produces. In general, a focused, alert, almost angry attitude promotes maximum generation of strength. The opposite of that mind state—a happy, giddy, or drowsy attitude—although perhaps enjoyable, does not produce maximum strength. This circumstance can be clearly seen when someone is being tickled. We all know that when we are tickled, it is as though our muscles have somehow been turned off. We can't generate any strength. The same is true immediately upon waking. Sleep turns off the nerves that control the muscles (or at least it normally does), and some time is needed to turn those nerves back on. Waking someone up and then immediately having the person max out in the bench press (or any lift) would not produce maximum results. Being fully awake, alert, focused, aggressive, and almost angry produces maximum strength. Elite weightlifters and powerlifters often yell, grunt, and appear to be fierce or intimidating as they prepare to lift. They are channeling their energy into that one action. Animals such as wolves and lions have a different demeanor when they are lounging around or playing compared with when they are hunting and fighting. Mind state is clearly related to force production on a basic, animalistic level. The purpose of having an optimal mind state is to prepare for maximal neuromuscular coordination.

CONCLUSION

A strong relationship exists between the function of the nervous system and human movement. It involves neuromuscular coordination and the steps involved in muscular contraction—from the brain to the myofilaments. Many factors can affect how much force is produced at a given time. Some of the variables are largely unchangeable, such as angle of pennation and joint structure. Some of the variables rely on certain movements, such as prestretching and preloading. And some of the variables are changeable over time, such as neuromuscular coordination, muscle size, and the ability to control mind state. The goal of the personal trainer and client should be to accept with grace the variables that cannot be changed, to fight with effort and constitution the variables that can be changed, and to be educated enough to know the difference.

Study Questions

1. What is the electrical impulse created by the brain called?

    a. neurotransmitter

    b. action potential

    c. synapse

    d. efferent nerve

2. What is the definition of a motor unit?

    a. one motor nerve and all the muscle fibers that it innervates

    b. one motor nerve and all the muscles that it innervates

    c. one muscle fiber and all the nerves that innervate it

    d. one muscle and all the nerves that innervate it

3. What does the all-or-none principle state?

    a. Either all the muscle fibers within one motor unit will contract or none of them will.

    b. Either all the muscle fibers within one muscle will contract or none of them will.

    c. Either you will be able to lift a weight or you will not be able to lift a weight.

    d. The contraction of each individual muscle fiber can be independently controlled with frequency of activation.

4. What are the two most important changeable factors that affect muscular strength?

    a. angle of pennation and muscle size

    b. preloading and neuromuscular coordination

    c. neuromuscular coordination and muscle size

    d. tendon insertion point and muscle length

5. What terms describes the direction of how the muscle fibers run in relationship to the direction of the tendon of the muscle?

    a. sarcopenia

    b. osteopenia

    c. angle of pennation

    d. angle of rotation

Energy Systems

Have you ever wondered why you can't sprint a marathon? Why you can't just start running at full speed and keep that going for more than 10 seconds? Or why when you start lifting weights, you can complete a set of 8 with a certain weight but can't perform a set of 20 with the same weight? Of course, you "get tired," but that answer is not specific enough. And no, the answer is not always because you can't breathe fast enough or because you run out of oxygen.

Our muscles need a steady supply of energy to keep working. Our bodies produce this energy through three distinct energy systems (figure 8.1). The end goal of an energy system is to produce adenosine triphosphate (ATP), which is the chemical form of energy (fuel) in the body. The body, through the process of digestion and absorption, breaks down the three macronutrients (carbohydrate, protein, and fat) into their building blocks (saccharides, amino acids, and fatty acids), which are converted into units of ATP. The ATP is then used as fuel to power the muscles and other systems in the body. What differentiates the three systems is the source and speed from which they derive the ATP and the process for replacing it (4).

There are three primary energy systems, one of which has two subsystems that operate almost as independent systems. When studying the energy systems, you should focus on these key points:

- Duration of the energy system
- Fuel source
- Ranking for power production
- Ranking for the most total energy produced
- Whether the system is aerobic or anaerobic
- Common examples of each system at work

PHOSPHAGEN SYSTEM

The phosphagen system is the most powerful energy system in the body. If you are trying as hard as you possibly can to run, swim, lift

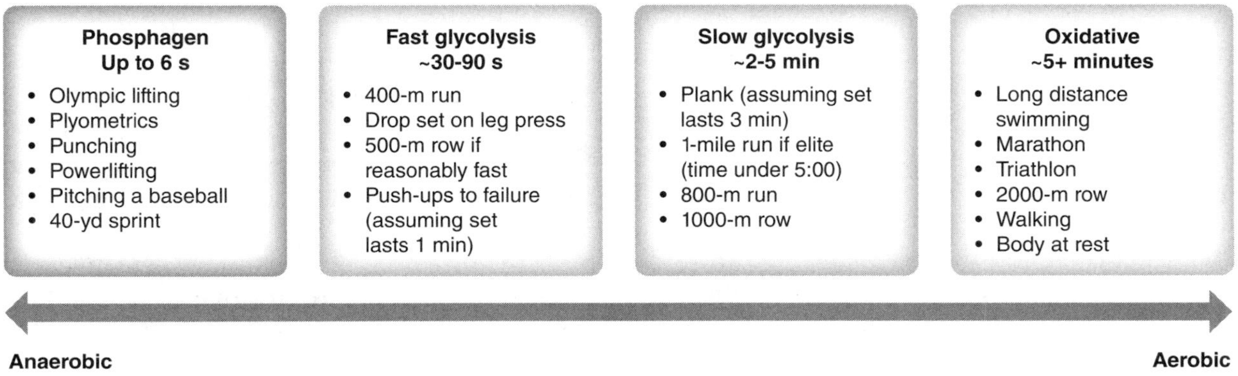

Phosphagen Up to 6 s	Fast glycolysis ~30-90 s	Slow glycolysis ~2-5 min	Oxidative ~5+ minutes
• Olympic lifting • Plyometrics • Punching • Powerlifting • Pitching a baseball • 40-yd sprint	• 400-m run • Drop set on leg press • 500-m row if reasonably fast • Push-ups to failure (assuming set lasts 1 min)	• Plank (assuming set lasts 3 min) • 1-mile run if elite (time under 5:00) • 800-m run • 1000-m row	• Long distance swimming • Marathon • Triathlon • 2000-m row • Walking • Body at rest

Anaerobic   Aerobic

Figure 8.1 Summary of the energy systems.

a weight, or do anything maximally, you are using your phosphagen system. The phosphagen system provides powerful, short-term energy, but the energy it provides doesn't last long—up to only 6 seconds—before it begins to fade. If you continue the activity, performance will drop, and after approximately 30 seconds this system will run out of fuel. Although the phosphagen system is the most powerful energy system, it produces the least amount of total energy because the duration is so short. Imagine that a client told you that he would pay you $600 per hour for personal training, an amount that almost all personal trainers would be pleased with. But if the client followed up that offer with the stipulation that the session would last only 1 minute, that proposal would not be so enticing. Your pay rate would be excellent at $10 per minute, but at the end of the session you would have earned only $10. Likewise, the phosphagen system can produce energy at a tremendous rate (the high pay scale), but it can create only a small amount of total energy (small total income) because of the short duration.

The phosphagen system is fueled by two substances, ATP and creatine phosphate (CP, from which the system derives its name). These two substances are located directly in the muscle cells in small amounts. They are readily available and don't have to be broken down or altered much, so no delay occurs in their use. If you need to jump for some reason or punch something hard immediately, you can. You don't need to wait for the system to charge up or chemicals to be converted to fuel. But the muscle has only small amounts of these substances, and the stores are quickly depleted. For that reason, the system works for up to only 30 seconds or so. If the activity is extremely hard, it won't last even that long (15, 23).

The longest distance that people can truly sprint, or run all out, is 200 meters. Highly skilled athletes need about 20 seconds to cover that distance. A 400-meter run, one lap around an outdoor track, takes most people about 60 seconds. Elite athletes can run that lap in as little as 45 seconds, which is still too long for the phosphagen system to provide full power throughout. Even elite athletes are unable to maintain a full-speed sprint throughout a 400-meter run; they must pace themselves at least a little bit.

After activity has stopped or decreased significantly in intensity, the body can begin to resynthesize ATP and CP. You do not need to eat food to do this. This energy system has the shortest duration of all energy systems, but it is the quickest to recover (60). Generally, ATP can recover to nearly full levels in about three to five minutes, and CP needs about five to eight minutes to recover to nearly full levels. The amount of time necessary to recover is related to how depleted the system is, which is related to how intense the activity was, how long it was performed, and the skill level of the person who performed it.

Athletes, because of their specialized skills, can more fully deplete the energy system and therefore need more time to recover fully. The greater a person's neuromuscular coordination is, the more completely that person can drain his or her energy systems. A layperson might assume that a well-trained athlete needs less rest between sets than an untrained person does, but to repeat a performance, this is not always the case. In addition, people often assume that any time spent resting in a personal training session is wasted time, but that is not necessarily true. If a client is training for maximal strength or power, he or she needs adequate rest to recover fully and produce maximal performance on each set. A client does not have to be physically active for every minute of the session for the workout to be productive. People must occasionally stop to sharpen the saw, which in this case can simply be rest (93).

Understanding the recovery of energy systems and its relationship to exercise intensity is crucial to understanding how to set up rest times correctly for your clients' fitness programs. Rest times (between sets) are extremely important in achieving the goals that you set for your clients.

The phosphagen system is the primary energy-providing system for the body in the following activities:

- Sprinting short distances (200 m or less)
- Olympic weightlifting

- Powerlifting
- Resistance training performed rapidly or using fewer than five reps or so
- Throwing something such as a ball, discus, or shot put
- Kicking something such as a football or soccer ball
- Hitting something with, for instance, a baseball bat or hockey stick
- Punching
- Jumping, such as when dunking a basketball or performing the long jump

The phosphagen system can be referred to as the high-intensity, short-duration system or the high-power-output system. Notice that when describing the fuel for this system, oxygen was not mentioned. A simple test to figure out whether an activity is in the phosphagen system is to imagine yourself performing it intensely while holding your breath. If you could still perform the activity pretty well while holding your breath, it is in the phosphagen system. If you couldn't, it is most likely not in this system. Note that it is not suggested that you actually hold your breath; just imagine whether you could do it. Because oxygen is not crucial to this system, it is considered an oxygen-independent system, which is sometimes called an anaerobic system (meaning "without oxygen") (111, 115, 131). See table 8.1 for a summary of the phosphagen system.

GLYCOLYSIS SYSTEM

The next energy system, the glycolysis system, has two subsystems in it—the fast glycolysis energy system and the slow glycolysis energy system. As the name implies, the fuel for both systems is glucose derived mainly from carbohydrate. The key difference between the two systems is their use of oxygen. The two subsystems are outlined below.

Fast Glycolysis

The fast glycolysis (FG) energy system is the second most powerful energy system in the body, behind the phosphagen system. As the phosphagen system begins to fade—and remember that it fades quickly—the fast glycolysis system is kicking into high gear. Its duration is from about 30 seconds up until about 90 seconds. It then also begins to fade, and by 2 minutes it will be drained. The FG system uses blood glucose for fuel. It takes a short time for the muscle cells to begin to metabolize glucose and turn it into ATP, which is why a slight delay (in seconds) occurs before the fast glycolysis system really starts to work. The FG system produces the third most total energy; it ranks above the phosphagen system in that regard.

Like the phosphagen system, FG is an anaerobic, or oxygen-independent, system. The result of using glucose for energy without using oxygen is that pyruvate, a by-product of glycolysis, is converted to lactate. The FG system is the only system that produces lactate (2). Lactate, and its role in exercise, has been studied extensively, and our ideas about it have shifted in the last several years. We used to think that lactic acid was produced by this energy system, and that term is sometimes still used, but technically the two substances, lactate and lactic acid, are different. We used to think that lactic acid was responsible for muscle soreness, but now we don't believe that either

Table 8.1 Key Points About the Phosphagen System

Duration	Up to 6 seconds, fades by 30 seconds
Fuel	ATP and CP found in small quantities directly inside the muscle cells
Ranking for power production	1st
Ranking for total energy production	4th
Aerobic or anaerobic	Anaerobic
Common examples	1RM bench press, shot put, baseball pitch, golf swing, knockout punch, high jump

lactic acid or lactate is responsible for soreness. Finally, we used to think that lactic acid caused the burning sensation in the muscles when people were fatigued. Now some scientists say that the human body can't even produce lactic acid and that the burning sensation is caused by unbuffered hydrogen ions released when certain compounds are used for energy (5, 10, 12, 42). But the burning sensation is still a good "feel test," and if you are experiencing a rapidly accelerating muscle burn, you are probably using primarily the FG system.

The FG system is the primary energy system used during intense exercises or activities that last about a minute. Performing push-ups or sit-ups for one minute is an example of this. If you are good at push-ups, you can bang out 30 or 40 as you settle into a groove, but as you continue you begin to get fatigued. The buildup of the unbuffered hydrogen ions interferes with the ability of the muscles to contract, and as you fatigue you must rely more on the phosphagen system, which can last only so long. In track, an athlete running the 400-meter race, which could require 45 seconds for athletes and 80 seconds for an untrained person, would use primarily the FG system. In competitive rowing, a well-trained male would be able to row 500 meters in less than 90 seconds, and that activity would be fueled primarily by the FG system (61). Table 8.2 contains a summary of the FG system.

Slow Glycolysis System

The slow glycolysis (SG) system is the second part of the glycolysis system. The big difference between the fast and the slow systems is that the fast system is anaerobic, or oxygen independent, whereas the slow system is aerobic, or oxygen dependent. When the mitochondria in the muscles have enough oxygen, the cells do not convert the pyruvate to lactate. Instead, the pyruvate is converted into acetyl-CoA, which then enters the citric acid cycle (Krebs cycle) and ultimately produces ATP.

We can visualize the use of oxygen in the energy systems as representing a cleaner and more efficient but less powerful method of producing energy. Imagine comparing a sports car with a gas–electric hybrid car. The sports car is fast and powerful but doesn't get good gas mileage and produces more emissions, whereas the hybrid car is slow in a race but can go for a long time and produces little waste. As the FG system begins to fade, which happens after 90 to 120 seconds, the SG system is kicking in. It is the third most powerful energy system. For fuel, it uses glucose in the blood and some glycogen in the muscles. It turns on after about 2 minutes and fades at 5 minutes. This system produces the second greatest amount of total energy (56).

An example of an activity that is powered primarily by the SG system is the mile (1.6 km) run for elite athletes (or half a mile for the rest of us). A fast mile can be completed in five minutes or less; the world record for the mile run is less than 3:45. Most people are able to run a half-mile in under four minutes. In competitive rowing, 1,000 meters should take about three to five minutes. The SG energy system is often the one that receives the least emphasis in a traditional exercise program. See table 8.3 for a summary of the SG system.

OXIDATIVE SYSTEM

The final energy system is the oxidative system; oxidative refers to oxygen. As you probably

Table 8.2   Key Points About the Fast Glycolysis System

Duration	30 to 90 seconds, fades by 2 minutes
Fuel	Glucose in the blood
Ranking for power production	2nd
Ranking for total energy production	3rd
Aerobic or anaerobic	Anaerobic
Common examples	400-m run, maximum push-ups

Table 8.3   Key Points About the Slow Glycolysis System

Duration	2 to 5 minutes
Fuel	Glucose from glycogen
Ranking for power production	3rd
Ranking for total energy production	2nd
Aerobic or anaerobic	Aerobic
Common examples	1-mile (1.6 km) run if highly trained, 800-meter run for most people, the plank exercise if in good shape

guessed, this is an oxygen-dependent aerobic system. The oxidative system is the weakest energy system in that it produces energy at the slowest rate, but it makes up for that shortcoming by being the longest lasting energy system; thus, it produces the most total energy. Think about sprinting and walking. Of course, when you sprint, you move the fastest, but you can sprint for only 100 meters or so. You will burn more total calories (use up more energy) by walking a mile (1.6 km) than you will by sprinting 100 meters.

The oxidative system has the ability to use all three nutrients as fuel. It can burn glucose, fatty acids, and amino acids. Fatty acids come from fat (such as the fat in the food that we eat), and amino acids come from protein (as in muscle tissue or protein in the food that we eat). The glucose comes from glycogen, which is stored in both the liver and the muscle tissue. The other energy systems use glycogen from the muscles; this energy system uses it from both the muscles and the liver. Note that fat has not previously been mentioned as a fuel source. Each of those fuel sources will ultimately be converted to ATP, and each fuel source will yield a certain amount of energy. Don't interpret this to mean that the only way to burn fat is to perform cardio because that is not the case, but performing cardio does actively burn fat minute after minute.

The intensity of the exercise determines whether glucose or fatty acids are the primary fuel source. Keep in mind that both of those fuels will be working together to power this energy system. The more intense your training is, the greater the percentage is of the fuel that comes from carbohydrate. Carbohydrate is considered a high-intensity fuel source. The less intense your training is, the greater the percentage is of the fuel that comes from fat. Fat is considered a low-intensity fuel source. Don't forget that the total number of calories burned always goes up, minute per minute, as intensity increases. As a rough guideline, when your heart rate is below 70 percent of its true maximum, fat is primarily fueling the exercise. If your heart rate goes above 70 percent of maximum, then the fuel source becomes primarily glucose. This glucose comes first from glycogen, and when the body starts to run low on glycogen, some glucose will be derived from amino acids. Although the body has the ability to turn amino acids into glucose, the procedure is complex, and it takes a while for this energy to become available to the muscles. The body gets amino acids from food or from the muscle tissue of the body (49).

You may have seen that 70 percent figure before, and you may have heard of cardiovascular exercise being divided into fat-burning zones and cardio training zones. That topic, and the appropriate zone for your training, is thoroughly discussed in chapter 22, "Aerobic Training Program Design."

The oxidative system kicks in fully when the glycolysis system is fatigued or if the intensity of the exercise never gets high enough to recruit the other energy systems. Any continual exercise that lasts longer than five minutes is fueled primarily by the oxidative system. Examples of this are jogging any distance longer than half a mile (.8 km), cycling, swimming long distances, cross-country skiing, using the treadmill or stair machine, or doing anything that lasts longer than five minutes (74).

The oxidative system is important in helping you recover between intense bouts of exercise, such as your recovery between sets during resistance training. The oxidative energy system is never turned off. Right now, as you sit and read this book, you are using the oxidative system. It may also surprise you to know that you are burning a very high percentage of fat just sitting there. Unfortunately, the total number of calories burned is low when you are at rest. Using any other energy system increases the demand on the oxidative system, which is why the other methods can be successful at burning fat. For example, a moderately fast but non-Olympic-level athlete might need 13 seconds to complete an intense 100-meter sprint. During those 13 seconds of activity, almost no significant amount of fat will be burned, but for the 5 minutes following that activity, the athlete's metabolism will be raised significantly. In those 5 minutes the athlete will burn a significant amount of fat. If the athlete completes five 100-meter sprints with 5-minute rest intervals, in a 30-minute workout the athlete might have worked for just over 1 minute, but the body will have been stimulated for the entire 30 minutes and will have burned a large amount of fat during that time. Indeed, that type of workout will likely create EPOC (see chapter 22 for more information), and the athlete's metabolism may remain elevated for several hours after the activity ends. Table 8.4 contains a summary of the oxidative system.

BLENDING OF THE ENERGY SYSTEMS

Understanding the energy systems becomes crucial because of the need to train in a specific manner to improve in a certain event.

First, recognize that all the energy systems are working together all the time. The body does not have a switch that turns one energy system off when another comes on. All the energy systems are working together, but knowing which energy system is contributing primarily to the activity can be useful. The intensity of the exercise is what determines the energy system being used. If a person (over the age of 21, of course) curls a beer for five reps, you might think that the person would be using the phosphagen system because only about five seconds are needed to perform the five reps. If a person curls 50-pound (22.7 kg) dumbbells for five reps, the phosphagen system would most likely be used, but a beer is so light that the person could curl it a hundred times or more, using primarily the oxidative system to power that activity. Don't think about how long the activity *was* performed; think about how long it *could be* performed. If intensity is high, you can use duration to separate out the energy systems, but intensity is the key determinant of which energy system is involved.

Going back to the car example, we can view different kinds of cars as representing different energy systems. A drag-racing car, with a huge engine, big tires in the back, and little tires up front, is the phosphagen system. This car can race a quarter mile (.4 km) in six seconds or less, but it has poor endurance and would not be good for any kind of long trip. A sports car is quite fast and performs exceptionally well on a track. It would be able to beat the drag-racing car on a road course type of track, but it would not beat the dragster on the strip. A sports car would represent the fast glycolysis system. An economy car would represent the SG system.

Table 8.4 Key Points About the Oxidative System

Duration	≥5 minutes
Fuel	Glucose, fatty acids, and amino acids
Ranking for power production	4th
Ranking for total energy production	1st
Aerobic or anaerobic	Aerobic
Common examples	Classic cardiovascular exercise—long-distance cycling, swimming, running, walking; the body at rest

It is not as fast as the dragster and does not do as well as a sports car on a track, but it still gets around pretty well and because the SG system uses oxygen, it is much more efficient (burns less gas to accomplish the same thing) than either of the other two cars. A hybrid car that combines an internal combustion engine and one or more electric motors would represent the oxidative system. It can't perform well in either a drag race or a race around a track, and it is even slower than the economy car, but if you were to drive across the country, a hybrid car would need the least amount of gas to make the trip.

An analogy can help you understand how the energy systems work in the body. Picture a lighter, such as a cigarette lighter. On most lighters you can adjust the size of the flame to make it larger or smaller. A lighter is your oxidative system. It is always running, but the more flame you produce, the more fuel you use and the quicker you run out of fuel. Imagine that the lighter is always on (because it represents the oxidative system and we are always breathing while we are alive), so it is always producing energy. The problem is that it doesn't produce much energy. If you need more heat than it can produce even when turned all the way up, you turn to something else. Imagine that you have a blowtorch right next to your lighter. If you want a significant amount of heat, you can turn on the blowtorch. The lighter stays on the whole time, but now it is overshadowed by the blowtorch, which will greatly increase the amount of energy produced. The blowtorch, however, uses up fuel a lot faster than the lighter does, so it doesn't last as long. Again, on most blowtorches you can adjust the amount of heat produced. The blowtorch is the glycolysis system. Finally, if you want a huge blast of heat, you have a flamethrower. This device emits an enormous amount of energy, but its duration is fleeting. When you use the flamethrower, the lighter and blowtorch stay on, but the flamethrower is the main producer of energy. The flamethrower is the phosphagen system. The key thing to remember is that all the energy systems are always in use, but the intensity determines which energy system is dominant.

REPLENISHMENT OF THE ENERGY SYSTEMS

The energy systems in our bodies help turn the food we eat into usable energy (ATP), but as that energy is depleted, it must be replaced. The rate and method of replenishment depends on the energy system.

Phosphagen System

ATP needs three to five minutes to return to near full levels, and creatine phosphate requires five to eight minutes to recover fully. This happens automatically if you are operating at an intensity that allows the muscles to recover—very light activity or nothing at all. For example, suppose that you are performing a chest press exercise. You perform one set of 10 reps with 100 pounds (45.4 kg) and then rest for two minutes. If that set was a maximal set (the most you could possibly do), you will not be fully recovered, so you might manage just 7 or 8 reps on the following set. If you rest 5 minutes or more, most likely you will be able to do 9 or 10 reps because you would have a near full recovery time. If you decide to jump rope for the 2 minutes that you were resting, you would likely not be able to get even 7 or 8 reps and instead might manage just 4 to 6 reps because the act of jumping rope is too strenuous to allow the phosphagen system to recover fully (19).

Glycolysis System

The fuel for the glycolysis system is glucose, which is derived from glycogen. For the glycolysis system to recover, your activity level must be greatly reduced, such as by taking a walking break after sprinting so that you can sprint again. In addition, more glycogen must be broken down so that blood glucose is continuously available. The body has a finite supply of glycogen; when it is depleted the performance of the glycolysis system will be compromised (68).

As mentioned previously, a high-functioning oxidative system facilitates recovery of the glycolysis system (and all systems). You will not fully deplete your glycogen levels in one bout using the glycolysis system alone, but repeated bouts can completely drain your glycogen storage levels. To get the idea, imagine running five 400-meter sprints with a two-minute rest after each. Glycogen levels can be restored by consuming carbohydrate. This process is more fully described later.

Oxidative System

The oxidative system uses all three fuel sources: carbohydrate, protein, and fat. To replenish those fuel sources, you must consume calories. Glucose comes from glycogen, and glycogen comes from carbohydrate. At the end of the exercise session, you should eat carbohydrate. This topic is covered in more depth in chapters 14 and 16, but a few guidelines are offered here. Try to eat within two hours of completing the exercise. The body is like a sponge after exercise, so feeding it early optimizes glycogen storage. You need to eat carbohydrate in this meal; the amount of carbohydrate depends on the intensity of the exercise. The National Strength and Conditioning Association (NSCA) recommends consuming .7 to 3.0 grams of carbohydrate per kilogram of body weight in a 24-hour period. A simpler recommendation is to eat 50 to 150 grams of carbohydrate in the first meal after working out (21).

The body can make glucose from stored glycogen, but when you are out of stored glycogen, you must replace it, and the body cannot synthesize glycogen from anything but food. Most people can store about 300 to 500 grams of glycogen in the body.

Remember that the energy systems can use protein in the form of amino acids to replace glucose, so you also need to eat protein after you work out and throughout your day. Recommendations vary about the amount of protein an athlete needs, but a simple recommendation for a postworkout meal is to include between 20 and 50 grams of protein. Protein will help with the recovery of your muscles and will help prevent possible muscle loss caused by exercise.

Finally, fat can be used for energy; fat should be included in each meal as well. Even if your goal is to lose body fat, you still need to eat some fat. A useful guideline suggests eating between 10 and 30 grams of fat in the post-workout meal. The majority of that fat should come from healthy fat sources (see chapter 14 for more information).

All energy systems generally require about 24 hours to recover fully from an activity or workout. The recovery time depends on how intense and exhausting the activity was, what the recovery factors were (that is, nutrition status before and after the event, amount of sleep before and after the event, and so forth), and what the fitness level of the person was. See table 8.5 for energy system contributions in many common sports.

CONCLUSION

All energy systems ultimately provide ATP to the body. The phosphagen energy system is the body's most powerful energy system. It is anaerobic, uses ATP and CP as fuel, and doesn't last longer than 30 seconds. Several minutes of rest is generally adequate to recharge this system. The glycolysis energy system has two subsets. The fast glycolysis energy system is the second most powerful energy system in the body. It is anaerobic, uses glucose from the blood as fuel, and lasts up to two minutes. This energy system turns pyruvate into lactate and produces the most unbuffered hydrogen ions; it is most associated with the burning feeling in the muscles. The slow glycolysis energy system is the third most powerful energy system in the body. It is aerobic because it uses oxygen, uses glucose broken down from glycogen as fuel, and lasts up to five minutes. Rest and food are necessary to replenish the glycolysis energy systems fully. The oxidative energy system is the least powerful energy system, but it produces the most total energy output. It is aerobic, is able to use all three macronutrients as fuel, and powers any activity that lasts longer than five minutes.

Athletes should know which energy systems and fuels are most important to them, and personal trainers should remember that a client's workout program will dictate which energy system adapts to the training. Intensity

Table 8.5 Energy System Contributions in Common Sports

Sport	Phosphagen and fast glycolysis	Slow glycolysis	Oxidative
Basketball	60	20	20
Fencing	90	10	0
Field events	90	10	0
Golf swing	95	5	0
Gymnastics	80	15	5
Hockey	50	20	30
Distance running	10	20	70
Rowing	20	30	*50
Skiing	33	33	33
Soccer	50	20	30
Sprints	90	10	0
Distance swimming	10	20	70
Tennis	70	20	10
Volleyball	80	5	15

is the number one variable that determines which energy system is primarily powering an activity.

Study Questions

1. What is the primary fuel for the phosphagen system?
   a. ATP and CP
   b. glucose
   c. fatty acids
   d. amino acids

2. Which energy system produces lactate?
   a. phosphagen system
   b. fast glycolysis system
   c. slow glycolysis system
   d. oxidative system

3. A person jogs at 60 percent of MHR for 30 minutes. Which energy system is primarily fueling that event, and which is the primary fuel source for that event?
   a. slow glycolysis, glucose
   b. slow glycolysis, fatty acids
   c. oxidative, glucose
   d. oxidative, fatty acids

4. Which is the primary energy system used to fuel a baseball pitcher pitching the baseball?
   a. phosphagen system
   b. fast glycolysis system
   c. slow glycolysis system
   d. oxidative system

5. About how long does it take creatine phosphate to achieve a nearly full recharge?
   a. less than 30 seconds
   b. 1 to 2 minutes
   c. 5 to 8 minutes
   d. about 24 hours

Endocrine System

The body is ruled by hormones, which are chemical messengers in the body that tell the body what to do. They are like directors in a movie. They may not perform the action themselves, they may not star in the movie, but hormones give orders to the cells in the body. Without hormones, very little is done. You can eat well and train hard, but your hormones stimulate the growth of new muscle tissue.

The endocrine system is made up of the endocrine glands, which store and secrete hormones. These glands are found all over the body including in the brain, throat, heart, liver, adrenal glands, and sex organs. Hormones are extremely complex, and this chapter cannot make you an expert on them. But arming yourself with some basic information about how hormones work and, more important, how to release them, will benefit you as a personal trainer.

Hormones have multiple roles, affect multiple tissues in the body, and often interact with each other. Sometimes one hormone will cause the release of another hormone, and sometimes the presence of one hormone will suppress the function of another. Hormones are thus difficult to study and understand (80). Because of these varied actions, interactions, and reactions, hormone therapy is complex. If a person is prescribed hormone replacement therapy, the doctor will experiment with the dosages during a trial period to determine the correct balance. This complexity is also why any use of synthetic hormones can have unintended consequences in the body.

LOCK AND KEY THEORY

Hormones can affect multiple tissues in the body, but they will not normally affect every single tissue in the body. This limitation is explained by the lock and key theory, which states that certain cells have certain receptor sites on them. Only the specific hormones that can bind with those receptor sites will be able to interact with that cell. For example, testosterone can have a powerful effect on muscle tissue, but it does not seem to have a similar effect on kidney tissue; that is, your kidneys do not become big, hard, and strong from testosterone. The effect differs because muscle tissue has receptor sites for testosterone but kidney tissue does not. In other words, the testosterone key is not able to fit into and open the lock on the receptor sites in kidney tissue (37). This theory is shown in figure 9.1.

ANABOLIC VERSUS CATABOLIC

Hormones are broken down into two categories: anabolic and catabolic (table 9.1). An anabolic hormone builds tissue (4). When we think of anabolic hormones, we tend to think of building muscle tissue (e.g., consider anabolic steroids), but any type of tissue in the body can be affected by anabolic hormones. A catabolic hormone breaks down tissue, and again that can be any kind of tissue in the body. In the fitness world, we tend to think of

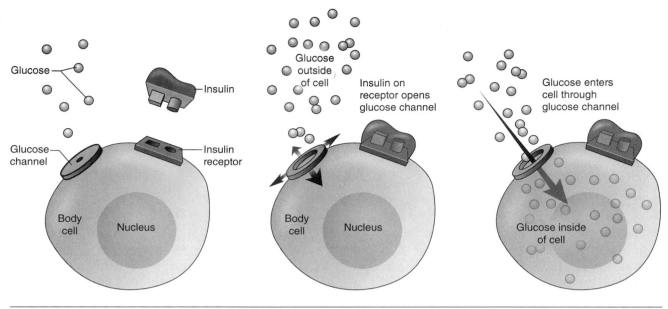

Figure 9.1 Illustration of the lock and key theory.

anabolic as good and catabolic as bad, but that simplification is not really accurate. Your body needs both types of hormones, just in certain amounts. A better perspective is to think of them as yin and yang rather than good and bad. Having said that, the goal of training is often to help maximize the anabolic hormonal response and minimize the catabolic hormonal response.

ANABOLIC HORMONES

Three primary anabolic hormones are within a personal trainer's scope of practice to understand (2, 113).

Testosterone

One of the body's primary anabolic hormones is testosterone. Although testosterone is the main male sex hormone, women have testosterone in their bodies as well. Adult men usually have about 15 to 20 times more testosterone in their bodies than adult females do, but these levels are not constant. Some men have significantly more testosterone than other men, and some women have more testosterone than other women. The release of testosterone becomes significant during puberty when a male starts to take on secondary sex characteristics. Men produce less and less testosterone as they age, and the decline usually begins around age 40. Men release testosterone from their testes, and women release it from their ovaries and adrenal glands (32, 34).

Testosterone, sometimes referred to as "test" for short, has several powerful effects on the body. First, testosterone is able to interact directly with skeletal muscle. The primary effect of testosterone is to make skeletal muscle grow bigger and stronger. Second, testosterone interacts with the motor neurons. It can increase the amount of neurotransmitters present and cause positive structural changes in the

Table 9.1 Key Anabolic and Catabolic Hormones

Key anabolic hormones	Key catabolic hormones
Testosterone	Cortisol
Growth hormone	Catecholamines
Insulin	Glucagon

neurons. In simple terms, testosterone can help increase neuromuscular coordination. This effect can be demonstrated by the increased physical ability in boys as they age, even with little or no training. A smaller and weaker 15-year-old will most likely demonstrate better coordination than a larger, stronger 11-year-old who has lower levels of testosterone in his system.

In addition, the rampant use of steroids in sport has not occurred solely because athletes want larger muscles. Neuromuscular coordination is the most important factor in sporting performance. For that reason, the use of the steroids as a performance enhancer is not limited to the strength sports; almost all sports can be touched by steroid use. Steroids are particularly prevalent in baseball, an exceptionally high-skill sport in which strength is not as crucial as it is in other sports. Certainly, being stronger does help players hit the ball a bit farther, but that improvement is not the primary reason for taking steroids to play baseball. Steroids directly affect the motor neurons—the nerves that control the muscles—and improve their operational effectiveness, which means that the athlete will connect with the ball more frequently. Steroids, when combined with practicing a specific activity, will normally increase neuromuscular coordination more than practicing the activity alone.

Third, testosterone can act on the pituitary gland and cause the release of growth hormone. These two hormones can have a synergistic effect on the body and generally help improve fitness levels. Anecdotal evidence also suggests that testosterone may increase metabolism and improve recovery ability. In addition, testosterone likely has a stronger effect on muscle tissue than it does on bones, ligaments, or tendons. Testosterone also seems to be more important in building strength than in maintaining it. Adult men who have lost their testes to cancer and take testosterone usually find their strength levels to be moderately similar to their precancer strength levels (57).

How to Release Testosterone

The body releases testosterone under certain situations, and exercise is one of those situations. If the goal is to release testosterone during training, then follow one or more of these guidelines:

- Train large-muscle groups. The bigger the muscle group is, the greater the amount is of testosterone released.

- Choose big, compound exercises. Likewise, the more of the body that is hit during the exercise, the greater the chance is for the release of significant testosterone. Squats, deadlifts, and cleans are likely good choices to release test, whereas seated calf raises and tricep kickbacks are not.

- Use heavy resistance. The training must be relatively intense to cause a test release, and one way to do that is to go heavy. Eighty-five percent of the 1RM is often given as a suggestion, but the bottom line is to challenge yourself or your clients in the gym.

- Use shorter rest periods. To release the most test, you want to recruit as much of the muscle as possible. You can accomplish this by limiting rest periods to less than 2 minutes; 30 to 90 seconds is the standard guideline. By completing additional sets when fatigued, you force your body to recruit additional motor units to complete the task. The more of the muscle that is fatigued, the more hormones are released.

- Make the workout short. Test levels are thought to drop off 45 to 75 minutes after the workout begins. Most authorities suggest keeping muscle-building workouts to an hour or less. If the workout is going to continue, the intensity should be reduced. For example, you could train hard with weights for 60 minutes and then walk for another 60 minutes. This idea is also part of the rationale for performing two or three shorter workouts spread throughout the day as opposed to one long 3-hour workout.

- Become experienced. Lifters continue to release test as they gain experience in the gym. Indeed, their ability to release test seems to improve with two or more years of training. With experience comes increased neuromuscular coordination, which enables lifters to take their muscles to a deeper level of exhaustion. That deeper level of fatigue promotes a stronger hormonal release.

The study of testosterone is in its infancy, and we are still learning much about it. We need to learn more about individual fluctuations in testosterone, daily fluctuations in testosterone in the same person, testosterone response to exercise, and synthetic drug use.

Growth Hormone

Growth hormone, sometimes abbreviated GH (or HGH for human growth hormone), is another powerful anabolic hormone. GH does play a role in the growth of a child to normal adult size, as the name implies, but after a person has stopped growing, additional GH will not cause any increase in height. GH still performs many significant functions in the body, often in conjunction with testosterone. Females have about the same levels of GH as males do (70).

GH has an effect on the fuel utilization of the body. GH causes an increase in lipolysis, which is a breakdown of fat, and it causes increased utilization of fatty acids as fuel. This in turn can cause a reduction in total body fat, because more of it is being used up as fuel. Because the body is burning a slightly higher percentage of fat for its fuel, it needs less fuel from carbohydrate, so glucose utilization decreases.

GH is anabolic, so it has a building effect on the body. It causes an increase in protein synthesis and collagen synthesis. GH is used to build bone, tendon, ligaments, and so forth, and it causes an increase in cartilage growth. GH also seems to have a positive effect on the immune system. It may increase the strength and recovery ability of skeletal muscles, cause a tightening effect on the skin, and improve joint health.

How to Release Growth Hormone

As we learned earlier, testosterone has the ability to release growth hormone, so the same things that release testosterone also release growth hormone. In addition, there is a strong correlation, but not necessarily causation, between feeling the burning sensation in the muscles from unbuffered hydrogen ions and a release in growth hormone. For that reason, there is some truth in the "go for the burn" goal during a workout. Essentially, using the fast glycolysis (FG) energy system should cause a release of growth hormone (18).

Outside the gym, growth hormone is released during sleep, particularly REM sleep, so getting a good night's sleep increases growth hormone levels. Some preliminary evidence indicates that consuming the proper pre- and postworkout meals can help with testosterone and growth hormone release in and out of the gym.

Anti-Aging Debate

Testosterone and growth hormone are being studied and used to help combat the effects of aging, although this activity is not without some controversy. Clearly, as people age, they start to release less and less testosterone and growth hormone. Some people take prescription hormones in an effort to duplicate the hormonal levels that they had in their 20s and 30s. But one theory is that there is a good reason that these two powerful anabolic hormones decrease as we age. The theory postulates that as people age, they develop a small number of cancerous cells, tumors, and other unhealthy tissue in the body. Test and GH have a powerful anabolic effect on the body, and tumors and cancer cells respond well to those hormones. A high level of GH in the body would feed and grow those harmful cells. The idea is that as we age, the body decreases output of the anabolic hormones to slow the growth of any unhealthy tissue, thus allowing us to live longer. In addition, if the rate-of-living hypothesis is correct—that lifespan is inversely correlated with the speed of metabolism—then taking these hormones, which would speed metabolism, could shorten the lifespan (16, 36).

Both testosterone and growth hormone are drugs, not supplements. A person cannot buy them legally over the counter in the United

States; a prescription is needed. Doctors are not legally allowed to give someone a prescription for test or GH just to look better or feel younger, although the law has a significant gray area. Doctors are allowed to give prescriptions if a person is deficient in those hormones, and therein lies the confusion. Clear levels of deficiency have not been identified for all ages. In addition, almost all males are deficient in testosterone at age 50 compared with what they had at age 25. So is that person deficient, even though he is in a normal range for his current age? The law does not address this point, so doctors are allowed to prescribe these drugs to bring patients up to "optimal" levels. A reasonable, logical question to ask is this: If these hormones can have some negative side effects, why would we want to release them through exercise? The amounts of these hormones released through natural methods (exercise, sleep, and so on) are small compared with what is taken artificially. In addition, the body has evolved to deal with any side effects for a natural hormonal release, but it has not evolved to deal with large amounts of exogenous hormones put into the body.

Insulin

The final primary anabolic hormone is insulin, which most people have heard about in conjunction with diabetes. Insulin metabolism is driven primarily by the diet; what you eat has a strong effect on insulin release. The main function of insulin is to serve as a shuttle by taking "stuff" from the blood and putting it into the cells. That stuff includes glucose, which can be turned into glycogen or fat; fatty acids, which can be turned into fat; and amino acids, which can become muscle or fat. Insulin ultimately lowers the blood sugar by removing glucose from the blood. It is mainly released after food is consumed (1).

Some release of insulin is necessary and generally beneficial, causing the synthesis of glycogen and muscle tissue, which is a good thing. But if the blood sugar rises rapidly or to a very high level, the body has to release a large amount of insulin. This discharge can promote the storage of fat and cause a large drop in blood sugar, which can leave the person feeling tired, sluggish, weak, or sleepy. Experienced occasionally, this rapid drop in blood sugar is probably not too detrimental, but if it happens too frequently, the person can become insulin resistant (desensitized to the effects of insulin). In insulin resistance, the insulin released is not doing its job, so the body must release even more insulin. Because the insulin is not effective in removing glucose from the bloodstream, the blood sugar levels stay unusually high. If this happens repeatedly and for a long time, it can lead to impaired fasting glucose levels and ultimately diabetes (24). The good news is that intense exercise serves to increase the number and sensitivity of the insulin receptors. Therefore, regular exercise can protect against diabetes and enhance blood sugar control.

As a personal trainer, you should have at least a basic understanding of this prevalent disease. Type 1 diabetes is the less common form. People with type 1 diabetes are unable to produce their own insulin; as a result, they have to monitor their blood sugar regularly and supplement with shots of insulin. They have a hard time gaining weight, especially muscle. Type 2 diabetes is more common. It is sometimes referred to as lifestyle diabetes because the lifestyle and eating habits of the person have a strong effect on it. Type 2 diabetes used to be referred to as adult-onset diabetes, but because of the rapid acceleration in childhood obesity, that term is no longer accurate. In type 2 diabetes, the person can still produce insulin, but not efficiently. People with type 2 diabetes are usually overweight, and if they monitor their diet, exercise, and lose weight, they can often rein in the effects of the disease. But if they continue to make poor food choices, the disease will progress. Diabetes is currently the sixth-leading cause of death in the United States, so it is a significant problem. Even when it isn't fatal, the disease can cause a host of complications, including the loss of toes, feet, and legs from circulation problems. The good news is that exercise uses glucose for fuel and thus helps keep blood sugar levels under control. Exercise can also promote the growth and improve the sensitivity of the insulin receptor cells, thereby reducing the likelihood of insulin insensitivity. Furthermore, exercise helps control body weight, and maintaining a healthy weight significantly lowers the risk of type 2 diabetes.

CATABOLIC HORMONES

A personal trainer should also be aware of the functions of the three primary catabolic hormones and the way in which exercise affects them (2, 113). The body needs to have anabolic hormones to help build up certain things, but at times it also needs catabolic hormones to help break down certain things.

Cortisol

Cortisol is one of the body's primary catabolic hormones. Cortisol is stored and secreted in the adrenal glands, which are small grape-sized glands that sit atop the kidneys. The primary function of cortisol is to help convert amino acids into glucose, which is then used as fuel. This hormone is released when the muscle glycogen stores are low and the body needs high-intensity energy. The body then releases cortisol to help break down amino acids and convert them to glucose to be used for that high-intensity energy (114).

Cortisol is sometimes referred to as the stress hormone because it can be released when a person is under chronic stress. Unfortunately, the body considers exercise as stress, so cortisol is released with exercise. Also, most of the factors that promote testosterone release also release cortisol. But there is some good news. The signal to release cortisol during exercise is a low glycogen level, and you can exercise for a while before your glycogen stores are depleted. Glycogen usually lasts one to four hours during intense exercise, assuming that you start with full glycogen levels. As glycogen levels begin to drop, your body releases cortisol.

You have a window approximately an hour long during which you can train hard, release testosterone, but still have enough glycogen to prevent a significant release of cortisol. If you

continue to train for much longer than an hour at an elevated intensity, then you may start releasing higher levels of cortisol. If you are working out to build muscle, you are in essence spinning your wheels. You are breaking down muscle to get energy to fuel the workout to build the muscle. Do you see the issue here? For that reason, among others, it is generally better to break down that long workout into shorter, smaller workouts. Instead of one 3-hour workout, perform two 1 1/2-hour workouts or three 1-hour workouts. Assuming that you rest and consume food during the break time, the body can recalibrate and return to normal levels. The second workout will then cause another testosterone spike. This concept can help explain the popularity of morning and evening workouts for bodybuilders and two- or three-a-days for football players.

Catecholamines

Catecholamines is a fancy name for what most of us would call adrenaline. Generally, epinephrine or norepinephrine is being released. Initially, we might assume that adrenaline is anabolic, but that is not the case. Adrenaline is all about the here and now because it tells your body to mobilize everything you have so that you can survive the moment. Something that is anabolic is all about the future (91). If somebody jumps out at you while you are walking down the street, the body is not worried about the vigorous chest workout you just had and how it wants to repair the pecs; it simply wants to survive the next few minutes. You release catecholamines, which prime the body for whatever activity is necessary. If you choose to run away, you want to do that as fast as possible, and if you choose to fight, you want to do that as effectively as possible. Specifically, catecholamines cause some of the following functions in the body:

- Increase neuromuscular coordination by improving the firing rate of the nerves
- Increase ability to recruit high-threshold motor units

- Release other hormones like testosterone and growth hormone
- Break down the storage form of the nutrients into their building blocks—glycogen to glucose, muscle to amino acids, and adipose tissue to fatty acids
- Increase pulse and blood pressure

The bottom line for adrenaline is that it is highly beneficial when necessary for performance—a maximal-effort lift, winning a competition, fighting for the end zone, and so forth—but you do not need to, nor should you, try to release all your adrenaline on every set in the gym (screaming during every set is a bad thing). You can get overstressed, and you can overtrain. You have only so much adrenaline, and you need to allow for recovery.

Glucagon

Glucagon is the opposite of insulin. Glucagon helps break down glycogen and turn it into glucose to be used for energy. A little saying that you can try to remember is, "When the glucose is gone, who are you gonna call? Glucagon." (15) Admittedly, the saying is a little corny, but sometimes those memory tricks work the best!

Glucagon helps raise blood sugar by sending glucose into the bloodstream. Glucagon also helps break down adipose tissue and turns it into fatty acids to be used for energy. Glucagon does not seem to have a catabolic effect on protein tissue. Like insulin, glucagon release is dependent on your diet, so the types and quality of the food that you eat have a significant effect on the release of insulin and glucagon.

OVERALL EFFECT OF HORMONES

The take-home point with hormones is that although they are complex, we can influence through exercise and diet how they act on the body. In general, we want to try to maximize the anabolic hormones, especially when trying to increase performance or change appearance. We can do this by choosing larger exercises, lifting relatively heavy weights, using moderate rest periods, and in general training relatively intensely.

Note that the hormones are going to affect only the tissues stimulated by exercise. If you don't train hard, you are going to stimulate only a small portion of the muscle. In turn, the hormones will act only on that small portion of the muscle, not the muscle in its entirety, and the results achieved will be relatively limited.

We also want to minimize the adrenal fatigue that results from too many catabolic hormones being in our systems, which is easier said than done, because we all seem to live in a stressful world. But we can help ourselves by getting a reasonable amount of sleep each night; eating a relatively healthy diet and consuming food at the proper times during the day; modulating the frequency, intensity, time, and type of exercise to avoid overtraining; and understanding that at advanced levels the nervous system will get and stay fatigued much longer than the muscular system will. Using tactics such as releasing adrenaline or using stimulants will significantly increase the adrenal fatigue, so those methods should be used sparingly.

CONCLUSION

Endocrine glands make and release hormones, which are chemical messengers that tell the body what to do. Hormones affect only specific tissues and cells because of the lock and key theory. Hormones are categorized as having either an anabolic (tissue building) or catabolic (tissue breakdown) effect on the body. Anabolic hormones include testosterone, growth hormone, and insulin. Intense training, proper nutrition, and adequate recovery can promote the release of anabolic hormones. Catabolic hormones include cortisol, catecholamines, and glucagon. Intense training, high levels of stress, and inadequate rest and recovery can promote the release of the catabolic hormones. Personal trainers and clients have to find a balance of work, exercise, and daily life that can promote or maintain the anabolic hormones while minimizing excessive release of the catabolic hormones.

Study Questions

1. What is the definition of an anabolic hormone?

   a. a hormone that helps the body break down tissue

   b. a hormone that must bind with a specific fatty acid carrier to travel in the body

   c. a hormone that operates on the lock and key theory

   d. a hormone that helps the body build up tissue

2. What is the definition of a hormone?

   a. a mineral with an electrical charge that controls water balance

   b. a chemical messenger

   c. a high-density lipoprotein that withdraws fat from the cells

   d. a substance that is only secreted from the adrenal glands

3. Which of the following are the anabolic hormones?

   a. testosterone, growth hormone, insulin

   b. cortisol, catecholamines, glucagon

   c. testosterone, growth hormone, glucagon

   d. cortisol, catecholamines, insulin

4. What type of exercise routine is most likely to release testosterone?

   a. circuit training, 10 to 15 reps, light to moderate intensity, two-minute rest between sets

   b. long, slow distance aerobic training

   c. resistance training, 8 to 12 reps, 50 to 60 percent of 1RM, one set per exercise, and two minutes of rest

   d. resistance training, 8 to 12 reps, 60 to 80 percent of 1RM, four sets per exercise, and one minute of rest

5. What is the primary function of cortisol?

   a. It turns fatty acids into glucose to yield high-intensity energy.

   b. It turns amino acids into glucose to yield high-intensity energy.

   c. It directly improves the motor neurons, thus increasing neuromuscular coordination.

   d. It increases fatty acid utilization and increases protein synthesis.

Biomechanics

One of your main priorities as a personal trainer is to help your clients strengthen and train their muscles. Skeletal muscles are responsible for nearly all our voluntary movements. To help people train their muscles more precisely for specific skills, kinesiologists have classified the different ways in which people can move. For instance, if you told 10 people to move forward, you might get 10 different movements. Some people might walk forward, others might bend forward, and some might raise their arms forward. Although all would have been following your directions, each movement has a different label and definition. Kinesiologists have created six specific categories to classify the majority of normal body movements. Besides these six primary movements, other joint-specific special cases exist.

To understand these movements, we need to refer back to anatomical position. In anatomical position, the body is facing forward, arms are by the side, palms are forward, and thumbs are out. The feet are just slightly apart. When we are thinking about how the body moves, we always start from this position, illustrated in figure 10.1.

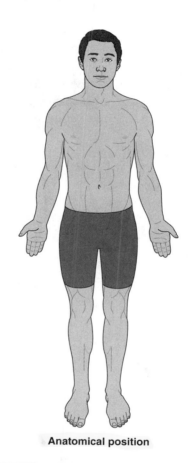

Anatomical position

Figure 10.1 Standard anatomical position of reference.

FLEXION

Decreasing an angle at a joint is called flexion. In anatomical position, most joints are in a straight line, which is 180 degrees. If you flex a joint, you are decreasing this angle (figure 10.2). The elbow and the knee are the easiest to visualize. When you bend your elbow, you are flexing your elbow, and the same applies to your knee. Almost all joints are capable of flexion. When the word *bend* or *curl* is applied to the movement, flexion is almost always occurring. Flexion usually involves a part of the body moving forward (with the exception of the knee) (28).

EXTENSION

Increasing an angle at a joint is called extension. In anatomical position, most joints are extended. So first, you need to flex a joint, such as by bending the elbow to 90 degrees. Now when you straighten your arm, you are extending your elbow (figure 10.3). When the word *straighten* is used to describe movement, it is normally referring to extension. Sometimes the word *extension* is used in the name of an exercise, such as the leg extension exercise (in which you sit down and straighten your legs) or the tricep extension exercise. Extension usually involves a part of the body moving backward (with the exception of the knee). Extension is the opposite of flexion (73).

A movement called hyperextension is a special case of extension. Hyperextension occurs when a joint is extended beyond 180 degrees, or anatomical position. For example, when you are standing straight with your neck extended, it is at a 180-degree angle to your body (a straight line). If you lean your neck back to look up at the ceiling, you have hyperextended your neck (figure 10.4). Sometimes hyperextension is not good for the body, such as when hyperextending the knee, elbow, or even the trunk under heavy resistance. Hyperextension is natural for other joints,

such as the shoulder, hip, or neck. Some joints are made to hyperextend, and some are not. Normally, during resistance training, we stick with a basic range of motion, which involves no hyperextension (77).

Flexion and extension movements take place primarily in the sagittal plane, an imaginary plane (a two-dimensional space, such as a sheet of paper) that extends forward and backward (34). Imagine standing with your shoulder next to a wall. Now imagine that you

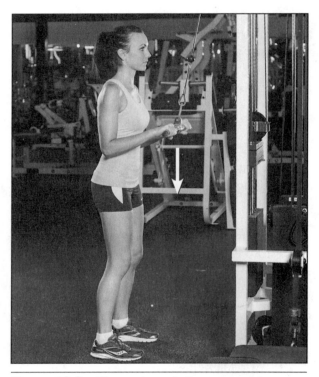

Figure 10.3 Illustration of elbow extension.

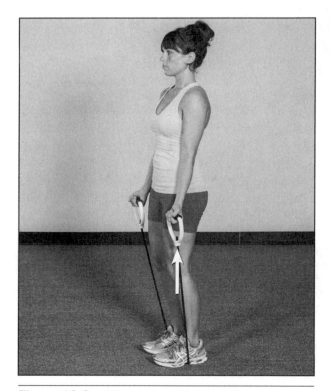

Figure 10.2 Illustration of elbow flexion.

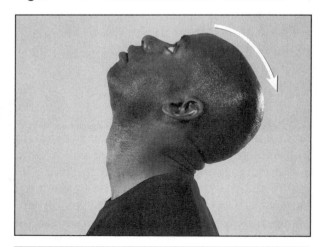

Figure 10.4 Illustration of neck hyperextension.

could phase yourself halfway into the wall. The wall itself represents the sagittal plane. (See figure 10.5 for an illustration of the different planes.) Now half of your body is on one side of the wall, and the other half is on the other side of the wall. One eye is on one side, the other eye is on the other side, one arm is on one side, the other arm is on the other side, and so forth. The sagittal plane divides the body into left and right sections (figure 10.5a). The sagittal plane doesn't have to be exactly in the middle of your body, but it normally is. The sagittal plane is also called the midline. The midline will be discussed in more detail shortly. Remember that a plane is a two-dimensional figure that continues forever in two directions, in this case forward and backward.

We are going to use a teaching trick to learn the planes. When an exercise takes place in a certain plane, the part of the body that is moving during the exercise stays in contact with that specific plane the entire time. When

examining the sagittal plane, you want to put your side against the wall (think *s* for "side" and "sagittal"). Now perform an exercise, such as a bicep curl. If what is moving (your forearm, in this example) can go through a normal range of motion and stay in contact with the plane, the exercise is in the sagittal plane. During the bicep curl exercise, the forearm stays in contact with the side of the wall. During the tricep push-down, leg extension, leg curl, sit-up, and hyperextension exercises—any movement that involves flexion or extension—you would stay in contact with the side of the wall. But you cannot do a lateral raise or bench press with your side up against the wall. Either you would have to bump yourself off the wall or, if you start with your hand against the wall, your hand would leave the wall as you perform the movement. Therefore, the lateral raise and bench press exercises are not performed in the sagittal plane.

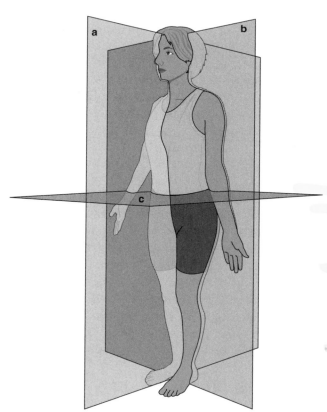

Figure 10.5 Illustration of the (a) sagittal plane, (b) frontal plane, and (c) transverse plane.

ABDUCTION

Abduction is movement away from the midline or away from anatomical position. Picture yourself back in that position with your side against the wall. If you were instructed to move your arms away from the wall, what would you do? Raise them out to the side. If you raise them out to the front, they would still be next to the wall. Remember that the midline runs forward and backward; moving your arms forward does not move you away from the midline; it keeps you next to it. If you abduct something, you take it away; for instance, when an alien abducts a person, they take the person away. Remembering this will help you remember the movement (19).

Not every joint is capable of abduction; notably, the elbow and the knee cannot abduct. The shoulder and hip are where abduction most commonly takes place. Abduction of the shoulder involves raising your arms out to the side. Abduction of the hip involves raising your leg out to the side. If you perform a jumping jack and stop when your arms and legs are out to the side, you are in an abducted position at the shoulder and hip. Another way to understand abduction is to think about moving away from anatomical position. In anatomical position, your limbs are next to your body. If you are going to abduct them, you will move them out to the side, away from anatomical position.

Note that after you begin a named movement, that movement has the same name throughout. One movement can't become another in the middle of the movement unless you pass through anatomical position during the movement. For example, as soon as you bend your elbow, you have flexed your elbow. Each time you bend it just a little more, that movement is still flexion. When you are in anatomical position and raise your arms out the side, you are abducting your shoulder. Abduction continues all the way through the range of motion, even after your arms have passed 90 degrees. Technically, the arms are returning to the midline after they pass 90 degrees, but changing the name makes no sense. The same muscle is working to create the same movement. When examining how the shoulder joint works (which is usually the hardest joint for most people to understand), thinking about where you are in relation to anatomical position is easier than visualizing the midline.

ADDUCTION

Movement toward the midline or movement toward anatomical position is called adduction. In anatomical position, your limbs are adducted. To perform adduction, first abduct the arms (or legs). From the stretched out, abducted position in the jumping jack, you produce adduction to return to anatomical position. When your leg is sticking out to the side and you bring it back to your body, that movement is adduction. Adduction is the opposite of abduction. Only joints that can abduct can also adduct (13).

As you can see, these two words differ by only one letter. When people are discussing these terms, they may spell out a-b-duction and a-d-duction to be extra clear about what movement they are referring to.

Abduction and adduction take place primarily in the frontal plane. To visualize the frontal plane, think of a wall again, but this time imagine that your front or back is against the wall before you phase yourself into the wall. The frontal plane is the wall itself, and it divides your body into front and back sections (figure 10.5b). Your whole face, pecs, abs, and quads are all on one side of the plane, and the back of your head, traps, lats, glutes, hamstrings, and calves are on the other side the plane. The frontal plane extends out to each side, theoretically continuing forever. Although it is not specifically stated, it is implied that if the term *abduction* or *adduction* is used by itself, vertical abduction or adduction is occurring, meaning that the movement is taking place in a vertical direction. This means that the movement is up and down. Performing jumping jacks or making snow angels is an example of regular abduction and adduction at the shoulder and hip (58).

The teaching trick for the frontal plane is similar to that used for the sagittal plane, but now you place your front or back against the wall. Perform the exercise or movement in question and see whether the part of the body that is moving is able to stay in contact with the wall. Now you can perform a lateral raise. A wide-grip lat pull-down, a pull-up, and a military press are all frontal plane exercises, because you can perform them while staying in contact with the plane. But if you try a bicep curl, a sit-up, or a bench press, none of those exercises work. For the bicep curl specifically, remember that the test is not whether you can keep your body up against the wall but whether the moving limb stays in contact with the wall. In this example, no, the forearm will move away from the wall as soon as you begin to curl if your back is on the wall, and if you are facing the wall, your hand will run into it right at the beginning of the movement.

HORIZONTAL ABDUCTION

Movement away from the midline, traveling parallel to the horizon, is horizontal abduction (figure 10.6). Visualize anatomical position. Now raise your arms out to the front, as if you were saying, "All rise." Now that your arms are sticking straight out in front of you, spread them to the side. This action is similar to a breaststroke in swimming (53).

What movement did you perform as you raised your arms forward? It may be confusing to determine, but it is shoulder flexion. They were at a 180-degree angle in anatomical position and now they are at a 90-degree angle (to your head). When your arms are sticking straight out, they are still next to the midline. In that position, to move away from the midline, you need to spread them out.

HORIZONTAL ADDUCTION

Movement toward the midline, traveling parallel to the horizon, is horizontal adduction. If you are in anatomical position and abduct your arms so that they are sticking out to the side, they are away from the midline. You want to return them to the midline and travel parallel to the horizon (visualize the ocean as the horizon; it goes side to side). Keep your arms high but bring them in front of you, as if you were clapping with your arms straight or hugging a tree. See figure 10.7 for a visual depiction of the movement (47, 49).

Horizontal abduction and adduction take place in the transverse plane, sometimes called the horizontal plane. We can't use a wall as our visual aid this time, but we can use a tabletop. Imagine that you are standing up with your hips next to a table, and you could meld yourself into the middle of the table. That tabletop represents the transverse plane. The transverse plane divides the body into top and bottom sections (figure 10.5c). The top part of your body is above the plane; the bottom part of your body is below the plane. If the part of your body that is moving would stay in contact with the tabletop (think *t* for "tabletop" and "transverse plane"), then that movement or exercise is in the transverse plane. For example, if you kneel down in front of a table and perform a bench press, you can simulate that motion and keep your upper arms against the tabletop; thus, a bench press is in the transverse plane, as is a 90-degree bent-over row, rear deltoid raise, and chest fly exercise. But exercises such as the shoulder press, bicep curl, sit-up, and lateral raise are not in the transverse plane (40).

The preceding are the six major movements of the body and the three planes in which those movements take place (table 10.1). If you put the planes next to each other, they make up real space (forward and backward, side to side, up and down) that we can move around in.

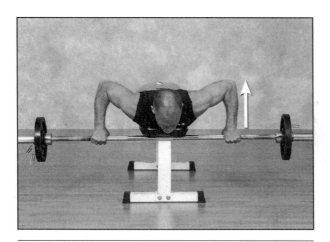

Figure 10.6 Illustration of shoulder horizontal abduction.

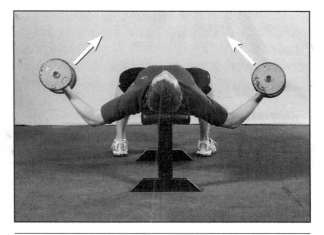

Figure 10.7 Illustration of shoulder horizontal adduction.

Table 10.1 Primary Movements and Their Planes

Movement	Plane
Flexion Extension	Sagittal
Abduction Adduction	Frontal
Horizontal abduction Horizontal adduction	Transverse (horizontal)

DETERMINING THE PRIMARY ANATOMICAL PLANE

When learning the planes, remembering two key points will help clear up a lot of confusion. The first is that the planes move with your body. Picture anatomical position and then picture the planes superimposed on that position—the sagittal plane going out to the front and back, the frontal plane going out to each side, and the transverse plane separating top from bottom. If you rotate your body (for example, by lying down on your back), the planes move with it. For example, standing and swinging your arms up and down out to the side would be movement in the frontal plane (just like the jumping jack example). Now, if you lie down on your back and perform the same movement (as in performing a snow angel), you are still in the frontal plane because the planes move with the body. Remember this idea as we think about which plane an exercise takes place in. For example, a chest press machine, a bench press, and a push-up (figure 10.8) all occur in the same plane (transverse) because the same movements occur in each exercise (horizontal adduction of the shoulder and elbow extension).

The second key point is that if two or more joints are moving in an exercise (a compound exercise), the movement at the primary joint determines the plane. For example, the movements occurring during a bench press are horizontal shoulder adduction and elbow extension. The horizontal movement is in the transverse plane, and the extension is supposed to be in the sagittal plane, but the exercise can't be in both planes. The primary joint in the bench press is the shoulder joint. That joint is used to determine the plane, so the plane for a bench press is transverse.

If you can't figure out what the primary joint is, determine which joint the primary mover (called the agonist) crosses. That joint is the primary joint. The pecs cross the shoulder joint. They are the agonist in a bench press, so the shoulder is the primary joint. In addition, the primary joint is the most proximal (close to the midline of the body) of the main joints involved. Most compound exercises involve movements at the shoulder and elbow or the hip and knee. In these cases, the shoulder and hip are proximal. Therefore, they are the primary joints, and the elbow and knee are the secondary joints.

ADDITIONAL MOVEMENTS

Besides the six major movements of the body, other movements are integral to sport and exercise activities and involve many of the same joints.

Internal Rotation

Rotation of the anterior aspect of a bone toward the center of the body is called internal rotation or medial rotation (figure 10.9). Rotation implies a swiveling motion in which the bone is rotating about its joint. This motion is separate and distinct from the six major movements of the body. The easiest way to visualize this movement is to bend (flex) your elbow so that your forearm is sticking out in front of you, as if you were in the halfway position of a bicep curl. Keep your upper arm by your side. Now, in that position, hit your belly with your

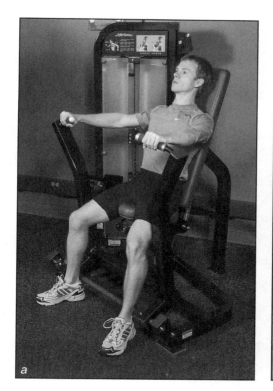

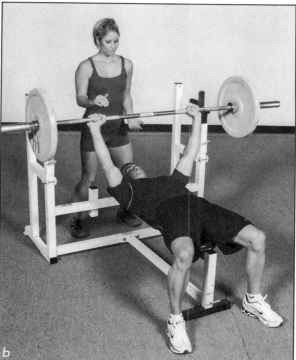

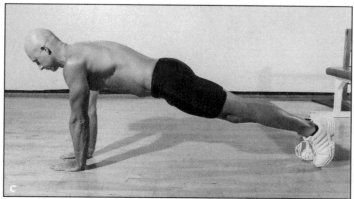

Figure 10.8 Three different chest exercises performed in the same plane: *(a)* chest press, *(b)* bench press, and *(c)* push-up.

hand. That motion is internal rotation that was caused by the humerus rotating and moving the lower arm. You can create this movement with your arm straight; it is just harder to see. When the winner drives the other person's arm down to the table in an arm wrestling competition, that movement is internal rotation.

External Rotation

The anterior aspect of the bone rotates away from the center of the body during external rotation or lateral rotation (figure 10.10), which is the opposite of internal rotation. Going back to the arm-wrestling example, the person winning is performing internal rotation, but the person losing is being forced into external rotation. Remember that external refers to something outside, so the movement is to the outside of the body. In racquet sports such as tennis, hitting a backhand shot involves external rotation. Rotation takes place mainly at the shoulder, hip, neck, and trunk. Several joints can't rotate or can perform it only

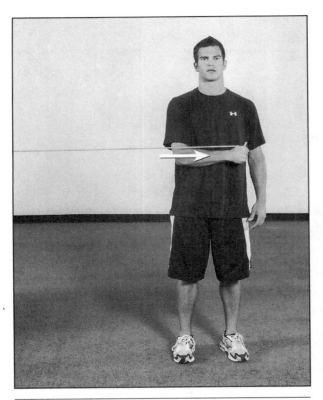

Figure 10.9 Illustration of shoulder internal rotation.

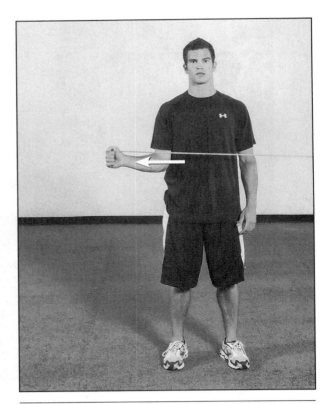

Figure 10.10 Illustration of shoulder external rotation.

minimally. Rotation normally takes place in the transverse plane.

Scapular Movements

Scapular movements can be performed only by the scapula (the shoulder blade). Remember that the scapula is a floating bone that lies on top of the rib cage but is not attached to it. It is attached to the clavicle and is only indirectly attached to the rest of the skeleton where the clavicle attaches to the sternum at the base of the neck, but it is not firmly anchored. The scapula thus has a lot of freedom to move in ways that other bones cannot. If you watch the back of a lean person in a tank top do a pull-up or the lat pull-down exercise, you will see that the scapula is capable of significant movement. See figure 10.11 for visual illustrations of the scapula-specific movements.

Elevation

Think of elevation like an elevator, something that lifts you up. To see elevation of the scapula,

shrug your shoulders as if you are saying, "I don't know." You are moving your scapula vertically, bringing your traps up to your ears. Elevation takes place in the frontal plane.

Depression

In anatomical position, your scapula is depressed. To see this movement, you must first raise the scapula. Shrug your shoulders and hold them there for a second. Now imagine using your muscles to pull the scapula back down, thereby making your neck extralong. That movement is depression of the scapula. Think of someone who is depressed; he or she is feeling down, and *depression* means "moving down." Depression is the opposite of elevation, and it also takes place in the frontal plane.

Protraction

The scapula moves forward along the ribs. If you were trying to touch your front delts to each other, you would have to roll the front of your shoulders together. That movement

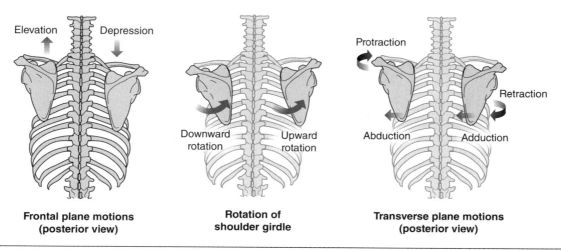

Elevation   Depression

Protraction

Retraction

Downward rotation   Upward rotation

Abduction   Adduction

Frontal plane motions (posterior view)

Rotation of shoulder girdle

Transverse plane motions (posterior view)

Figure 10.11   Illustration of the movements of the scapula.

is protraction. Someone who has bad posture with rounded shoulders might be permanently protracted. Protraction takes place in the transverse plane.

Retraction

The scapula moves through retraction when it moves backward along the ribs when you pull your shoulders back, as if you were trying to touch your shoulder blades together. Retraction is the opposite of protraction. Good resistance training form normally involves having the scapula retracted because this position helps keep the spine in a normal arch. When we sit for long periods, especially if we are driving, reading, or working at a computer, our shoulders tend to become protracted, but we should try to keep them a little retracted. Retraction takes place in the transverse plane.

Upward Rotation

During upward rotation, the scapula travels upward and the inferior angle (the bottom point) rotates outward at the same time. This movement occurs whenever you lift your arms over your head. If you perform a shoulder press, your scapula moves up but it also moves outward, which is upward rotation. Upward rotation takes place in the frontal plane.

Downward Rotation

Downward rotation involves the scapula traveling downward and the inferior angle of the scapula rotating inward at the same time. To see this, you first have to perform upward rotation. If you lift your arms over your head and then pull your arms back to your body, as in a lat pull-down, you are performing downward rotation. This movement is the opposite of upward rotation. Downward rotation takes place in the frontal plane.

Wrist-Specific Movements

The following two movements occur in the wrist but originate at the top of the forearm, near the elbow joint. The bone that makes up the elbow itself is the ulna, and this bone cannot rotate. Put your finger on your elbow and then move your wrist around. You will discover that your elbow doesn't move. But the other bone in the forearm, the radius (the bone on the thumb side in the forearm), is able to swivel back and forth. Put your finger on the radius and move and twist your wrist; you should feel that bone move. Figure 10.12 depicts pronation and supination, the two wrist-specific movements.

Pronation

When you rotate the wrist so that the palms face down, you are performing pronation. In anatomical position, if you pronated the palms they would face your back (i.e., you would see your palms from the back). When you type at your keyboard or perform the bench press exercise, your palms are pronated.

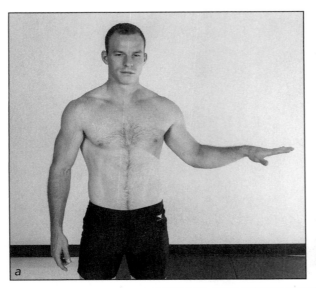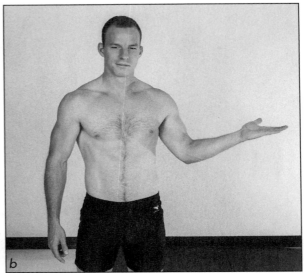

Figure 10.12 Illustration of *(a)* pronation (palm down) and *(b)* supination (palm up).

Supination

Supination involves rotating the wrist so that the palm faces up or forward. In anatomical position, your palms are supinated. When you perform a bicep curl or a chin-up, your palms are supinated. An easy way to remember this is that you "carry the soup supinated," meaning that you would carry a bowl of soup with your palms facing up. If you turned your palms down, you would spill the soup.

Ankle-Specific Movements

The ankle, like the wrist, performs unique movements. First, no extension of the ankle occurs. In anatomical position the ankle is in a neutral position; it is not extended as most joints are. A starting position is thus more subjective. Movements up and down are both described as flexion, just special cases of flexion. In addition, you can roll inward or outward on your ankle. See figure 10.13 for visual illustrations of the ankle-specific movements.

Dorsiflexion

Dorsiflexion involves lifting the end of your foot up (not just your toes). Examples of dorsiflexion are lifting your foot off the gas pedal in your car and lifting your foot up as if you are trying to scratch your knee with your big toe. You can remember that *dorsi* is a form of *dorsal*, which in this case means "up" or "back." You can remember that a shark's dorsal fin is the fin that you see cutting through the water. The dorsal fin points up, which is what your foot does when you dorsiflex it.

Plantar Flexion

When you are pointing the end of your foot down, your ankle is moving through plantar flexion. Examples of plantar flexion include stepping on the gas pedal in your car and pushing your foot down when you perform calf raises. If you are standing and do this movement, say to look for someone in a crowd, you would rise up on the balls of your feet. When you "plant" your feet, you perform this movement. In addition, you might remember that *p* means "point," as in to point your toes down. You can also remember that the bottom of your foot has plantar fascia, so plantar refers to going in that direction.

Inversion

Rolling your ankle to make the bottom of your foot point inward is inversion. If you did this with both feet, the soles of your shoes would face each other. Generally, this movement is more comfortable to perform than its opposite motion. Some people can sit or even stand with one or both feet inverted. When people sprain

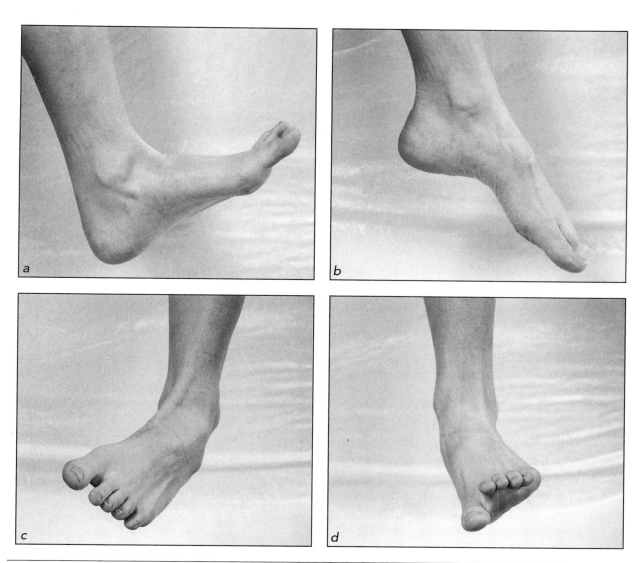

Figure 10.13 Illustration of the movements of the ankle joint: *(a)* dorsiflexion, *(b)* plantar flexion, *(c)* inversion, and *(d)* eversion.

an ankle, they have usually inverted the ankle beyond a normal range of motion.

Eversion

Eversion is rolling the ankle to make the bottom of the foot point outward. If you did this with both feet, the soles of your shoes would face away from each other. This position is less natural, and people rarely sit or stand with their feet heavily everted.

Circumduction

One additional movement has its own name, although it is a combination of several move-ments put together. Circumduction describes something moving in a circular motion. If you put your arms out to the side and then move them in circles, circumduction is occurring at the shoulder. But circumduction is really the six main movements performed together, so it is not considered a separate movement.

EXERCISES, MOVEMENTS, AND PLANES

The body contains hundreds of joints. Some are capable of significant movement, but many are not. Exercise and resistance training programs target only some of those joints. The following is a list of these main joints and their primary movements.

- Neck—The neck actually has several joints within it, but taken as a whole it functions as a ball-and-socket joint that is capable of the six major movements as well as rotation.
- Shoulder—The shoulder is the most flexible joint in the body. It is capable of the six major movements as well as rotation. It is a ball-and-socket joint (10).
- Elbow—The elbow is primarily a hinge joint, meaning that it can perform only flexion and extension.
- Wrist—The wrist can perform most movements, including flexion, extension, abduction, and adduction. The wrist can rotate (supinate and pronate), but that movement occurs because the radius swivels near the elbow. Hold your forearm and try to rotate your wrist; you will see that you cannot rotate it.
- Fingers—Fingers can flex, extend, abduct, and adduct.
- Trunk—The trunk is a series of joints in the vertebral column and hip that work together. Taken as a whole, the trunk functions as a ball-and-socket joint and is capable of the six main movements as well as rotation.
- Hip—The hip is the second most flexible joint in the body. It is less flexible, but more stable, than the shoulder joint. It is a ball-and-socket joint and it can do the six main movements as well as rotation.
- Knee—The knee is similar to the elbow in that it functions mainly as a hinge joint, so it performs flexion and extension. It can perform a little bit of rotation, but rarely is that motion targeted in the gym (2).
- Ankle—The ankle is like the wrist in that it can flex and extend, but those movements are called plantar flexion and dorsiflexion. It can also rotate, a movement that is initiated near the knee joint, and it can invert and evert.
- Toes—The toes can flex, extend, abduct, and adduct. Personal trainers rarely train this joint intentionally.

Why are the movements so important? Remember that muscles move the body. If you want to understand how muscles work, you need to know how the body moves. With this information and the information about muscles in the following chapters, you can look at any movement, break it down into its parts, and figure out whether a certain muscle is particularly important to that movement. This analysis will also solve any persistent questions about whether a muscle is working during an exercise. As a personal trainer, you may not end up telling your clients what specific movement they are performing (although some will be curious and will want to learn as much as possible), but you should still know what is happening. Your doctor may not tell you everything that is happening when he or she operates on you, but you certainly want your doctor to know about the subject in depth. The same applies to training.

Having a solid knowledge of the planes is beneficial for several reasons. If you can figure out what plane the exercise is taking place in, you have a good guess as to what movement is taking place. In addition, according to the principle of specificity, you want to train in the plane that you or your client plays or competes in. For example, sprinting is mainly flexion and extension in the sagittal plane, so most of a sprinter's training will take place in that plane. Tennis involves a lot of side-to-side movement, so tennis players want to make sure that some of their training is in the frontal plane, particularly for the lower body. And using a bat or a racquet involves a lot of twisting movements that happen in the transverse plane, so athletes who use that equipment need to train in that plane (16).

Some movements take place in more than one plane. The incline bench press exercise, for example, takes place between the frontal and transverse planes. A complex action like pitching a baseball occurs in all three planes. But resistance training exercises are generally performed in one plane. Listed here are five things to know about each exercise.

- Name of the exercise
- Agonist of the exercise
- Synergists of the exercise
- Movements of the exercise
- Plane of the exercise

First, know the name of the exercise. Second, know the agonist for the exercise. That muscle is the primary reason that you are performing the exercise. Third, know the important synergist for the exercise. What other muscles are helping the agonist? Fourth, know the movement of the exercise. This should confirm the agonist and synergist involvement. Finally, know the plane that the exercise takes place in. Although this item is last on the list, it is still important.

Table 10.2 contains common resistance training exercises classified by their name, movement, and anatomical plane. The agonist and synergists are not listed, but you should be able to determine them from movement anatomy. For a more complete list, consult appendix B.

LEVERS

The final piece in the puzzle that will help you develop a deeper understanding of human movement is having a basic grasp of how levers work. The body is a system of levers, and levers can be complicated. The goal here is to gain a basic understanding of levers and understand how modifying some properties of levers can affect how an exercise is performed. First, a few terms must be defined:

- Lever—a semirigid body that rotates when a force acts on it. In the body, this is a bone.
- Fulcrum—the pivot point of the lever system. In the body, this is a joint.
- Muscle force (mf)—the muscle generating the force producing the movement. In an exercise, this is the agonist, synergist, or both.

Table 10.2 Exercises, Movements, and Planes

Exercise	Movement	Plane
Bench press	Shoulder horizontal adduction Elbow extension	Transverse
Fly	Shoulder horizontal adduction	Transverse
Wide-grip lat pull-down	Shoulder adduction Elbow flexion	Frontal
Chin-up	Shoulder extension Elbow flexion	Sagittal
Pull-up	Shoulder adduction Elbow flexion	Frontal
Barbell shoulder (military) press	Shoulder abduction Elbow extension	Frontal
Lateral raise	Shoulder abduction	Frontal
Bicep curl	Elbow flexion	Sagittal
Tricep push-down	Elbow extension	Sagittal
Squat	Trunk extension Hip extension Knee extension	Sagittal
Leg press	Hip extension Knee extension	Sagittal
Leg extension	Knee extension	Sagittal
Leg curl	Knee flexion	Sagittal

- Resistance force (rf)—the resistance generating the force that the muscles are working against. In an exercise, this is commonly the weight being lifted, and the resistance force usually comes from gravity.
- Moment arm of the muscle force (mmf)—the perpendicular distance from the muscle (usually its insertion point) to the fulcrum.
- Moment arm of the resistance force (mrf)—the perpendicular distance from the resistance (usually its center of gravity) to the fulcrum.

A seesaw is a good example of a simple lever system because most people intuitively understand how it works. The lever is the seesaw itself, the long board that people sit on. The fulcrum is the midpoint of the seesaw at the top of the triangle or axis. A person sitting on the seesaw generates force from his or her body weight pushing the seesaw down (muscle force). If another person sits on the other end of the seesaw, that person works against the first person to generate resistance (resistance force). The distance of each person from the fulcrum affects the moment arm of the forces (4, 5). A seesaw is depicted in figure 10.14.

Most people know that if two people of equal weight sit on a seesaw at equal distance from the center (fulcrum), the seesaw will be balanced. When the moment arms are the same length, then it is just a matter of which force is stronger (muscle force versus resistance force). Most people also know that if one person moves significantly toward the center of the seesaw, that person will lose leverage, causing the seesaw to tip down toward the person who is sitting farther from the fulcrum. The force that has the longer moment arm has the advantage, and that advantage is often relatively significant. To calculate the difference, we can use simple math. If one person is 6 feet (183 cm) away from the fulcrum on a seesaw and another person is 3 feet (91 cm) away from the fulcrum, the person who is 3 feet away needs to weigh twice as much (because 6 is twice as much as 3) to balance the seesaw. Otherwise, the seesaw is going to tip toward the person who is 6 feet away, even if he or she is lighter.

Three Classes of Levers

There are three classes of levers, and they are determined by the location of the muscle force and resistance force in relation to the fulcrum, as well as the comparative length of the moment arms.

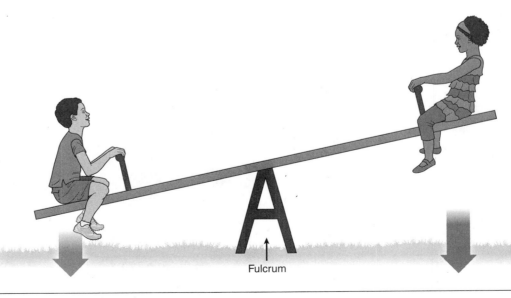

Figure 10.14 Seesaw: a basic lever system.

First-Class Lever

In this lever the muscle force and resistance force are on opposite sides of the fulcrum. The seesaw example is an illustration of a first-class lever (figure 10.15a). In the body the triceps and quads are generally considered first-class levers (32).

Second-Class Lever

In this type of lever the muscle force and the resistance force are on the same side of the fulcrum and the moment arm of the muscle force is longer than the moment arm of the resistance force (figure 10.15b). The setup creates mechanical advantage, which means that the amount of muscle force necessary to move the resistance can be less than the resistance force. Many tools that people use such as wheelbarrows and crowbars are second-class levers, but second-class levers are rare in the body. The heel raise exercise is an example of a second-class lever. Here a relatively small muscle is able to generate significant force. You can probably rise up on your toes using just one leg while standing. You just lifted your body weight for that exercise without a warm-up and likely without a struggle. What other muscle group in your body is capable of the same feat? Think of attempting to curl a dumbbell equal to your body weight with just one arm, and the challenge becomes more apparent. The calves can perform this movement not because of some magical property of that specific muscle but because they are a part of a second-class lever (57).

Third-Class Lever

In this type of lever the muscle force and resistance force are on the same side of the fulcrum and the moment arm of the resistance force is longer than the moment arm of the muscle force (figure 10.15c). This setup creates the opposite effect of a second-class lever; it creates mechanical disadvantage (21). Unfortunately for us, most muscles in the human body operate at a mechanical disadvantage. Exercises that isolate the deltoids, biceps, rectus abdominis, and hamstrings are examples of third-class levers. If, for example, your biceps inserts 2 inches (5 cm) from the elbow joint and you

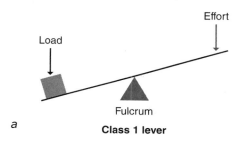

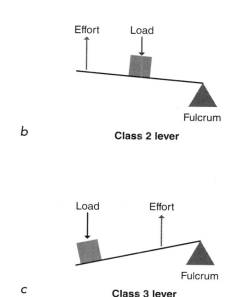

Figure 10.15   *(a)* First-class lever, *(b)* second-class lever, and *(c)* third-class lever.

are holding a 20-pound (9.1 kg) dumbbell 12 inches (30 cm) from the elbow, when the arm is curled to 90 degrees, the biceps would be generating 120 pounds (54.4 kg) of force (20). Your biceps don't seem so weak now, do they?

Role of Levers in Training Clients

By understanding these variables, you will be able to explain what is happening in the gym and manipulate them to provide clients with better workouts and better results.

The two key things to examine in an exercise are the length of the moment arm of both forces (muscle and resistance). Remember that the moment arm is determined by the perpendicular distance, not the total distance, to the fulcrum. This means that the moment arms of both the muscle and the resistance change during the range of motion. This concept is called the strength curve of an exercise, and it helps explain why during some exercises a certain portion of the range of motion can be easy and another portion can be much more challenging. When the moment arm of the resistance force is the longest, that part of the exercise is usually the hardest. The most challenging part of the range of motion of an exercise for a client is called the sticking point, which is where he or she is most likely to fail. The personal trainer should carefully watch and spot the client at all times, but particularly during the sticking point. The sticking point can vary during exercises because the moment arm of the resistance changes. It is in the middle of the range of motion for exercises such as the bicep curl, sit-up, and bench press; at the end of the range of motion for exercises like the lateral raise and the leg extension; and at the beginning of the concentric movement in exercises like the dumbbell pullover or ab wheel. Of course, removing the sticking point, which might occur when using partials or when cheating to use momentum to get through the sticking point, makes the exercise easier to perform.

A personal trainer has only some control over the variables in a lever system. The moment arm of the muscle force, for example, is determined by the insertion point of the muscle on the bone, and this is unchangeable (at least without surgery). But the moment arm of the resistance force is determined by where the resistance force is, and this is changeable. Shortening the moment arm of the resistance force to make the exercise easier is sometimes desirable. This may be done to help a client break through a plateau, to make the exercise safer, to use more weight and thus possibly stimulate the muscle fibers more, or perhaps to increase the performance of the exercise. This technique is most commonly applied to the use of dumbbells for the upper body. The moment arm of the resistance force can be shortened significantly by bending the elbows (up to 90 degrees) on exercises such as the lateral raise, rear deltoid raise, and chest

fly. This modified form is traditionally called a power form; a lateral raise performed in such a fashion would be labeled a power dumbbell lateral raise. Although this form is definitely easier, it should not be thought of as cheating or a waste of time because the primary muscle is going through the same range of motion as it does in the standard form. The muscle is simply able to lift more weight with this technique, and that method can be effective in increasing the size or strength of the muscle. If a client is unable to cross the minimal essential strain necessary to build the muscle one way, modifying the exercise to allow more weight to be lifted is appropriate (62).

At other times a personal trainer may want to make the exercise harder, not easier. Suppose that a client is in the middle of a set of the dumbbell fly exercise and the personal trainer realizes that the set is too easy. Instead of stopping the set or asking the client to perform a large number of reps, the personal trainer can ask the client to use a stricter version of the form by straightening the elbows (without locking them out). This modification makes the exercise harder because the weight is moved farther from the fulcrum.

Personal trainers often like the idea of making an exercise harder, but the real goal should be to make it more effective. Sometimes making it harder is a good idea. For example, push-ups on the toes are more effective than push-ups on the knees. But sometimes making an exercise easier is appropriate. The client is often able to lift more weight or ultimately get better results from the exercise. If a client cannot perform any push-ups at all on the toes, choosing the modified version might be wise. Performing a strict pull-up with full extension of the arms is often ideal, but if you wait until the person is capable of performing that exercise, you might end up waiting a long time, particularly with females. You may want to allow the client to use a modified version of the exercise, such as a partial range of motion pull-up that eliminates the sticking point, a kip involving some body English, or a chin-up to reduce the moment arm of the resistance, which allows the person to accomplish more work on the desired area.

This approach often gets the person to the desired form faster. Allowing clients to perform partial pull-ups for a while may help them reach that perfect strict pull-up quicker than requiring them to struggle with the strict pull-up all the time (24).

The final point to discuss when it comes to levers and moment arms is recognizing that people vary in their tendon insertion points, which can explain some of the differences seen in the world of performance. All humans have moderately similar insertion points. For example, the biceps inserts primarily on the bicipital tuberosity of the radius, which is a prominent bump on the radius usually about 2 inches (5 cm) from the elbow. But the bicipital tuberosity is not located in the same position for everyone. One person's bump might be 1 inch (2.5 cm) from the elbow, another person's might be 2 inches (5 cm), and yet another person's could be 3 inches (7.6 cm). Those different locations affect the moment arm of the muscle force and the subsequent force and strength generated by that muscle.

We might logically think that the ultimate goal is to have the moment arm of the muscle force as far from the fulcrum as possible, but that is not always the case. This issue highlights a difference between strength and speed. If the goal is pure strength as measured by maximal weight lifted, then the goal is to have the moment arm of the muscle force as long as possible. In the previous example, the person with an insertion point 3 inches (7.6 cm) from the fulcrum would have the advantage. This factor is not the only important one; length of forearm, size of muscle, neuromuscular coordination in the muscle, and stability of the involved joints would all affect the person's strength in this example. If the goal is pure speed, however, having the insertion point closer to the fulcrum is often more advantageous. This helps generate a longer range of motion, which helps focus on speed. Littler people demonstrate a good example of this contrast. Little people often have tendinous insertions that are advantageous for lifts such as the bench press, and they are often able to lift a tremendous amount of weight for their size (or sometimes for any size). But that same characteristic that is a benefit when it comes to strength production is a hindrance in speed production. When pitching a baseball or throwing a punch, a little person will not normally be able to generate the speed that a normal-sized person can. Some of that difference is a result of simple limb length, but some of it is because of the insertion points of the muscles.

This concept can help explain what we see in the sporting world. The strongest athlete in the gym is not always the best athlete in all sports. In sports such as football (particularly for some positions), strength is extremely important, but for other sports (tennis, golf, pitching in baseball), speed is much more important. A combination of the two will usually yield the best all-around performance.

CONCLUSION

The six primary movements of the body are flexion, extension, abduction, adduction, horizontal abduction, and horizontal adduction. There are also several special cases of movement. The three planes of movement are sagittal, frontal, and transverse. Personal trainers should be able to look at movements or exercises and identify the movements taking place and the plane in which the movement is occurring. They will then be able to identify the muscles working in a movement.

The body works as a series of levers that operate in conjunction with each other. Personal trainers should have familiarity with lever systems, including the lever, fulcrum, muscle force, resistance force, and moment arms for each force. First-class levers have force on either side of the fulcrum, as seen in a seesaw. Second-class levers create mechanical advantage, as exemplified by a wheelbarrow. Third-class levers, the most common type in the body, create mechanical disadvantage, as seen in a bicep curl. By understanding the lever system, personal trainers will understand why some exercises are harder than others, know how to manipulate an exercise to help a client get optimal results, and be able to explain why certain body types perform better at certain activities.

Study Questions

1. What movement is performed in a sit-up?
   a. trunk flexion
   b. trunk extension
   c. trunk abduction
   d. hip flexion

2. What movement is performed at the shoulder in a dumbbell row?
   a. shoulder flexion
   b. shoulder extension
   c. shoulder horizontal abduction
   d. shoulder horizontal adduction

3. What movement is performed at the shoulder in a dumbbell military press?
   a. shoulder abduction
   b. shoulder adduction
   c. shoulder horizontal abduction
   d. shoulder horizontal adduction

4. Which class of lever is a leg curl?
   a. first class
   b. second class
   c. third class

5. Why can a client lift more in a power dumbbell lateral raise than in a standard dumbbell lateral raise?
   a. The moment arm of the muscle force is doubled.
   b. The moment arm of the muscle force is shortened.
   c. The moment arm of the resistance force is lengthened.
   d. The moment arm of the resistance force is shortened.

Upper-Body Anatomy

Chapters 11 through 13 present one muscle at a time and describe the origin (where a muscle starts on the body, almost always a part of a bone), insertion (where a muscle ends on the body, also almost always a part of a bone), and primary action or actions (when the muscle is contracted concentrically). Some muscles cross and cause action at one joint (a single-joint muscle), whereas others cross two joints in the body and cause action at one or both joints (a two-joint muscle).

In this chapter we look at all the major muscles in the upper body. We review their origins and insertions, but our focus is on practical information that you can use to create more effective and efficient routines for your clients. Just understanding the anatomy of a muscle doesn't allow you to do that; you have to spend time training the muscle and learning how it responds to exercise.

Many muscle names have an abbreviated way that they are referred to or written. Common examples are pecs (pectoralis major or pectoralis minor), lats (latissimus dorsi), delts (deltoids), and traps (trapezius). The shortened version can also be written in singular form.

PECTORALIS MAJOR

The pec major is a large, fan-shaped muscle in the upper body (figure 11.1, *a* and *b*). No muscle is on top of this one, so it is a superficial muscle. When people are talking about their chests, they are talking about this muscle. This is a single-joint muscle.

- Origin—lateral sternum and medial half of the clavicle

- Insertion—lateral lip of the bicipital groove of the humerus
- Action
  - Overall—horizontal adduction, adduction (when internally rotated), internal rotation
  - Upper chest—flexion
  - Lower chest—extension from a flexed position

The pecs are known for their pushing motion, as performed in a push-up and the bench press. Almost all pressing motions and almost all flying motions work the pecs through horizontal adduction. This action is its most common. To train the pecs in regular adduction, you need to lean forward a little bit, internally rotate the humerus, and have the palms pointing down, such as in the cable crossover exercise. Leaning back and allowing the upper arm to rotate externally, which allows the arm to go well above 90 degrees (such as in the lat pull-down exercise), and then performing adduction, significantly decreases the involvement of the pecs.

In two other movements the pecs are involved but are of secondary importance. These are flexion and extension of the shoulder. The upper chest assists with flexion of the shoulder, such as in front raises. The lower pecs (figure 11.1*a*) assist with extension of the shoulder from a flexed position. The best example of this is a chin-up. As you lift yourself up, you are extending the shoulder. After your humerus is parallel to the ground, the pecs do not assist as much. For that reason, people often pull themselves almost halfway up on a chin-up and then fail. A pullover is

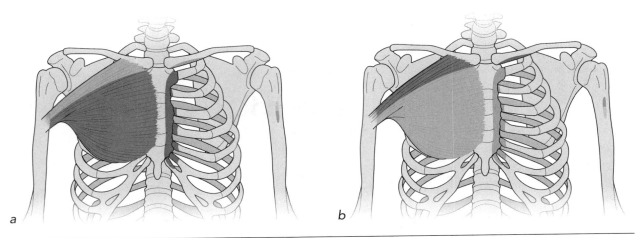

Figure 11.1 Illustrations of the *(a)* lower and *(b)* upper pectoralis major muscle.

another example of extension from a flexed position (2, 9).

The pec is divided into three main sections: upper, middle, and lower. The middle section is the largest, and it is targeted when your arms work at a 90-degree angle to your body, as in horizontal adduction. The upper chest is called the clavicular head of pec major (figure 11.1*b*) because it starts on the clavicle. This section of the muscle is worked when the exercise is performed on an incline, such as an incline press or incline dumbbell fly. You want your arms to extend at about a 45-degree angle to your body, or about eye level if you are standing. The lower chest is the smallest section of the pecs, and it is emphasized by performing decline actions. The hands should finish down low close to the hips to target this area of the pecs.

Clients can be confused about what part of the pec they are emphasizing during the chest fly or cable crossover exercise. Here is an easy way to remember it. If you are standing up relatively straight, where your hands are at the finish of the movement—up high, down low, or in the middle—is the part of the chest that you are working. If you start with your hands out by your side and bring them up across your chest to about chin height, you are working your upper chest. If you start with your arms high and end with them low in front of your waist, you are working your lower chest.

The front deltoid usually works with the pecs; it is hard to work the pecs without using the front delt. The wider your grip is, the more stress you place on the shoulder joint. If your shoulders are sensitive, try a narrower grip. Do not lift heavy weights with an extrawide grip until you are used to that movement, and even then use caution (26).

In some people, particularly males who overemphasize the bench press or people who sit at a desk and type on a keyboard all day, the pecs tend to get tight. Such people need to stretch this muscle so that they don't lose flexibility. Stretches such as a wall or floor glide, shoulder dislocations, and the open book stretch are good stretches for the pecs (68).

When training the chest, using proper form is important. Key points include touching the chest and using a full range of motion; stopping short of the chest significantly reduces its involvement during a press. For maximal strength and shoulder health, another important point is to tuck the humerus slightly when pressing; a good angle to aim for is a 45- to 60-degree angle between the humerus and the body (a 90-degree angle would have the humerus sticking straight out to the side).

You need to follow some simple guidelines when lining up machines or free weights to make sure that everything is set up correctly for your clients. For the incline bench press exercise, you want the bar or the handles to line up just below the start of the clavicle. As stated, the incline bench press targets the upper chest, so you are lining up the machine with the part of the chest that you are hitting. When a client is performing the decline bench press exercise, the handles or the bar should line up with the lower chest. This is below nipple level, right at the bottom of the sternum. Many people go too high when performing the decline bench press; the lower the bar is, the better the result will be, assuming that the bar is not on the abdomen. Finally, when you are using a regular (flat bench) bench press to target the middle chest, the machine or the bar should line up with the midchest, which is normally the nipple line. This is where the bar should touch on a bench press. Females generally touch the highest point on the chest when they lie down (highest means the part of the chest that is the farthest from the floor, not up toward the chin) (91).

When the chest is working, several synergist muscles work with it. The front deltoids usually work with the chest, and in any press the front deltoids are receiving a lot of stimulus. In compound exercises the triceps work with the chest. Depending on the exercise, the lats can also work with the pecs. In isolation exercises such as flies, the biceps can work with the pecs. The chest is not significantly involved in the shoulder press exercise in which the bar goes straight over the shoulders.

Exercises for the Pectoralis Major

- Bench press
- Incline and decline press
- Fly
- Machine press
- Push-up

PECTORALIS MINOR

The pec minor is a small muscle that sits deep under the pec major (figure 11.2). This muscle is not visible superficially. The insertion of pec major and the insertion of pec minor are on different bones, so the two muscles have little relationship with each other. They are so named because they have a similar location, but the two muscles do not really work together.

- Origin—anterior surface of ribs 3, 4, 5
- Insertion—coracoid process of the scapula

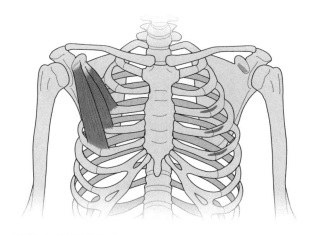

Figure 11.2 Illustration of the pectoralis minor muscle.

- Action—protraction, depression, and downward rotation of the scapula

Most people do not perform specific exercises for the pec minor. Maintaining flexibility in this muscle is important because tightness will contribute to rounded shoulders. Sometimes the pec minor is recruited when it should not be that active. One of the most common instances when this happens is during a pressing motion. When you press, the shoulder blades should stay retracted the whole time; do not roll your shoulders forward at the end of the press. Rolling your shoulders recruits the pec minor. When you perform a lat pull-down, if you round your shoulders at the end of the movement, you are recruiting the pec minor. You want to lift your chest and pinch your shoulder blades together to leave the pec minor out of the movement. If you are rounding your shoulders, try leaning back a little more, another 10 degrees or so, and lift your chest. You can fix this problem in a few weeks, and ultimately you will be able to lift a lot more weight that way (63).

Exercises for the Pectoralis Minor

- Protraction
- Push away

SERRATUS ANTERIOR

The serratus anterior is a medium-sized muscle that covers most of the ribs (figure 11.3). It is

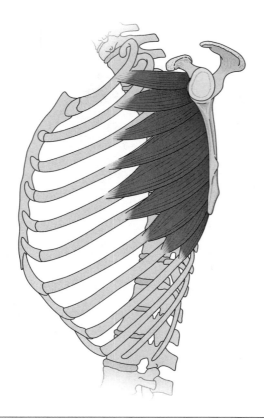

Figure 11.3 Illustration of the serratus anterior muscle.

under several muscles, mainly the pec major, although part of this muscle is visible in most people. If you raise your arm and look about 5 or 6 inches (12.7 or 15 cm) below your armpit, you might see some ridges that most people mistake for ribs. If you are lean, you will probably see them. Or touch that area and you will be able to feel them. The *serratus* part of the name comes from the fact that the muscle has many fingers that look serrated, like a knife, and *anterior* means "anterior part of the scapule." This muscle looks like four or five ribs, but it is really a muscle.

- Origin—upper eight ribs
- Insertion—anterior surface of scapula (vertebral border)
- Action—protraction, slight upward rotation, and stabilization of scapula

This muscle starts on the ribs and goes backward to latch on to the front of the scapula. You can't see this at all. The muscle pulls the scapula forward, so it works with the pec minor to produce protraction. As mentioned earlier, this movement is not commonly performed in the gym. The main function of this muscle is to stabilize the scapula, and it generally gets adequate stimulus during normal exercises for the chest, back, and shoulders. But if it or the pec minor is weak or injured, training it directly may be necessary (15). A possible sign of a weak serratus anterior is a winged scapula whereby the scapula sticks out in the back in anatomical position.

Exercises for the Serratus Anterior

- Protraction
- Push away
- Pullover if finished in a protracted position
- Serratus cable pullover

LATISSIMUS DORSI

The latissimus dorsi is a broad, strong muscle in the middle back (figure 11.4). The word *dorsi* means "dorsal," or "relating to the back," like a dorsal fin. Sometimes the lats operate opposite, antagonistic, to the pecs, and sometimes they work with the pecs. The lats are a pulling muscle, meaning that they help to pull the arm back to the body.

- Origin
  - Thoracolumbar aponeurosis
  - Lower six thoracic spinous processes
  - Sacrum and iliac crest
  - Lower three or four ribs
  - Inferior angle of the scapula
- Insertion—bicipital groove of the humerus
- Action
  - Overall—extension, adduction (when externally rotated), horizontal abduction, internal rotation of the humerus
  - Special case—flex the humerus when in an extended position

The lats produce many actions, five specifically. Not coincidentally, the pecs are respon-

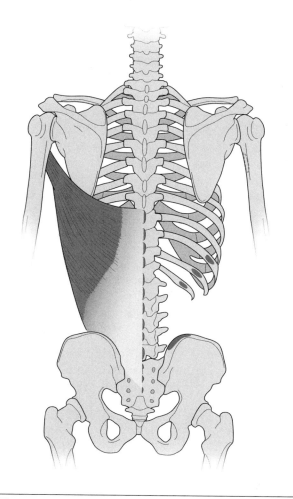

Figure 11.4 Illustration of the latissimus dorsi muscle.

sible for five movements. The lats perform extension of the shoulder, specifically pulling the arm back to the body from an extended position while keeping the elbows at the side. This action is performed in most close-grip rows and chin-ups. The lats perform adduction, pulling the arms back into anatomical position. The best example of this is a wide-grip lat pull-down. The lats work best when the body is leaning slightly back, the arms are pointing straight up or close to it, and the humerus is externally rotated. Remember that the pecs perform adduction when the humerus is internally rotated. The lats perform horizontal abduction in rows using a wide grip with the elbows flared out to the side. In addition, the breaststroke in swimming is an example of horizontal abduction powered mainly by the

lats. The lats perform internal rotation. They perform this movement because the lats come around the inside of the arm and insert on the front of the humerus. If the lats went around to the outside of the humerus, they would produce external rotation. If that were the case, when you put your arm out to the side, you literally would have wings and your body would look quite different. So if you remember that they attach on the inside of the arm, it makes sense that they rotate the humerus internally (42).

The last action for the lats is a special case. Most people are unaware of this action, but it is important. As previously mentioned, the lats insert on the front of the arm, right at the top of the biceps, not the back of the arm, as most people think. Therefore, after your arm is next to your body, the lats will stop pulling it into the body, because in that position, the insertion of the muscle is behind the origin. So if you pull your arm as far back as you can go, the front of your humerus is behind your body. If you contract the lats in this position, they function to pull the arm forward a few inches but cease to contribute to that motion after the insertion is past the origin. This action is the opposite of the pecs' production of extension in a flexed position. When a client is performing a bench press, the lats are crucial in the beginning of the lift. Similarly, when a person throws an uppercut punch, the lats initiate the movement (which is part of the reason that boxers have extremely strong lats) (78).

Exercises for the Latissimus Dorsi

- Pull-up and chin-up
- Bent-over barbell row (45 or 90 degree)
- Dumbbell row (one or two arm)
- Lat pull-down
- Cable row
- Inverted row
- Pullover machine
- Straight-arm lat pull-down

Table 11.1 shows a comparison of the actions of the lats and the pecs, along with an exercise example.

Table 11.1 Comparison of the Pectoralis Major and Latissimus Dorsi Muscle Movements and Related Exercises

Movement	Pecs	Lats	Exercise
Extension*	Slight involvement	Heavy involvement	Cable row
Flexion*	Heavy involvement	Slight involvement	Close-grip bench press
Horizontal adduction	Heavy involvement	Very slight involvement	Chest press
Horizontal abduction	No involvement	Heavy involvement	Wide cable row
Adduction (externally rotated)	Slight involvement	Heavy involvement	Pull-up
Adduction (internally rotated)	Heavy involvement	Slight involvement	Cable crossover
Internal rotation	Heavy involvement	Heavy involvement	Arm wrestling
External rotation	No involvement	No involvement	Backhand in tennis

*Remember that at the end of these movements, the special cases kick in. These are minimal for the cable row because the arm is not high enough (unlike in a chin-up) but are somewhat significant in a close-grip bench press because of the angle of the humerus in the bottom position.

TERES MAJOR

The teres major is a small muscle that sits directly superior to the lats (figure 11.5). Both the lats and the teres major are superficial, meaning that nothing but skin is on top of them.

- Origin—inferior angle of the scapula
- Insertion—medial lip of the bicipital groove of the humerus

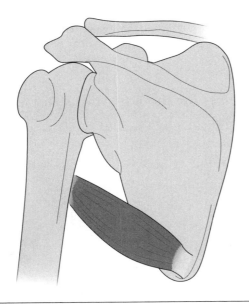

Figure 11.5 Illustration of the teres major muscle.

- Action
  - Overall—extension, adduction when externally rotated, horizontal abduction, medial rotation of the humerus
  - Special case—flexion in an extended position

The teres major and the lats work together. Note that the five actions of the teres major and the five actions of the lats are the same. They have a synergistic relationship, and the lats produce the most force. Separating the lats and the teres major in an exercise is almost impossible. If you were to reach around your body and scratch your back, you would be scratching some of your teres major. Just like the lats, the teres major goes from the back to the inside of the arm to attach at the front of the upper arm. The insertion for pec major, lats, and teres major are all right next to each other. The pec's insertion covers up the other two, and the front delts also cover it up somewhat. The teres major is called major because it is big compared with the teres minor, although it is small compared with the lats. To keep it simple, whenever you are working the lats, you are working the teres major. Using a wider grip with lat exercises emphasizes the teres major (63).

Exercises for the Teres Major

- Pull-up
- Wide-grip lat pull-down

- V-grip lat pull-down
- Pronated one-arm dumbbell row

RHOMBOIDS

The rhomboids are a deep muscle in the upper back that sit right between the shoulder blades (figure 11.6). They are targeted during most back exercises. The two rhomboids, major and minor, are right next to each other and are basically inseparable when it comes to training, so the rhomboids are considered one muscle for our purposes.

- Origin—spinous processes of C7–T5
- Insertion—vertebral border of the scapula
- Action—retraction, downward rotation of scapula

The rhomboids start at the seventh cervical vertebrae (C7), which is the lowest of the cervical vertebrae, the vertebrae in your neck. C7 is the easiest one to feel. If you feel the back of your neck, you'll find a bony knob right at the base of your neck where the top of a T-shirt might be. That is C7. The rhomboids run down five more vertebrae. Because each vertebra is about 1 inch (2.5 cm) high, this muscle is about 6 inches (15 cm) wide. It is higher up than most people realize. When you perform squats, the bar is normally sitting on your

rhomboids. The rhomboids then angle down at about a 45-degree angle and attach to the vertebral border of the scapula. The vertebral border is the side of the scapula that is closest to the spine (vertebral column). The rhomboids are completely hidden from view because they are underneath the traps. The rhomboids look like a square on a diagonal slant, which amazingly is called a rhomboid.

Note that the lats begin almost where the rhomboids leave off, at the seventh thoracic vertebrae (T7), which is right about where a bra strap or a heart rate monitor strap would be.

The rhomboids produce retraction; they pull the shoulders back. In good lifting posture, the shoulders are in a retracted position, and the end point of almost all back exercises involves retraction. In addition, the rhomboids produce downward rotation of the scapula. This action occurs when the arms are up over your head and you pull them back to your body, as in a lat pull-down or a pull-up. Because you are retracted during any rowing motion exercise or pull-down, the rhomboids generally work with the lats. The rhomboids do not insert on the humerus, so they do not perform movements like internal rotation. In most back exercises, separating the rhomboids and the lats is difficult. The lats are normally the agonist because they are large and strong, and the rhomboids are a synergist, much like the teres major (79).

Exercises for the Rhomboids

- Pull-up
- Wide-grip lat pull-down
- Bent-over barbell row (45 or 90 degree)
- Cable row (wide or V-grip)
- Inverted row
- Retraction

TRAPEZIUS

The traps are a large, superficial muscle in the upper back (figure 11.7, *a–c*). When well developed, they make a person's neck look thick, but they are not properly called the neck muscles. The traps are the second largest muscle in the back after the lats. The traps are normally separated into three parts: the upper

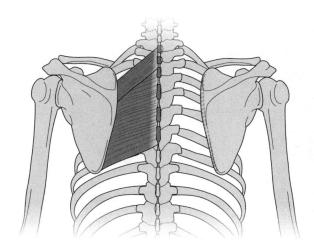

Figure 11.6 Illustration of the rhomboids muscle.

(figure 11.7*a*), the middle (figure 11.7*b*), and the lower (figure 11.7*c*). This distinction is fabricated because clear lines do not divide those sections of muscle.

- Origin
  - Upper—occipital bone and ligamentum nuchae
  - Middle—C7–T3 spinous processes
  - Lower—T4–T12 spinous processes
- Insertion
  - Upper—lateral third of clavicle, acromion process of scapula
  - Middle—spine of the scapula
  - Lower—root of the spine of the scapula
- Action
  - Upper—elevation, upward rotation of the scapula
  - Middle—retraction of the scapula
  - Lower—depression, upward rotation of the scapula

The traps have a broad origin. The occipital bone is the bone that makes up the bony knob on the back of your head; you can normally see this on a person who has a shaved head. The ligamentum nuchae is a fancy name for a ligament in your neck that covers up the spinous processes of C1 through C6. So the traps really start on the occipital bone and then go from the first spinous process all the way down to the bottom of the ribs, probably about 6 inches (15 cm) higher than the waistline. Part of the traps originate above the insertion, and part originate below the insertion. For that reason, the traps have many actions.

The upper traps are the most visible section of the traps and receive the most attention in the gym. They are also the strongest part of the muscle. Their function is to elevate the scapula, as when performing shrugs. They also help the scapula perform upward rotation, but that is not a major action. When you perform a lateral raise, you should try to relax your traps and not involve them too much. You should not actively shrug your shoulders when you perform a lateral raise. The upper traps do not really work with any other major muscle when they perform elevation, so a separate exercise for this area is often included in a workout program.

The middle traps have fibers that run parallel to the ground. They start in the middle of the upper back and go to the spine of the

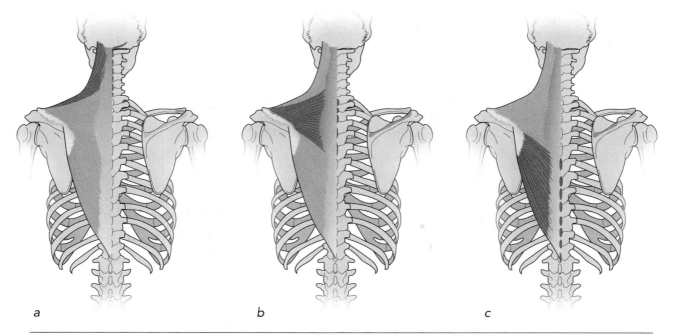

a   b   c

Figure 11.7 *(a)* Upper, *(b)* middle, and *(c)* lower trapezius.

scapula, which is that ridge of bone that you can feel when you reach back and feel your shoulder blade. They produce retraction, but they are usually not specifically trained. They contribute to many other exercises, namely back exercises. The middle traps work with the rhomboids (10).

The lower traps have fibers that run at an upward angle. They start in the middle and lower section of the back and then run up to the scapula, specifically the root of the spine of the scapula. The root of the spine of the scapula is where the spine of the scapula begins. This part of the trap performs depression, which is lowering of the shoulder blades. This action is not commonly trained in the gym, but it receives some stimulus during most exercises, particularly back exercises such as the lat pull-down and pull-up. When you perform those exercises, you want to keep your shoulders depressed for at least most of the range of motion. The lower traps also produce upward rotation, such as when you press something over your head. They work with the upper traps in that action.

The traps are one of just a few muscles in which one part of the muscle is the antagonist to another part of the same muscle. The upper trap is often the antagonist to the lower trap. Therefore, finding one exercise that hits all the traps at once is difficult. The serratus anterior and the pec minor are the antagonist to the middle traps and the rhomboids.

Although shrugs are the most common exercise for the traps, the deadlift exercise is also an excellent and underused exercise for this muscle. The traps are not normally a prime mover, but they are a stabilizer in most actions and a holder when carrying something. Isometric contractions of the traps are normal in everyday life, in actions such as carrying suitcases while walking. The deadlift is an example of an isometric contraction of the traps because the traps keep the upper body in position as you perform the deadlift. The large amount of weight used in the deadlift produces a lot of stimulus on the traps.

Exercises for the Trapezius

- Barbell shrug—upper
- Dumbbell shrug—upper
- Trap bar shrug—upper
- Farmer's walk—upper
- Retraction—middle
- Depression—lower

DELTOIDS

The delts are the shoulder muscles (figure 11.8, a–c). They are the superficial muscles that cap the shoulder joint. Some part of the deltoid is involved in almost every upper-body exercise. For aesthetics and performance, the delts should be relatively evenly developed; one part should not be much larger and stronger than another. The delts are broken up into three sections: the anterior deltoid (front; figure 11.8a), the medial deltoid (middle; figure 11.8b), and the posterior deltoid (rear; figure 11.8c).

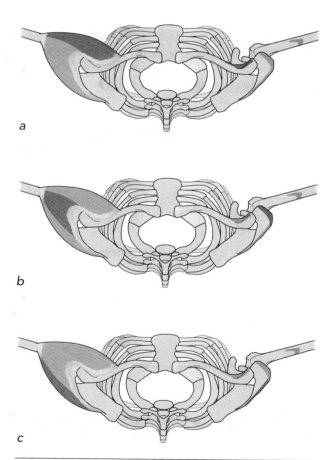

a

b

c

Figure 11.8 (a) Anterior deltoid, (b) medial deltoid, and (c) posterior deltoid.

- Origin
  - Anterior—lateral third of clavicle
  - Middle—lateral acromion process of the scapula
  - Posterior—spine of the scapula
- Insertion—deltoid tuberosity of the humerus
- Action
  - Front delt—flexion, horizontal adduction, abduction (when externally rotated), internal rotation of humerus; special case—adduction (when internally rotated)
  - Middle delt—abduction of humerus
  - Rear delt—extension, horizontal abduction, adduction (when externally rotated), external rotation of humerus

The delts, like the traps, are unusual in that one part of the delts is the opposite of another part. The front and rear deltoids have an antagonistic relationship. The middle delt is kind of out there by itself; its opposites are the pecs and the lats for most actions. Looking at the individual sections of the delts is the best way to understand them (9).

The front delt is the strongest part of the deltoid. It is involved in any pressing motion, either pressing your arms out in front of you or up over your head. It is also involved in raising your arms straight out in front of you. To keep the stimulus mainly on the front delts and to go easy on your shoulders when performing front raises, use a neutral grip the whole time. Using a pronated grip places more stress on the shoulder joint and a slightly greater emphasis on the middle delt. The front delt is usually working when the pecs are working; they are closely related. Performing inclines shifts even more emphasis to the front delt. In addition, bench pressing with the elbows out (not recommended) puts more emphasis on the shoulders (19).

The middle delt is one of the few muscles to produce abduction of the shoulder. Hitting the middle delt without using some sort of lateral raise is hard. When performing lateral raises, raise your arm until your elbow is level with your shoulder; going higher can place unnecessary stress on the shoulder joint. The middle delt is a synergist in a shoulder press, and the front delt is the agonist. Some people like the idea of training the middle delt to make their shoulders look wider, which in turn makes the waist look smaller, adding to the V-taper that is often desired. Shoulder pads in a suit provide the same effect (7, 9).

The rear delt is the part of the delt that is most often neglected. Few exercises target the rear delt, and you can't see it looking in the mirror as you can your front or middle delt. The rear delt does receive some stimulus when you train your lats, but generally you should target it with a specific exercise. When training your back, the rear delts are most emphasized by having a wide grip and keeping your elbows up as opposed to tucking them in next to your body. You will be weaker in this position, but it will hit your upper back more effectively.

One important note: Performing the behind-the-neck military (shoulder) press does not effectively target the rear delts. The front delts are still the agonist in that exercise, and the rear delts are not that heavily involved. Additionally, this exercise is not recommended because it places high stress on the shoulder joint. Instead, perform the shoulder press exercise with the bar moving in front of the face.

When training the delts with free weights, use this simple way to identify which delt is working. Whichever delt is facing the ceiling when you are lifting is the delt that is receiving the most stimulus. A bench press is mainly front delts, a lateral raise is middle delts, a shoulder press is front delts (your middle delts are facing backward, and your rear delts are facing down), and a rear delt raise obviously targets your rear delts (48).

When performing the isolation movements for the delts, weight can often be a limiting factor. Many people reach a plateau of 12, 15, or 20 pounds (5.4, 6.8, or 9.1 kg) on most of the raises and can't go much higher. If your goal is bigger or stronger delts, this plateau will limit your results. Using power form for the isolation exercises, which is bending your arms up to 90 degrees, is acceptable and sometimes desirable. This technique works particularly well with the lateral and rear delt raises. You can use much heavier weight, often double what you were using before, and still put a lot of stimulus on the delts. As you get stronger, slowly straighten your arms. Over time you can become stricter with your form. This approach is an effective way to add size and strength to the delts and to overcome a plateau in that area (39, 44).

Exercises for the Deltoids

- Barbell shoulder press—anterior
- Dumbbell shoulder press—anterior
- Handstand push-up—anterior
- Front raise—anterior
- Dumbbell lateral raise—middle
- Power lateral raise—middle
- Leaning lateral raise—middle
- Dumbbell rear delt raise—posterior
- Power dumbbell rear delt raise—posterior
- Rear delt machine—posterior

ELBOW FLEXORS

Three main muscles flex the elbow: the biceps brachii, brachialis, and brachioradialis. Each of these important muscles can be targeted using specific exercises. Most people just refer to them as the biceps, but that label is an over-simplification.

Biceps Brachii

The biceps is a prominent muscle on the anterior part of the upper arm (figure 11.9). It is called biceps brachii because it has two heads (*bi* means "two") and because *brachii* means "upper arm" in Latin, so together the name means "two-headed muscle of the upper arm." The biceps is a two-joint muscle, and this has interesting ramifications for training it.

- Origin
  - Long head—supraglenoid tubercle of the scapula
  - Short head—coracoid process of the scapula
- Insertion
  - Bicipital tuberosity of the radius

- Bicipital aponeurosis (goes to both radius and ulna)
- Action
  - Flex the elbow
  - Supinate the forearm
  - *Long head →* Assists in flexion of the shoulder

The biceps helps to flex the elbow and to twist (supinate) the forearm so that the palm is facing up. The biceps receives the greatest stimulation when the palm is facing up during a curl or when you twist on the way up, so the palm should be fully facing up by the halfway point. In addition, keeping the palm up on the way down during the exercise maintains tension on the biceps.

The biceps has two heads, and some people try to target one more than the other. You can place more emphasis on one head or the other depending on your grip. If you take a wide grip,

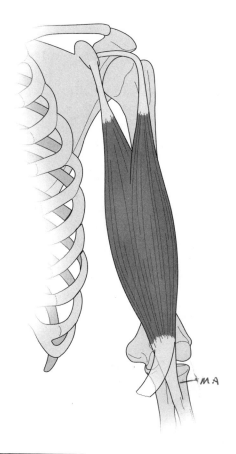

Figure 11.9 Illustration of the biceps brachii muscle.

wider than shoulder-width, you will emphasize the short head, which is the inner head (the one next to your pecs). A close grip, narrower than shoulder-width, will place more emphasis on the long head (the outer head). Most clients, however, should just take a grip that suits them and where they are the strongest and mainly use that one. Lifting an extra 20 to 30 pounds (9.1 to 13.6 kg) is more beneficial than using a grip that feels awkward just to try to hit one head a little more than the other (12).

Many people want to know a specific exercise to help build the peak of their biceps. The peak of the biceps comes from the development of the long head of the biceps. No exercises will train just the peak, but you can perform exercises to emphasize the long head. Narrow-grip supinated curls, straight-bar curls (preferably strict or on a preacher bench), perfect curls, cross-body supinated curls, and double dumbbell curls are all good at hitting the long head. In addition, if you want to focus on the peak, you want to work primarily the biceps, not the other elbow flexors, so choose exercises in which your palms are up and be strict with that position.

As mentioned before, the biceps is a two-joint muscle. It starts on the shoulder and goes down past the elbow. Although it fully covers the humerus, it doesn't originate or insert on that bone. The main action of the biceps is at the elbow, but it also helps to flex the shoulder. Remember, however, that the front delt is the main muscle that flexes the humerus. Some people have misinterpreted this information and exaggerate shoulder flexion while they are performing curls. That technique is incorrect. What this information means is that the elbow naturally moves forward a little bit when you are doing a curl, somewhere between 3 and 6 inches (7.6 and 15 cm) for most people, or up to 45 degrees. But if you end with your elbow up around shoulder height, you have performed the exercise incorrectly. You usually do not want to restrict elbow movement totally either, because doing that will unnecessarily limit the power of the biceps.

Because the biceps is a two-joint muscle, the position of the muscle at one joint (the shoulder) can affect the power of the muscle at the other joint (the elbow). Your biceps is in the strongest position when your upper arm is by your side or it has moved forward somewhat. If your upper arm is at 0 degrees when it is by your side (anatomical position) and at 90 degrees when your elbow is even with your shoulder, it would be the strongest somewhere between 0 and 35 degrees. If your elbow moves far forward, past 90 degrees, the biceps becomes weaker and cannot contract as forcefully (61).

An example of this is the seated cable curl exercise in which you keep your arms out in front of you and curl to your face. In addition, if you stretch your upper arm past 0 degrees, moving it behind your body, the biceps will be weaker. The incline dumbbell curl exercise is an example of this weaker position. Training in those weaker positions is not necessarily bad, but you want to spend more time training in the strong position, using exercises such as the standing EZ-bar curl or the dumbbell curl.

Exercise for the Biceps Brachii

- EZ-bar curl
- Power curl
- EZ-bar preacher curl
- Strict curl
- Supinated dumbbell curl
- Supinated cross-body dumbbell curl

Brachialis

The brachialis sits underneath the biceps (figure 11.10). It is hard to see unless you know what you are looking for; it pokes out underneath each side of the biceps and is easier to see on the lateral aspect of the upper arm. Although most clients will not have heard of this muscle, it plays an important role in flexing the elbow.

- Origin—lower half of anterior shaft of the humerus
- Insertion—coronoid process and tuberosity of the ulna
- Action—flexes the elbow

Compared with the biceps, the brachialis is a straightforward muscle. It starts on the humerus, goes to the ulna (note that it is the

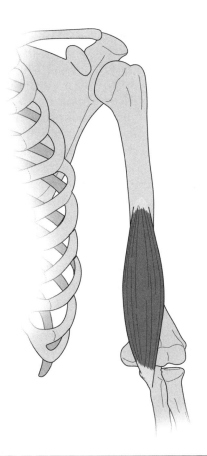

Figure 11.10 Illustration of the brachialis muscle.

brachialis is quite strong and can contribute to the overall strength of your arm. In addition, if you look at your biceps when they are relaxed and then push them up with your other hand, they look much larger. Training the brachialis can have this effect to some degree. Because the brachialis sits under the biceps, as it gets bigger it pushes the biceps up, making them look bigger. In this way, the brachialis adds to the size and aesthetics of the overall arm.

Exercises for the Brachialis

- Dumbbell hammer curl
- Parallel bar curl
- Cross-body neutral grip curl

Brachioradialis

The brachioradialis is the last main elbow flexor (figure 11.11). Although it is the smallest and weakest of the three, it is still important. It

only main elbow flexor to go to the ulna), and bends the elbow. Some books note that the brachialis is the strongest elbow flexor, even stronger than the biceps. That statement may be correct, but the biceps shows a greater ability to hypertrophy, and in well-trained people the biceps may become stronger than the brachialis.

The brachialis muscle is always working when you bend your elbow. Because it inserts on the ulna, you can't deactivate it the way you can the biceps by using different hand positions. To place the most stimuli on the brachialis, you should perform curls in a neutral position (also called the hammer position), which means curling with the thumbs up the whole time. Really, the way that you emphasize this muscle is by altering the emphasis on its neighbors, the biceps and the brachioradialis.

Although isolating the brachialis is difficult, you still need to train it. As mentioned, the

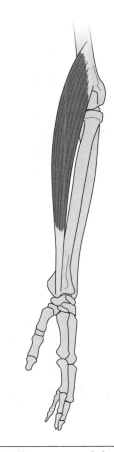

Figure 11.11 Illustration of the brachioradialis muscle.

contributes more to the size and shape of the forearm than it does to the size and shape of the upper arm.

- Origin—lateral supracondylar ridge of the humerus
- Insertion—styloid process of the radius
- Action—flex the elbow with hand neutral or pronated

The brachioradialis is so named because it starts on the brachium (upper arm) and ends on the radius. This long muscle runs the entire length of the forearm. You can find the origin if you feel for it. Start by crossing your right arm across your belly. Touch your elbow with your left hand. Now go up (toward the ceiling) about 1 inch (2.5 cm) and press in; you should find a bumpy part of the bone. That is the epicondyle of the humerus. The brachioradialis starts just above that and runs all the way down the radius. The muscle turns into a long tendon about halfway down the forearm, which is one reason why the forearm gets thin as you get to the wrist. But the tendon goes all the way to the end of the radius. You can find this by putting your thumb up as in a hammer curl and then bending your wrist down, as if you were dipping a fishing rod down. Stay in that position, find the base of your thumb, come up a little bit, and press in. You will feel nothing right at your wrist, and then you will feel the point of the radius. *Styloid process* means "sharp point," and it actually is a relatively sharp point on the bone (16).

The brachioradialis helps bend the elbow, but as noted, hand position greatly influences how this muscle works. When your hand is in the neutral position, this muscle is at its strongest. You might think that to work this muscle, the neutral position would be best, but remember that the brachialis is strong in this position and the biceps isn't too bad either. This muscle is weak, so for it to get the most stimuli, we have to emphasize it as much as possible. To do that, perform the reverse curl exercise. It is similar to the standard bicep curl, but the bar is grasped with the palms facing down. This position emphasizes the brachioradialis and basically takes the biceps out of it. This exercise also places a good amount of emphasis on the forearm extensors because the wrist has to resist falling into flexion during the exercise.

Exercises for the Brachioradialis

- EZ-bar reverse curl
- Zottman dumbbell curl
- Rotating barbell curl

Table 11.2 describes the effect of changing the hand (grip) position on the bar on the primary muscle being trained and the muscles that assist the agonist in performing each exercise.

The elbow flexor muscles are involved when a client is performing exercises for the back. Table 11.3 lists the primary elbow flexor and the synergists for various hand (grip) positions of common back exercises.

TRICEPS BRACHII

The triceps is a three-headed muscle in the back of the arm (figure 11.12). The difference between a three-headed muscle and three separate muscles is that separate muscles have separate origins and insertions, whereas a muscle with multiple heads has multiple origins but just one insertion. The triceps mainly work to straighten the arm, and thus is the antagonistic muscle to the biceps. A working familiarity with the three heads of the triceps is important; each triceps head can be targeted and specifically trained.

Table 11.2 Hand Position and Elbow Flexor Involvement During Biceps Exercises

Hand position	Exercise	Agonist	Synergist 1	Synergist 2
Palms-up grip	Barbell bicep curl	Biceps brachii	Brachialis	Brachioradialis
Thumbs-up grip	Hammer curl	Brachialis	Biceps brachii Brachioradialis	–
Palms-down grip	Reverse curl	Brachioradialis	Brachialis	Biceps brachii

Table 11.3   Hand Position and Elbow Flexor Involvement During Back Exercises

Hand position	Exercise	Agonist	Primary elbow flexor	Synergist 1	Synergist 2
Palms-up grip	Chin-ups	Lats	Biceps brachii	Brachialis	Brachioradialis
Thumbs-up grip	V-grip cable row	Lats	Brachialis	Biceps brachii Brachioradialis	–
Palms-down grip	Wide-grip lat pull-down	Lats	Brachioradialis	Brachialis	Biceps brachii

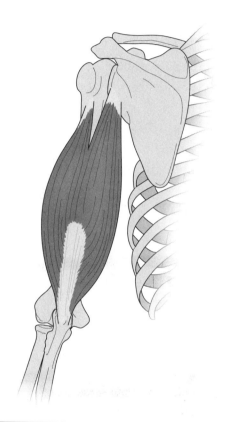

Figure 11.12   Illustration of the triceps brachii muscle.

- Origin
  - Long head—infraglenoid tubercle of the scapula
  - Lateral head—posterior humerus above the spiral groove
  - Medial head—posterior humerus below the spiral groove
- Insertion—olecranon process of the ulna
- Action
  - Overall—extends the elbow (all heads)

- Long head—assists in extension of the shoulder

The long head of the triceps is the most interesting head, so we start there. The long head is the only section of the triceps that is a two-joint muscle. It helps extend the elbow and the shoulder. It helps extend the shoulder significantly only when the arm is straight or virtually straight. If the elbow is bent during shoulder extension (as in a cable row), the triceps is not working to any significant degree.

The long head is the largest head of the triceps and is the most visible on the back of the arm. To target the long head, you should perform exercises with your elbows tucked in in relation to your hands; the goal is for the hands to be wider than the elbows. A useful exercise for this is a reverse-grip tricep push-down. That exercise is particularly good because you cannot cheat by flaring out your elbows, although it can be hard on some people's wrists and forearms. Skull crushers (also called the lying tricep extension) are also a good exercise for the long head, but it is easy to cheat by flaring the elbows out on that exercise, thus decreasing the stress on the long head. The long head is stressed during bench press, depending on the form (more with an elbows-tucked position) (27).

If you have to hold your arm out isometrically while performing a triceps exercise, the long head also gets a good workout. Examples include the overhead rope tricep extension, overhead dumbbell tricep extension, and cable skull crushers. Performing exercises in which the shoulder is flexed up with the arm overhead recruits the long head because it is placed in a stretched position. The pullover and straight-arm lat pull-down exercises also place significant stress on the long head because of its role in shoulder extension.

The back of the arm, where the long head is located, can become flabby. Excess body fat accumulates there. Clients often comment that they want to improve that area aesthetically. You are not going to be able to make the fat disappear in that area by training it, but there are two main ways to improve the way that an area looks. The first method is to reduce the total amount of fat by reducing overall body fat (achieved through good nutrition and a proper workout program). The second method is to improve the muscle in that specific area by training it and building it. You probably can't achieve spot reduction, but you can achieve spot improvement.

The lateral head of the triceps is the second biggest head. It is a single-joint muscle; its only action is to extend the elbow. To target the lateral head, you want the hands to be relatively close in relation to the elbows; the elbows should be wider than the hands. The best exercise to target the long head is a simple one—the V-grip tricep push-down. The lateral head is easy to target and is often the most developed triceps head. If you cheat on some triceps exercises and allow your elbows to flare out (as in skull crushers), you are shifting emphasis from the long head to the lateral head. Although the long head is the biggest head, it is often underdeveloped, particularly in people with long arms.

The medial head of the triceps, also a single-joint muscle, is the smallest head. With your arms at your sides, you can't really see this muscle; you have to put your arms up as if you were flexing your biceps. The part of your triceps near your inner elbow is the medial head. It is more difficult to target the medial head. To place the most emphasis on this head, you need to flare out your hands at the end of the range of motion. This is most easily accomplished with the rope. You want to get a full flare and really lock out your arms when you are training the triceps. Locking out the joints is typically not recommended, but with the triceps muscle you should fully extend the elbows to a point just short of hyperexten-

sion. When you are lifting with cables, the resistance isn't going directly through your joints, so fully extending the elbows presents little danger. The medial head is the smallest and therefore the weakest head. You will use less weight with it than with any of the other heads (65).

Exercises for the Triceps Brachii

- Tricep push-down
- Lying dumbbell tricep extension
- Skull crusher
- Overhead dumbbell tricep extension
- Dip (body vertical)
- Bench dip
- Diamond (close-grip) push-up
- Close-grip bench press
- Dumbbell tricep pullover

ROTATOR CUFF

The rotator cuff is composed of four muscles. Its purpose is to help move and stabilize the shoulder joint. Remember that the shoulder is the most flexible joint in the body and that flexibility comes with a price—lack of stability. Because the humerus is not solidly locked into a bone, it needs muscles, among other soft-tissue supports, to help stabilize it and hold it in place. Rarely is the rotator cuff the main muscle working during an exercise. Normally, it is a synergist or stabilizer in almost all upper-body exercises (33). The downside of this is that when the rotator cuff is injured, almost any movement of that shoulder hurts. Specific exercises can target the various sections of the rotator cuff. As you might guess from the name, some of these exercises involve rotation. People who have injured the rotator cuff often perform these exercises for rehabilitation and rehab, but they are also useful in preventing injury. Most of the rotator cuff muscles are relatively small compared with the other muscles in the upper body, so you will use a light weight for these exercises.

You can use the acronym *SITS* to remember the names and location of the rotator cuff muscles:

S—supraspinatus
I—infraspinatus
T—teres minor
S—subscapularis

Supraspinatus

The supraspinatus is a relatively small and thin muscle, about the size of two fingers side by side (figure 11.13). It starts on the scapula, in the depression just above the spine of the scapula (the spine is the ridge that you feel if you rub your upper back). In anatomy, we use the word *supra* (superior) to mean "above or higher," and the word *fossa* means "depression." So the origin, supraspinous fossa of the scapula, is the depression above the spine of the scapula. This muscle is hidden from view. It starts under the traps and goes under the flat part of the scapula (the acromion process) to attach to the humerus under the delts.

- Origin—supraspinous fossa of the scapula
- Insertion—greater tubercle of the humerus
- Action—abduction and stabilization of the humerus

The supraspinatus (named for its place of origin) helps the middle delt abduct the shoulder, or raise it out to the side. To emphasize the supraspinatus in that movement, begin with your hands by your sides and pronate your hands so that your thumb and pointer finger face your thigh. Staying in that position, raise your arm out to the side, keeping your pinky high; raise it to just 90 degrees. If you have sensitive shoulders this action will often feel uncomfortable even with no weight.

The supraspinatus helps stabilize the shoulder, mainly by holding the humerus in place when a weight is in your hand. For example, when you pick up your briefcase or a suitcase, that object pulls on your shoulder. The supraspinatus holds the humerus in place. If you were to cut the supraspinatus while you were holding something heavy, your humerus would likely dislocate. For that reason, just carrying something for a long time can bother your shoulders, even though your delts are not involved in that activity.

The supraspinatus is the rotator cuff muscle that is most commonly injured in the gym (67). It is in a tight spot in the body, so it is easy to rub it the wrong way. Some people have more subacromial space than others do; those with a smaller space are more likely to suffer from impingement. This inflames the muscle, which makes the tight spot even tighter. To keep the supraspinatus healthy, people need to maintain at least normal flexibility in the shoulders and avoid performing exercises that are often contraindicated, such as the behind-the-neck military press and upright row exercises.

Exercises for the Supraspinatus

- Dumbbell lateral raise
- Lateral raise with the pinky held high

Infraspinatus

The infraspinatus is the one rotator cuff muscle that is relatively easy to see, if you know where to look. It is found just under the spine of the scapula (figure 11.14). Its name, like that of many other muscles, comes from its origin. *Infra* means "inferior (below)," so it is in the depression below the spine of the scapula. No muscle covers this one. If you can watch a lean person train his or her back, you may see a triangular muscle that appears to be right

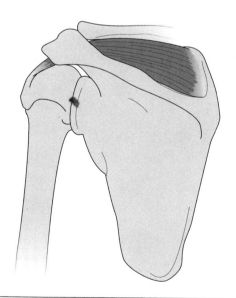

Figure 11.13 Illustration of the supraspinatus muscle.

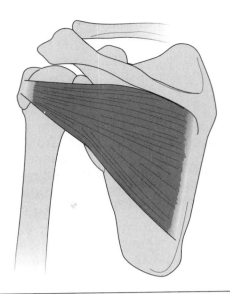

Figure 11.14 Illustration of the infraspinatus muscle.

on the scapula moving up and down with the scapula. That muscle is the infraspinatus. It is surrounded by the traps on top of it and to one side, the rear delts to another side, and the lats (and teres major) below it.

- Origin—infraspinatus fossa of the scapula
- Insertion—greater tubercle of the humerus
- Action—external rotation of the humerus; extension, horizontal abduction, adduction (when externally rotated) of the humerus

When you are training your back, you are generally giving this muscle some stimulus. It normally works with the lats, the one notable exception being that the infraspinatus performs external rotation and the lats perform internal rotation. External rotation against a cable or band, one of the most effective rotator cuff exercises, specifically targets the infraspinatus.

Teres Minor

The teres minor is the smallest of the four rotator cuff muscles (figure 11.15). It sits just lateral to the infraspinatus, but it tends to get lost in the midst of that muscle, teres major, and the rear delts. It does essentially everything

that the infraspinatus muscle does. It starts on the lateral border of the scapula. *Axilla* means "armpit," so it is on the side that borders the armpit. Together, this muscle, the infraspinatus, and the rear deltoid are the three muscles that produce external rotation. All these muscles are relatively small, which is why the force generated in external rotation is nothing compared with that generated in internal rotation. Have you ever seen two people try to arm wrestle by starting with the backs of their hands placed next to each other? The strength generated would be extremely weak compared with normal arm-wrestling position. The teres minor is trained using the same exercises as those used for the infraspinatus; these are sometimes called the IT muscles.

- Origin—upper two-thirds of axillary border of the scapula
- Insertion—greater tubercle of the humerus
- Action—external rotation of the humerus; extension, horizontal abduction, adduction (when externally rotated) of the humerus

Note that the teres minor sits on top of the teres major and is obviously smaller than the teres major. In addition, the teres major inserts

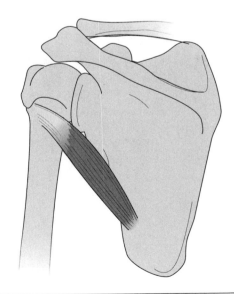

Figure 11.15 Illustration of the teres minor muscle.

on the front of the humerus, whereas the teres minor goes around the back of the humerus, so the actions are not exactly the same for these two muscles. Again, these muscles are named because of their size and location, not because of their similar actions.

Exercises for the Infraspinatus and Teres Minor

- Cable external rotation
- Band external rotation
- Band pull-apart
- Shoulder horn external rotation
- Lying dumbbell external rotation
- Pull-up and other lat exercises

Subscapularis

The subscapularis is the final and largest of the rotator cuff muscle (figure 11.16). It is located on the anterior side of the scapula, which is the side that runs along the ribs. If you were lying on your belly, you would have to go through the scapula to get to this muscle. It helps with internal rotation and is the only rotator cuff muscle involved in that action. Remember, though, that pecs major, lats, front delts, and teres major also perform internal rotation, so five strong muscles contribute to that action. Subscapularis works most closely with the front deltoid (36).

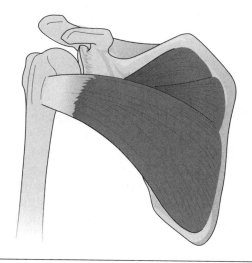

Figure 11.16 Illustration of the subscapularis muscle.

- Origin—subscapular fossa of the scapula
- Insertion—lesser tubercle of the humerus
- Action—internal rotation of the humerus; adduction and horizontal adduction of the humerus

The subscapularis is named for where it sits. It rests in the subscapular fossa, the depression under the scapula. It is the only rotator cuff muscle to insert on the lesser tubercle of the humerus (which is medial); the other three rotator cuff muscles insert on the greater tubercle of the humerus (which is lateral).

The subscapularis is directly trained with internal rotations. Holding a cable in your hand with your elbow bent at 90 degrees and then patting your belly is an example of internal rotation. The subscapularis almost gets some stimulus through pressing motions.

Exercises for the Subscapularis

- Cable internal rotation
- Band internal rotation
- Lying dumbbell internal rotation
- Shoulder abducted internal rotation
- Bench press and other chest exercises

As a personal trainer, you can benefit from understanding the relationship between the deltoids and the rotator cuff muscles. Table 11.4 lists the deltoid heads, the rotator cuff partners, and large-muscle partners that are trained with the specific deltoid, and their primary collective action.

FOREARM MUSCLES

The forearm flexors and forearm extensors (figure 11.17) are two main groups of muscles in the forearms. These muscles contain mostly slow-twitch muscle fibers that are capable of repetitive, continuous movement. Think of how many reps the fingers perform to write a letter!

Forearm Flexors

The forearm flexors are the larger of the two groups (figure 11.17, *a* and *b*). They are on the anterior (smooth) side of the forearm. There

Table 11.4   Relationship Between the Rotator Cuff and Other Movers of the Humerus

Deltoid head	Rotator cuff partner	Large-muscle partner	Primary action
Front deltoid	Subscapularis	Chest	Internal rotation
Middle deltoid	Supraspinatus	NA	Abduction
Posterior deltoid	Infraspinatus Teres minor	Lats*	External rotation

*Note: The lats do not perform external rotation, but the lats, rear delts, and IT muscles work to extend the shoulder, which is how those muscles are commonly trained.

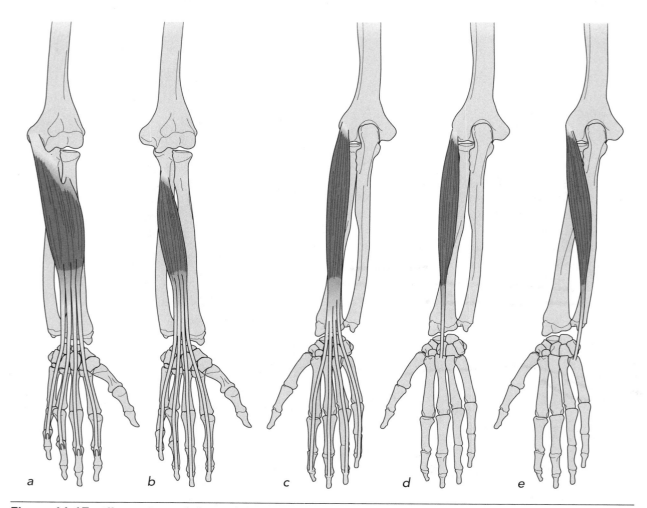

a   b   c   d   e

Figure 11.17   Illustrations of the *(a, b)* anterior and *(c–e)* posterior forearm muscles.

are multiple muscles in that area. Remember that muscles create movements. The more possible movements you can do, the more muscles you need to have. Our hands possess great dexterity and can perform many movements, so it follows that our hands and forearms contain many muscles. The muscles in the forearm are responsible for wrist flexion, finger flexion, and grip strength.

Training the forearms is important for those who want larger forearms, want to improve their grip strength, or think that their wrists or hands give out on other activities. Using lifting aids such as straps (which attach you to the weight so that you don't have to grip it) allows you to lift more weight but ultimately weakens your grip. A general rule is to use straps only on a few exercises—namely, bent-over rows, shrugs, and romanian and stiff-legged deadlifts. In those exercises the strength of the muscles normally exceeds grip strength. The grip is working a lot when training back muscles and to a much lesser extent when training the biceps.

There are two primary types of grip strength: concentric and isometric. Concentric grip strength refers to crushing grip strength, which is developed by using grippers, holding extrathick bars (fat bars) while lifting, performing plate pinches, and using the wrist roller, among other exercises. Isometric grip strength refers to holding grip strength, which is more commonly developed in most training programs. Holding on to a deadlift or pull-up bar or dumbbell in a row will all develop isometric grip strength. The principle of specificity correctly predicts that these two abilities are distinct, and concentric grip strength has a better transfer to isometric grip than vice versa. Grip strength is important to anyone who participates in racquet sports, martial arts, rock climbing, or contact sports that require grabbing and holding another person.

Forearm Extensors

The forearm extensors are on the posterior (hairy) side of the forearm (figure 11.17, *c–e*). The extensors are not as large or as strong as the flexors. Their two main actions are wrist extension and finger extension.

Something to be aware of is that the muscles that control the fingers are located more in the forearms than in the hands. The muscles turn to tendons, and then those tendons run to the fingers and move them. The forearm flexors are much stronger and more powerful than the forearm extensors. To verify this, make a fist and then grab that fist with your other hand. Now try to open up the fist while trying to keep it closed with the other hand. Keeping it closed is easy (77).

Exercises for the Forearms

- Barbell or dumbbell wrist curl
- Barbell or dumbbell wrist extension
- Cable row forearm curl

- Cable wrist flexion
- Wrist roller
- Grippers
- Farmer's walk
- Pronated shrug without straps
- Fat-bar exercises
- Pull-up and row with limited fingers
- Plate pinch
- Fingertip push-up

OTHER UPPER-BODY MUSCLES

The upper body contains several smaller muscles. Most training programs do not specifically address these muscles, but personal trainers should be familiar with them.

Levator Scapulae

A relatively small muscle in the upper back is called the levator scapulae (figure 11.18). It runs from the side of the neck (near the skull) to the top of the scapula and helps lift the scapula. It is so named because *levitate* means

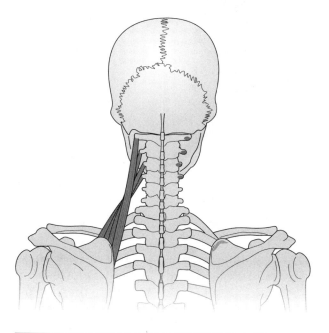

Figure 11.18 Illustration of the levator scapulae muscle.

"lift up," so *levator scapulae* means "lift (elevate) the scapula." It works with the upper traps to perform shrugging motions.

Coracobrachialis

The coracobrachialis is a thin muscle in the upper arm (figure 11.19). It is named for its origin and insertion. It starts on the coracoid process (where the pec minor and the short head of the biceps originate) and goes out to the humerus. The coracobrachialis helps flex and adduct (both vertically and horizontally) the shoulder. If someone has his or her arm up to flex the biceps, you can see this muscle under the front delt and above the triceps long head. It looks almost like the bone itself, but you can't see the humerus. You can often see the coracobrachialis when someone is performing the bench press or shoulder press exercise; it appears to go into the armpit (49).

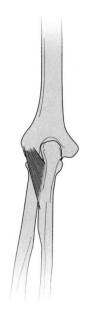

Figure 11.20   Illustration of the anconeus muscle.

CONCLUSION

This chapter provided a comprehensive overview of the muscles found in the upper body. The origin, insertion, and action of each of the main muscles in the upper body were described. A comprehensive list of exercises for those muscles and tips and techniques for optimally training them were presented. This information helps personal trainers understand how these muscles function, how to train them properly, and how an injury to a particular area might affect a client.

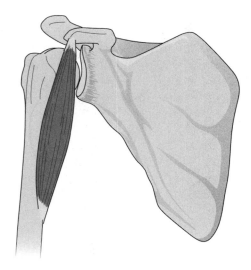

Figure 11.19   Illustration of the coracobrachialis muscle.

Anconeus

The anconeus (figure 11.20) is a very small muscle just below the elbow. It helps extend the elbow so that it works with the triceps. The muscle is very small and therefore cannot generate much force.

Study Questions

1. List two muscles that insert on or near the bicipital groove of the humerus.

   a. biceps brachii and pec minor

   b. teres major and pectoralis major

   c. latissimus dorsi and posterior deltoid

   d. pectoralis major and anterior deltoid

2. Which rotator cuff muscle works with the middle deltoid to produce abduction?

    a. supraspinatus

    b. infraspinatus

    c. teres minor

    d. subscapularis

3. In which of the following exercises would the rhomboids and middle traps receive the most training stimulus?

    a. bench press

    b. dumbbell military press

    c. dips

    d. wide-grip cable row

4. Which of the following choices represents the actions of the pectoralis major?

    a. shoulder extension, shoulder horizontal abduction, shoulder external rotation

    b. shoulder flexion, shoulder horizontal adduction, shoulder internal rotation

    c. shoulder abduction, shoulder flexion, shoulder external rotation

    d. scapular protraction, scapular downward rotation, scapular elevation

5. List the muscles that can produce shoulder extension.

    a. latissimus dorsi, teres major, infraspinatus, posterior deltoid

    b. pectoralis major, pectoralis minor, subscapularis, anterior deltoid

    c. latissimus dorsi, rhomboids, teres major, erector spinae

    d. pectoralis major, triceps brachii, posterior deltoid, brachialis

Lower-Body Anatomy

This chapter is devoted to the anatomy of the lower body, which refers to the hips and below. The focus is on the glutes (gluteus maximus or gluteus minimus), quads (quadriceps), hamstrings, adductors, and calves. Also included is a brief description of some of the smaller muscle groups.

GLUTES

Three muscles make up the glutes: gluteus maximus, gluteus medius, and gluteus minimus. *Gluteus* comes from a Greek word that means "rump." The glutes are the muscular part of the butt.

Gluteus Maximus

The gluteus maximus is a large, powerful muscle (figure 12.1). It is usually the thickest and strongest muscle in the body, although that can vary from person to person. Most people can lift more weight on exercises involving the glutes, such as a leg press or squat, than on exercises involving any other muscle group. Think of the gluteus maximus as the motor for the body. It contributes significantly in standing up from a squat, climbing stairs, sprinting, and jumping.

- Origin—posterior sacrum
  - Superior gluteal line of the ilium
- Insertion—gluteal tuberosity of the femur
  - Iliotibial tract
- Action—extends the hip, extends the trunk
  - Externally rotates the hip

The gluteus maximus is a superficial muscle, meaning that the only thing covering it is skin and fat. It begins on the back of the pelvis and goes to the back of the femur. It also attaches to the iliotibial tract, a large thick tendon named for the fact that it starts on the ilium, runs down the leg, and inserts on the tibia. This is sometimes called the IT band, and it can become problematic for runners and cyclists (78).

The gluteus maximus helps extend the hip, meaning that this muscle draws the thigh backward. This action occurs in walking, more so in jogging, and even more in running, sprinting, and jumping. If the feet are fixed in position and one is bent over, contracting the glutes will help extend the trunk by pulling the pelvis down and back. This action occurs when you stand up after taking a bow. Remember this action when you want to train the gluteus without also training the quads, because that

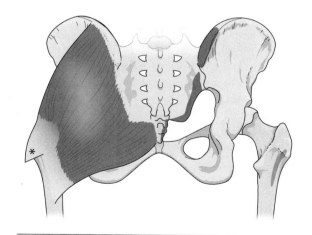

Figure 12.1 Illustration of the gluteus maximus muscle.

movement (trunk extension) is one of the primary ways to accomplish that (35).

When the glutes are involved, they are usually the agonist in the exercise. Exercises that work the glutes by hip extension include all variations of squats, leg press, all variations of lunges, and hip thrusts. Exercises that work the glutes by trunk extension include all variations of deadlifts, good mornings, and hyperextensions. As noted earlier, the gluteus maximus also performs external rotation of the hip. This action occurs mainly when the leg is straight. The motion of lateral rotation is not often trained in the gym, but the easiest way to see this is to stand with your leg straight and then rotate your foot outward. You are accomplishing this movement by using your glutes to rotate the femur, which in turn rotates the foot. Externally rotating the feet slightly while squatting can increase hip stability (124).

Exercises for the Gluteus Maximus

- Squats
- Leg press
- Lunge
- Step-up
- Sumo deadlift
- Hip thrust
- Butt blaster
- Bridge
- Smith machine squat

Gluteus Medius

The gluteus medius, also a superficial muscle, is the second-largest muscle of the gluteals (figure 12.2). It is located where you find the hip pockets on a pair of pants—the outer, upper part of the butt.

- Origin
  - Iliac crest
  - Ilium—between superior and middle gluteal lines
- Insertion—greater trochanter of the femur
- Action—abduction (horizontal and vertical) of the hip, stabilizes the leg when moving

The gluteus medius is an abductor, which means that it raises the leg to the side. Note that it is not a strong hip extensor, so it does not work that closely with the gluteus maximus. Compared with the gluteus maximus, the gluteus medius starts more anteriorly and more laterally on the hip bone. It inserts on the greater trochanter. *Trochanter* means "big bump" on a bone (*tuberosity* just means "bump" on a bone), so the greater trochanter is a really big bump on a bone. The greater trochanter is easy to feel. If you stand up, put your hands on your hips, press in, and then run your hands down your legs a couple of inches (5 cm) to approximately the bottom of your butt; you should feel a hard knob of bone. If you lie on your side on the floor, the greater trochanter is what is digging into the floor. The gluteus medius has a closer relationship with the gluteus minimus than it does with the gluteus maximus (80, 104).

In the gym we train this muscle using abductor exercises, but in real life it has an interesting function. When you walk, the glute medius contracts with every step to keep your hip stable as the other leg moves forward (91). If this muscle isn't working well, your hip tilts with every step, which throws off your posture as you walk. Good exercises for this muscle group include the abductor machine, cable hip abductions, lying lateral leg raises, X-band walks, penguin walks, fire hydrants, lateral leg kicks, and step-downs. Training the legs singly (unilaterally) also increases recruitment of the abductors.

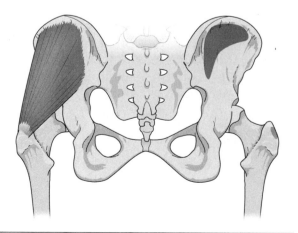

Figure 12.2 Illustration of the gluteus medius muscle.

Gluteus Minimus

The gluteus minimus is the smallest glute muscle that works closely with the gluteus medius (figure 12.3). It is also the only one that can't be seen; it is hidden under the medius.

- Origin—posterior ilium between middle and inferior gluteal line
- Insertion—greater trochanter of the femur
- Action—abduction of the hip (horizontal and vertical)

The gluteus minimus is another abductor, just like the medius. Again, it does not perform extension, so it does not work closely with gluteus maximus. When performing compound leg exercises, such as squats and the leg press, these two muscles work mainly as stabilizers. As you can guess from the name of this muscle, it is relatively small, which means that it is rather weak (82).

The abductors and adductors (discussed later) are sometimes considered women's muscles, but that viewpoint is uneducated. Men and women have the same muscles in their legs, and the hip adductors and abductors are important knee stabilizers.

Exercises for the Gluteus Medius and Gluteus Minimus

- Abductor machine
- Penguin walk

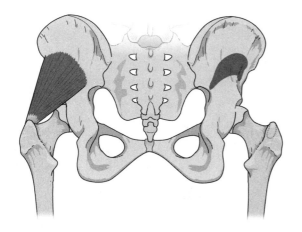

Figure 12.3 Illustration of the gluteus minimus muscle.

- X-band walk
- Lateral sled drag
- Side jump
- Fire hydrant
- Lying leg raise
- Cable hip abduction
- Side kick
- Step-down

ILIOPSOAS

The iliopsoas is often called the hip flexor muscle. It is actually two muscles—the psoas major (figure 12.4a) (the *p* is silent in iliopsoas and psoas) and the iliacus (figure 12.4b). The muscles are located in a similar place and do the same thing, so generally they are studied as one muscle, although some experts prefer to teach them separately for the sake of accuracy.

- Origin
  - Lumbar vertebrae T12–L5 (psoas major)
  - Anterior, inner surface of ilium (iliacus)
- Insertion—lesser trochanter of the femur
- Action
  - Flexes the hip
  - Flexes the trunk if the legs are fixed

The hip flexor is a deep muscle. To see it, you would look at a person's front and go through the abdominal muscles, through the stomach, and behind the intestines and then stop in front of the vertebral column. The bulk of the hip flexor starts there, but part of it starts on the inside of the ilium, the hip bone. It then goes down and attaches to the lesser trochanter on the proximal part of the femur. If you remember the glutes, the abductors are attached to the greater trochanter of the femur, a really big bump on the bone. The hip flexor goes to the lesser trochanter, which is only a relatively big bump on the bone. The lesser trochanter is similar in location to the greater trochanter, but it is on the opposite side of the bone, medial as opposed to lateral. This is right where your groin is and where your leg attaches to your body.

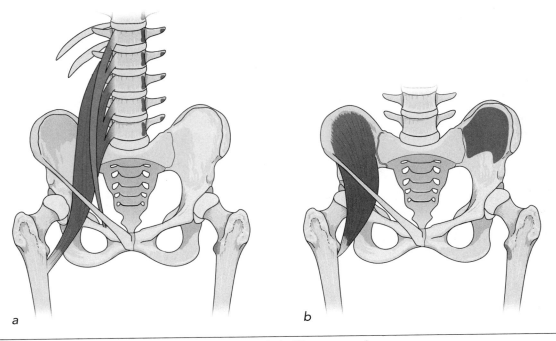

a

b

Figure 12.4   Illustration of the *(a)* psoas major and *(b)* iliacus muscles.

The iliopsoas is the muscle opposite the gluteus maximus. It is not nearly as powerful as the maximus because the maximus was designed to lift heavy weights against gravity, such as body weight, whereas the hip flexor was designed to lift the leg. The iliopsoas helps pull the leg forward in walking and running, and it is particularly involved in sprinting and hurdling. If people want to improve their speed, they need to train this muscle (104).

If the goal is to focus on the hip flexors when training the abdominal muscles, lock your feet in a fixed position during the sit-up exercise or keep your knees straight during the leg raise exercise. To place less emphasis on the hip flexors, keep them freely moveable, place them on top of a bench (for sit-ups and crunches), or keep your knees flexed during leg raises. But if sprinting speed is important, exercises for the hip flexors need to be part of the training program.

The iliopsoas can get tight on some people, particularly cyclists, runners, and people who sit all day. A tight iliopsoas can tilt the pelvis forward and contribute to back injury, so the iliopsoas should be stretched regularly. A good stretch for the hip flexor is to get in lunge position, allow the knee to rest on the ground, and then shift forward and push the front leg forward as much as possible, keeping the front foot flat on the ground. After attaining that position, sit up tall with the chest and lean back. Both the hip and trunk should be in a position of hyperextension, which is the best way to stretch the hip flexor. Try to keep the glutes and the abs "on" (meaning contracted), so that the spine doesn't hyperextend too much, which can cause pain in the lower back for some people.

Exercises for the Hip Flexor

- Banded mountain climber
- Hip flexor sled drag
- Hip flexor machine
- Decline sit-up
- Hanging leg raise
- Inverted sit-up
- L-hold

QUADRICEPS

The quadriceps is a large, powerful muscle in the leg, commonly called the thigh muscle. The muscle is so named because it has four heads, just as the biceps has two heads. Many people treat the quads as though they are four separate muscles, but that is not correct. Most textbooks list the quads as four heads of one muscle because of the similar insertion point for all of them. The muscles that make up the quads are the rectus femoris, vastus medialis, vastus lateralis, and vastus intermedius.

When studying the quads, you should look at rectus femoris separately because it is a two-joint muscle capable of hip flexion and then study the three vastus muscles together. A nickname for them can be the three vastus brothers. All the vastus muscles originate on the femur, insert on the tibia, and extend the knee, which is the only thing they do. In general, during compound leg exercises, the deeper you go, the more you emphasize the glutes, and the shallower you go, the more you emphasize the quads. Because of the weight used and the emphasis placed on the quadriceps muscle, the leg press is an excellent exercise to build up the quads. In everyday activities, the quads work with the glutes to allow people to stand up from a sitting position and to provide power for running and jumping.

Exercises for the Quadriceps

- Squat
- Leg press
- Leg extension
- Lunge
- Step-up
- Front squat
- Hack squat
- Single-leg squat

Rectus Femoris

The most central quadriceps, which runs straight down the middle of the leg, is the rectus femoris (figure 12.5). Among the quads, it is unique in that it is a two-joint muscle, crossing both the hip and the knee joint. The other quads are one-joint muscles.

- Origin—anterior inferior iliac spine (AIIS), lower ilium

- Insertion—patella to the tibial tuberosity through the patellar ligament
- Action
  - Extends the knee
  - Flexes the hip

The rectus femoris is the only quad to start on the hip bones, and thus it helps flex the hip. It works with the iliopsoas in this motion, although the iliopsoas does most of the work. It addition, like all quads, it can extend the knee. The rectus femoris is easy to see on a lean person; it is the middle quad among the three that you can see, and it sits right on the top of the femur. Good exercises for the rectus femoris are any that hit the quads such as squats, leg press, lunges, and leg extension (11, 127). In addition, anything for the hip flexor involves the rectus femoris as a synergist. The rectus femoris is commonly tight, and this tightness can contribute to knee pain. To stretch the rectus femoris, get in the position

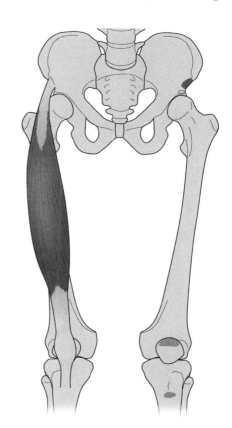

Figure 12.5 Illustration of the rectus femoris muscle.

described earlier for the hip flexor, but pull the foot up to the hip at the same time. A partner or a stretching strap can make this stretch much easier to perform. A good stretch for the rectus femoris require both of its joints to be stretched; hip extension and knee flexion are simultaneously required (35).

Vastus Medialis

The vastus medialis is the inside part of the quadriceps (figure 12.6). *Medialis* means "medial," referring to the part of your thigh that is closest to the midline. The medialis is relatively low on the thigh; most of it is just above your kneecap. Do not confuse your medialis with your adductors, which are much higher up your leg. The vastus medialis is called the teardrop in the gym because it looks like a teardrop when developed, starting narrow and then getting wider going down.

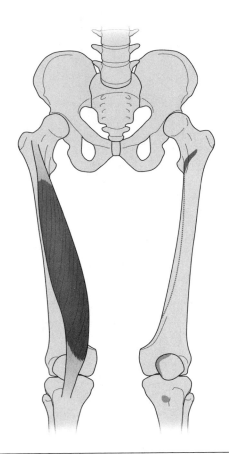

Figure 12.6 Illustration of the vastus medialis muscle.

- Origin—linea aspera of the femur (medial aspect)
- Insertion—patella to the tibial tuberosity through the patellar ligament
- Action—extends the knee

To train the medialis, you need to target the quads. Squats, lunges, leg press, and leg extension all hit the medialis. To place extra emphasis on this muscle, place your feet wider than normal, significantly wider than shoulder-width, and point your toes out at about a 45-degree angle during those exercises. This stance shifts more emphasis to the inner part of the thigh. In addition, the medialis receives more stimulus as the legs lock out, so focusing on the last half of the concentric range of motion is particularly good for emphasizing the medialis. When using the leg extension machine, you do not want to point the toes in or out. That orientation is not good for the knee because the muscle pulls the patella in an unnatural position. When using the leg extension machine, just keep the feet in the neutral position.

Vastus Lateralis

The vastus lateralis muscle is the outer quad; *lateralis* means "lateral" (figure 12.7). If you slap the outside of your thighs, you will hit this muscle. In the gym this part of the quad is called the sweep because a well-developed lateralis goes up and out from the knee and can add significant size to the overall quad.

- Origin—linea aspera of the femur (lateral aspect)
- Insertion—patella to the tibia through the patellar ligament
- Action—extends the knee

Any exercise that involves straightening the leg against resistance works the quads and, therefore, the lateralis. But to emphasize the lateralis during those exercises, you want to keep your toes straight ahead and keep your feet relatively close together, narrower than shoulder-width. Doing this is hard with a free-weight squat, but it is easy to do using the hack squat, leg press, and Smith machine.

In addition, the lateralis receives more stimuli the lower you go in a squatting motion, so make sure to go all the way down to emphasize this muscle. Sometimes you can just perform bottom-quarter squats, in which you squat all the way down, come up only about a quarter of the way, and then go down again. You can use that technique on almost any major leg exercise. When you go extra low, your form can easily deteriorate, so work hard on keeping your form correct—feet flat and planted on the floor and lower back slightly arched.

Vastus Intermedius

The vastus intermedius muscle, the smallest of the quads, is not visible (figure 12.8). It sits under and is covered completely by the rectus femoris. The vastus intermedius is the only one of the quads to originate on the front of the femur.

- Origin—upper anterior shaft of the femur
- Insertion—patella to the tibia through the patellar ligament
- Action—extends the knee

This muscle starts up high on the thigh and turns into tendon about halfway down the leg. It has a larger tendon than any other quad. The vastus intermedius is not emphasized specifically by any exercise. It receives the most stimuli with the feet in normal position during leg exercises, and in that way, as part of the quad, it works the most closely with the rectus femoris (130, 131).

HAMSTRINGS

The hamstrings are a group of three separate muscles that make up the back of the leg. They are the antagonistic muscles to the quads.

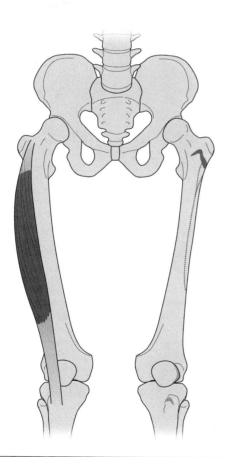

Figure 12.7 Illustration of the vastus lateralis muscle.

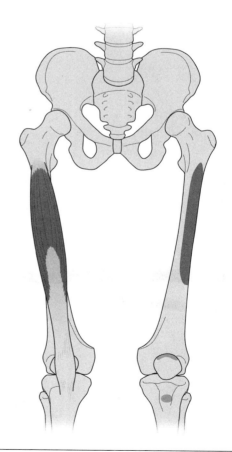

Figure 12.8 Illustration of the vastus intermedius muscle.

Every hamstring muscle is a two-joint muscle, whereas only one quad muscle is a two-joint muscle. The muscles that make up the hamstrings are the biceps femoris, semitendinosus, and semimembranosus.

Because the hamstrings can produce three significant actions, all those actions should be trained at some point. The basic function of the hamstring is knee flexion. Exercises that train that movement are a variety of leg curls such as seated, prone, dumbbell, and ball leg curls along with the glute–ham raise (GHR), a more challenging variation. The hamstrings (in tandem with the glutes) produce hip extension in such exercises as the squat, leg press, lunge, step-up, and reverse hyperextension exercises. The hamstrings also cause trunk extension and are particularly emphasized when the knees are held relatively straight during this motion. Examples include the stiff-legged deadlift, romanian deadlift, and good morning exercises.

Exercises for the Hamstrings

- Seated leg curl
- Prone leg curl
- Glute–ham raise
- Ball leg curl
- Dumbbell leg curl
- Stiff-legged deadlift
- Romanian deadlift
- Good morning
- Reverse hyperextensions

Biceps Femoris

The largest muscle of the hamstrings is the biceps femoris (figure 12.9). It gets its name because it has two heads (like the biceps brachii in the upper arm) and sits on the femur. The biceps femoris is the most lateral of the hamstrings.

- Origin
  - Long head—ischial tuberosity
  - Short head—linea aspera of the femur
- Insertion—head of the fibula
- Action

- Flexes the knee
- Long head only—extends the hip or trunk

The biceps femoris is the only two-headed hamstring muscle. The short head is unique among the hamstrings because it is a one-joint muscle; it flexes only the knee. The long head is a two-joint muscle that acts on the hip and knee. When the hamstrings perform hip extension, they are synergists with the glutes. The hip is the fulcrum of the body, so as with the glutes, hip extension can work two ways. Generally, the upper leg is moved backward as in running or squatting, but if the legs are fixed and this muscle contracts, it pulls the pelvis down and back, which leads to trunk extension, as in a deadlift or hyperextension (75, 77).

The biceps femoris is the strongest hamstring on most people. When performing the leg curl

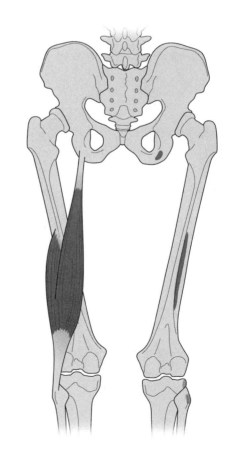

Figure 12.9 Illustration of the biceps femoris muscle.

s
tu
us
foo
the i
If you
you c
you pe
should
knee, bu
that can t
safely poir
a leg curl. II
while stretc
for any hams

Semitendi

The semitendin is a simple, classic hamstring muscle (figure 12.10). It gets its name

because it has a long tendon of insertion. Unlike the biceps femoris, which inserts on the fibula, the semitendinosus inserts on the tibia. You can think of *f* for "femoris" and "fibula," and *t* for "tendinosis" and "tibia." The semitendinosus comes around the inside of the upper tibia and inserts on the front of the tibia, about inches (7.6 cm) below and one inch (2.5 cm) side the kneecap. It is a two-joint muscle, so oth flexes the knee and extends the hip or ik (75, 77).

- Origin—ischial tuberosity
- Insertion—anterior proximal tibial shaft
- action—extends the hip or trunk, flexes the knee

Semimembranosus

The semimembranosus is similar to the semitendinosus in location and action (figure 12.11). Indeed, just as we had the three vastus brothers

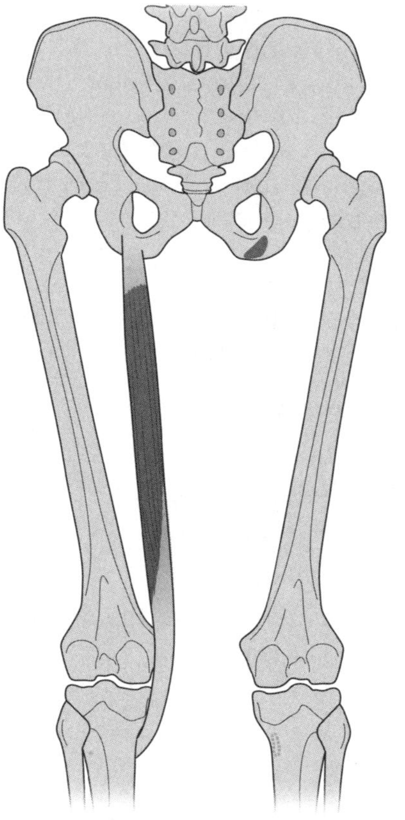

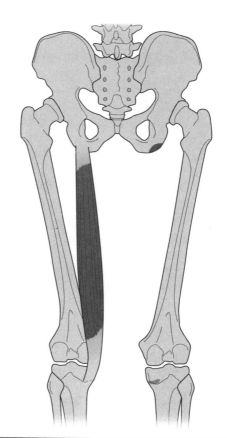

Figure 12.10 Illustration of the semitendinosus muscle.

Figure 12.11 Illustration of the semimembranosus muscle.

of the quads, we have the two semi sisters of the hamstrings. The only notable difference between the two is that the semitendinosus has a longer tendon and inserts on the front of the tibia whereas the semimembranosus inserts on the back of the tibia (44). The semitendinosus sits on top of the semimembranosus. At the bottom of the leg, the semimembranosus is the most medial hamstring. You can think of the two *m*s in *membranosus* as standing for "most medial." The semitendinosus is right next to it, and then biceps femoris is the most lateral. The two semi sisters insert on the tibia, and the biceps femoris inserts on the fibula. If you are thinking that having two hamstring muscles going to the inside of the leg and just one to the outside might be uneven, remember that biceps femoris has two heads and is the largest, so the size difference between the sides is small.

- Origin—ischial tuberosity
- Insertion—posterior medial tibial condyle
- Action—extends the hip, flexes the knee

As discussed with biceps femoris, a personal trainer can tell a client's strength or weakness in the hamstrings by how the toes point during a heavy set of the leg curl exercise. Usually they point out to indicate a stronger biceps femoris and weaker semi sisters. If they point in, then the reverse is likely to be true. People who walk pigeon toed often experience this. If someone wants to emphasize the semi sisters while stretching, pointing the toes in toward each other will place extra emphasis on the semi muscles of the hamstrings.

ADDUCTORS

The adductor muscles of the leg make up the inner thigh. They are a cluster of five muscles that make up a relatively large-muscle group when taken as a whole. The bulk of this muscle group starts where the leg meets the body and travels about halfway down the lower leg. All the adductor muscles originate on the pubic bone, at least in part, and all but one insert on the femur. As the name implies, they all perform adduction of the hip, both horizontal

and vertical. A memory trick to remember the insertion points is to think of "peanut butter loves mashed grapes" (mashed grapes is jelly). Going from top to bottom, the insertion of the muscles are pectineus, brevis, longus, magnus, and gracilis.

The five muscles originate on the pubic bone, and all except the gracilis insert on the femur. Even in very lean people separating out the individual adductors is difficult; they tend to look like a lump of muscle in the inner, upper thigh. Most of the mass of the adductors is above the halfway point in the thigh. If a client wishes to monitor the change in the size (girth) of the adductors, the best way is to measure the thigh at its thickest point, right where the leg meets the body. Using a measurement halfway down the thigh, a common location, usually focuses on the quads and hamstrings.

A client can emphasize the adductors in the gym by using a wide stance on most compound bilateral exercises. Going extra low also emphasizes the adductors. Using single-leg variations works both the adductors and abductors more. The adductor machine and cable hip adduction can also be effective, as is having to hold something weighted (such as a dumbbell or medicine ball) between the feet while performing a movement. If a client is dealing with a strained adductor (pulled groin), bringing in the stance significantly and slightly reducing the range of motion of the exercise should limit the involvement of the adductors.

Exercises for the Adductors

- Adductor machine
- Cable hip adduction
- Lying hip adduction
- Sumo deadlifts
- Wide-stance squats and leg press
- Medicine ball leg raise (ball held between feet)

Adductor Magnus

The adductor magnus is the largest adductor muscle, as the name implies (think of *magnificent* for "magnus"; see figure 12.12). It is also the deepest adductor, so many other adductors sit on top of it. In addition, it has the lowest insertion point of any adductor muscle that inserts on the femur.

- Origin
  - Pubic bone (inferior ramus of the pubis)
  - Ischium (ischial tuberosity and ramus of the ischium)
- Insertion—linea aspera of the femur
  - Adductor tubercle of the femur
- Action
  - Overall—adduction of the hip
  - Anterior part—assists in hip flexion
  - Posterior part—assists in hip extension

The adductor magnus is the strongest adductor muscle (56). Its lowest point of insertion is the adductor tubercle, which is on the distal, medial part of the femur close to the patella. This muscle has a relatively broad origin; it originates on both the pubic and ischium bones. It is the only adductor that originates on two bones. The word *ramus* in the origin means "bridge," so it is the part of the bone that bridges out to meet another part of the bone. Because of its broad origin, the front part of the muscle, sometimes referred to as the anterior head, can help flex the hip. The back part of the muscle, sometimes referred to as the posterior head, can help extend the hip. As with the hamstrings, tight adductors can significantly limit the range of motion of the leg.

Adductor Longus

The adductor longus is, ironically, not as long as the adductor magnus, although it sits on top of the magnus (figure 12.13). In fact, it is about half as long as the magnus. It is longer than the next muscle that we discuss (brevis),

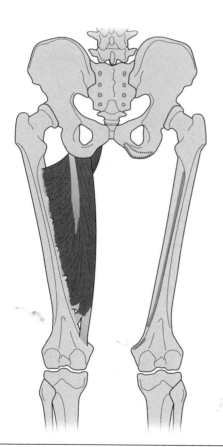

Figure 12.12 Illustration of the adductor magnus muscle.

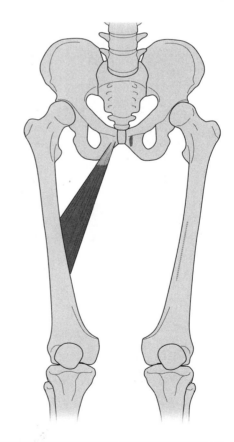

Figure 12.13 Illustration of the adductor longus muscle.

so that is where the name comes from. It is a relatively simple one-joint muscle. Because of its somewhat anterior origin, it helps flex as well as adduct the hip.

- Origin—pubic bone
- Insertion—linea aspera of the femur
- Action—adduction of the hip, helps with hip flexion

Adductor Brevis

The adductor brevis is the shortest of the three main adductor muscles (figure 12.14). The word *brevis* means "brevity" or "brief," so the name makes sense. The adductor brevis sits somewhat superior and deep to the adductor longus, but it is superficial compared with the adductor magnus. The origin, insertion, and action are the same for the adductor brevis and adductor longus muscles.

- Origin—pubic bone
- Insertion—linea aspera of the femur
- Action—adduction, helps with hip flexion

Pectineus

The pectineus muscle is the most superior adductor at its insertion point (figure 12.15). It starts on the pubic bone, close to the ilium. Because of its anterior origin it is a relatively strong hip flexor, working with the iliopsoas. It inserts in a similar place to the adductor brevis. The upper adductor muscles (pectineus, brevis, and longus) are often thought of as groin muscles, and when people say that they pulled a groin muscle, it is often one of these muscles (32).

- Origin—anterior pubic bone
- Insertion—proximal femur between lesser trochanter and linea aspera
- Action—adduction and flexion of the hip

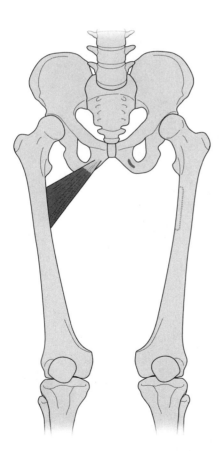

Figure 12.14 Illustration of the adductor brevis muscle.

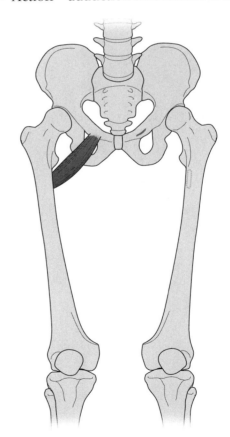

Figure 12.15 Illustration of the pectineus muscle.

Gracilis

The gracilis is the final adductor muscle (figure 12.16). It is long and thin, about the width and thickness of a man's belt. It runs from the pubic bone all the way down the inside of the leg to the tibia. It is the only two-joint adductor muscle. Because it inserts on the tibia, it can help flex the knee, but it is weak in that action. This muscle is the most medial of the adductors. If your thighs rub together when you walk, your gracilis muscles are touching.

- Origin—pubic bone
- Insertion—medial proximal tibia
- Action
  - Adduction of the hip
  - Assists with knee flexion (very weak)

ABDUCTORS

The two main abductors of the hip, the gluteus medius and gluteus minimus, were already covered. The other two muscles that help perform abduction are the sartorius and the tensor fascia lata. Keep in mind that most of the muscles that perform abduction are located on the outside of the hip (not on the outside of the thigh) and the muscles that perform adduction are located on the inner thigh. They are not exactly opposite each other in terms of location on the body.

Sartorius

The sartorius is the longest muscle in the body; it covers the complete length of the longest bone in the body, the femur (figure 12.17). It is a long, thin muscle and relatively weak.

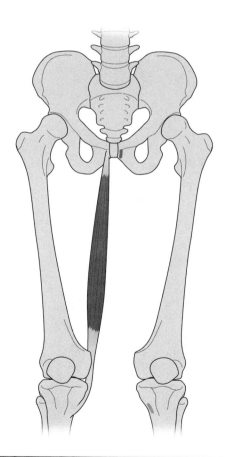

Figure 12.16   Illustration of the gracilis muscle.

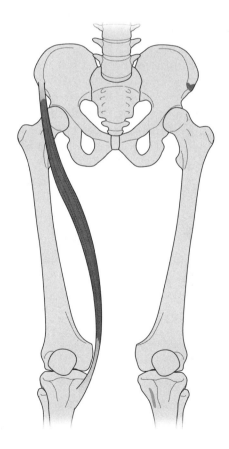

Figure 12.17   Illustration of the sartorius muscle.

- Origin—anterior superior iliac spine (ASIS)
- Insertion—upper medial shaft of the tibia
- Action
  - Assists in hip flexion and hip abduction
  - Assists in knee flexion

The sartorius is a two-joint muscle that acts at both the hip joint and the knee joint. It helps flex the hip (with the iliopsoas and rectus femoris), abduct the hip (with the gluteus medius and gluteus minimus), and flex the knee (with the hamstrings). The sartorius is weak in most of those actions, notably abduction. If you perform those three actions all at once, the result is what this muscle really does, which is cross your leg so that one foot is over your other knee.

The sartorius is not generally emphasized in the gym; it is trained as a stabilizer during most leg exercises. It is a superficial muscle but can be hard to see unless the person is extremely lean (32). The origin of this muscle can be found by locating the iliac crest (the top of the hip bone), walking the fingers forward until the bone begins to dive downward (this is just under the waist line), firmly pressing in at that spot, and then bringing the leg forward (hip flexion). This muscle comes down the leg and heads inward to go to the inner part of the upper shin. It perfectly divides the quads and adductors of the leg, and it is lateral to the adductors and medial to the quads.

Tensor Fascia Lata

The tensor fascia lata (abbreviated as TFL) is another abductor; although it sounds like something that you order at Starbucks (figure 12.18).

- Origin—lateral iliac crest
- Insertion—iliotibial tract
- Action
  - Assists in abduction of the hip
  - Helps stabilize the knee when walking

The TFL is a relatively small muscle that inserts onto the big IT band that runs down the outside of the leg. It is involved in almost all hip actions and some knee actions but is mainly a stabilizer. It sits on the outside of the hip just above the greater trochanter; the meat of this muscle would usually be covered up by underwear. The TFL is rarely emphasized in the gym. Like the sartorius, it is a stabilizer that normally gets enough stimuli during regular leg workouts and cardio (56).

CALVES

The calf muscles are made up of two main muscles (the gastrocnemius and soleus) and several smaller ones. Just as the muscles in the forearms control the fingers, the muscles in the calves can control the feet and the toes. The group name for the calf muscles as a whole is triceps surae. Because the gastrocnemius and soleus have a common insertion point and share the insertion tendon, they can be thought of as a single muscle with three heads.

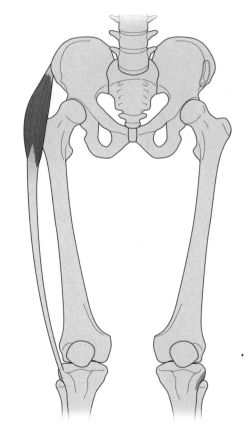

Figure 12.18 Illustration of the tensor fascia lata muscle.

Gastrocnemius

The gastrocnemius, or gastroc for short, is the most superficial calf muscle, so it is easy to see (figure 12.19). When someone goes up on his or her toes, the ball of the calf is the gastroc. It is a two-joint muscle that has two heads, much like the biceps brachii.

- Origin—medial and lateral epicondyle of the femur (two heads)
- Insertion—the calcaneus through the Achilles tendon
- Action
  - Plantar flexes the ankle
  - Flexes the knee

The gastroc is a two-joint muscle that acts on the knee and the ankle. It can help flex the knee, so performing a leg curl works the gastroc, although it would be classified as a relatively weak synergist in that movement (124). To emphasize this action, point the toes down (plantar flex) while performing a leg curl. This movement sometimes causes a cramp to

occur in the calf. To de-emphasize the gastroc during the leg curl exercise, bring the toes up (dorsiflex) during the movement. The goal is normally to work the hamstrings during that exercise, so keeping the feet in neutral position is generally best. If you feel the calves working or if they cramp during leg curls, then slightly dorsiflex the foot.

The gastroc is most powerful at the ankle in producing plantar flexion, which is the motion of pointing the foot down. This action occurs when you step on the gas pedal or when you jump. The calves are working when you jump, but their importance is overrated. The glutes and quads are more important in jumping. The gastroc is primarily involved when performing a calf (heel) raise with the leg straight. Because it is a two-joint muscle, bending the knee and performing calf raises (as in a seated calf raise) weakens the muscle (57).

Soleus

The soleus muscle lies underneath the gastroc (figure 12.20). You can see parts of it on either side of the leg, but it is generally covered up. It gets its name from the Latin word *sole*, which means "flat fish."

- Origin
  - Soleal line of the tibia
  - Posterior head and upper shaft of fibula
- Insertion—the calcaneus through the Achilles tendon
- Action—plantar flexes the ankle

The soleus is a single-joint muscle, so it does not act on the knee. The area of the soleus muscle has a large section of tendon, much larger than the tendon area of the gastroc. The soleus muscle on most people generally has a high percentage of slow-twitch muscle fibers. The soleus is always working in any calf raise, but if emphasizing it over the gastroc is a priority, then the seated calf raise exercise (which places the knee in a 90-degree flexed position, thereby reducing the involvement of the two-joint gastroc muscle) is a better choice (18, 42).

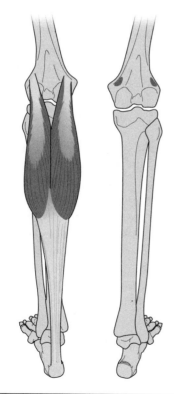

Figure 12.19   Illustration of the gastrocnemius muscle.

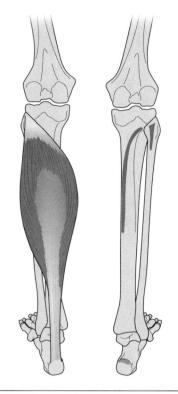

Figure 12.20 Illustration of the soleus muscle.

The soleus and the gastroc attach to the Achilles tendon, the large, thick tendon that runs down the back of the ankle. This tendon gets its name from Greek mythology. Achilles was an ancient Greek hero who could not be hurt by weapons because, as the story goes, as a baby he had been held by his ankles and dipped into the river Styx, a magical river that made his skin invulnerable to weapons. But his mom was holding him, and because she was a mortal she would die if she touched the water. To submerge as much of his body as possible, she held him by his feet and ankles and turned him upside down to dip him in the water. She did not submerge his feet and ankles, so they remained vulnerable. When Achilles was later in a fight, someone shot an arrow through his tendon, severing it, which rendered him immobile, and he was killed. In real life, an injury to the Achilles tendon is debilitating; surgery is often required to repair it, and it may not fully recover. Now we use the term *Achilles heel* as a generic term for a person's weak spot.

People are often frustrated because the calf muscles are slow to respond to training. Calf muscles, like most muscles in the body, are somewhat predetermined by genetics, but people can make significant improvements in their calves. But the calf is small in general and can be slow to respond. The ancient Greeks believed that the ideal male form would have equal measurements in the neck, upper arm, and calf and that those measurements should indicate moderate muscularity by being at least 15 inches (38 cm) (2).

Exercises for the Calves

- Standing calf raise
- Seated calf raise
- Donkey calf raise
- Calf raise on the leg press
- Barbell calf raise
- Single-leg calf raise
- Single-leg dumbbell calf jump
- Pushing or pulling a prowler or sled on the balls of the feet

TIBIALIS ANTERIOR

The tibialis anterior is the shin muscle (figure 12.21). It is a relatively small muscle that sits right next to, or lateral to, the shinbone in the lower leg. It is the antagonist muscle to the calves. The tibialis anterior produces inversion of the foot, which rolls the foot so that the sole (bottom) faces inward. Its additional purpose is to lift the foot during walking so that it doesn't drag on the ground. Shin splints are often felt in the area of this muscle. A weakness in this muscle or related lower-leg muscles often contributes to shin splints. The pain might be caused by fatigue in this muscle or by its pulling on part of its origin, the interosseous membrane. The interosseous membrane is the membrane that connects the tibia and fibula. *Inter* means "between," and *osseo* means "bone," so it is a membrane between bones.

- Origin
  - Proximal lateral shaft of the tibia
  - Interosseous membrane

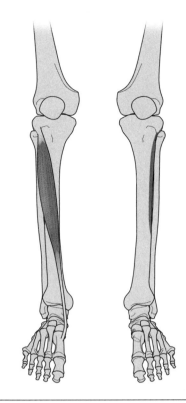

Figure 12.21 Illustration of the tibialis anterior muscle.

- Insertion
  - Base of first metatarsal, plantar surface
  - First cuneiform, plantar surface
- Action
  - Dorsiflexes the foot
  - Inverts the ankle

An effective flexibility exercise for the tibialis anterior is based on a version of the classic quad stretch. First, stand and bend the knee as though you are trying to kick your butt, grab the ankle, and pull the lower leg to your butt. Then, to stretch the tibialis anterior, move the hand holding the ankle to hold the end of the foot at the toes and pull the bottom of the foot toward your butt. This version should feel significantly different from the classic quad stretch. Propping the top side (where the shoelaces are located) of the tip of your foot on something sturdy (like the railing of a treadmill) can work well to mimic this stretch. A flexibility exercise is the child's pose in yoga.

Kneel down and place your hips on your ankles. Point the feet away from you and let your weight push you down. Depending on your level of flexibility, you can begin to lean backward. Some people can lie all the way to the floor in this position, but many people with tight tibialis anterior muscles will find that just kneeling in the basic start position provides a big stretch for this muscle.

Exercises for the Tibialis Anterior

- Tibialis anterior machine
- Barbell dorsiflexion (barbell held vertical)
- Banded dorsiflexion
- Heel walks
- Plate lifts (plate on top of foot)

OTHER LOWER-BODY MUSCLES

The muscles listed in the preceding sections are the main lower-body muscles and the ones that people will have some interest in improving for fitness or appearance. But other muscles in the lower body are worth mentioning. The following sections contain short descriptions of what each muscle does and where it is located in the body.

Deep Lateral Rotators of the Hip

Similar to the rotator cuff muscles of the upper body that keep the shoulder joint stable, a group of lower-body muscles help keep the hip joint stable (figure 12.22). Because the hip is surrounded by bone (the pelvis), the deep lateral rotators of the hip are not as crucial or as likely to be injured as the rotator cuff muscles are. The deep lateral rotators sit deep under the glutes, attach to the femur, and laterally rotate the hip (as the name implies). The muscles, listed from superior (top) to inferior (bottom), are the following:

1. Piriformis
2. Gemellus superior
3. Obturator internus

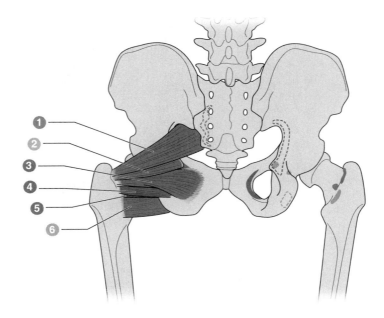

Figure 12.22 Six deep lateral rotators of the hip.

4. Gemellus inferior

5. Obturator externus

6. Quadratus femoris

Of the six muscles, the piriformis receives the most attention. The sciatic nerve, a huge nerve that runs from the lower back down to the feet, normally runs next to this muscle, but in some people it goes right through this muscle. If this muscle is injured or aggravated, it will inflame, which in turn will put pressure on the sciatic nerve.

A common stretch for the piriformis is to bring the knee up to the chest and at the same time grab the outside of the foot and pull that to the opposite shoulder. That action should flare out the knee and place the piriformis in a position to receive a good stretch. If this muscle is tight, some soft-tissue work can also be of value. Foam rolling can work well; sit on a foam roller or smaller object like a tennis ball or lacrosse ball. Place the ball right in the center of the glute so that you are sitting just on the ball, cross the leg on the side being stretched, and roll around until you feel the pain; it usually doesn't take long.

Plantaris

The plantaris is an extremely small muscle that works with the calves (figure 12.23). It is about the size of the pinky and has a superlong tendon. Not everyone has this muscle; it is kind of a leftover muscle from our evolution.

Popliteus

The popliteus is another small muscle located behind the knee (figure 12.24). This muscle functions to unlock the knee. When your leg is straight and you then unlock it, you work this muscle. Poorly performed squats are sometimes referred to as popliteal squats because instead of going all the way down, the person just unlocks the knees and comes back up. It is gym slang for a weak squat.

Other Plantar Flexors of the Ankle

Although the soleus and the gastroc are the main muscles that plantar flex the ankle, other deeper muscles assist in plantar flexion:

- Tibialis posterior
- Flexor digitorum longus
- Flexor hallucis longus

These muscles are referred to as the Tom, Dick, and Harry muscles as a way to remember their names. The tibialis posterior (Tom) helps plantar flex the ankle, the flexor digitorum

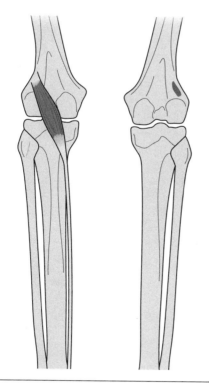

Figure 12.23 Plantaris muscle.

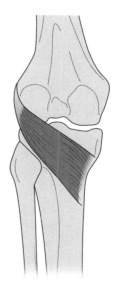

Figure 12.24 Popliteus muscle.

longus (Dick) helps flex the ankle and toes, and the flexor hallucis longus (Harry) flexes the big toe. *Hallucis* means "great toe." Some people think that doing calf raises with bare feet is important because otherwise these muscles are inactive. Arnold Schwarzenegger was a big proponent of this practice. You can try it and see whether you like it, but get permission from your gym manager first. Wearing finger shoes is a good way of replicating being barefoot without having the hygiene issues of going barefoot indoors (52).

Other Dorsiflexors of the Ankle

Several muscles assist the tibialis anterior in producing dorsiflexion. These muscles either sit under the tibialis anterior or are in the top of the foot:

- Extensor hallucis longus—extends the big toe
- Extensor digitorum longus—extends other toes
- Extensor digitorum brevis—extends other toes

Peroneal Muscles

The peroneal muscles (figure 12.25, *a–c*) produce eversion of the foot, which rolls the foot so that the sole faces outward. This movement is not as natural for most people as inversion is. Often visible in lean people, the three peroneal muscles are located on the lateral side of the calf on the outside of the fibula:

- Peroneus longus
- Peroneus brevis
- Peroneus tertius

If a person regularly strains or sprains the ankles, the recommendation might be made to train those muscles. Wearing finger shoes and performing ankle circles in both directions is a good way to help improve or at least maintain the strength of some of the smaller muscles surrounding the ankle joint. Unfortunately, some of the stability of the ankle comes from ligaments, and after those are overstretched or torn, tightening them back up is harder (54).

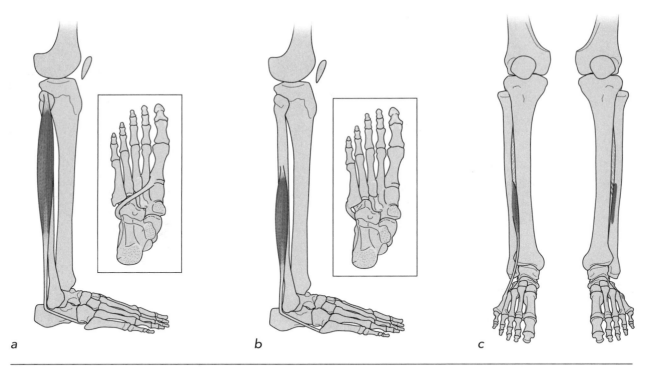

Figure 12.25   *(a)* Peroneal longus, *(b)* peroneal brevis, and *(c)* peroneal tertius.

In addition, the foot contains many muscles (about 15), but they are beyond the scope of this book. Generally, they function to help move and stabilize the toes and feet.

CONCLUSION

This chapter provided a comprehensive overview of the muscles found in the lower body. The origin, insertion, and action of each of the main muscles in the upper body were described. A comprehensive list of exercises for those muscles was presented, as were tips and techniques for optimally training them. This information will help personal trainers understand how these muscles function, how to train them properly, and how an injury to a specific area might affect a client.

Study Questions

1. Which of the following groups of muscles performs knee flexion?

   a. rectus femoris, sartorius, semitendinosus, soleus

   b. biceps femoris, pectineus, gastrocnemius, gracilis

   c. semimembranosus, gastrocnemius, gracilis, sartorius

   d. gluteus medius, vastus lateralis, adductor longus, soleus

2. Which of the following squats would most emphasize the gluteus maximus, assuming that equal weight was used on all exercises?

   a. quarter squat

   b. half squat

   c. three-quarter squat

   d. full squat

3. Which exercise would be effective at targeting the short head of biceps femoris?

    a. prone leg curl

    b. hyperextensions

    c. leg extensions

    d. stiff-legged deadlift

4. Which of the following exercises most stimulates the soleus?

    a. seated calf raise

    b. standing calf raise

    c. donkey calf raise

    d. squats

5. Which of the following muscles inserts on the tibia?

    a. gluteus medius

    b. biceps femoris

    c. gastrocnemius

    d. semimembranosus

Anatomy of the Core

The anatomy of the core (the front, side, and back of the torso, or trunk) includes the abdominal muscles, obliques, lower back, and all the smaller muscles in that area.

RECTUS ABDOMINIS

The rectus abdominis is the main muscle of the abdomen (figure 13.1). People often try to improve the appearance of this muscle by doing crunches, sit-ups, and other similar exercises.

- Origin—pubic symphysis
- Insertion
  - Costal cartilage of ribs 5, 6, 7
  - Xiphoid process
- Action
  - Flexes the trunk
  - Compresses the abdominal contents

The rectus abdominis runs in a straight line from the groin to the rib cage. It gets wider as it goes up; you can visualize it as a man's tie upside down. The rectus abdominis functions to fold the trunk forward. If your hips are held in place, the upper torso is pulled forward, and if the upper torso is held in place, the rectus abdominis will pull the hips toward the chest, so it can operate in two directions. Note that the rectus abdominis does not attach to the femur, so lifting the legs up is not an effective concentric abdominal exercise. To target this muscle, you need to raise the hips when doing leg raises. A personal trainer can choose to emphasize the upper or lower part of the abs, although true isolation of either section

is not possible. Exercises that effectively target the upper rectus abdominis are incline sit-ups, crunches, sit-ups, decline sit-ups, cable crunches, and ball crunches. Resistance can be added to all those exercises to increase the difficulty. Exercises that effectively target the lower rectus abdominis generally involve bringing the hips toward the chest. These exercises include reverse crunches, leg thrusts, incline knee or leg raise, roman chair knee or

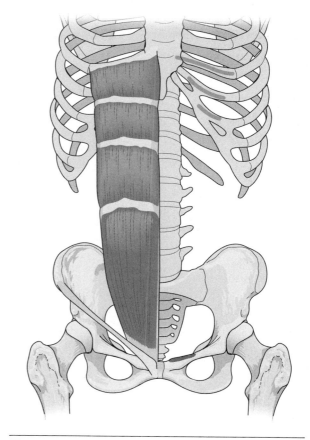

Figure 13.1 Rectus abdominis muscle.

leg raise, hanging knee or leg raise, and dragon flags. Exercises that target the entire rectus abdominis through flexion are harder to come by but include clams, dead bugs, and inverted sit-ups (28, 46).

Another important function of the rectus abdominis, implicit in its regular action, is its role in antiextension of the spine. A muscle is always capable of resisting the opposite of its action; the biceps could be classified as muscles that can resist extension of the elbow. During an exercise the challenge or goal is often to hold the spine stable while movement occurs. Several exercises to train the rectus abdominis have this goal, including the plank (the progression for the plank exercise is plank from the knees; to the toes; to the hands; to using a ball, rings, or suspension device; to weighted; and finally to spread eagle), the ab wheel (the progression for the ab wheel is on the knees at an incline, on the knees, on the knees at a decline, on the knees with weights, on the toes at an incline, on the toes, on the toes at a decline, and finally using just one arm), and wood chops.

Exercises for the Rectus Abdominis

- Crunch
- Reverse crunch
- Clam
- Sit-up
- Decline sit-up
- Inverted sit-up
- Ab wheel
- Plank

When personal training first became popular, clients were often taught they could target certain sections of their muscles. As the study of kinesiology progressed, people realized that a muscle could rarely be worked in isolation and that targeting specific parts of certain muscles was likely not possible because of the fiber and neural arrangements of the muscle. With this information, the pendulum likely swung too far in the other direction. Some fitness experts scoff at the idea of targeting the upper or lower abs, despite loads of evidence that it can be done. The muscle fibers of the rectus abdominis are not continuous from

origin to insertion; they stop and start along the tendinous insertion points of the obliques. Some research has failed to show a difference in upper versus lower ab firing in exercises, but other research has shown significant differences in the electromyography (EMG) of the muscle during different exercises. In this instance one well-designed study would be all that is necessary to confirm what most people can feel happening: The upper abs work more in some exercises, usually involving bringing the insertion to the origin, and the lower abs work more in other exercises, usually involving bringing the origin to the insertion. Here is a statement from one such study:

> The reverse curl resulted in the greatest amount of lower rectus activity, the V-sit and reverse curl exercises resulted in the greatest amount of external oblique activity, and the trunk curl, reverse curl, trunk curl with a twist, and V-sit all resulted in similar amounts of upper rectus EMG activity. (140)

EXTERNAL OBLIQUE

The external oblique is the only superficial oblique muscle (figure 13.2). It starts on the outside of the rectus abdominis and is often called the love handles. The muscle fibers run diagonally in a downward direction, so they head down and in. The meaty part of the muscle turns into tendon as it hits the rectus abdominis, and this tendon then envelops the rectus abdominis and goes to the linea alba, a ligament that runs from the pubic symphysis to the xiphoid process. This ligament is right in the middle of the rectus abdominis; it goes right through the belly button (108, 118).

- Origin—lower eight ribs
- Insertion
  - Linea alba
  - Pubis
  - Anterior iliac crest
- Action
  - Bilateral—flexes the trunk, compresses the abdominal contents

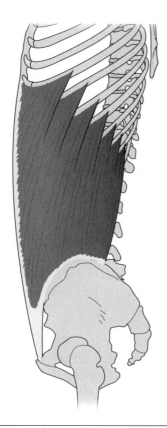

Figure 13.2 Illustration of the external oblique muscle.

- Unilateral—abducts the trunk, rotates the trunk to the opposite side

The part of the muscle that originates on the higher ribs runs in a more diagonal fashion. It is specifically involved in any sort of rotational movement, and adding a twist to sit-ups emphasizes the obliques. The part of the muscle that originates on the lower ribs runs downward in almost a straight line, so it is heavily involved in abducting (bending to the side) the trunk. Side bends and the like are good exercises for that muscle. When you are doing a side bend, the side that the weight is on is not the working side. Do not hold a weight in each hand when doing side bends, because one will balance the other and offset the effectiveness of the exercise.

INTERNAL OBLIQUE

The internal oblique sits deep to the external oblique, as the name implies (figure 13.3).

It is also lower than the external oblique. Its fibers run in a diagonal direction upward and inward. The inguinal ligament begins at the pubic symphysis and goes to the front of the iliac crest. You cannot see a person's internal oblique.

- Origin
  - Inguinal ligament
  - Anterior iliac crest
  - Thoracolumbar aponeurosis
- Insertion
  - Costal cartilages of lower four ribs (9–12)
  - Abdominal aponeurosis and linea alba
- Action
  - Bilateral—flexes the trunk, compresses the abdominal contents
  - Unilateral—abducts the trunk, rotates the trunk to the same side

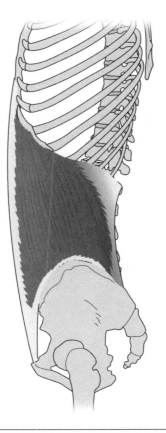

Figure 13.3 Internal oblique muscle.

The exercises that work the external oblique also work the internal oblique. The only difference is that in rotations, one side of the external oblique is working and the opposite side of the internal oblique is working; the two working sides form an X on the midsection. But because you would perform rotations in both directions, this will balance itself out (81).

In the gym we don't usually separate out exercises for the external oblique from those for the internal oblique. We simply train the oblique muscles as a whole. Just as the abs can resist the extension of the spine, so too can the obliques resist the lateral movement of the spine.

Exercises for the Obliques

- Dumbbell side bend
- Hyperextension side bend
- Suitcase deadlift
- Medicine ball rotation
- Sword swing
- Diagonal wood chop
- Landmine
- Side plank
- Windshield wiper
- Human flag

TRANSVERSE ABDOMINIS

The transverse abdominis, sometimes abbreviated as the TA, is the deepest abdominal muscle (figure 13.4). It sits under the rectus abdominis, external oblique, and internal oblique muscles. If you went deeper, you would hit your stomach and intestines. Think of this muscle as acting like a corset for your body; it wraps around your whole midsection and, when functioning normally, keeps everything tight. You cannot see a person's transverse abdominis.

- Origin
  - Inguinal ligament
  - Iliac crest
  - Thoracolumbar aponeurosis
  - Internal surface of costal cartilage of ribs 7 through 12

- Insertion
  - Abdominal aponeurosis and linea alba
  - Pubis
- Action
  - Compresses the abdominal contents

The transverse abdominis does not produce any specific movement such as flexion or extension because its fibers run parallel to the horizon, not up and down or diagonally. Its main purpose is to provide support and protection for the abdominal contents. To activate this muscle, suck your abdomen in. You can visualize this by imagining that you are drawing your belly button in to your spine.

This muscle has received more attention than it deserves because of the increased focus on core training. Sucking in the belly button during resistance training is sometimes appropriate, but it should not be done all the time.

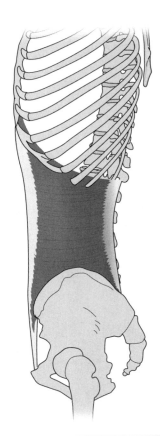

Figure 13.4 Transverse abdominis muscle.

For example, it should never be done during the squat exercise. In general, the best way to keep the core engaged is to brace it. Imagine that someone was going to punch you in the abdomen. How would you react? That action is bracing your core.

This muscle is trained with heavy compound structural lifts such as squats and deadlifts, as well as with exercises in which movement is resisted such as a plank or ab wheel (81). Martial artists often actively brace the core and then allow it to be hit by a partner or a medicine ball to learn how to deal with punches to the midsection. Bodybuilders used to practice a movement called the vacuum in which they would suck their belly in as tightly as possible.

Exercises for the Transverse Abdominis

- Vacuum
- Plank
- Ab wheel
- Braces
- Absorbing hits

ERECTOR SPINAE

The erector spinae muscles are the main lower-back muscles. That term is a little misleading because these muscles run the whole length of the spine. The erectors are really three muscles put together—the spinalis, longissimus, and iliocostalis.

The erector spinae muscles are responsible for extending both the spine and the trunk. If a person is slouched over, as in the finish of a crunch position, and then straightens up, that action would be extension of the spine. Extension of the trunk refers to the torso as a whole. When you lean forward to touch your toes and then straighten up, you are using your lower-back muscles to bring yourself up, even if you do not round over to touch the toes. They are heavily involved in exercises such as the deadlift and are important stabilizers in exercises such as the squat and bent-over row. Each of the three muscles has the same action, so they are trained together as a group. When both sides of the lower back are work-ing, they are the antagonistic muscle group to the abs. When training this muscle with heavy loads, keeping the lower back relatively flat or slightly arched is important to protecting the back (143).

The erector spinae muscles are not arranged like other muscles in the body. If you snipped the origin and the insertion of many muscles of a cadaver, you could then lift that muscle out of the body. The erector spinae can be visualized as a frayed rope extending from the pelvis up to the back of the head. The frayed parts of the rope are similar to the parts of the muscle that originate and insert on the various parts of the vertebral column and surrounding areas. To lift the erector spinae out of a body, you would have to snip all those various frays to separate it from the body (25).

Exercises for the Erector Spinae

- Lower-back machine
- 45-degree hyperextension
- 90-degree hyperextension
- Reverse hyperextension
- Conventional deadlift
- Sumo deadlift
- Stiff-legged deadlift
- Romanian deadlift
- Good morning

Spinalis

The spinalis is the most medial erector spinae muscle (figure 13.5). It starts and inserts on the spinous processes of the vertebral column, hence the name. The origin is always inferior to the insertion. This muscle starts at one point on the spine, travels up several vertebrae, and then reattaches itself. It leapfrogs up the spine in this manner until it finally attaches itself to the back of the skull (at the occipital bone). The ligamentum nuchae is a ligament in the neck that covers the spinous processes of C1 through C6 (32).

- Origin
  - Ligamentum nuchae
  - Cervical and thoracic spinous processes

- Insertion
  - Cervical and thoracic spinous processes
  - Occipital bone
- Action
  - Bilateral—extends the spine or trunk
  - Unilateral—abducts the spine or trunk

Longissimus

The longissimus is so named because it is the longest erector spinae muscle, starting in the lower back and going all the way up the mastoid process (figure 13.6). If you move your fingers backward an inch or so (2 to 3 cm) from your ear, you will come to a bump on your skull, which is the mastoid process. The longissimus is the middle erector spinae muscle; it is lateral to the spinalis. It is the muscle most associated with the transverse processes of the vertebrae. Like the spinalis this muscle starts low and then leapfrogs up until it reaches the head (16).

- Origin
  - Thoracolumbar aponeurosis
  - Lumbar and thoracic transverse processes

- Insertion
  - Thoracic and cervical transverse processes
  - Mastoid process of the skull
- Action
  - Bilateral—extends the spine or trunk
  - Unilateral—abducts the spine or trunk

Iliocostalis

The iliocostalis is the most lateral erector spinae muscle (figure 13.7). It is named for the origin (ilium) because the thoracolumbar aponeurosis attaches to the ilium and because this muscle both originates and inserts on the ribs, the costals. It starts on the ribs, leapfrogs up a few ribs, and then reattaches. As it gets higher it veers back in and ultimately attaches to the transverse processes in the neck. It is the only erector spinae muscle that does not attach to the skull.

- Origin
  - Thoracolumbar aponeurosis
  - Posterior ribs
- Insertion
  - Posterior ribs
  - Cervical transverse processes

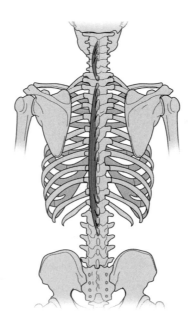

Figure 13.5 Spinalis muscle.

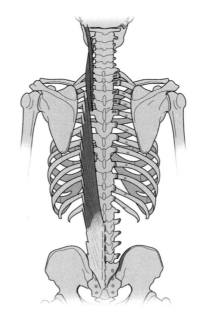

Figure 13.6 Longissimus muscle.

- Action
  - Bilateral—extends the spine or the trunk
  - Unilateral—abducts the spine or the trunk

QUADRATUS LUMBORUM

The quadratus lumborum, or QL as it is often called, is a small muscle in the lower back (figure 13.8). It sits deep to the erector spinae and the thoracolumbar aponeurosis. It is called the quadratus because it inserts on four parts of the lumbar vertebrae. If it inserted on the fifth part, the muscle would actually head downward instead of upward. The *lumborum* part of the name comes from *lumbar*, meaning "lower back." This muscle works with the erector spinae; you can think of it as the little brother (a synergist) of the erector spinae. It does everything that the erectors do, just not as well.

- Origin—posterior iliac crest
- Insertion
  - L1 through L4 transverse processes
  - 12th rib

- Action
  - Bilateral—extends the trunk
  - Unilateral—abducts the trunk or raises the hip

The QL muscle is also sometimes called the hip hiker because it can also elevate the hip. When both sides of the hip are lifted, the QL arches the lower back and makes it look as if you are trying to stick your butt out. When only one side is lifted, the QL raises one part of the hip. The spine ends up bending to correct that shift, possibly causing postural problems. Maintaining flexibility in this muscle helps prevent those problems. When people strain their lower back, sometimes they have actually strained their QL (63).

DIAPHRAGM

The diaphragm is an unusual muscle that is usually not heavily studied by personal trainers or actively trained by people in the gym. It is included here both for completeness and because of its importance in the body. It is a relatively large muscle that when contracted looks like a large pancake (figure 13.9). The diaphragm separates the abdominal cavity, which holds the stomach, intestines, liver, kidneys, and bladder, from the thoracic cavity, which holds the heart and lungs. When the diaphragm contracts, it pulls down and creates more space in the thoracic cavity. This causes a

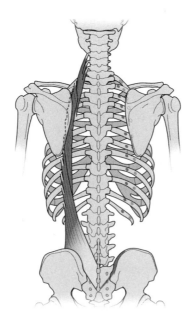

Figure 13.7 Iliocostalis muscle.

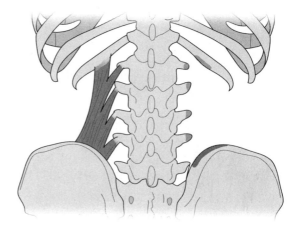

Figure 13.8 Quadratus lumborum muscle.

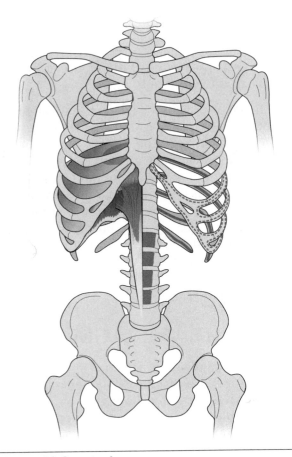

Figure 13.9 Diaphragm.

vacuum to occur in the lungs and air is drawn into them. When the diaphragm relaxes, it draws back up and air is exhaled from the lungs. The diaphragm generally operates without our conscious intention, but we can control this muscle for a short while to either breathe more forcefully or hold our breath.

- Origin
    - L1 through L3
    - Costal cartilage of ribs 7 through 12
    - Xiphoid process
- Insertion—central tendon of the diaphragm
- Action—flattens central tendon, increasing thoracic space and causing respiration

The diaphragm has three holes in it to allow the passage of blood and food from the thoracic cavity and above to the abdomen and beyond.

One hole is for the esophagus for food, one is for the aorta for delivering blood to the body, and one is for the inferior vena cava for draining blood from the body.

OTHER MUSCLES OF THE CORE

Several other small trunk muscles are not normally trained in the gym or considered important to movement. They are generally deep muscles that help move or stabilize the spine or assist with respiration.

Muscles That Perform or Assist With Respiration

In addition to the diaphragm, multiple layers of muscles are involved with breathing.

- Serratus posterior superior—four finger-like muscles in the upper back that raise the ribs during breathing
- Serratus posterior inferior—four fingerlike muscles in the lower back that depress the ribs during breathing
- Levatores costarum—12 pairs of small muscles that lift the ribs during breathing
- Transversospinalis—five deep muscles that help move the spine (107)
- Semispinalis—starts in the upper back and neck, goes to the neck and head, and helps extend and rotate the spine; similar to spinalis muscle
- Multifidus—starts on the sacrum and runs all the way up the back to the neck, helps extend and rotate the spine (often the location of a small knot in the back or a small pull of the muscles in the back)
- Rotatores—small muscles that start on the transverse processes of each vertebrae and run to the spinous processes of the vertebrae above it; help extend and rotate the spine
- Interspinales—small segmental muscles that go from one spinous process to another; help extend the spine

- Intertransversarii—small segmental muscles that go from one transverse process to another; help extend and abduct the spine; have some crossover with the levatores costarum
- Intercostals—located between the ribs; contain three sections: external, internal, innermost; help with breathing and maintaining posture (when you eat ribs you are eating these muscles!)

OTHER MUSCLES OF THE BODY

The neck and face are not commonly considered part of the core, but their muscles are often involved or contracted during exercises that train the muscles of the core.

Neck

Four primary muscles support and protect the neck. None of them is very long, but they are quite strong and allow the neck to move with a significant range of motion.

Sternocleidomastoid

This muscle is relatively large and easy to see. It is named for its origin, sternum and clavicle, and its insertion, mastoid process. It runs up and down the side of the neck. It is easier to see when the muscle is contracted, as when straining. It helps flex the neck, abduct the neck, or rotate the neck to the opposite side.

Scalene

The scalene muscles are several small muscles broken up into sections: anterior, medius, and posterior. They start on the anterior part of the cervical vertebral column and run down to the first two ribs. They help lift the ribs during breathing or flex or abduct the neck. They are hard to see on a person unless the person is extremely lean.

Splenius

The two splenius muscles are the splenius capitis and the splenius cervicis. The cervicis is longer and thinner, and the capitis is short and thick. They both start on the back of the spine in the upper back and neck region, insert on the skull, and help extend and abduct the neck and rotate the head.

Platysma

The platysma is a broad, thin, superficial muscle that covers the entire anterior neck surface and is easy to see when contracted. If you tighten your neck muscles and grimace at the same time, the platysma comes alive. It looks as if the skin is pulling up off the neck and chest (23).

Face

The face includes many muscles. People make a large variety of subtle movements in the face, and muscles must contract to cause those movements. For example, 6 muscles move the eye, 20 muscles create facial expression, 6 muscles are used for chewing, and 7 muscles are involved in swallowing—a total of 39 muscles.

CONCLUSION

This chapter provided a comprehensive overview of the muscles of the core. The origin, insertion, and action of each of the main muscles were described. A comprehensive list of exercises for those muscles was presented, and tips and techniques for optimally training those muscles were offered. This information will help personal trainers understand how these muscles function, how to train them properly, and how an injury to a specific area might affect a client.

Study Questions

1. What is the agonist in a conventional deadlift?

   a. quadriceps

   b. hamstrings

   c. rectus abdominis

   d. erector spinae

2. The rectus abdominis inserts on the _____.

   a. pubic symphysis and costal cartilages of ribs 5 through 7

   b. xiphoid process and pubic symphysis

   c. xiphoid process and costal cartilage of ribs 5 through 7

   d. inguinal ligament and thoracolumbar aponeurosis

3. Which erector spinae muscle does not insert on the skull?

   a. spinalis

   b. longissimus

   c. iliocostalis

   d. quadratus lumborum

4. True or false: The external oblique muscles produce trunk rotation to the opposite side.

   a. true

   b. false

5. True or false: The majority of the muscles in the trunk (abs, obliques, erectors, QL) originate superiorly and insert inferiorly.

   a. true

   b. false

Macronutrients

A book about personal training is incomplete without detailed information about nutrition. Clients who wish to gain or lose weight, alter their body composition, or improve their health must devote significant attention to their nutritional habits. Body composition is one of the five components of fitness, and providing nutritional advice is within the established scope of practice for personal trainers. Indeed, combining personal training with sound nutritional advice is a necessity, not just a nicety.

Three chapters in this book are devoted to nutrition. This chapter explains the key elements of the macronutrients; chapter 15 discusses micronutrients, water, metabolism, and the way in which nutrients are digested and absorbed; and chapter 16 provides practical guidance on nutrition, such as when and what to eat to improve athletic performance and ways to change a client's body weight and body composition.

The science of nutrition is the study of both the food that people eat and the way in which the body uses that food. The highest level of education in the nutrition field is a registered dietitian, or RD. This degree requires college work at the undergraduate and graduate level. Certified personal trainers are not RDs unless they have significant additional education. RDs are trained in the specifics of nutrition for special populations. A personal trainer who has a client whose nutritional needs fall outside his or her scope of practice should refer the client to an RD for nutritional guidance. For example, instead of giving a client with diabetes specific nutritional information, the personal trainer should instead refer the client to an RD for more comprehensive advice. Some, but not all, RDs are well versed in the field of sports nutrition, and many work with patients in a clinical (hospital) setting. For personal trainers, sports nutrition is of primary importance, and that is the focus of this book.

Only a cursory glance at the population is needed to indicate that significant nutritional intervention is necessary. As of a 2010 CDC report, 68 percent of the U.S. population is either overweight (a BMI of 25–29.9) or obese (BMI ≥30.0), split evenly down the middle in terms of proportions (34 percent are overweight and 34 percent are obese). BMI is not a perfect method for measuring body fatness, but it does work when looking at large populations. Interpreted another way, the number of people with a healthy BMI is a minority (32 percent) (17, 29). Approximately 20 percent of children age 6 to 19 are obese. We have become so accustomed to seeing overweight people that being 20 pounds (9.1 kg) overweight seems normal. Only when people are 100 pounds (45.4 kg) or more overweight do they start to feel obese or does the public begin to consider them fat. The staggering health care costs associated with excess weight and obesity, particularly in an aging population, are just now becoming apparent. The good news is that America is ready for a change. As a highly qualified certified personal trainer, you can be at the forefront leading the charge for a healthier nation.

The macronutrients are carbohydrate, fat, and protein. Together these nutrients make up half of the six essential nutrients for the human body. The other three—vitamins, minerals, and water—are discussed in the next chapter. In the field of nutrition, the word *essential* indicates that the body is unable to produce this nutrient on its own; it must be consumed for normal, healthy functioning. When deprived of an essential nutrient for a prolonged period, the body becomes ill, functioning is impaired, and death ultimately results.

The term *macronutrient* refers to big (*macro* means "large") nutrients. These nutrients are measured in grams and can easily be seen with the naked eye. You can look down at your plate and see the carbohydrate, fat, and protein found there; that is not the case with calcium or vitamin C. All macronutrients contain kilocalories; micronutrients do not. A kilocalorie is a unit of energy that is abbreviated as kcal (or referred to as calorie). It is the amount of heat necessary to raise one liter of water one degree Celsius. Human nutrition is measured in kilocalories, and attention is paid to both the kilocalories consumed in food and drink and the kilocalories expended, or "burned," by the body during activity and metabolism. For each macronutrient, you need to know its building blocks, storage form, fuel factor, recommended daily allowance (RDA) and suggested intake, key functions, and common food examples.

CARBOHYDRATE

Carbohydrate is composed of three primary elements from which its name is derived: carbon, hydrogen, and oxygen. Carbohydrate is sometimes abbreviated as *CHO* for this reason. Carbohydrate usually comes from plants. Plants, unlike animals, use photosynthesis to receive and convert energy from the sun. A plant receives sunlight and turns that energy into a form of energy that animals can consume and use.

Carbohydrate is consumed in significantly greater quantities than the other macronutrients in most diets across cultures and around the globe. Three primary reasons explain this pattern. First, carbohydrate is widely available, and it can be grown in some form almost anywhere humans reside. Second, carbohydrate is easy to store and does not spoil as rapidly as protein or fat does. Third, calorie per calorie,

carbohydrate is usually the cheapest of the three macronutrients. A few dollars can buy a good amount of rice or noodles but not a lot of steak or oil.

Types of Carbohydrate

The building blocks of carbohydrate are saccharides, which are a unit of sugar. There are three categories of saccharides—monosaccharides, disaccharides, and polysaccharides. Monosaccharides and disaccharides are collectively referred to as simple carbohydrates or simple sugars because they are simple, or easy, for the body to digest.

Monosaccharides

Monosaccharides are single sugar units, which are the simplest form of carbohydrate. There are three types of monosaccharides.

Glucose Glucose is the fundamental unit of a carbohydrate in the body. It is rarely eaten directly, but most foods containing carbohydrate are broken down into glucose through digestion. Glucose is found in the human body in the blood, and the blood contains approximately 5 to 10 grams of glucose in all, which is a small amount. Glucose in hospital settings is often referred to as dextrose (42).

Fructose The sweetest form of carbohydrate, which is found in fruit, is fructose. It is digested slightly differently from glucose; it goes to the liver first, thus slowing the rate at which it raises the blood sugar.

Galactose Galactose is rarely eaten, but it comes from milk. It is the monosaccharide used to create breast milk; it is used by all mammals to create milk for their young.

Disaccharides

Disaccharides consist of two monosaccharides joined together. The prefix *di* is similar to *bi* in that it means "two." Disaccharides are always made up of glucose plus another single sugar unit.

Sucrose Sucrose is a widely consumed carbohydrate, and it is commonly known as table sugar. Sucrose is composed of glucose and fructose; the fructose component provides its pleasing flavor, especially when it is combined with other foods.

Lactose Lactose is the sugar found in milk. Milk and dairy products are among the few animal products that are high in carbohydrate. Lactose is made up of glucose and galactose. People who are lactose intolerant are not able to produce enough of the proper enzyme, lactase, to digest lactose.

Maltose This sugar is rarely consumed independently (even in malt beverages), but it comes from the breakdown of starch. Maltose is made up of two units of glucose.

Polysaccharides

The final category of carbohydrate is polysaccharides. The prefix *poly* indicates that many, usually 22 to 30, sugar units are bound together. There are three main types of polysaccharides.

Starch Starch is the main type of carbohydrate that humans consume. Starch is usually composed of strings of maltose, so a single starch unit will yield many units of glucose. Starch is found in significant quantities in rice, cereal, grains, pasta, and potatoes and in smaller quantities in vegetables and fruit. As a rule, foods closer to their natural form contain forms of starch that are more beneficial (105).

Glycogen This carbohydrate is rarely eaten, but the body stores carbohydrate in this form for later use. The body packages up the glucose units into glycogen molecules which are then stored in the liver and muscles. When full, the liver contains about 100 grams of glycogen, and the muscles collectively contain about 200 to 400 grams of glycogen. Therefore, the human body contains 300 to 500 grams of glycogen. Body size, amount of lean tissue, and training status can affect the ability to store glycogen. Given that the fuel factor of carbohydrate is 4 kilocalories per gram, the body has approximately 1,200 to 2,000 calories of stored energy in the form of carbohydrate. This storage form will last approximately 12 to 48 hours if a person is engaged in light to moderate activity and 1 to 4 hours if the person is engaged in high-intensity activity.

Fiber This polysaccharide is indigestible to humans; we lack the appropriate enzymes to digest it. Your initial reaction might be, "Why should we consume something if we don't digest it?" In fact, in its indigestibility lies its usefulness. Fiber is beneficial to many bodily processes, but the typical American diet is low in fiber. Fiber binds with bile and cholesterol, provides antioxidants, holds water, provides bulk to the stool, cleanses the intestines, and creates a feeling of fullness in the stomach. Fiber can be water soluble (which means that it dissolves in water), or it can be insoluble in water (5, 7, 14). Table 14.1 describes the various types of fiber, where they are found, and their main function in the body.

Higher levels of fiber are found in natural, unprocessed plant foods. The closer a food is

Table 14.1 Understanding Fiber

Type of fiber	Solubility	Where found	Main function
Cellulose	Insoluble	Green framework of plants	Holds water, provides bulk to the stool, helps absorb minerals
Hemicellulose	Insoluble	Framework of brown plants (bran and grains)	As above; binds with bile
Lignin	Insoluble	Woody part of plants, seeds	Antioxidant, binds with bile and cholesterol
Gums	Soluble	Secretions of plants and seeds	Slows rate of digestion, may help with irritable bowel syndrome (IBS)
Mucilage	Soluble	As above; flax seeds	Helps with digestion
Algae	Soluble	Algae, seaweed	Binds with bile and cholesterol
Pectin	Soluble	Connecting material in fruit	Provides feeling of fullness, may fuel intestinal flora

to the way it naturally occurs in nature, the less processed it is. The RDA for fiber for men under 50 is 38 grams per day; for men over 50, it is 30 grams per day. For females under 50, the RDA is 25 grams per day; females over 50 require 21 grams per day. Men need more fiber because they consume more calories.

Other Carbohydrates

Aside from the common carbohydrates listed earlier, there are other types of carbohydrate. Sweeteners have become increasingly common; sweeteners can be both nutritive and nonnutritive. Nutritive sweeteners have calories and are often called sugar alcohols, the most common being sorbitol. Sugar alcohols do not raise the blood sugar quite as rapidly as other carbohydrate does, but they can cause diarrhea and are often found in highly processed foods. Nonnutritive sweeteners do not have any significant calories. The most common nonnutritive sweeteners are aspartame, saccharin, and sucralose. These sweeteners are often found in diet soda or low-calorie foods.

Although sweeteners are low in calories, a positive correlation is not found between the use of sweeteners and healthy body weight. Indeed, some studies suggest an inverse correlation. Some authorities believe that artificial sweeteners prime the sweet tooth and make the cravings stronger rather than satisfy them. Other experts believe that ingestion of sweeteners causes the body to think that it is consuming carbohydrate, to release insulin, and to promote the storage of fat. Although the Food and Drug Administration (FDA) has declared all major artificial sweeteners safe for human consumption, these sweeteners are anecdotally associated with significant health issues such as headaches, mental disturbances, and cancer. Sweeteners are often found in nonnutritious, highly processed food, so people would likely improve their health by eliminating or significantly moderating the intake of sweeteners.

Functions of Carbohydrate

Carbohydrate serves many important functions in the body. Glucose is the primary fuel for the brain and the central nervous system, so changes in blood glucose levels can affect the way that a person thinks or acts. Carbohydrate provides a high-intensity energy source. At rest, the body gets approximately 30 percent of its energy from carbohydrate, but as intensity increases, that percentage increases significantly. Carbohydrate is stored in the liver as glycogen, and that storage form helps the liver function normally. Finally, carbohydrate has a protein-sparing effect. Protein can also yield high-intensity energy, but the body prefers to use carbohydrate for energy and to spare (save) the protein for its primary function, which is tissue building and repair (10, 15).

Recommended Intake of Carbohydrate

Carbohydrate should make up 45 to 65 percent of the day's total caloric intake; any diet that is below 40 percent carbohydrate is considered a low-carbohydrate diet. The recommended maximum intake for simple sugars is 25 percent of the day's total intake if the diet includes fruit or 10 percent if it is does not include fruit (i.e., if the percentage applies only to added sugars). The fuel factor, the amount of energy provided per gram, for carbohydrate is four kilocalories per gram.

Quality of Carbohydrate

Much confusion exists about carbohydrate. Some carbohydrate is labeled good, and some is considered bad. Carbohydrate is often ranked on how rapidly it affects a person's blood sugar. The glycemic index (GI) and glycemic load (GL) are the two most popular tools used for this purpose. The GI ranks how rapidly 50 grams of carbohydrate raises a person's blood sugar. White bread is the standard, yielding a score of 100. All foods are given a score; the higher the score is, the more rapidly the food raises the blood sugar. The GL is a similar test, but it compares how the standard serving size of the food affects a person's blood sugar. This score is useful because it relates more closely to how people consume foods. Carrots, for example, have a relatively high GI, but a typical serving of carrots does not contain much carbohydrate. Therefore, the glycemic load of eating carrots is low. Eating a standard serving of carrots will have little effect on a person's blood sugar.

Role of Insulin in Carbohydrate Metabolism

As noted in the chapter about the endocrine system, insulin acts like a shuttle that takes the building blocks—glucose, protein, and fat—to the cells of the body. This action is beneficial and necessary, but if blood sugar rises rapidly, a large amount of insulin will be secreted to handle the increased level of glucose in the blood and a large number of building blocks will be deposited around the body, which can contribute to undesired weight gain. In addition, if the body is subjected to repeated spikes in insulin, regularly for months and years, the body may become insulin resistant, in which case the insulin does not work as it should and the blood sugar remains elevated beyond its normal range for extended periods. This circumstance can be a precursor to type 2 diabetes (13, 20).

Food Sources of Carbohydrate

Many approaches to nutrition and weight control can be successful, and clients can have success with both higher and lower carbohydrate options. The type and quantity of carbohydrate selected can have a big effect on both performance and health. Clients should remember the original guideline of selecting carbohydrate that is as natural and unprocessed as possible and then eat it in the proper quantity. Clients often don't know the standard serving size for carbohydrate, and eating too much is easy. Portion control is important for weight loss. One slice of bread, half a cup of cooked rice, and 1 ounce (28 g) of cereal are standard serving sizes, but many people eat two to four servings of those foods in just one sitting.

A good rule of thumb when shopping for carbohydrate is to focus on the perimeter of the store, which is usually where the fresh fruit and vegetables, as well as the more natural sources of starch such as yams and potatoes, are located. Healthy, high-energy sources of carbohydrate include all fruit, all vegetables, sweet potatoes, rice, potatoes, and natural oatmeal. Grains like wheat, pasta, and whole grains can also be healthy sources of carbohydrate, but for weight loss and body-fat reduction, they are best eaten in moderation. Some people are mildly intolerant of gluten.

FAT

Fat is made up of the same elements as carbohydrate is—carbon, hydrogen, and oxygen—but the chemical complexity is greater. The group name for fats and their related substances is lipids, and the chemical name for the fat that we ingest from the food we eat is triglycerides (75).

Types of Dietary Fat

The building blocks of fat are fatty acids. A triglyceride is one glycerol chain with three fatty acids attached to it. There are four primary types of dietary fat.

Saturated Fatty Acids

Saturated fatty acids are found predominantly in animal sources. The word *saturated* indicates that this fat is full; specifically, it means that all the available hydrogen bonds in the fatty acid are full. The fat thus has certain characteristics; namely, it is solid at room temperature (think of the texture of butter at room temperature). These types of fats have been labeled bad fats, but research on that topic has evolved. It now appears that certain saturated fats may be beneficial to health, although others may be detrimental.

Monounsaturated Fatty Acids

Monounsaturated fatty acids come mainly from plant sources. A monounsaturated fat has one hydrogen bond open, so the fat remains liquid at room temperature. The most common food item that is high in monounsaturated fat is olive oil. Peanuts are also high in monounsaturated fatty acids.

Polyunsaturated Fatty Acids

Polyunsaturated fatty acids also come primarily from plants, although fish is a good source of polyunsaturated fats. Polyunsaturated fatty acids have two or more hydrogen bonds open. Polyunsaturated fatty acids are liquid at room temperature, and they contain what are known as the essential fatty acids (EFAs). The body is unable to make the EFAs; those fatty acids must be consumed. Note that plants can provide these fats, so a vegetarian diet could adequately provide the fat necessary for health.

The two main essential fatty acids are linolenic acid (omega-3s) and linoleic acid (omega-6s). The EFAs have received a lot of press lately, and they seem to be involved in a host of body functions, including maintaining healthy skin, strengthening cell membranes, and sustaining proper brain activity. Diets deficient in EFAs can lead to hair loss, blood-clotting problems, visual problems, and learning disabilities. The recommended intake for linoleic acid is 17 grams per day for men and 12 grams per day for females. The recommended intake for linolenic acid is 1.6 grams per day for men and 1.1 grams per day for females, although not all experts agree with the omega-3 recommendations. An easy way to differentiate the two is to remember that 3 is lower than 6, and you need fewer omega-3s than omega-6s. The current recommended intake suggests approximately a 10:1 ratio of omega-6s to omega-3s, although many authorities believe that increasing the amount of omega-3s to a ratio that is closer to 3:1 would be optimal for health (121, 122).

Omega-6 fatty acids are found in vegetable oils and plants; the traditional American diet is usually not low in omega-6s. Omega-3s are found in fish, eggs, milk, red meat, wild game, soybeans, and flaxseed. Note that the quality of the food source has an effect on the type of fatty acids that it provides. Wild fish, cage-free and free-roaming hens, and cows fed a diet of grass provide significantly higher levels of omega-3s than farmed-raised corn-fed fish and hens that are contained and rarely, if ever, see sunlight. This circumstance is true even if the general carbohydrate, protein, and fat ratios are similar to that found in more naturally raised animals.

Encourage your clients to buy organic, natural, wholesome foods whenever possible.

Trans-Fatty Acids

A final type of fat is called a trans-fatty acid. Human-made trans fat was created when reports suggested that high levels of saturated fat might have negative health implications. In response, food manufacturers started to look to unsaturated fat as a substitute for lard and butter. Because the unsaturated fats were liquid at room temperature and their hydrogen bonds were not full, they did not behave like the saturated fats and were harder to work with. Food manufacturers got around this problem by superheating the unsaturated fatty acids and adding hydrogen to them, thus creating a trans-fatty acid. This fatty acid had a pleasing taste, was easier to use in foods, and had a good shelf life. Initially it was thought that this fat might be healthier than the original natural saturated fat, but that turned out not to be the case (8, 18, 22, 135).

As the principle of unintended consequences often predicts, trans-fatty acids were found to be significantly worse for the body than any type of natural fat, saturated or not. Public awareness has been increasing about this type of fat, and businesses are responding to their demands, but people have spent decades consuming a rather large amount of this type of fat. The negative health consequences of trans fat are still being studied, but it appears that it might have the following effects:

- Raise total cholesterol
- Raise LDL cholesterol
- Weaken cell membranes
- Decrease essential fatty acid utilization
- Increase risk of atherosclerosis
- May be more permanently stored as fat

Moderation is often a good policy to follow with nutrition. Research has shown that regular consumption of as little as two grams per day of trans fat can have long-term negative health effects, so abstinence is a good goal when dealing with trans fat. Commonly consumed foods that contain trans fat include the following:

- Most premade hot chocolate
- Cookies, brownies, and cake mixes
- Most pancake and waffle mixes
- Taco mix
- Flour tortillas
- Candy bars
- Many high-sugar breakfast cereals
- Potato chips
- Goldfish and animal crackers
- Most peanut butters
- Margarine
- Cool whip
- Marshmallow fluff
- Nondairy creamer
- Doughnuts

Types of Lipids

The form of fat in the bloodstream is lipids. When you have your blood lipid profile tested, your blood is drawn and the levels of lipoproteins and cholesterol are measured.

Lipoproteins

Fat is not water soluble, meaning that it does not dissolve well in water. Blood is mainly water, and it is the major transportation highway in the body. For fat to travel effectively in the blood, which is necessary, it must be wrapped up and packaged for the trip. Lipoproteins enter the scene here. A lipoprotein is a combination of a fat and protein, and its main function is to transport fat in the blood. Fat adheres to other fat molecules if they come in contact with each other, so a lipoprotein is essentially a protein envelope for the fat to keep it separate from other fats. There are two main types of lipoproteins.

Low-Density Lipoproteins These lipoproteins, also called LDLs, contain more fat and less protein. The primary function of LDLs is to take fat from the blood and shuttle it to the cells. Although sometimes referred to as the bad type of lipoprotein, LDLs are necessary and not inherently bad—you just do not want to have an excessively high level in your blood. LDL values above 130 milligrams per deciliter are considered a risk factor for coronary artery disease.

High-Density Lipoproteins These lipoproteins, also called HDLs, contain more protein and less fat. The primary function of HDLs is to take fat from the cells and put it in the blood where it can be used up or excreted by the body. HDL values less than 40 milligrams per deciliter are considered a risk factor for coronary artery disease, whereas values greater than 60 milligrams per deciliter are considered a protective factor.

Cholesterol

Cholesterol is a nonessential, naturally occurring product in animals. It is a sterol and is related to the hormone family. Cholesterol is naturally synthesized in the body, primarily by the liver along with other tissues, and because the body can produce cholesterol, it is not classified as essential. Cholesterol in food is found only in animal products; plants do not contain cholesterol. Cholesterol helps build cell membranes, facilitates nerve function, is part of the cell signaling process, can be converted to bile (which helps digest fat), serves as an important precursor to vitamin D formation, and may have antioxidant capabilities (38).

Public and professional opinion on cholesterol has changed over the years. A maximum intake for cholesterol is no longer recommended (it used to be 300 milligrams per day), and some people may not have to avoid high-cholesterol foods, such as seafood and eggs, that are otherwise healthy. Some experts are even beginning to question the role of cholesterol in heart disease, especially when it is examined as a stand-alone factor. For those wishing to lower their cholesterol, the task is more complicated than just avoiding certain foods. Consuming a high-fiber diet rich in the EFAs and getting plenty of exercise seems to help lower total cholesterol, lower LDL levels, and increase HDL levels a moderate amount. Drugs are available to lower cholesterol, but their protective value to health is unclear.

Functions of Fat

Fat has several key functions. Fat is a key energy source for the body, but it is a weak fuel and provides mainly low-intensity energy in contrast to carbohydrate, which is a high-intensity energy source. At rest, the body burns approximately 70 percent fat. As intensity increases, that percentage goes down even as the total amount of fat used goes up.

Fat provides essential nutrients to the body, including the EFAs and the fat-soluble vitamins (A, D, E, and K). Fat adds flavor to foods and helps keep people feeling full, or satiated. Fat in the body is stored as adipose tissue, which tends to have a yellowish, spongy texture similar to chicken fat. Adipose tissue is not all bad; it protects and cushions the internal organs, maintains body temperature, and provides a protective barrier for the bones and muscles. Fat also covers motor nerves in a protective sheath called myelin. Because fat is a good conductor of electricity, the nerves that are covered with myelin are more efficient than those that are not. Fat is used to build cell membranes, which are the walls of the cell. Just as the walls of a house keep certain things inside the house and certain things outside, the walls of a cell keep the necessary things inside the cell and the not-so-good things outside. If a cell's membrane fails, the cell dies.

Recommended Intake of Fat

Fat should account for 20 to 35 percent of the daily total caloric intake. The typical American diet is 35 to 45 percent fat, and that fat often comes from poor-quality sources. Fat is a calorically dense nutrient; its fuel factor is nine kilocalories per gram, over twice that of carbohydrate or protein. Fat is easy to overeat because it is dense in calories and tastes good. Consuming too much fat can have a variety of negative consequences. Excess fat is stored as adipose tissue, and too much fat can lead to obesity. Obese clients are at higher risk for heart disease, high blood pressure, stroke, type 2 diabetes, sleep problems, joint problems, cancer of the breast, prostate cancer, colon cancer, and gallbladder disease (42).

People can consume too little fat, and this happens with some regularity in the fitness world. People strive to get lean, and they believe that they need to go on a very low fat diet to become lean. That approach can work, but it is usually not ideal. Diets below 20 per-

cent total fat fail to provide the appropriate amount of EFAs for optimal body health. Little research supports low-fat diets for increased performance, and diets below 20 percent fat often cause the body to produce less testosterone, which slows metabolism and leads to muscle loss.

Food Sources of Fat

Vegetables and natural starches provide small amounts of fat to the diet. Good healthy fat sources include whole eggs, fatty fish, humanely raised animals, wild game, nuts and seeds, avocados, coconuts, and dairy products (milk, cheese, butter, and yogurt) from grass-fed cows.

PROTEIN

Unlike carbohydrate and fat, protein is composed of five fundamental elements: carbon, hydrogen, oxygen, nitrogen, and sulfur. These five elements are considered fundamental to life. Protein is the only macronutrient that provides nitrogen and sulfur; for that reason, among others, protein is essential. Because these five elements are found in anything living, some protein is found in all natural foods, but the highest concentrations of protein are found in animal sources.

Types of Amino Acids

The building blocks of protein are amino acids. The foods we eat contain 20 common amino acids (table 14.2). Amino acids can be classified as indispensable, sometimes called essential, which means that they cannot be manufactured by the body but must be consumed as part of the diet. Some amino acids are dispensable. This term does not mean that they are unimportant; rather, it means that the body can manufacture these amino acids by modifying the indispensable amino acids. There are 9 indispensable amino acids and 11 dispensable amino acids. Of the 11 dispensable amino acids, 6 are considered conditionally indispensable. Although the body can create those amino acids, under certain conditions

Table 14.2 Amino Acids

Indispensable amino acids	Dispensable amino acids	Conditionally indispensable amino acids
Histidine Isoleucine* Leucine* Lysine Methionine Phenylalanine Threonine Tryptophan Valine*	Alanine Aspartic acid Asparagine Glutamic acid Serine	Arginine Cysteine Glutamine Glycine Proline Tyrosine

*A branched-chain amino acid (BCAA).

the body is unable to make enough of them to meet its demand (42).

Types of Protein

A food that contains all nine of the indispensable amino acids is considered a complete protein. Complete protein is generally found in all animal products such as milk, eggs, chicken, steak, fish, and seafood. Soy, which comes from plants, is also a complete protein. An incomplete protein is a protein that is missing one or more of the indispensable amino acids. The significant majority of plant products are incomplete proteins. For example, apples, broccoli, peas, corn, grapes, rice, and bread all contain incomplete proteins. It is possible to combine two incomplete proteins to form a complete protein. Each of these is called a complementary protein because the two protein sources complement each other. It used to be thought that these protein sources had to be consumed at the same meal, but now the belief is that as long as the two complementary protein sources are consumed within approximately 24 hours of each other, the body can use them together.

Quality of Protein

Not all protein, whether complete or incomplete, is the same quality. Several tests are used to measure the quality of the protein found in food (32). See table 14.3 for a summary.

- Chemical score (CS)—This test measures the amino acid profile of the food compared with an ideal standard for the amino acids. The more closely the food matches the standard, the higher the score is.

- Biological value (BV)—This test is based on how the protein in the food affects the body's nitrogen balance. A higher number indicates a higher-quality protein.

- Net protein utilization (NPU)—This test measures the biological value of the food combined with its digestibility. No food is perfectly digested, so the scores for this test will always be lower than the BV. A higher number indicates higher-quality protein.

- Protein digestibility corrected amino acid score (PDCAA)—This score is a ranking of protein based on the amino acids and the digestibility of the food. A higher number indicates a higher-quality protein.

- Protein efficiency ratio (PER)—This test measures the rate of weight gain that an animal experiences when fed this type of protein. A higher number means that the animal gained proportionally more weight with this type of protein.

Protein Balance

A person is said to be in a state of protein balance if the protein being consumed is adequate to meet the body's daily need for protein. Protein is the only macronutrient that provides nitrogen to the body, so protein balance is often called nitrogen balance. This indicator is not normally measured by personal trainers, but other health professionals can measure a person's nitrogen balance, usually by testing

Table 14.3 Protein Scores for Various Foods

Source	CS	BV	NPU	PER
Whey isolate	>100	159	92	3.60
Whey concentrate	>100	104	92	3.60
Egg	100	100	94	3.92
Human milk	–	95	–	–
Cow's milk	95	93	82	3.09
Veal	94	–	–	–
Egg white	–	88	–	–
Unpolished rice	67	86	59	2.59
Cheese	–	84	70	–
Tuna	–	83	–	–
Chicken, turkey	91	79	80	–
Pork	–	79	68	2.57
Fish	71	76	72	3.55
Beef	69	74	67	2.30
Egg protein powder	69	74	61	2.20
Soybeans	47	73	61	2.32
Corn	49	72	36	1.20
Casein protein powder	82	71	76	2.50
Oats	57	65	–	2.19
Whole wheat	53	65	49	1.53
Polished rice	57	64	57	2.18
Peas	37	64	55	1.57
Sesame seeds	42	62	53	1.77
Peanuts	65	55	55	1.65
Lentils	33	50	30	0.93
Red kidney beans	52	50	39	1.40

the urine. If a body is in a state of positive nitrogen balance, more protein is coming in than is being used up. This state is necessary during phases of childhood, as the child grows into an adult, during pregnancy and lactation, and for a person seeking to add muscle mass (hypertrophy) (6).

The opposite state is termed negative nitrogen balance. This circumstance occurs when the body does not take in enough protein to meet daily need, particularly over a period of several days or weeks or longer. When the body does not consume enough protein, it turns to its own sources of stored protein to meet the mandatory daily need. Effects of negative nitrogen balance can include loss of lean tissue and decreased muscle mass and strength,

compromised immune system, impaired organ functioning, and impairment of other bodily functions. In children, prolonged negative nitrogen balance might lead to a slowing in the normal growth rate or growth retardation. It can also lead to kwashiorkor, which is a protein deficiency characterized by the edema in the belly, usually a swollen stomach that results from an enlarged liver. Kwashiorkor is thankfully rare in the United States, but unfortunately it occurs in some third world countries (69).

Functions of Protein

Protein has a variety of important functions in the body. Its primary function is to repair and build tissue. Tissue, in this case, does not refer only to muscle. Essentially all the tissues in the body—hair, skin, nails, organs, muscles, and so forth—are made from protein. You literally are what you eat, so eating good-quality foods is important.

Although there are only 20 main amino acids, the body can build an amazing array of tissues with those amino acids. A reasonable analogy is to look at the alphabet. From the 26 letters in the English alphabet, hundreds of thousands of words can be created, and a subtle change such as adding or subtracting a single letter can completely change the word. The vowels are the most important letters in the alphabet and are necessary to make sense of the word; they are analogous to the indispensable amino acids. The body can construct the various tissues it needs by recombining the necessary amino acids into various formations.

Most of this work goes to repair the tissues of the body. The cells of the body are constantly dying and being replaced. Even if you are not actively growing or building muscle, a moderately active turnover rate is ongoing, which means that protein is essential in all stages of life. If the goal is to build new tissue, protein will be used for that as well, and the protein requirements will likely increase.

Protein can also provide energy for the body. Protein backs up carbohydrate and as such provides high-intensity energy. When the body has enough of both resources, the body prefers to use carbohydrate for energy and protein for tissue building and repair, but energy production takes precedence over tissue building and repair. If the body is low on carbohydrate and needs high-intensity energy, protein will be used as an energy source. The fuel factor for protein is four kilocalories per gram.

Protein helps regulate the metabolism by producing enzymes to aid in the digestion of nutrients. Protein is used to create enzymes in the body. Specific enzymes are made up of specific proteins, and those enzymes are necessary to digest food. Certain hormones that have an effect on metabolism are made up of protein as well; examples are insulin and glucagon. Protein is also used to help control water balance. Protein helps hold water, and the plasma protein found in the blood helps ensure that enough water is always present in the blood. Protein can help neutralize the acidity in the blood. If blood pH levels rise significantly, the body can use protein as a buffering agent to balance the increase in hydrogen ions. Protein assists with the transport of a variety of nutrients; it particularly helps transport fat in the blood by lipoproteins. Finally, protein aids in the immune system of the body. Protein is used to build the white blood cells, or T-cells, in the body that help fight off illness and disease (21).

Storage of Protein

Protein is stored as muscle. It is not stored *in* muscle, as glycogen is; it is stored *as* muscle. Unlike the stored forms of the other nutrients, which are relatively inert, the stored form of protein contributes to everyday life, because the additional muscle tissue is able to help perform work. If protein is needed for energy, this muscle can be broken down into amino acids that can then be used for energy production. Protein will not be stored as muscle unless the necessary hormonal stimulus instructs the body to do so. In simple terms, a client must work out hard and consume protein, as well as the other nutrients, if the goal is to gain significant muscle without adding a lot of fat. Common sense tells us that simply eating a lot of protein alone is not sufficient stimulus to add large quantities of muscle.

If excess protein is consumed, the extra protein can be stored as fat. This path goes in just one direction. After the additional calories have been stored as fat, the body can't break down the fat and turn it back into protein (amino acids). The body usually has more excess fat than excess muscle, but that is not always the case with some people in the fitness world. The body burns first whatever nutrient it has the largest store of. For a normal client, the body burns primarily fat and generally a small amount of muscle as the client loses weight. But for a larger, leaner, more muscular person, the body burns a significant amount of protein unless there is a strong stimulus (hormones) to direct it otherwise.

Recommended Intake of Protein

A common question asked by a client is, "How much protein should I consume?" The answer is related to a number of factors. As discussed previously, protein varies in quality. In general, a person who eats primarily lower-quality protein sources needs to consume more grams of protein to compensate for the poor quality. If a person is in a state of tissue growth, either as part of the natural lifecycle (a child or a pregnant or lactating female) or because of personal goals (adding significant muscle), additional protein is required for optimal results. Also, the state of a person's health will affect how much protein is needed. People with chronic illness, burns, or degenerative diseases usually need more protein than healthy people do. Other factors that can affect protein requirements include body size and body composition, physical activity level, and the amount of the other macronutrients consumed in the diet.

Debate continues about how much protein people need. There are three main schools of thought when it comes to protein consumption (table 14.4). The first is represented by the RDA, which recommends that protein should make up 10 to 35 percent of the diet. The recommended intake for protein based on body weight is .8 gram per kilogram per day. This number is the basis for the common recommendation that adults consume 50 grams of protein per day. This number often aligns with about 10 percent of the caloric total coming from protein (72).

The NSCA suggests that approximately 20 percent of an active person's diet should come from protein. Using a body-weight ratio, the NSCA recommends consumption of 1.4 to 1.7 grams per kilogram per day. Because the RDA suggests .8 gram per kilogram per day, which aligns with about a 10 percent protein intake, it makes sense that moving to a 1.6 grams per kilogram per day recommendation (twice .8) aligns with a 20 percent intake recommendation. The range provided is to encompass all athletes. The general guideline suggests that aerobic athletes most likely need numbers on the lower end of the range (1.4 to 1.5 grams per kilogram per day) because they will use protein primarily as fuel during long bouts of exercise, whereas strength athletes most likely need numbers on the higher end of the range (1.6 to 1.7 grams per kilogram per day) because they will use additional protein primarily to aid in muscle building and repair (134).

A third school of thought contends that both of those protein recommendations are too low. Common recommendations that emerge from the bodybuilding and fitness media are that active people should consume 30 percent or more of their diet from protein. Thirty percent is still within in the RDA range, so the figure isn't crazy or outlandish, although 30 percent is high for protein. A number significantly higher than that, such as 50 percent or even 70 percent, should raise an eyebrow, and recommending a diet that differs radically from the RDA would be unwise.

As with the other recommendations, the fitness media also provides a guideline based on body weight in pounds: 1 to 2 grams per pound per day. One gram per pound tends to align with approximately 30 percent of the diet coming from protein, although that can certainly vary. Two grams per pound would almost certainly take a person over the upper RDA limit of 35 percent. This group argues that anything below 1 gram per pound per day is not optimal for people who are doing hard training and that those who advocate the RDA are underestimating the increased need for protein by athletes who train intensely on a regular basis. The response to this argument would be that because carbohydrate has a protein-sparing effect, consuming higher levels of carbohydrate saves the body from using protein as energy. Therefore, consuming extrahigh levels of protein is unnecessary if a person eats enough carbohydrate.

Food Sources of Protein

To apply the recommendations effectively, the personal trainer should have an idea of how many grams of protein per day the client is currently consuming. The most accurate way to calculate this is to have the client keep a food log and then analyze that information. A

Table 14.4   Protein Intake Recommendations

	RDA	NSCA	Fitness media
Percentage of daily caloric intake	10–35%	about 20%	≥30%
Amount based on body weight (per day)	0.8 g/kg	1.4–1.7 g/kg	1–2 g/lb
Sample female* daily intake	48 g	84–102 g	132–264 g
Sample male* daily intake	72 g	126–153 g	198–396 g

*Sample female is 132 pounds (59.9 kg); sample male is 198 pounds (89.8 kg).

simpler way is to learn some of the common values of protein in food, because significant patterns exist. With this information you, as the personal trainer, can estimate approximately how many grams of protein are in each meal that is consumed. Then, by adding the values for the meals together, you can approximate how many total grams of protein the client consumes each day. Here is the protein content of various foods:

- 1 fluid ounce (30 ml) of milk—1 gram
- 1 ounce (28 g) of meat*—6 to 8 grams
- 1 whole egg—6 to 7 grams
- 1 serving of carbohydrate—2 to 5 grams
- 1 serving of vegetables—3 to 5 grams
- 1 slice of cheese—4 to 5 grams
- 1 serving of peanuts—4 to 6 grams
- 1 egg white—3 grams
- 1 serving of fruit—trace amount to 2 grams
- 1 protein bar—15 to 30 grams
- 1 protein shake—20 to 40 grams (each scoop usually has about 20 g)

*Meat includes red meat, chicken, turkey, fish, seafood, and pork. The leaner the meat is, the more protein and less fat it has; the fattier the meat is, the less protein and the more fat it has.

There is more variability in the group listed, but these are common guidelines. For most clients engaged in regular personal training, a starting point of 20 percent protein intake seems logical and usually yields good results.

As the personal trainer gains a better understanding of how the client's body responds to exercise and diet, that number can be modified to reach the appropriate goal.

CONCLUSION

The macronutrients are three of the six essential nutrients for humans and provide energy in the form of calories. Carbohydrate comes primarily from plants, and its building blocks are monosaccharides. Carbohydrate provides the body with high-intensity energy. Carbohydrate can be stored as glycogen, and the excess can be stored as fat. Carbohydrate has a fuel factor of four kilocalories per gram, and the recommended intake is 45 to 65 percent of the daily caloric intake.

Fat is found in both plant and animal sources, but it is often more highly concentrated in animal sources. Its building blocks are fatty acids. Fat provides the body with a low-intensity energy source. Fat also provides essential fatty acids, helps build cell membranes, and helps in hormone construction. Excess fat is stored as adipose tissue. Fat has a fuel factor of nine kilocalories per gram, and the recommended intake is 20 to 35 percent of the daily caloric intake.

Protein tends to travel with fat, and thus it too is found in both plant and animal sources. Protein is more concentrated in animal sources. The building blocks of protein are amino acids. The primary function of protein is to build and repair tissue. Protein also backs up carbohydrate as a high-intensity energy source. Protein can be stored as muscle, and excess protein can be stored as fat. Protein has a fuel factor of four kilocalories per gram, and the recommended intake is 10 to 35 percent of the daily caloric intake.

Study Questions

1. What is the RDA for protein?
   a. 10 to 35 percent
   b. 20 to 35 percent
   c. 45 to 65 percent
   d. less than 25 percent

2. What is sucrose composed of?
   a. glucose plus glucose
   b. glucose plus fructose
   c. glucose plus galactose
   d. polysaccharides plus fatty acids

3. What are the fuel factors of the macronutrients?
   a. carbohydrate 4, fat 9, protein 4
   b. carbohydrate 4, fat 4, protein 9
   c. carbohydrate 9, fat 4, protein 9
   d. carbohydrate 4, fat 7, protein 4

4. Which of the following is a function of fat?
   a. provides high-intensity energy
   b. provides the largest share of energy for the central nervous system
   c. helps build cell membranes
   d. helps build collagen tissue

5. Which of the following foods is likely to provide a complete protein?
   a. broccoli
   b. peanuts
   c. salmon
   d. peach

Metabolism, Water, Digestion, and Micronutrients

In this chapter we look at the three components of metabolism, the role and requirements of water in the body and in the diet, and the steps of digestion and the structures of the body that are involved in the process. Further, we consider the many micronutrients that are critically important in maintaining a healthy body, despite the fact that their recommended intake levels are much smaller than those of the macronutrients described in the previous chapter.

METABOLISM

Metabolism is defined as the sum of all chemical processes, both anabolic and catabolic, in the body. The body has trillions of cells, and each one produces chemical reactions. Taken individually each cell is relatively insignificant, but taken as whole the body uses a moderate amount of energy each day (24, 36, 37). The body expends energy in three main ways: basal metabolism, physical activity, and food digestion.

Basal Metabolism

The number of calories that the body burns at rest is called the basal metabolic rate (BMR). This energy expenditure pathway has several other names, including resting metabolic rate (RMR), resting energy expenditure (REE), and basal energy expenditure (BEE). The BMR is affected by a variety of factors:

- Body weight—The single most significant factor in calculating BMR; the bigger the body is, the more total calories it expends.

- Organ size—Organs are metabolically expensive, meaning that they expend a large number of calories every day. The larger a person's organs are, the more calories they burn. See table 15.1 for the relative contributions of organs and tissues to body weight and BMR.

- Lean mass—Muscle is more metabolically active than fat mass, although fitness publications tend to overestimate how much more active it is. One pound (.45 kg) of muscle burns six calories per day, 1 pound (.45 kg) of fat burns two calories per day, so lean mass (muscle) is three times more metabolically active than fat.

- Growth periods—during periods of growth (children becoming adults, pregnancy, lactation), metabolism increases. Pound for pound, children have faster metabolisms than adults do; the metabolic rate usually peaks at age two and then begins to slow slightly through the remainder of the lifecycle. Pregnant females usually need another 300 calories per day in the second and third trimesters, and women need an extra 500 calories a day when lactating.

- Age—As the body begins to age, the metabolic rate usually slows down. This decrease normally occurs around age 30, and the metabolic rate tends to decrease 3 percent through age 49, 7.5 percent from 50 until 69, and 10 percent at age 70 and older (8).

- Body temperature—Core body temperature has a strong effect on the overall metabolic rate. For every 1-degree increase, the metabolic rate increases by 7 percent (14). If a person's normal body temperature is 98.6 degrees Fahrenheit (37 degrees Celsius) and he or she gets a fever that drives the temperature to 102.6 degrees Fahrenheit (39.2 degrees Celsius), the person's metabolism will increase by 28 percent. This higher metabolism is one reason that people tend to lose significant weight when they are sick.

- Hormones—The various hormones have different effects on the metabolism; some speed it up, and others slow it down. The thyroid hormone has a particularly strong effect; testosterone can also affect the metabolism. This factor, combined with increased organ size and increased lean mass, is the reason that males usually have faster metabolism than females do.

Many formulas have been designed to estimate BMR. One of the most popular, easiest to remember, and still highly accurate is the simple formula of taking weight in kilograms, multiplying it by a coefficient, and then multiplying it by time:

Males: weight (in kg) × 1.0 kcals/hour × 24 h = BMR (calories burned at rest per day)

Females: weight (in kg) × 0.9 kcals/hour × 24 h = BMR (calories burned at rest per day)

The 1 or .9 is the coefficient; the coefficient is about 10 percent lower for females because of the factors previously discussed. From this we can also deduce the following:

Calories burned per hour = weight in kg × 1 for males; weight in kg × 0.9 for females

Table 15.1 Relative Contributions of Organs and Tissues to Body Weight and BMR

Organs	Total weight in kg	% body weight	Metabolic rate (kcal × kg/day)	Total kcal burned by organ/day	% total metabolism
Average male (154 lb [70 kg])					
Liver	1.8	2.57%	200	360.0	21%
Brain	1.4	2.00%	240	336.0	20%
Heart	0.33	0.47%	440	145.2	9%
Kidneys	0.31	0.44%	440	136.2	8%
Muscle	28.0	40.00%	13	364.0	22%
Adipose tissue	15.0	21.43%	4.5	67.5	4%
Other*	23.16	33.09%	12	277.9	16%
Total	70 kg	100%		1686.8	100%
Average female (127.6 lb [58 kg])					
Liver	1.4	2.41%	200	280.0	21%
Brain	1.2	2.07%	240	288.0	21%
Heart	0.24	0.41%	440	105.6	8%
Kidneys	0.28	0.47%	440	123.2	9%
Muscle	17.0	29.31%	13	221.0	16%
Adipose tissue	19.0	32.75%	4.5	85.5	6%
Other*	18.89	32.58%	12	226.7	19%
Total	58 kg	100%		1330.0	100%

*Includes bones, skin, intestines, and glands.

Reprinted, by permission, from J. Kang, 2008, *Bioenergetics primer for exercise science* (Champaign, IL: Human Kinetics), 132.

Calories burned per minute =
(weight in kg × 1) ÷ 60 for males;
(weight in kg × 0.9) ÷ 60 for females

For simple generalizations, at rest most people burn between 1 and 1.5 calories per minute, approximately 50 to 90 calories per hour, and approximately 1,200 to 2,200 calories per day.

Physical Activity Level

The second significant way for the body to burn calories is related to physical activity level (PAL), sometimes known as voluntary work (BMR is considered involuntary because it must occur; it can't be shut off). This energy expenditure pathway includes activities of daily living (ADLs) and exercise.

In general, people are ranked in one of four categories depending on how active they are. Each category has a corresponding coefficient, which is used in the next chapter to calculate energy expenditure:

- Sedentary—These people participate in normal daily life but have little mandatory activity, and they do not exercise. The average daily activity would be the equivalent of walking 1 mile (1.6 km) or less. This level of activity yields a coefficient of 20 percent.

- Lightly active—These people engage in some extra physical activity outside the standard ADLs. A sedentary person who exercises two to three times a week with a personal trainer and a person who has a job that involves some extra activity fall into this category. Being a full-time personal trainer or a waiter or waitress would likely put a person into the lightly active category. The average daily activity would be the equivalent of walking 2 to 3 miles (3.2 to 4.8 km) per day at a reasonable speed (3.5 to 4 mph or 5.6 to 6.4 km/h). This level of activity yields a coefficient of 30 percent.

- Moderately active—These people engage in physical activity on a regular basis and would classify themselves as active. A person in this category likely has a full-time job that involves some activity and participates in a regular exercise program three to five times per week. The average daily activity would be the equivalent of walking 4 to 6 miles (6.4 to 9.7 km) per day at a reasonable speed (3.5 to 4 mph or 5.6 to 6.4 km/h). This level of activity yields a coefficient of 40 percent.

- Heavily active—These people are not likely to be personal-training clients. A heavily active person has a demanding physical job or engages in several hours of intense training every day. Marathon runners and triathletes fall into this category, as do collegiate athletes who train for several hours a day. The average daily activity would be the equivalent of walking 10 to 15 miles (16 to 24 km) per day at a reasonable speed (3.5 to 4 mph or 5.6 to 6.4 km/h). This level of activity yields a coefficient of 50 percent.

The most common mistake that people make when assessing themselves is ranking the intensity level of their workouts as their overall activity scale. People might think to themselves, "I work out hard four times a week for an hour. I must be heavily active." This ranking does not measure workout intensity alone; it also looks at how people spend most of their time each week. A week contains 168 hours. How is the person spending that time? In the previous example, the person who works out four times per week would likely be classified as moderately active or perhaps lightly active. If you, as a personal trainer can't decide which category a client falls into, splitting the difference is OK. In this example, you could use 35 percent (between light and moderate). If a client is trying to lose weight but can't be easily categorized, you could use the lower category. If a client is trying to gain weight but can't be easily categorized, you could use a higher category. Finally, you should realize that when you ask clients to recall their activity level over the previous week, they tend to exaggerate how active they are for fear of looking bad. Most clients will fall into the lightly active category after they begin working with you a few times per week.

Thermic Effect of Food

The final factor in calculating metabolism is to know the thermic effect of food (TEF), which is an estimate of the number of calories required to burn and digest food. As you will see from the digestion and absorption section in this chapter, those activities are complex processes that require energy. The more food we eat, the more energy we need to digest it. Each specific food item has its own thermic effect of food score, but calculating each individual food item consumed would be time consuming and cumbersome. Instead, we use an average of all food, which is 10 percent. That means that approximately 10 percent of the energy that people consume in terms of total caloric intake is spent on digestion. Protein and natural, complex carbohydrate like vegetables have a relatively high thermic effect of food. Simple carbohydrate, processed carbohydrate, and most fat have a relatively low thermic effect of food (24).

The total metabolic rate can be determined by adding BMR, PAL, and TEF together to yield the number of calories that a person expends per day. That number can then be manipulated to cause weight loss or weight gain, which is a key theme in chapter 16.

WATER

Of the six essential nutrients, water is the most essential, if that term is defined by how rapidly the body stops working (dies) without that nutrient. Oxygen is essential, of course, but it is not a nutrient. On average, most people can go about four to seven days without water, about a month without food (macronutrients), and months or years without certain micronutrients.

Water makes up 45 to 55 percent of an average adult female body and 55 to 65 percent of the average adult male body; the difference is mainly because of differences in the quantity of muscle tissue. Muscle tissue has the second highest water content of any tissue in the body, behind blood (it might surprise you to learn that blood is considered a tissue). The water in the body is part of a continuous system, meaning that at one time some part of the water could be in the arm, later in the leg, and then later in the torso. Although the body is divided into compartments, no waterproof barriers completely restrict water flow. Therefore, the water tends to stay where it is. Key particles in the water—electrolytes and plasma proteins—control where the water flows. Unlike an aquarium, the body does not have an active pump that forces the water to circulate in the body. Movement is one key way to force the water to move through the body.

As with most aspects of the body, homeostasis (the body's state of dynamic balance; *dynamic* means "changing" in this definition) dictates water balance. Things in the body are always changing, but the body generally seeks to stay the same. It functions a bit like a captain who is guiding a sailboat across the water. The goal is to sail in a straight line, but the wind and the water force the captain to turn the wheel many times, in both directions, to maintain that nearly straight line. Homeostasis affects body temperature, body weight, energy level, pH level, blood sugar, and water balance.

Water has many significant functions in the body. It is a universal solvent, and it provides the environment for many cellular reactions to take place. Water is a key transporter; blood transports many nutrients as well as the lymph fluid. Water helps the body regulate its temperature; we can consume hot water to help heat us up and we shed water, as sweat, to cool us down. Water is an important lubricant in the body. Water makes up the synovial fluid found in the joints, and it helps lubricate the wet tissues of the body in the gastrointestinal tract.

Water Requirements and Stores

Our need for water varies. The average sedentary female is thought to need 9 cups (2.1 L) of water a day. An equivalent male needs 12 cups (2.8 L) a day. This water need is affected by many variables, including how active we are. The more activity we do, the greater our need is for water. The environment also affects the need for water. Working out in an air-conditioned gym requires less water than playing American football outside in the middle of August. Health status affects water need. A person who has a fever, is vomiting, or has diarrhea has an increased need for water (58). Age also affects water need. Younger children, particularly infants, fluctuate in their water levels more easily than adults do. A person's total metabolism affects water need; a simple guide is that 1 liter (4.2 cups) of water is needed for every 1,000 calories burned. Taking drugs such as diuretics can also affect how much water is needed. A common recommendation for water intake is eight large glasses (16 fluid ounces [473 ml] of water per glass) a day. That recommendation likely is adequate, but scientific evidence behind that guideline is lacking.

The short-term goal of water intake is to prevent dehydration, which is a state of less than optimal water volume. The effects of dehydration are often noticed when a person loses 1 to 2 percent of his or her body weight in water. Some decrease in physical performance may occur. As the body loses more water, the person will likely become ill and have a hard time focusing. If the person starts to vomit, the loss of water increases, of course, intensifying the process. At 6 to 7 percent water loss, the body may not be able to control its temperature, and if the person stays in a hot environment, heat stroke could occur. A 10 percent loss of water affects kidney function and slows blood circulation.

People can also consume too much water. This process can lead to hyponatremia, which occurs when the blood doesn't contain enough sodium. As a person sweats or excretes water, sodium is lost. If a person consumes large amounts of pure water, the sodium in the system is further diluted with the new water that has been consumed. This excess water can cause swelling, weakness, and even death. This circumstance most commonly happens to people who are hypersensitive to water loss, to those who actually drink too much water, and to those who play drinking games that involve alcoholic beverages but substitute water for the alcohol (23).

Water in the body is located in one of two places. Most of the water is located inside the cells; this water is called intracellular fluid

(ICF). Visualize a cell as a snow globe. The snow globe is a glass sphere (the glass being the cell wall) that contains water inside it and some other things like some fake snow and a representation of Santa Claus. Inside the cell are the organelles, which sit in a pool of water, held in by the cell wall. If the glass sphere of the snow globe were to break, the water would spill out and the snow globe would no longer work. It could be thrown out. If the cell wall breaks on a cell, the fluid leaks out and the cell dies.

The cells of the body are all sitting in a giant bed of water. Continuing with the snow globe analogy, imagine that a thousand snow globes were all in a pool. Each snow globe has its own water, the intracellular fluid, but it is sitting in the pool. The pool represents the total body of water, called extracellular fluid (ECF), which is the fluid outside the cells. Intracellular fluid makes up approximately two-thirds of the total water in the body; extracellular fluid makes up approximately one-third of the total. In reality, the water in the pool (water inside the body) can flow in and out of the water in each snow globe (water inside the cells).

Water Balance

Water balance is managed by two relatively simple systems, at least when looked at broadly. Water is taken into the body, and water is excreted from the body. Water is taken in and made available for the body by three main methods. Water can be consumed in liquid form (i.e., a person drinks a glass of water) or solid form (i.e., a person eats food that contains water such as potatoes, rice, pasta, fruits, and vegetables), and water can come from a product of cell oxidation. The latter method is the least significant contribution to total water intake, but when nutrients are burned for energy, some water is released in that chemical reaction and the body attempts to use that water as well.

The body can get rid of water relatively easily. It can be excreted by kidneys in the form of urine, from the intestines in the form of feces, from the skin in the form of sweat, and from the lungs as part of breathing. Significant water is found in your breath; it is water that fogs up a mirror when you breathe onto it, not heat from your breath.

Particles in Water

As previously mentioned, particles in the water, such as electrolytes, help control the flow of water in the body. Electrolytes are a category of inorganic substances, usually minerals, that have an electrical charge. There are two types of electrolytes (48).

- Cations—positively charged ions. Examples include sodium, potassium, calcium, and magnesium, although there are many cations.
- Anions—negatively charged ions. Examples include chloride, fluoride, phosphate, and sulfate, although there are many anions.

Because these particles have electrical charges, they can interact with each other, similar to the way that one magnet can either push or pull another magnet without ever touching it. These particles are on both sides of the cell walls (some inside the cell in the intracellular fluid, some outside the cell in the extracellular fluid). The amount of electrolytes in either position will determine the flow of water, which can flow through the cell membrane (see figure 15.1). For example, sodium helps retain water. When people eat a high-sodium meal like pizza or Chinese food, they will have extra sodium in their system. Therefore, they will hold on to their water, and they will often feel thirsty as the body perceives

an increased need for water. People may weigh an additional pound or kilogram the following day because of water retention (59).

In addition to electrolytes, plasma proteins in the blood ensure that enough water is maintained in the blood to assist with normal blood flow. As the body loses water (through sweat, for example), some of that water will be drawn from the blood, causing the blood to thicken. But the blood must not become so viscous (thick) that it will not be able to flow properly. Plasma proteins help make sure that the blood has enough water in it to flow freely.

The body relies on hormones to help maintain water levels. The body produces antidiuretic hormone (ADH), which has the opposite function of a diuretic in that it helps keep water in the body. As an interesting side note, the consumption of alcohol suppresses the release of this hormone, which in turn causes the body to secrete more water than normal when alcoholic drinks are consumed, especially in higher quantities.

The body also releases aldosterone, a hormone that tells the body to conserve sodium. By saving sodium, which draws water to it, the body can hang on to its water longer than normal.

Acid–Base Balance System

One function of water is to help balance the acid–base system in the body. Personal trainers should have a fundamental understanding of how this system works. All substances can be ranked in terms of how acidic or basic they are, using a pH scale. The pH scale measures the

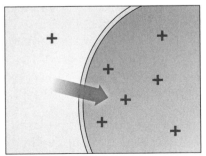
Hypotonic solution

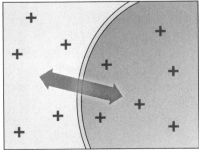
Isotonic solution

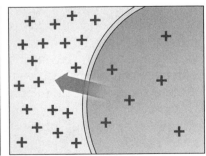
Hypertonic solution

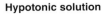

Figure 15.1 Particles affecting the flow of water across a cell membrane.

power of hydrogen. The more acidic something is, the more hydrogen ions it contains; and the less acidic it is, the fewer hydrogen ions it contains. On the opposite end of the spectrum is something that is basic, or alkaline. Substances can be ranked on the pH scale. A score of 7.0 is neutral. Anything less than 7.0 is acidic, and the lower the number is, the higher the level of acid is. Anything higher than 7.0 is basic, and the higher the number is, the more basic the substance is. The human body needs to maintain a pH of 7.35 to 7.45 (which is slightly basic) in the extracellular fluid for it to operate optimally.

The body balances out this system through breathing. Breathing faster helps fight acidosis (more common); breathing slower helps fight alkalosis (less common). The body can also excrete more or less hydrogen ions in the urine depending on need. The body is generally more susceptible to acidosis because of the environment and the types of foods that we eat, so it

tends to work hard to balance out the extra acids. The use of Alka-Seltzer helps explain this. A person eats too much acidic food, starts feeling poorly, and then takes Alka-Seltzer to help balance out the extra acid with a more alkaline substance.

DIGESTION

Digestion is the process of breaking down food, usually into its building blocks, and absorption is the process of up taking the nutrients into the bloodstream (72). Both are key steps that must happen to turn food into energy. See figure 15.2 for a diagram of the whole digestive tract.

Two main types of digestion occur in the body. Mechanical digestion is the process of breaking down food into smaller chunks of itself. If you grab a cookie and then crumble it up in your hands, you are left with smaller bits of the same cookie. You would not able to crumble up the cookie enough to separate out

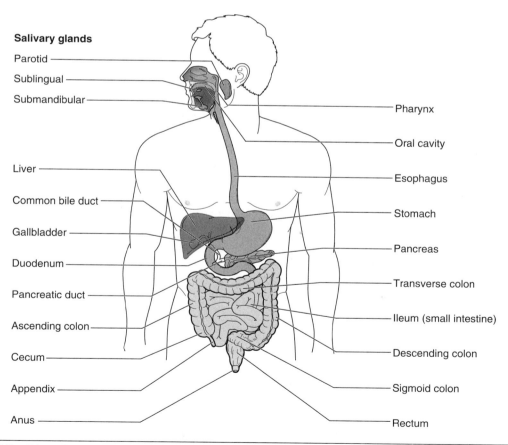

Figure 15.2 Digestive tract.

the carbohydrate, protein, and fat. Mechanical digestion generally takes place first. Chemical digestion is the process of using chemicals to break apart, and break down, the food into its building blocks. If you poured a digestive acid over the cookie, the acid would eat away at the cookie and leave not just smaller bits of the cookie itself but also new substances such as the glucose and fatty acids in the cookie.

Mechanical digestion is usually caused by muscles. Peristalsis is the name for the rhythmic, wavelike contraction of the muscles that move food along the intestinal tract. The movement is similar to the action that a snake uses to swallow its food. These muscles are in the gastrointestinal tract (GI tract). Remember that these muscles are made up of smooth muscle cells and that their contraction occurs involuntarily. Nerves detect the presence of food, and the process of digestion begins automatically (8).

Chemical digestion occurs through several means. One example is the use of acid. The stomach releases hydrochloric acid (HCL) to break down the food. This acid has a pH of nearly 1, so it is very strong.

The body relies on many digestive enzymes to break up food. Enzymes are made up of protein, and specific enzymes are used for specific foods. For example, the body needs the enzyme lactase to digest the nutrient lactose. Herbivores have many enzymes that people do not. Horses and cows can feed off grass, but we cannot. Carnivores lack enzymes that herbivores and omnivores have. For example, cats do not have the same level of enzymes to digest plants as people do because their systems are set up to consume just meat.

Mucus is used to help lubricate and protect the GI tract, and it helps break up the food mass. Water is a solvent that helps digest food and move it along the digestive tract. Bile is made in the liver and stored in the gallbladder. Its function is to help break down fat by emulsifying it. Think of bile as a hammer that smashes fat into smaller pieces. Fat is a complex molecule that takes a while for the body to break down, so bile aids in that process. People who have had their gallbladder removed may be more sensitive to the amount and type of fat

that they consume, but usually the liver adapts by sending more or less bile out as needed.

Digestive Process

Four key stages of digestion take place at certain points within the digestive tract. The goal of this section is to trace the path that food takes in the body and highlight what is occurring at each section.

Mouth

The first stop in the digestive process is the mouth. The food is chewed, which is a form of mechanical digestion called mastication (produced by the masseter muscle on the side of the jaw). In addition, enzymes in saliva can work to digest simple carbohydrates. Food like hard candy will therefore disappear if you suck on it on long enough, but more complex food like meat or broccoli will not disappear, even if you hold it in your mouth for a long time (chicken breast lollipops are unlikely to be the next big hit for nutritional supplements). The action of the enzymes is why consuming large amounts of sugar can lead to cavities. The enzymes hack away at the sugar to break it down, the sugar is stuck on the teeth, and the enzymes accidentally damage the teeth in the process.

After the mouth does its work, the food is swallowed and it heads down the esophagus. No real digestion occurs here. The esophagus is simply a tube that leads the food down into the stomach. Food generally spends little time in the esophagus.

Stomach

Food then enters the stomach, which can be thought of as a holding pot for the food. Some animals stuff food in their cheeks, but we store our food in our stomachs for digestion. The stomach then uses mechanical digestion to mix and mash up the food into a liquid food mass called chyme. Note that at no point does the body divide food into certain categories. For example, all the protein is not sent to one place in the stomach and all the carbohydrate sent to another. The food is all mixed up together. (People who are squeamish about one food touching another on the plate seem a little silly now, don't they?)

The stomach employs chemical digestion to begin to break down the food. Hydrochloric acid is released. This substance is particularly powerful in affecting protein, which is hard to break down. Mucus attaches to the food, helps it move along, and helps protect the stomach from its own acid. The stomach releases various enzymes, which work on the process of breaking down the food. Note that little to no absorption of food takes place in the stomach; absorption is covered later in the chapter.

Small Intestine

The small intestine, not the stomach, is really where all the action happens. Part of the job of the small intestine is to get the food fully ready for absorption, so it must finish the process of digestion. It employs both mechanical and chemical digestion to accomplish this. The small intestine uses five methods of mechanical digestion:

- Peristaltic waves—This rhythmic contraction helps move the food along the GI tract and break it up into smaller chunks.

- Pendular movements—The muscle cells contract with movements that mimic a pendulum, moving the food mass back and forth and mixing it up.

- Segmentation rings—Muscle cells shaped in a circle close when they contract. As the food goes through the ring, the ring closes down on it, dividing it into smaller quantities.

- Longitudinal rotation—Muscle cells arranged in a long arc move the food in a spiraling motion. This motion is similar to that of a cement truck spinning the wet cement.

- Surface villi—The wall of the small intestine has villi, which are like little finger protrusions that help move the food along. A simple visualization would be a centipede flipped over and held on its back; its legs would move as it tried to escape. The villi in the intestine move in a similar way to move the food along the length of the intestine.

The small intestine also employs strong chemical methods of digestion to break down the food. A large number of enzymes, released from the pancreas and intestines, are used to break down all types of nutrients, including carbohydrate, protein, and fat. The intestine uses mucus to move the food and help protect its own walls from the acid that came from the stomach, and it uses additional bile to help break up the fat. Hormones control the rate at which the enzymes are released into the intestine (34).

Large Intestine

Little actual digestion of food occurs in the large intestine. Food that makes it to the large intestine will likely escape the digestive tract, and the body will be unable to use it. The large intestine serves more as a way station for waste as it builds up and is prepared for excretion by the body.

Absorption

A key aspect in nutrition, and one likely not studied enough or given enough attention, is how the body absorbs food, particularly at an individual level. Food must first be digested before it can be absorbed. Bits of chicken and rice and broccoli do not float around in the blood; instead, amino acids, glucose, and fatty acids are in the blood. If a food is not properly digested, it cannot be absorbed. And even a food that is digested may not be absorbed.

Small Intestine

Little food absorption takes place in either the mouth or the stomach. Most absorption takes place in the small intestine. The SI (small intestine) is approximately 22 feet (6.7 m) long. Special structures inside increase the surface area and help with absorption. The internal walls have mucosal folds, or ridges, so the inside of the intestine is not smooth like a straw but ridged. Those ridges have villi on them, the fingerlike projections mentioned earlier, and the villi have microvilli, which are very small projections on the villi that help grab and absorb the food.

It has been estimated that if the entire surface area of the small intestine were spread out, it would be half the size of a basketball court! Essentially, a person has a giant net, half the size of a basketball court, stuffed inside the abdomen in an area that is likely smaller than 1 cubic foot (.03 cubic m).

To absorb the food, the food must come in contact with the walls of the intestine. If the food were to stay right in the middle of the intestine, it would not be absorbed. The body tries to ensure that the food contacts the walls by mixing, mashing, and flipping it all around. An analogy would be the cooking of ground beef. The goal is to take the ground beef and have all sides of it touch the frying pan. You do not just plop a pound (.45 kg) of ground beef in the frying pan, turn the burner on high, and then come back in 10 minutes to find it cooked properly. You have to mash up the meat, divide it into smaller sections, flip it over, and move it around so that all the meat is cooked evenly. The body is trying to do that to the food. You have to push the meat up against the frying pan for it to cook well, just as the body has to push the food up against the walls of the intestines for it to be absorbed.

Large Intestine

Not much digestion occurs in the large intestine, and little absorption of nutrients occurs there either, with the exception of water. The main job of the large intestine is to recapture and reabsorb the large amount of water that was used in the process of digestion. An analogy could be a water slide. A water slide needs water to help people slide down it (our GI tract needs to be wet to allow food to move through it), but without a mechanism to reuse the water, a tremendous amount would be wasted because the system is running constantly. So water parks have pools that collect the water, recycle it, and then use it again. Water is too precious to be wasted, so the body tries not to let water escape. The large intestine reabsorbs the water, which then is purified and used again. If a person gets ill and the large intestine does not function properly, it will not absorb water from the waste. Diarrhea is usually the result, which can give us an idea about the significant amount of water commonly reabsorbed from the digestive process (6).

Of course, this process is not perfect, and people must regularly excrete the remains of the process of digestion and absorption. The frequency with which a person defecates can vary significantly. Normal rates vary from as low as three times a week to as high as three times a day. A person who regularly has bowel movements more frequently than three times a day might be suffering from irritable bowel disease or another disorder. If a person experiences bowel movements less than three times a week, he or she might be constipated, but the normal range of bowel movements does vary greatly between individuals.

MICRONUTRIENTS

The micronutrients consist of vitamins and minerals. Like the macronutrients, they are essential to the body. They function primarily to build and repair tissue and to help regulate metabolism. But unlike the macronutrients, vitamins and minerals do not provide energy because they do not have any kilocalories. Therefore, the fuel factor for all vitamins and minerals is zero kilocalories per gram. In addition, the micronutrients are consumed and used in much smaller quantity than the macronutrients (hence the name). The macronutrients are measured in grams; there are 454 grams in 1 pound and 1,000 grams in 1 kilogram. A gram of a substance is typically visible to the naked eye; it is about the size of a pea or a raisin. The micronutrients are measured in either milligrams (1/1000 of a gram) or micrograms (1/1,000 of a milligram). Therefore, something as small as a multivitamin can contain, at least in theory, all the necessary micronutrients for the body. Cramming all the essential macronutrients into such a small package would be impossible, at least with current technology.

Vitamins

The word *vitamin* means "essential (vital) to life." Vitamins are small, organic compounds; therefore, vitamins come from something living or that was alive. Discovery of vitamins occurred in relatively recent history given how long humans have been consuming them. The first acknowledgement of vitamins or something similar occurred in the Age of Sail hundreds of years ago. Sailors in those years often got scurvy, which is a deficiency of vitamin C that made their gums bleed and their teeth fall out. Sailors travelled for long periods on slow boats and had minimal ability to store fresh food. Some sailors got scurvy, and some did not. Initially, they thought that scurvy was some sort of contagious disease, but it always went away when the sailors returned home. Ultimately, someone did an experiment in which one group of sailors ate limes and lemons on their trip and another group did not. Those in the group that consumed the limes and lemons did not get scurvy; those in the group that did not eat the fruit got it. Although the sailors didn't know exactly what it was in the fruit that was keeping them healthy, they knew that there was something in there different from standard carbohydrate, protein, and fat. This is where the term *limey* came from; the sailors consumed limes to stay healthy (3, 43).

Vitamins are either fat soluble or water soluble. This distinction indicates how the vitamin is stored and what the best carrier of that vitamin will be. Refer to the section later in this chapter for specific details about each fat- or water-soluble vitamin.

Guidelines for Intake

A variety of recommendations apply for vitamin intake, depending on their definitions:

- RDA (recommended dietary allowance)—an amount that in theory should meet the needs of most healthy people. The percentages on food labels are based on the RDA.

- EAR (estimated average intake)—the least significant guideline for the fitness world, EAR is the average requirement for the nutrient.

- AI (adequate intake)—an amount that seems to provide adequate levels and functioning. This recommendation is given if information on a vitamin or a particular group (infants, elderly) is insufficient to give an RDA.

- UL (tolerable upper intake level)—an amount that the American Dietetic Association (ADA) recommends that people not regularly exceed. This guideline and the RDA are the most debated in the fitness world.

Overall Functions

The understanding of what vitamins do is influenced by a common misconception. Vitamins do not provide energy. A nutrient must contain calories to provide energy, and vitamins do not contain calories. What vitamins can do is make the system of energy production run more smoothly. To use an analogy, if a car had a clogged fuel line, it would perform sluggishly. If a mechanic fixed the problem, the driver might believe that the car now had much more power. But the mechanic did not improve the engine or add more horsepower to the car. Instead, the mechanic simply got the car to function the way it was supposed to in the first place, resulting in the boost in performance.

Vitamins have several broad functions in the body:

- Regulate metabolism—Vitamins can be coenzymes in energy production. A coenzyme is a substance that works with an enzyme to help break down something. The most common example of this is the B vitamins. Collectively, they are coenzymes that help break down glucose and turn it into energy.

- Serve as an antioxidant—An antioxidant is a substance that inhibits (prevents) oxidation in plant and animal cells. As cells use oxygen as part of the process of living, that oxygen can damage those tissues. A half-eaten apple that is abandoned will turn brown; that process is an example of oxidation. The rusting of a metal object is also oxidation. In simple terms, oxidation happens inside the body, and because we are oxygen-dependent beings, oxidation is a fact of life. But we can try to slow this process as much as possible. Antioxidants fight the free radicals produced by the process of oxidation. Free radicals can damage or destroy cells; we know that cancer produces many free radicals. Antioxidants help fight off and kill some of the bad stuff in the body. In simple terms, they are like police officers trying to fight off the robbers. Each of the many kinds of antioxidants is best suited to fight off a different kind of free radical. For that reason, among others, eating a variety of foods is important. A blueberry might be high in antioxidants that are effective in fighting off one type of problem. A pineapple might have antioxidants better suited to fight off a different problem. All fresh living things provide some level of antioxidants because antioxidants are necessary for life. Processed food and food that has been dead a long time have much lower levels of antioxidants (6).

• Build and repair tissue—Many vitamins are associated with tissue building and repair. Vitamin C helps hold gums together, vitamin E is good for the skin, and vitamin A is good for the eyes.

• Prevent deficiency disease—Having proper levels of vitamins helps the body function optimally. If low levels of a vitamin are consumed, particularly over a long period, the body can develop a deficiency disease. Each vitamin is associated with a deficiency disease. In the world of personal training, a vitamin deficiency disease is rare, but in areas of the world where food is scarcer, deficiency diseases are unfortunately more common.

Fat-Soluble Vitamins

Fat-soluble vitamins (A, D, E, and K) are carried in fat, although eating an excess amount of fat is not required to get the appropriate levels of vitamins. Fat-soluble vitamins are more easily stored in the human body than water-soluble vitamins are. The benefit of this is that the body is less likely to run out of fat-soluble vitamins because it can draw on body fat to provide them. On the other hand, the body is slightly more likely to store excessive amounts of fat-soluble vitamins. This problem is most common with vitamin A.

Vitamin A Vitamin A is most known for its function in maintaining eye health, particularly its role in helping the eye adjust to various levels of light. Vitamin A also helps strengthen epithelial tissue, an example of which is the skin, and it can help the skeletal tissue and soft tissue during periods of growth. The chemi-

cal name of vitamin A is retinol. In foods it is commonly referred to as beta-carotene (53).

• RDA—for males it is 900 micrograms per day; for females it is 700 micrograms per day.

• Sources—beta-carotene helps provide color to foods, namely orange, yellow, or green, so foods that have those colors have high levels of vitamin A (specific food examples are sweet potatoes, Chinese cabbage, carrots, and liver).

• Deficiency—night blindness is an early sign of deficiency. Xerosis (inflamed eyes) and xerophthalmia (blindness) are full-deficiency diseases.

• Toxicity—hypervitaminosis A is the term for excessive intake of vitamin A, which is probably the vitamin most commonly taken in at excessive levels. An early sign of hypervitaminosis A is the skin taking on an orange hue. The UL for vitamin A is 3,000 micrograms per day.

Vitamin D Vitamin D has the chemical name cholecalciferol. Technically, vitamin D is not a vitamin because the human body can produce it when exposed to sunlight. Vitamin D is more of a prohormone, but a name change is unlikely. Vitamin D has a large number of functions. It works with phosphorous and calcium to build bone, helps modulate cell growth, works with the immune system, can help promote neuromuscular function, and can help reduce inflammation.

• RDA—15 micrograms per day or 600 IUs (1 microgram = 40 IU).

• Sources—fatty fish, fish oil, fish livers, and fortified foods (such as milk or cereal); exposure to sunlight (the body can produce several thousand IUs of vitamin with 15 minutes of sunlight exposure at peak times during the day).

• Deficiency—rickets, a disease characterized by weak bones in children in which the leg bones tend to bow under body weight.

• Toxicity—exceedingly rare with vitamin D and generally not a concern; the

UL for vitamin D is 2,000 IU a day (50 micrograms).

Vitamin E   Also known as tocopherol, vitamin E has several significant functions. It is an antioxidant, the most common one in the body for fat-soluble vitamins, and it protects the polyunsaturated fatty acids from oxidation. It has a partner that it primarily works with, the mineral selenium. It helps the immune system, helps cells interact with each other, and it can help with blood flow by keeping blood vessels healthy. Initially, vitamin E was thought to be an effective treatment for infertility, but little evidence supports that conclusion in humans (14).

- RDA—15 milligrams per day.
- Sources—nuts, vegetable oils, seeds, green vegetables, and some fortified foods.
- Deficiency—rare in adults; might interfere with myelin production or vision.
- Toxicity—exceedingly rare and generally not a concern; the UL for vitamin E is 1,000 milligrams per day.

Vitamin K   Vitamin K has two forms: a dietary form and an intestinal form. The intestinal form, produced by the bacteria in the intestines, contributes approximately half of the total amount of vitamin K needed by the body. Vitamin K is most known for its role in blood clotting, and it can help with bone development.

- RDA—has not been established; the AI is 120 micrograms per day for men and 90 micrograms per day for females.
- Sources—green leafy vegetables such as kale, parsley, brussels sprouts, spinach, and mustard greens.
- Deficiency—rare in adults; infants are often given a shot of vitamin K at birth to help with their blood clotting.
- Toxicity—has not been observed, so no UL has been established.

Water-Soluble Vitamins

The water-soluble vitamins (B vitamins and vitamin C) are stored in the water of the body, which experiences regular turnover. The benefit is that the body is less likely to store toxic levels of these vitamins because most are excreted in waste, although the body will run out of these vitamins sooner.

Vitamin B$_1$ This vitamin, also known as thiamin, is a coenzyme for energy production (8).

- RDA—1.2 micrograms per day for men, 1.1 micrograms per day for women.
- Sources—beef, pork, liver, whole grains, and enriched foods; small amounts are found in most foods.
- Deficiency—beriberi, which is common in Asia. Beriberi translates to "I can't, I can't," which represents the low energy level of the affected person. A deficiency in America is associated with alcoholism.
- Toxicity—has not been observed, so no UL has been established.

Vitamin B$_2$ Also known as riboflavin, this vitamin is a coenzyme for energy production and can help in the creation of antioxidants.

- RDA—1.3 micrograms per day for men, 1.1 micrograms per day for women.
- Sources—liver, beef, chicken, fish, milk, enriched foods, spinach, mushrooms, and avocados.
- Deficiency—usually occurs with other deficiency diseases; no specific riboflavin deficiency disease exists.
- Toxicity—has not been observed, so no UL has been established.

Vitamin B$_3$ This vitamin, also called niacin, is a coenzyme for energy production and DNA repair. Niacin is made from tryptophan, an amino acid, and requirements are given in terms of a niacin equivalent; 60 milligrams of tryptophan can provide 1 milligram of niacin. Niacin supplementation might help reduce total cholesterol.

- RDA—16 milligrams NE for men, 14 milligrams NE for females.
- Sources—liver, chicken, beef, fish, nuts, and fortified foods.

- Deficiency—pellagra, which causes weakness, poor appetite, skin and nervous system problems; it was common in the United States in the early 1900s, but food is now fortified with niacin.
- Toxicity—can cause skin flushing; UL has been set at 35 milligrams per day.

Vitamin B₆ Also known as pyridoxine, this vitamin is a coenzyme that works with amino acids and protein metabolism and is stored in muscle tissue.

- RDA—1.3 milligrams per day.
- Sources—liver, meats, chicken, potatoes, and fortified foods.
- Deficiency—rare in the United States.
- Toxicity—rare with food, but it can occur from taking supplements because it is stored; associated with nerve problems; UL is 100 milligrams per day.

Folate This vitamin is a coenzyme that works with DNA synthesis and gene expression (16, 57).

- RDA—400 micrograms per day.
- Sources—liver, beans, chickpeas, fortified foods, green leafy vegetables, and orange juice.
- Deficiency—can cause a specific anemia that primarily affects pregnant females and can cause neural tube defects in fetuses and children. All women of child-bearing age should supplement their diets with folate, which is called folic acid in supplement form.
- Toxicity—rare; very high levels might interfere with vitamin B₁₂; UL has been set at 1,000 micrograms per day.

Vitamin B₁₂ This vitamin is also known as cobalamin. It acts as a coenzyme that helps with blood formation and gene expression.

- RDA—2.4 micrograms per day.
- Sources—widespread in animal products.
- Deficiency—rare but can happen with a vegan diet; deficiency can lead to pernicious anemia; long-term deficiency can lead to nerve damage.
- Toxicity—has not been observed, so no UL has been established.

Pantothenic Acid This vitamin has many functions in the body; it acts primarily as a coenzyme for cellular metabolism and protein use.

- RDA—no RDA established; the AI is 5 micrograms per day.
- Sources—found in all food, particularly liver, yogurt, milk, fruits, and vegetables.
- Deficiency—has not been observed.
- Toxicity—has not been observed, so no UL has been established.

Biotin This vitamin functions as a coenzyme for energy production.

- RDA—no RDA has been established; the AI is 30 micrograms per day.
- Sources—found in most foods, particularly in corn, soy, egg yolk, liver, meat, and tomatoes.
- Deficiency—has not been observed.
- Toxicity—has not been observed, so no UL has been established.

Vitamin C This vitamin is also called ascorbic acid, and it may be the most common vitamin consumed as a supplement, likely because of its antioxidant properties and its use to reduce the duration and frequency of the common cold. Vitamin C also has important roles in tissue building and repair and serves as a type of cement for the wet tissues in the body, notably in the gums and GI tract (it aids in the production of collagen). Vitamin C is a strong antioxidant that helps in fighting the production of free radicals.

- RDA—90 milligrams per day for men, 75 milligrams per day for women; smokers should consume an additional 35 milligrams per day.
- Sources—citrus fruits such as oranges, lemons, limes, and strawberries and peppers, broccoli, and, in smaller amounts, potatoes.

- Deficiency—scurvy and its symptoms (bleeding and swollen gums, loss of teeth, fatigue, depression, and joint pain) can appear after one month without consuming vitamin C; deficiency is not common in developed countries that have adequate access to fresh foods.
- Toxicity—2,000 milligrams per day; symptoms commonly include upset stomach, diarrhea, and other gastrointestinal disturbances; some authorities believe that the UL should be raised.

Choline It is unclear whether this micronutrient is essential to humans or not. Choline helps maintain cell membranes and helps with the creation of acetylcholine (Ach), the neurotransmitter involved in muscular contraction.

- RDA—no RDA established; the AI is 550 milligrams per day for men, 425 milligrams per day for women.
- Sources—milk, eggs, liver, and nuts; widespread in foods.
- Deficiency—has not been observed with normal diets.
- Toxicity—rare without supplementation; UL is 3.5 grams per day; excess choline can cause low blood pressure, fishy body odor, sweating, and excessive salivation.

Minerals

Minerals make up the second category of the micronutrients. They are essential to the diet, are used in small quantities, and do not contain calories. But unlike vitamins, minerals are not organic. A rock might contain important minerals, but it will not contain vitamins. Minerals have some of the same broad functions as vitamins do. They help build and repair tissue and help regulate metabolism. Minerals are broken into two categories—major minerals and trace elements (18).

Major Minerals

The body requires seven major minerals in reasonably high amounts—100 milligrams or more per day.

Calcium Calcium is the most abundant mineral in the human body; approximately 2 percent of total body weight is calcium. Calcium has a broad array of important functions. It helps build bone and teeth, helps with blood clotting, helps the muscles contract, helps the nerves fire, and helps with other broad metabolic reactions (28, 38).

- RDA—1,000 milligrams per day.
- Sources—fish (with bones), dairy products, green vegetables, fortified foods.
- Deficiency—osteoporosis (a disease of bone) is associated with low calcium intake, poor calcium absorption, and lack of physical activity; osteoporosis causes the bones to become brittle, a condition that commonly affects older adults, particularly females.
- Toxicity—unlikely with food; too much supplemental calcium can lead to kidney stones or the decreased use of other minerals; the UL is set at 2,500 milligrams per day.

Phosphorous This mineral works with calcium to build bone and teeth, helps with energy metabolism as the building blocks of the nutrients are turned into ATP, and controls the pH of the body.

- RDA—700 milligrams per day.
- Sources—widespread; liver, yogurt, animal products, nuts, dairy products, and potatoes.
- Deficiency—rare with a normal diet.
- Toxicity—rare, but excess phosphorous may lead to bone loss; the UL is 4,000 milligrams per day.

Sodium This mineral, which is also an electrolyte, is the mineral that people usually eat the most of each day in the form of salt. Sodium helps maintain water balance, helps maintain normal blood pressure, helps muscles contract, and helps nutrients be absorbed (60).

- RDA—no RDA has been established; an AI has been set at 1,500 milligrams per day.

- Sources—widespread in natural foods but not found in large amounts; can be added to food by salting food; often found in large amounts in processed and packaged foods, preserved food, and junk food.
- Deficiency—rare for adults in America, but it can happen with athletes who sweat excessively; deficiency causes cramping and improper water balance (note that water alone does not replace sodium levels).
- Toxicity—most people can excrete excessive sodium through the urine, which can cause hypertension; the UL is set at 2,300 milligrams per day; people who sweat excessively even at rest may need more than this amount.

Potassium   Potassium is another electrolyte that has widespread functions in the body. Sodium is prevalent, but the body contains about twice as much potassium as it does sodium. Therefore, the general recommendation is to consume twice as much potassium as sodium in the diet. Potassium helps maintain water balance, convert glucose to glycogen, contract muscles, release insulin, and maintain blood pressure.

- RDA—no RDA has been established; an AI has been set at 4,700 milligrams per day.
- Sources—found in many foods, particularly natural unprocessed foods such as prunes, potatoes, yogurt, orange juice, bananas, milk, meats, and beans.
- Deficiency—more likely to occur in a chronically ill person or someone on diuretics or antihypertension medication; symptoms include weakness, breathing difficulties, heart problems, and bloating.
- Toxicity—rare without medical intervention; UL has not been established.

Chloride   Chloride is most commonly found in the body in the extracellular fluid. It helps with digestion by aiding the body in producing hydrochloric acid. Also, chloride helps red blood cells function properly by maintaining the electrical balance within cells and water balance in the body.

- RDA—no RDA established; AI set at 2.3 grams per day.
- Source—table salt.
- Deficiency—rare under normal conditions; can occur if excessive fluid is lost through vomiting or diarrhea, which could cause acidosis.
- Toxicity—rare; UL has not been established.

Magnesium   Magnesium has many important functions in the body. It helps aid in general metabolism (it is a common cofactor in many enzymatic reactions), protein synthesis, muscle contractions (by allowing the sarcoplasmic reticulum to function), and secretion of the thyroid hormone.

- RDA—420 milligrams per day for males, 320 milligrams per day for females.
- Sources—common in many foods; good sources include nuts, seafood, beans, and green vegetables.
- Deficiency—rare; symptoms can include weakness, cramps, and hypertension.
- Toxicity—rare from food; UL for supplemental intake only is 350 milligrams per day.

Sulfur   An extremely prevalent mineral found in protein (and thus anything living), sulfur helps with hair, skin, and nail creation; is a cofactor in metabolic reactions; helps create vitamins thiamin and biotin; and helps create collagen.

- RDA—none given because sulfur comes with protein.
- Sources—good protein sources such as chicken, beef, eggs, dairy products, beans, and nuts.
- Deficiency—not observed.
- Toxicity—no toxicity has been observed; no UL has been established.

Trace Elements

Eighteen trace elements, which are minerals, are required by the body in small amounts of less than 100 milligrams per day. The nine most important trace elements are listed here.

Iron Likely the most significant trace element, iron has been extensively studied. Iron is used to help build heme, which is part of a red blood cell (RBC). The RBCs carry oxygen in the body. Iron is also used to help build myoglobin, which is a protein that carries oxygen inside the muscle cell. Iron is also involved in many metabolic reactions including energy production, detoxification, and collagen synthesis (63, 78).

- RDA—8 milligrams per day for males, 18 milligrams per day for females (8 milligrams per day after age 50); females need more iron because of frequent blood loss during the menstrual cycle.
- Sources—a variety of foods such as liver, meat, eggs, vegetables, and fortified foods; aids in absorption of iron.
- Deficiency—anemia, which is a low level of RBCs or RBC hemoglobin in the blood that leads to feelings of tiredness, low energy, and fatigue, and can ultimately lead to death. In developing countries across the world, anemia is considered the most common nutrition problem by the World Health Organization, and it is usually a top 10 cause of death in those countries. For personal-training clients, anemia is unlikely to lead to death, but it can occur, more often with female clients who are on calorie-restricted diets.
- Toxicity—toxicity can be a real problem; an extremely large amount of iron can be fatal in a single dose. This tragedy more commonly affects children who find and eat a bottleful of pills. Adults who chronically consume high levels of iron can also damage their bodies over time. Short-term symptoms include illness. Long-term problems include organ damage and central nervous system problems that can lead to death. The UL for iron is 45 milligrams per day.

Iodine The primary function of iodine is to help the body build the hormone (thyroxine) that is related to the thyroid hormone that helps control the basal metabolic rate (79).

- RDA—150 micrograms per day.
- Sources—seafood and salt.
- Deficiency—goiter, an enlargement of the thyroid gland, which can become very large. If females experience a deficiency in iodine during adolescence and pregnancy, their children may have cretinism, which may cause a child to have a physical deformity, dwarfism, or mental challenges. Iodine can also affect the function of the thyroid gland, leading to hypothyroidism or hyperthyroidism.
- Toxicity—unlikely from food; excess from supplements may lead to acne or similar problems; the UL has been established at 1,100 micrograms per day.

Zinc Zinc is widely present in the body. It functions broadly as part of enzymes, maintains the immune system, helps with the storage of insulin, acts as an antioxidant for the RBCs, and is involved in sensual perception, particularly of taste and smell. Zinc is especially important during periods of growth and physical development.

- RDA—no RDA established; AI is 11 milligrams per day for men, 8 milligrams per day for women.
- Sources—meat and seafood.
- Deficiency—rare, but symptoms can include poor wound healing, hair loss, diarrhea, and skin problems; important for pregnant and breastfeeding females.
- Toxicity—rare from food; excessive supplementation may cause illness and decreased immune function; can lead to a copper deficiency; UL has been established at 40 milligrams per day.

Selenium Selenium works with ~~vitamin~~ E and is an important antioxidant. It is found in all tissues in the body except fat.

- RDA—55 micrograms per day.
- Sources—organ meats, meat, and seafood are good sources; grains vary.

- Deficiency—compromises the immune system and, if severe, can affect the functioning of the heart.
- Toxicity—rare but can lead to brittle hair and nails and upset stomach (11); the UL has been set at 400 micrograms per day.

Fluoride This mineral is best known for its relationship to calcium and the idea that it helps protect the teeth and properly form bone. Fluoride is commonly added to water in the United States, and it is often an ingredient in toothpaste. The prudence of adding fluoride to water is subject to debate; some countries ban it.

- RDA—no RDA established; an AI has been set at 4 milligrams per day for men and 3 milligrams per day for women.
- Sources—fish and tea.
- Deficiency—an increase in dental carries and possibly poor bone development.
- Toxicity—fluorosis, which can negatively affect the teeth by causing spots, pitting, or molding; the UL for fluoride is 10 milligrams per day.

Copper This mineral works with iron and has similar functions, including working as a coenzyme and helping build components of red blood cells.

- RDA—900 micrograms per day.
- Sources—organ meats, seafood, nuts, legumes, and grains.
- Deficiency—rare; usually associated with an iron deficiency or excess zinc; can contribute to anemia.
- Toxicity—the UL has been set at 10 milligrams per day.

Manganese Manganese is an important component of cell enzymes.

- RDA—no RDA has been established; an AI has been set at 2.3 milligrams per day for men and 1.8 milligrams per day for women.
- Sources—plants.

- Deficiency—rare; can be associated with diabetes.
- Toxicity—rare from food; UL has been set at 11 milligrams per day.

Chromium Chromium works with insulin and is commonly marketed as a supplement that will increase insulin sensitivity and fight insulin resistance, although scientific backing for those claims is lacking (25).

- RDA—no RDA has been established; the AI is 35 micrograms per day for men and 25 micrograms per day for women.
- Sources—grains and cereals.
- Deficiency—rare without medical intervention.
- Toxicity—has not been observed; no UL has been established.

Molybdenum Molybdenum is similar to manganese in that it is a component in cell enzymes.

- RDA—45 micrograms per day.
- Sources—organ meats, eggs, milk, grains, and vegetables.
- Deficiency—very rare.
- Toxicity—rare with food; UL is 2,000 micrograms per day.

Phytonutrients

In addition to vitamins and minerals, substances called phytonutrients occur in plants and animals. Phytonutrients are needed in small amounts; the absence of most is unlikely to cause deficiency diseases, but they are important to health. These phytonutrients are just beginning to be studied. The number of phytonutrients reportedly exceeds 25,000, and their absence may be associated with chronic health problems. This information is important to personal trainers in terms of the food choices that their clients make. Whole foods are better than supplements because they likely contain elements or aspects that make the foods work together and be easier to absorb. To get the proper phytonutrients from food, the suggestion is to eat a healthy variety of food that covers a broad range of colors, particularly in plant foods. Good colors to look for include red, green, white green, orange yellow, orange, yellow green, and red purple foods.

Vitamin and Mineral Supplementation

After studying vitamins and minerals and their beneficial effects on health, a logical question to ask is, "Should people take supplements?" As with most topics on nutrition, the answer is not clear-cut.

In general, people have attitudes when it comes to supplement use. All parties generally agree on the first point. A person who is found to be deficient in a vitamin or mineral (self-diagnosis is not preferred; blood tests or other tests conducted by a doctor are the best way to tell) should take a supplement to help correct the deficiency. Most also agree that the person should seek to fix or correct his or her diet so that the deficiency can be corrected through food intake. Even so, taking a supplement is recommended to provide additional protection against a deficiency. Clients should consult a health care professional before adding a supplement if any risk factors are present.

The second part of the debate about supplements is the value of megadoses, and this area provides significantly more fire for the debate. Two schools of thought weigh in on the issue. On one side are those who believe that the RDAs may be able to maintain adequate levels of health and fitness but cannot provide optimal levels of health and fitness. This group also usually argues that athletes or those engaged in hard training programs need more nutrients than their sedentary counterparts do. They point to evidence in support of this position in studies that suggest the following: People who take supplements live longer; antioxidants may help fight free radicals that can be produced by intense training; soil quality is not what it was hundreds of years ago, so the food consumed today is less nutritionally dense than the same food of an earlier time; and people need extra nutrients to help counteract the greater stress and more environmental toxins in today's society. These people tend to argue

for megadoses, or large quantities of vitamins and minerals, particularly for active people. They also point out that many of the studies on vitamins (which tend to show little positive benefit) were conducted in the 1950s or around that time and that supplement technology has improved since then. Vitamin and mineral remedies are more common in the East than in the West and have been around a long time. Current medicinal strategy often involves using high levels of vitamins or minerals to treat certain problems. This group also points out that although the more conservative group is against supplements for active people, they often suggest supplements for pregnant and lactating females, kids, and people who are suffering from significant health problems.

The ADA (American Dietetic Association), which puts forth the RDAs, most registered dietitians, and medical doctors are usually against megadoses. They cite the following evidence: The bulk of supplement studies show no positive effects; some supplements can be taken in toxic levels that can have significant negative health effects; although studies do show that those who take supplements live longer, no supplement, when isolated, seems to have that effect, so the type of person who takes a supplement (concerned about health) is what causes the person to live longer—not the supplement. They argue that the RDAs have been set above the EAR and should be enough for all people, even if they are active, and they point out that active people consume more calories and thus more nutrients anyway. A strong placebo effect often accounts for the anecdotal evidence heard when people talk about what taking a certain vitamin or mineral did for them. In addition, food can act like a drug, and although a vitamin or mineral might produce a certain effect (for example, calcium builds bone), an excess of that substance does not necessarily produce an even stronger effect (excess calcium does not necessarily make bones extrastrong) (2).

The bottom line is that a consensus has not been reached. Many athletes take additional vitamins and minerals as a way to cover their bases, figuring that it probably won't hurt and might help. Bill Starr, author of the classic text

The Strongest Shall Survive, provided guidelines for those who wish to consume higher levels of vitamins and minerals than suggested by the RDA (62).

CONCLUSION

Metabolism is measured by the number of kilocalories burned per day by a person. Three key factors are combined to calculate total metabolism. Basal, or resting, metabolic rate is most affected by weight and gender, and it constitutes most of the metabolic expenditure. Physical activity level also affects the quantity of kilocalories burned, as does the thermic effect of food.

Adults are made up largely of water; about one-half to two-thirds of a client's weight comes from water. Water helps regulate the metabolism and transport nutrients. It is a lubricant and a solvent. It provides form and structure, and it carries water-soluble vitamins. Particles in the water determine where it flows in the body.

Digestion is the process of breaking down food into its building blocks; absorption is the process of taking up those building blocks into the body. Digestion occurs in two primary ways: mechanical and chemical. Food travels along the GI tract, and digestion occurs at four primary sites: the mouth, the stomach, the small intestine, and the large intestine. The small intestine is the primary site for absorption.

The micronutrients are vitamins and minerals. They are essential to the body but are used in small amounts. Vitamins are classified as either fat soluble (A, D, E, and K) or water soluble (Bs, C). Minerals are inorganic compounds and are further classified as major minerals (calcium, phosphorous, sodium, potassium, chloride, magnesium, and sulfur) or trace elements. Vitamins and minerals collectively serve to build and repair tissue as well as regulate metabolism, but they do not provide energy to the body because they lack kilocalories.

Study Questions

1. What is the normal pH of the extracellular fluid in the human body?
   a. 5.4
   b. 6.4
   c. 7.4
   d. 8.4

2. Which of the following factors contributes the most to a normal person's caloric output per day?
   a. basal metabolic rate
   b. physical activity level
   c. thermic effect of food
   d. age

3. Approximately how many calories does 1 pound (.45 kg) of lean muscle burn per day?
   a. 6 kilocalories per day
   b. 20 kilocalories per day
   c. 50 kilocalories per day
   d. 150 kilocalories per day

4. Which vitamin is most associated with eye health?
   a. A
   b. B_3
   c. C
   d. D

5. What two minerals have primary roles in bone growth?
   a. selenium and choline
   b. iodine and iron
   c. sodium and potassium
   d. calcium and phosphorous

Practical Application of Nutritional Knowledge

Working with clients who are overweight, overfat, or need to gain weight is certainly worthwhile. Many, if not nearly all, clients have goals or at least questions surrounding this topic. Clients use (or will want to use) many weight-loss practices, but the personal trainer needs to guide and advise clients to follow safer and more effective strategies for fat loss and weight gain. One of the central approaches is calculating the client's metabolic rate and applying the concept of energy balance to make changes in body composition. The personal trainer should understand the types of food that are ideal to consume before and after a workout and provide clients with examples of sample diets that can help them reach their nutritional goals.

OVERWEIGHT AND OVERFAT

To understand these terms, we must first define them. Overweight is defined as having a BMI score of 25 or greater or being 10 percent over the recommended weight for height. Obesity is defined as having a BMI score of 30 or greater (see table 3.2) or being 20 percent over the recommended weight for height (11). Note that this guideline applies to Americans; other countries have their own standards (for example, obesity in Japan is a BMI of over 25).

Remember that BMI does not consider body fat; it simply compares weight with height. BMI is useful when looking at populations as whole,

but it is not as useful when looking at individual clients. Height and weight charts should be one tool among many that personal trainers use to evaluate and assess their clients; charts should not be followed religiously or applied blindly. People vary significantly in frame size, physical activity, age, desired weight, natural weight, and the necessity for body fat (36).

Definitions of overfat and obesity in terms of body fat percentages can be vague. In general, an unhealthy level of body fat is over 25 percent for males and over 35 percent for females. See table 16.1 for more classifications for men and women based on percent body fat.

A multitude of health problems are associated with excess weight and excess body fat. Those problems include increased risk of heart disease, hypertension, stroke, and type 2 diabetes. Excess weight also contributes to insulin resistance, joint problems, sleep problems, and reflux disease (22). Carrying large amounts of extra fat also worsens the risk for certain cancers such as breast, colon, and prostate cancer. A social stigma against those who are overweight places significant social pressure on people of both genders, particularly females, to be thin.

Why people are obese is not completely understood. Energy balance clearly plays a large factor. At some level, if positive energy balance is maintained for too long, the body will store significant extra weight. But exactly how certain factors affect the energy balance scales, on both sides of the equation, remains to be clearly understood. Genetic factors appear

Table 16.1 Classifications of Percent Body Fat for Men and Women

Body type	Men	Women
Athlete	<10%	<17%
Lean	10–15%	17–22%
Normal	15–18%	22–25%
Above average	18–20%	25–29%
Overweight	20–25%	29–35%
Obese	>25%	>35%

Data from William's Basic Nutrition and Diet Therapy.

to have a role in obesity, and people can be predisposed to becoming obese. Predisposition is not a guarantee; it simply means that a person is more likely to have that issue happen (34). A person can be predisposed to becoming an alcoholic if alcoholism runs in the family, but if the person never consumes alcohol, he or she will never become an alcoholic. A person who knows that obesity tends to run in his or her family can be extravigilant in fighting against weight gain. Preventing weight gain is much easier than causing weight loss. Family reinforcement teaches a person how to eat. Unfortunately, many people simply don't know how to eat in a healthy way, but education can change that. Hormones can affect weight gain, metabolism, lean mass, and appetite, so factors like testosterone, insulin, thyroid, and ghrelin can play a role in obesity. Physiological factors such as the number of fat cells that a person has or perhaps even the food that the mother ate in utero can affect obesity. Psychological factors might affect a person's relationship with food; a person who is surrounded by tasty but unhealthy food needs a lot of energy to restrain him- or herself from eating that food. Studies have shown that willpower is finite. A person has only so many resources to devote to various matters. Finally, environmental factors might play a role in obesity. Exposure to or consumption of plastics, pesticides, preservatives, additives, or other chemicals might adversely affect how a person handles and stores fat. Some people have even suggested that being overweight could be linked to some sort of virus that might be contagious. The theory is just a speculation at this time, but the point is that obesity is a complex issue. The simple recommendation to eat less doesn't work for everyone. In addition, a noticeable rise in obesity has occurred since 1980 (see figure 16.1), and why the increase has occurred during the intervening years is not clear (44, 52).

WEIGHT-LOSS PRACTICES

Because no one wants to be obese and because so many people are obese, people have resorted to some extreme practices to cause weight loss.

Fad Diets

People can choose from a plethora of fad diets that range on a continuum from being completely ludicrous to moderately helpful. Fad diets usually have two flaws. First, they don't teach a person how to eat for the long term and they don't provide a maintenance strategy. True, someone can lose weight by eating cabbage soup for a week, but what happens after that? A good diet should teach clients how to eat for the rest of their life. Second, many fad diets offer information that is simply incorrect; most are not scientifically sound. Someone with some knowledge might be able to write a book or article that seems to put a lot of scientific information behind a diet. This promotion can convince a layperson, but when a person who understands how the system works examines the data, the argument falls apart. An author might declare that squeezing grapefruit juice over food releases enzymes that destroy all the calories in food, but a person who spends a week squeezing grapefruit juice over pizza and chocolate cake

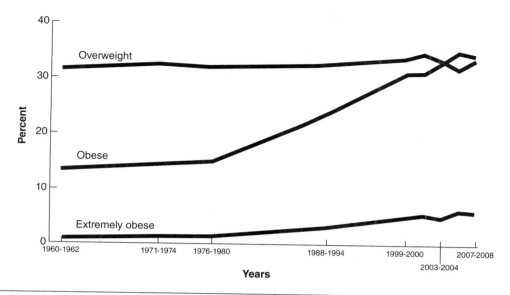

Figure 16.1 BMI data for the U.S. population from 1960–2008. Note: Age-adjusted by the direct method to the year 2000 U.S. Census Bureau estimates, using the age groups 20-39, 40-59, and 60-74 years. Pregnant females were excluded. Overweight is defined as a body mass index (BMI) of 25 or greater but less than 30; obesity is a BMI of greater than or equal to 30; extreme obesity is a BMI of greater than or equal to 40.

Reprinted from C.L. Ogden and M.D. Carroll, 2010, *NCHS health E-stat: Prevalence of overweight, obesity, and extreme obesity among adults: United States, trends 1960–1962 through 2007–2008* (Hyattsville, MD: Division of Health and Nutrition Examination Surveys). Available at www.cdc.gov/nchs/data/hestat/obesity_adult_07_08/obesity_adult_07_08.htm.

might not be pleased with what happens to his or her waistline.

Yo-Yo Dieting

Fad diets tend to lead to yo-yo dieting, sometimes referred to as chronic dieting syndrome. Here is an example. A female weighs 155 pounds (70.3 kg) and wants to lose some weight. She goes on a fad diet, does not exercise, and loses 25 pounds (11.3 kg). A reasonable estimate is that with that weight loss, especially if it is rapid, coupled with no exercise, she will lose 40 to 50 percent muscle and 50 to 60 percent fat. If she lost 25 pounds, she likely lost 10 to 12.5 pounds (4.5 to 5.7 kg) of muscle and 12.5 to 15 pounds (5.7 to 6.8 kg) of fat. She now weighs 130 pounds (59.0 kg), but she may not like the way she looks. She is likely just a smaller version of herself, but she is not lean and fit, and her metabolism is now even slower because of the low food intake and loss of muscle. The fad diet did not teach her how to eat. Now that she is at her goal weight, she goes off her diet and eventually returns to her previous eating habits. Over the course of several months or a year, she regains all the weight (95 percent of dieters regain weight lost within a year). When gaining weight without exercising, a person will likely add 10 to 20 percent muscle and 80 to 90 percent fat. She ends up regaining approximately 5 pounds (2.3 kg) of muscle and 20 pounds (9.1 kg) of fat. She is back to 155 pounds (70.3 kg) but looks and feels worse than she did originally at this weight because she now has less lean tissue. She is not happy with her weight and resumes the fad diet to repeat the process, which gets harder each time she does it. She needs to break the cycle, sign up with a personal trainer, begin resistance training, start eating a healthy diet, build up her muscle and fitness level, and reduce her body fat. She might lose less weight with the personal trainer than she did on the fad diet. For example, she might lose only 15 to 20 pounds (6.8 to 9.1 kg) because she will retain or perhaps even build lean mass. She might ultimately weigh 138 pounds (62.6 kg), but she will look, feel, and perform much better than she did at 130 pounds (59.0 kg) (95).

Fasting

Some clients resort to an extreme method of weight loss, which is fasting. Contemplating fasting for religious or moral reasons is beyond the scope of this book, but fasting for weight-loss reasons is generally not recommended for personal-training clients. Of course, a person cannot fast forever, and fasting doesn't teach a person how to eat. Fasting does allow fat to burn, but it also causes a significant loss of muscle tissue and other lean mass. It can cause a loss of electrolytes and a decrease in blood pressure. Metabolism can slow, and if fasting continues for a long time, it can produce acidosis. From a personal-training point of view, if a client is truly fasting (eating no food and consuming only water), the person's energy will be so low after a day or two that any type of physical activity is likely to be too hard or will produce hypoglycemia (low blood sugar, which leads to weakness, nausea, difficulty concentrating, and shaking). Intermittent fasting or fasting for periods of 8 to 20 hours might have some benefits, but more research is needed in that area. Prolonged fasting for days or weeks is not recommended for personal-training clients.

Macronutrient Restrictions

Some clients follow diets that suggest a severe restriction of a macronutrient, usually carbohydrate or fat. These diets can work but are hard to follow long term. Moreover, chapter 14 clearly demonstrated that each of the macronutrients has important roles to play in the body. Balancing their ratios is generally better than seeking to place severe limits on one or the other. The Atkins diet (restricting carbohydrate) and the Ornish diet (restricting fat) are examples of these types of diets.

Special Clothing or Body Wraps

Some people use clothing or wrap part of the body in an attempt to burn fat. People do not sweat fat out of the body (if we did, reusable gym towels would not be socially acceptable); instead, we sweat water out of the body. The body must burn fat to get rid of it after it has been stored as adipose tissue. Wrapping an area to raise its temperature and the amount that it sweats might possibly increase the number of capillaries in that area, and some research shows that certain areas in the body with poor blood flow have a hard time using that fat after it is stored (sometimes called cold fat), but that is just speculation at this stage. If clothing or body wraps had a powerful effect, they would be more popular. Any excess water loss caused by these methods is simply stored again as soon as the person consumes food and drink, so those methods are not suggested for personal-training clients.

Drugs

Clients might look to drugs as a quick fix to obesity, but there are no quick fixes. Recommending any of these drugs would be outside the scope of practice for a personal trainer. Most have negative consequences and are only partially effective, so they are generally not worth the tradeoff. Taking up smoking is an effective way to lose 5 pounds (2.3 kg) or so, but who could justify recommending that course of action given how harmful cigarettes are to health?

Thermogenics

The goal of thermogenics is to increase metabolism by increasing body temperature. The drugs that cause that reaction in the body can put undue stress on the heart, which may lead to medical problems. The body adapts to these drugs quickly, and the dosage needs to be increased regularly to maintain effectiveness. Also, long-term use of these drugs may negatively affect the thyroid gland.

Fat Blockers

These drugs bind with fat when it is in the digestive tract, reducing the absorption of fat. They also block the absorption of the essential fatty acids and fat-soluble vitamins. The body does not know how to process this fat that it is now unable to absorb, and the result is that these drugs often cause diarrhea or anal leakage (15).

Appetite Suppressants

These drugs attempt to suppress appetite, but they don't teach clients how to eat or how to know when they are satisfied. Reports of significant side effects such as pulmonary hypertension, which can be fatal, have occurred in a significant minority of users, so these drugs are not worth the risks.

Surgery

Two main types of surgery are now available to clients to help with weight loss and physical appearance. Liposuction literally sucks the fat cells out of a certain area. This procedure does work, but it is expensive and painful, requires some recovery time, carries certain risks (anesthesia and infection), and can remove only a small amount of weight. If the client continues to overeat, the body will store fat in other places, sometimes in abnormal locations.

Gastric banding involves using a band or other device to shrink the stomach so that only a small amount of food can be eaten. This type of surgery is appropriate only for significantly overweight people. Treatment and therapy are required before the surgery, and lifestyle modification is required after the surgery. This kind of surgery can work, but the client needs to consider it seriously for a long time and consult with a doctor. Gastric banding is not a permanent fix, and the client can regain weight if old eating habits return (24).

UNDERWEIGHT

Some clients go in the other direction and become underweight. Underweight is defined as being 10 percent or more under the goal weight for height or having a BMI below 18.5 (table 16.2). A person must be quite thin to reach a BMI that low. In terms of health, being underweight is generally considered a greater risk than being overweight, particularly as people age. When people are underweight, they have no reserves. If they become sick or develop a health problem, they have no resources to draw on.

Table 16.2   BMI Classification and Associated Health Risk

BMI	Health risk
Obesity ≥30	Greatest
Underweight <18.5	High
Overweight 25–29.9	Moderate
Healthy 18.5–24.9	Lowest

People can be underweight for a variety of reasons, some of which can be controlled and some of which cannot. Wasting disease, malabsorption problems, and the inability to afford food are difficult to control. Psychological issues, excess activity level, and lack of education are easier to correct.

EATING DISORDERS

The main cause of being underweight in otherwise healthy clients is the presence of an eating disorder. Eating disorders most commonly affect women, but men are susceptible as well. Eating disorders most commonly appear among people in their teens and 20s and then often subside in incidence among those in their 40s. In general, however, eating disorders are more prevalent than many people recognize. Estimates of prevalence vary, but 3 to 10 percent of females likely have an eating disorder. The three most common eating disorders are anorexia nervosa, bulimia nervosa, and compulsive overeating (142).

All eating disorders are complex psychological issues that require professional help. If a personal trainer is working with a client suspected of having an eating disorder, after establishing some trust the personal trainer should suggest that the client speak to a psychologist or psychiatrist to receive help. Eating disorders are not cured overnight, and the client is likely to struggle with them for a long time. If left unchecked, eating disorders can negatively affect a client's physical and mental health and can even be fatal. Anorexia is particularly dangerous. According to the National Association of Anorexia Nervosa and Associated Disorders, 5 to 10 percent of anorexics die within 10 years of developing the disorder, 20 percent die within 20 years, and only 30 to 40 percent recover fully. As the body is starving, it breaks down its own lean tissue for amino acids, and one of those tissues that is broken down is the heart. If this occurs on a regular, long-term basis, the heart will weaken and fade prematurely.

Anorexia Nervosa

Anorexia nervosa is characterized by self-imposed starvation. The person eats a very small amount of food and often combines that with excessive aerobic exercise that may take on a slightly obsessive–compulsive behavior (same elliptical machine, same time of the day, same routine, and so on). People with anorexia are often noticeably thin. Generally, they are attempting to exert control over this aspect of their life because they think that other aspects are out of control. People with anorexia tend to be Caucasian, affluent, intelligent females, although about 10 percent are males. This eating disorder poses an immediate threat to short- and long-term health (8).

Bulimia Nervosa

Bulimia nervosa is characterized by bingeing on food and then engaging in some form of purging. The person consumes a large quantity of food in an almost uncontrollable, addictive state. The person then feels intense guilt over his or her actions and attempts to purge to correct the binge. Purging involves either vomiting or using laxatives. Regularly vomiting is hard on the tissues of the throat and tends to discolor the teeth. Continual use of laxatives can make people dependent on them to excrete their waste. People with bulimia tend to be closer to a normal weight.

Compulsive Overeating

Compulsive overeating is characterized by bingeing without purging. This type of eating is often done in private, so the person may appear to eat little. Compulsive overeaters tend to be significantly overweight, although not all overweight people are compulsive over-eaters (16).

Reverse Anorexia

Another disorder worth mentioning is found only in the fitness world. It is reverse anorexia, also known as bigorexia, the Adonis complex, or body dysmorphia. People who have this disorder are large and muscular, and most often are males, but they see themselves as smaller and weaker than they really are. This disorder may be associated with steroid use, but that is not mandatory. The person obsesses over building up muscles so much that the obsession negatively affects his or her daily life.

BEHAVIORAL ASPECTS OF WEIGHT MANAGEMENT

As personal trainers, we don't want our clients to follow fad diets or yo-yo diets, fast, develop eating disorders, or use any of the extreme practices mentioned earlier. Instead, the goal is to provide clients with sound weight management guidelines. Initially, you start by helping the client understand and ultimately modify his or her behavior. Look for the cue, or stimulus, that causes the behavior. Then see what the response is to that cue. What action does the client take next? Finally, think about the consequences of that behavior. What happens when the person performs that behavior regularly? Two examples can highlight this thought process.

Example 1. A client wishes to engage in evening workouts. But she finds that after getting home from work, relaxing on the couch, and watching some TV, her motivation to exercise is gone for the day. She skips the gym that evening.

Example 2. A client is on a diet and hopes to lose weight. He works hard and is often hungry on the ride home from work. The sight of a fast-food restaurant that he always passes on the drive home is often enough to cause him to pull in and get dinner there instead of making dinner at home.

What are the cues in the examples? In the first, it is arriving at home and sitting on the couch. In the second, it is seeing that fast-food restaurant. What is the response? The client relaxes on the couch and skips the gym in the first example. In the second example, the client orders a fast-food dinner. What are the consequences? Neither client is a bad person for making those choices, but neither choice, made regularly, will do much to improve the person's health and fitness. The client who skips the workout sessions will not achieve her goals or see results. The client who eats the fast food is likely to continue to gain weight, which may negatively affect his health. So what can we do?

To help those clients modify their behavior, we should first define and analyze the behavior. What is really going on? Make it as specific as possible. The first client isn't lazy; she simply has a hard time getting to the gym after going home at night. The second client isn't weak for eating fast food; he simply made a poor food choice that conflicts with his weight-loss goals. Don't generalize. Instead, define the specific behavior. A workout log or a food diary can be helpful in accurately assessing the extent of the problem.

After the specific problem is isolated, a new strategy can be developed. Doing this in the middle of the issue is difficult. Instead, during a more neutral time you can role play the scenario and identify some possible new approaches that might work. The first client might try to work out in the morning. Studies show that people who work out early are more likely to stick with their fitness routine. Or the client might drive straight to the gym after work and not go home at all. If the client has to go home, maybe she can promise not to turn on the TV at all during that time. The second client might decide to drive a different route home, even if it takes him five minutes out of the way, to avoid seeing the fast-food restaurant. Or the client might pack a small snack, such as an apple. When he sees the fast-food restaurant, he eats the snack to take the edge off the cravings and continues home. He might eat a bigger lunch so that he is not as hungry on the drive home, or he could prepare dinner the day before so that he knows he can eat as soon as he gets home and doesn't have to cook for an hour after a full day of work. Any one of those methods could work, but none is

guaranteed to work. The trick is to find the one that works with the specific client.

Good nutritional plans involve realistic weight-change goals (1 percent loss of body weight per week or a .5- to 1-pound [.23 to .45 kg] gain of muscle per week) and an adequate minimum number of calories per day (at least 1,200). They are nutritionally adequate so that the person consumes enough of the macronutrients and micronutrients to meet daily needs. The food is moderately pleasing to the taste so that the person will eat it. Finally, a good plan has an energy readjustment and maintenance period after the client reaches the goal weight. To help achieve those goals, personal trainers should follow the guidelines presented in the next section of the chapter.

CALCULATING A CLIENT'S METABOLIC RATE

Several formulas can be used to estimate metabolic rate. This quantity is defined as a person's total metabolism, which indicates how many calories that person burns per day at his or her current activity level and food intake. This number is useful to figure out because after it is known, it can be modified to help the client achieve body-weight and body-composition goals.

NPTI Metabolism Formula

The National Personal Training Institute (NPTI) uses the same formula as the International Sports Sciences Association (ISSA) does, developed by Dr. Fred Hatfield, to estimate a client's basal metabolic rate (BMR). After the BMR is known, the client's physical activity level and the thermic effect of food (TEF) can be calculated. Those three key factors—BMR, physical activity level (PAL), and TEF—are necessary to calculate a person's total metabolism. The information needed includes the following:

- Sex
- Weight
- Activity level
- Calories eaten per day
- Age (optional)

Step 1: Find the BMR (number of calories burned at rest)

Find weight in kilograms (weight in pounds divided by 2.2)

Example: 198 lb ÷ 2.2 = 90 kg

Weight in kg × 1.0 (male) × 24 = BMR; weight in kg × 0.9 (female) × 24 = BMR

Example: 90 kg × 1.0 (male) × 24 = 2,160 kcals/day BMR

Step 2: Find calories burned through physical activity level (PAL)

Estimate activity level:

Sedentary, 20 percent—rarely works out, job involves little movement

Light, 30 percent—sedentary job but works out a few times a week, or more active job but does not work out

Moderate, 40 percent—somewhat active job and works out regularly

Heavy, 50 percent—rare; very active job involving constant physical labor, or long-distance aerobic athlete

BMR (from step 1) × activity percentage (20 percent through 50 percent) = activity calories

Example: 2,160 × 40 percent (moderate) = 864 activity calories

Step 3: Find the thermic effect of food (TEF)

Calories eaten per day × 10 percent = TEF

Example: 3,250 × 10 percent = 325 TEF calories

Step 4: Sum BMR, PAL, and TEF to find total metabolism

BMR + PAL + TEF = total metabolism

Example: 2,160 + 864 + 325 = 3,349 total metabolism

Total metabolism is the number of calories that a person burns each day at his or her activity level.

Step 5: Adjust for age

30–49 years old: −3 percent

50–69 years old: −7.5 percent

70 or more years old: −10 percent

Example: 3,349 − 3 percent (35 years old) = 3,248.5 calories per day

If a client does not know his or her caloric intake per day and the personal trainer does not feel comfortable estimating it, the following formula can be used to calculate the total metabolism for that person:

(BMR + PAL) ÷ 0.9 = total metabolism

A client's total metabolism should be recalculated for every gain or loss of 10 pounds (4.5 kg) or for a significant change in activity level (up or down).

This formula is based on averages, so the number is an estimate. Human metabolic rates, however, do not vary much, and this number usually serves as a solid starting point. If you know the client's height, weight, and percent body fat, you can also calculate total metabolism, which takes into account the metabolic rate of all the tissues in the body and provides a more accurate estimation of the metabolic rate.

ENERGY BALANCE

The variance between caloric intake and caloric expenditure (from BMR, PAL, and TEF) is called energy balance. If intake exceeds expenditure, the client is in positive energy balance, which leads to increases in body tissue (e.g., overall physical growth or body fat, which increases the tendency to becoming overweight and obese). Negative energy balance occurs if expenditure exceeds intake. The body will use its reserves of fat and protein (muscle), which can lead to physical wasting and undernutrition.

Note that if resistance training is performed when an adult enters a state of positive energy balance, the body doesn't have to create reserves of fat. Instead it can and often does add muscle mass. In addition, if resistance training is performed during negative energy balance, the body uses more fat and conserves protein, thus minimizing any wasting effect.

WEIGHT LOSS

Most Americans are overweight, and many want to lose weight. An even greater majority of personal-training clients want to lose weight and improve their body composition. Personal trainers should explain to clients that when they wish to lose weight (which would be measured solely on the scale), in reality they often wish to lose body fat, which is similar but not the same thing (95).

To lose body fat, the client needs to create a caloric deficit. This circumstance can be created by eating a reduced number of calories, increasing the PAL, increasing the metabolic rate, or using a combination of those methods. Ideally, the client is already engaged in regular physical activity that is enough to create excess postexercise oxygen consumption (EPOC) and further stimulate his or her metabolism. EPOC measures the amount of additional oxygen (and energy) used up after exercise has ceased. Creating EPOC is a powerful method for inducing weight loss. In addition, if the client is engaged in resistance training, he or she should be building and maintaining lean tissue, which was shown in the previous chapter to increase the metabolic rate slightly. Other methods of increasing the metabolic rate (drugs) are outside the scope of a personal trainer and are not without side effects. Thus, the primary method for inducing weight loss for clients is caloric manipulation.

Quantity and Rate of Weight Loss

One pound (.45 kg) of body fat contains 3,500 kilocalories. Note that 1 pound is 454 grams and that number multiplied by the fuel factor of fat (9 calories) is greater than 3,500. The discrepancy occurs because 1 pound of body fat contains only 388 grams of fat; the rest is water and other substances. Losing 1 pound of body fat in one day is difficult. (Most people do not have a metabolic rate of 3,500 calories a day, so they could not burn that many calories even if they did not consume any food at all.) The common recommendation is to focus on losing weight and fat at a certain rate per week.

Realistic weight-loss and fat-loss guidelines are 1 to 2 pounds (.45 to .91 kg) per week or 1 percent body fat per week (which is aggressive but realistic). The second guideline means that a heavier person could lose more than 2 pounds of fat per week (many extremely obese people also carry a significant quantity of extra water in their tissues, which helps explain the rapid weight loss that they can achieve), whereas a lighter person might not be able to lose 2 pounds of fat per week. The lighter and leaner a person is, the harder it is to lose body fat.

> Example 1: A 275-pound (124.7 kg) client who loses 1 percent body fat per week drops 2.75 pounds (1.25 kg) of fat, which is a maximum realistic goal for a week.

> Example 2: A 125-pound (56.7 kg) client who loses 1 percent body fat per week drops 1.25 pounds (.57 kg) of fat, which is a maximum realistic goal for a week.

Personal trainers usually recommend that clients lose anywhere from .5 to 2 pounds (.23 to .91 kg) of fat per week. Certainly, people can lose more weight than that per week, but it will not be primarily fat for a person of normal weight.

Changes in Caloric Intake

To create a negative caloric balance, clients can reduce their caloric intake (table 16.3). But personal trainers should not recommend that clients eat less than 1,200 calories per day. Any diet that includes less than that amount is a very low calorie diet (VLCD), which is outside the scope for a personal trainer. At that caloric

Table 16.3 Daily Caloric Adjustments to Lose Fat

Desired fat loss per week	Daily caloric adjustment needed to create a negative caloric balance
−.5 lb (.23 kg)	−250 calories
−1 lb (.45 kg)	−500 calories
−1.5 lb (.68 kg)	−750 calories
−2 lb (.91 kg)	−1,000 calories

Note: Do not recommend a caloric intake below 1,200 calories per day.

level, receiving the proper amounts of the essential nutrients for the body is difficult, and such diets should be recommended only by a registered dietitian. Clients themselves should be aware than a VLCD rarely leads to long-term success because metabolism is stressed and generally slows as a result, significant protein is lost, intense exercise is difficult to perform, hormone production is suppressed, and cravings tend to become difficult to control. A better approach is to feed the body adequate amounts of the right fuel, create a slight caloric reduction, and exercise hard to lose weight and stay fit. People forced to consume low-calorie diets regularly because of imprisonment or lack of food availability rarely look lean and fit. Instead, they tend to look skinny and sickly. The body needs moderate amounts of healthy fuel if it is to look and perform optimally.

Clients can lose weight by reducing the number of calories, and they can have success with many kinds of diets. Clients often slightly reduce their percentage of carbohydrate when trying to get lean. In addition, clients should focus on eating the healthiest and most natural sources of carbohydrate when on a diet. Most clients see success with their weight loss by keeping their carbohydrate intake close to or fewer than 100 grams per day, which in turn is likely to be about 40 percent of the diet. The rest of the diet will be made up of protein and fat. People often slightly increase the protein percentage when on a diet to consume enough grams per day for tissue building and repair (109).

Listed below are common dietary recommendations for weight and fat loss:

- Carbohydrate: 40 to 60 percent
- Protein: 20 to 35 percent
- Fat: 20 to 35 percent

Note that these guidelines do not radically differ from the recommended intake described in chapter 14.

Practical Recommendations

Losing weight is not easy, especially in a society that surrounds us with a surplus of convenient, tasty food, and in a technologically advanced world that requires little physical activity. Clients should be aware of the four common keys to losing weight or preventing weight gain:

- Portion control. Many clients are uneducated about what a portion is, particularly when it comes to carbohydrate and meats. When attempting to lose weight, people must eat smaller portions of food, and they should not feel stuffed or full on a diet. Eating in this way can be visually unappealing because the brain is used to seeing a certain proportion of food on the plate, but after eating the smaller portions and waiting for the food to digest, people are often pleasantly surprised about how satisfying the smaller meal can be.

- Restaurant eating. In this day and age, particularly in the life of the affluent client, restaurant eating occurs with high frequency. Gone are the times when a family or individual might eat out once a month as a special treat. Now many busy clients are getting the majority (or at least a significant minority) of their meals on the run or at a restaurant. But the idea that eating at a restaurant is a special treat still lingers, and people tend to splurge more when they are there. Restaurants need to keep people happy and keep customers coming back, and they have to compete with other restaurants. They do this by providing large amounts of food (huge portions) that is tasty (with lots of added sugar, fat, and salt), often making it as cheaply as possible (using cheaper food that is not natural or organic because it can be too expensive). In addition, restaurants rarely emphasize fruits and vegetables and instead focus on processed foods and less healthily grown meats.

- Processed food. The type of food that humans eat has changed radically in the last hundred years. The consequences of this change are unknown, but the preliminary evidence is not encouraging. We are eating a huge amount of processed food, food products, and fake food. Food designed for children is often some of the worst because it is quick, easy, cheap, and tasty. Parents are happy, and so are the kids, at least in the short term. But long term, that type of food does not benefit either party. Nutrition has become so complicated that some people don't even know what healthy food is anymore. They choose the heavily processed "health" food that resembles cardboard more often than they do a naturally occurring product like rice, sweet potatoes, or eggs that humans have been eating for thousands of years and that our bodies have evolved to digest properly. Processed foods often have high levels of food additives such as fat, sugar, salt, trans fat, and preservatives. When trying to lose weight, people should significantly limit, avoid, or abstain from processed food, which includes but is not limited to bread, pancakes and waffles, cereals, fruit bars and breakfast bars, chips, candy, french fries, hot cocoa, desserts, and so on. If the food is not close to its natural form, people are better off not eating it when trying to lose weight.

• Physical activity. The final piece of the equation is physical activity. The average work capacity of people has dropped significantly as activities of daily living (ADLs) have decreased. This reduction on activity has caused the average person to gain weight and decrease his or her $\dot{V}O_2max$, which in turn has decreased work capacity, so these factors create a negative snowball effect. Take away the car, the washing machine, the dishwasher, and the refrigerator, and a person's level of activity will increase significantly. The goal is not to advocate the banning of technology or rid ourselves of those conveniences, but simply to make clients aware that formal exercise was less important a hundred years ago because daily life forced most people to perform a moderate amount of exercise on a regular basis. As technology has advanced and daily life has become more comfortable and sedentary, clients need to be aware that formal exercise is now important because the ADLs in today's society are no longer enough to maintain even baseline levels of fitness necessary for health. Looking into the future, we can assume that technology will only advance more, that lifestyles will become even more sedentary, and that exercise will thus play an even more important role in maintaining health. The silver lining in this is that the need for well-qualified and properly educated personal trainers will increase as time goes by.

Awareness of the previous keys (portion control, restaurant eating, processed food, and physical activity) to losing and controlling weight can be a positive step in the right direction. Sometimes clients also need more simple, practical, and immediately applicable tips that they can begin to use right away in their journey toward a healthy weight. Clients might find the following tips useful. The goal is not for clients to use and incorporate every tip listed, nor should they stress about seeing how many tips they can follow. Instead, the goal is for clients to pick a few tips that might be useful in making the daunting task of losing body fat seem just a bit more attainable.

Listed here are additional practical recommendations to follow when on a weight-loss program:

- Plan what you are going to eat a day in advance.
- Prepare your meals ahead of time (for example, cook everything on Sunday).
- Weigh your food.
- Serve the food on smaller dinner plates.
- Wait at least 15 minutes after eating before getting seconds.
- Avoid or limit foods that you have a problem eating in moderation.
- Avoid or limit desserts for a certain time (one to three months, for example).
- Avoid or limit alcohol from the diet, particularly beer and hard liquor.
- Avoid or limit eating at restaurants.
- Avoid or limit trans fats.
- If you are eating out, decide what you are going to order before you enter the restaurant and write it down or tell someone.
- If you are served a larger meal, immediately divide it in half and eat only half of it at that time. Put the other half in a box or move it off your plate or out of your sight.
- Try to have a serving of vegetables or fiber with every meal.
- Avoid or limit fast food.

- Avoid heavily processed food.
- Eat a piece of fruit like an apple or banana before you eat your main meal.
- Eat on a regular schedule; don't allow yourself to become extremely hungry.
- Eat relatively small amounts. You should never get full or stuffed when trying to lose weight.
- If you do fall off track and eat a meal that is not on the meal plan, don't give up. Pick up where you left off and begin again. One meal will not ruin a diet plan; a week of poor eating will have a much more negative effect.
- Temporarily eliminate gluten for two to three weeks and see how your body responds to that period and a period of reintroduction.
- Keep a food journal. Having to record what you eat helps you learn what you are eating, when you eat, how your body responds to food, and what you need to work on. In addition, your diet is likely to improve simply by recording your food intake.
- Drink more water, including one big glass before every meal. Sometimes people confuse thirst with hunger and eat to satisfy their thirst.
- Weigh yourself daily (or even multiple times during the day). View the scale as an educational tool that teaches you how foods affect your body, not a judgment tool that tells you whether you have been good or bad.
- Allow yourself to have one cheat meal a week or one cheat day per week to help relieve the mental stress of dieting and make it easier to be social.
- Carbohydrate cycling can be an option to incorporate to help change body composition. This approach is better for those with advanced nutritional knowledge.

WEIGHT GAIN

To lose weight, a client must enter a state of negative energy balance. To gain weight, the opposite is true. The client must enter a state of positive energy balance. Additional calories must come in over and above what was spent on metabolism, activity, and the processing of food eaten. When clients talk about gaining weight, most want to increase their lean mass. In simple terms, they want to add muscle. For most people, gaining fat is not that difficult, so clients rarely seek advice on that topic. But adding muscle is a different story. Traditionally, this goal is more common with men, but women have recently been seeking to add lean muscle mass to their frames as well. The preferred female form has changed from a thin, underfed runway model to a female athlete who is lean and fit and has clearly visible muscles.

Approximately 2,200 calories are needed to build 1 pound (.45 kg) of muscle. Note that the number is not the same as the number given for a pound of fat because the fuel factors for the tissues are not the same. That number is not as universally agreed upon as the fat number is, but both science and anecdotal evidence are behind it. A pound contains 454 grams, and the fuel factor for muscle (protein) is 4, which yields 1,800 calories. Extra calories are required to build muscle, which takes the number to approximately 2,200. In addition, significant anecdotal evidence reinforces this number. When athletes add 500 calories a day over their maintenance level, they gain weight too fast and too much of it is fat. Most health and fitness experts recommend adding approximately 300 calories to the diet per day to gain muscle. NPTI uses the following specific guidelines.

Changes in Caloric Intake

A realistic weight gain is .5 to 1 pound (.23 to .45 kg) of muscle per week. Approximately 2,200 calories are needed to build a pound of muscle. To create a positive caloric balance, clients can increase their caloric intake (table 16.4).

Example: A male needs 3,300 calories per day to maintain current weight. The goal is to gain 1 lb (.45 kg) of muscle per week.

3,300 calories per day + 315 calories = 3,615 calories per day

Table 16.4 Daily Caloric Adjustment to Build Lean Tissue

Desired muscle gain per week	Daily caloric adjustment needed to create a positive caloric balance
+.5 lb (.23 kg)	+157 calories
+1 lb (.45 kg)	+315 calories

Realistic weight gain in the form of muscle is .5 to 1 pound (.23 to .45 kg) per week. Repeated consistently, a gain of 1 pound per week is aggressive, and clients should be happy with that rate of lean tissue gain. A gain of .5 pound per week is more conservative and easier to achieve, particularly for females. Athletes who take anabolic steroids and similar products will be able to exceed this guideline. Note that people can add significantly more weight than this amount per week, but most of that weight will not be muscle. In addition, note that the rate of weight loss will exceed the rate of weight gain at maximal levels. All things being equal, the body can lose weight faster than it can put it on (26).

Adding 315 calories a day is not an excuse to gorge at every meal, but the body does need to consume more calories than it spends. Some clients, particularly smaller and leaner people, and most often males in their teens and 20s, will report that they have a hard time gaining weight or maintaining any weight that they gain. All clients who are attempting to gain weight, especially those just mentioned, should regularly include some or all of the following foods: whole organic eggs, whole organic milk, wild fish, potatoes, nuts (any), red meat, and rice. The addition of some of the following high-calorie foods can also be helpful: sour cream, butter, peanut butter (preferably natural), oils, meal replacements, protein bars and shakes, and even organic ice cream on occasion. The leaner that people are, the less strict they need to be with their diet when trying to put on size.

Practical Recommendations

Attempting to gain quality lean mass without adding significant fat can be almost as chal-lenging as attempting to lose weight. Listed here are some tips that might help clients gain weight. Note that some of these tips are the same as the weight-loss guidelines. These tips simply help clients get on track and become more aware of what they are eating, so they work well for either goal.

- Plan what you are going to eat a day in advance.
- Prepare your meals ahead of time (for example, cook everything on Sunday).
- Weigh your food.
- Try to have a serving of vegetables or fiber with every meal.
- Eat on a regular schedule; don't allow yourself to get extremely hungry.
- Keep a food journal. Having to record what you eat helps you learn what you are eating, when you eat, how your body responds to food, and what you need to work on. In addition, your diet is likely to improve simply by recording your food intake.
- Weigh yourself daily (or even multiple times during the day). View the scale as an educational tool that teaches you how foods affect your body, not a judgment tool that tells you whether you have been good or bad.
- Allow yourself to have one cheat meal a week or one cheat day per week to help relieve the mental stress of dieting and make it easier to be social.
- Carbohydrate cycling can be an option to incorporate to help change body composition. See the sample food days later in this chapter for examples.
- Add in small amounts of extra food to your normal diet to cause a caloric increase (have a small bowl of oatmeal in addition to a normal breakfast, add a yogurt with lunch, and add a banana and peanut butter to a protein shake).
- Reduce or eliminate additional physical activity that may not help you reach your goal (excess cardio or conditioning).

- Substitute higher-calorie foods for lower-calorie options. For example, have a yogurt smoothie instead of water or choose full-fat options instead of light foods.
- Add protein or meal replacement powder to normal food like oatmeal and pancakes.
- Consume sports drinks during workouts.
- Eat as soon as possible after completing a workout.
- Don't eat a gigantic meal. Many people think that they can binge because they are trying to gain weight. They eat one big meal but are then stuffed for several hours. They have no desire to eat again, and they actually eat fewer total calories for the day and do not maximize hormonal release.
- Combine food with healthy, high-calorie options like olive oil and guacamole.
- Drink a certain amount of whole milk every day. Guidelines range from 16 ounces (473 ml) to a gallon (3.8 L) per day. A gallon will almost assuredly add fat; a quart (liter) is a good starting point.

Note that the additional calories required to build muscle do not have to come only in the form of protein. Because carbohydrate is protein sparing, if the client is eating an adequate amount of protein, consuming extra fat or carbohydrate can help ensure that the protein goes to building lean tissue.

PREWORKOUT MEAL

Generally, each meal should have a purpose. The primary purpose of the preworkout meal, or precompetition meal for athletes, is to provide energy for the upcoming activity. The most important nutrient in the preworkout meal is carbohydrate, ideally natural, unprocessed, complex carbohydrate. Consuming some protein is important (to maintain blood amino acid levels, reduce carbohydrate absorption rate, and provide a possible backup for carbohydrate if necessary), as is consuming some fat (to add taste to the food, provide lower-intensity

energy, and reduce the absorption rate of the carbohydrate).

Guidelines for the preworkout meal include the following:

- Eat two to four hours before activity if possible. Eat a large meal if it is closer to four hours; eat a smaller meal if it is closer to two hours. If you must eat within one hour of the activity, cut the recommendations in half.
- Choose primarily complex, nonprocessed, natural forms of carbohydrate when possible.
- Eat foods that you like that you believe will benefit your performance.
- The more intense the exercise is, the longer you will need to digest the food.
- The more intense the workout is, the more important the preworkout meal becomes.
- Aim for 50 to 200 grams of carbohydrate, 20 to 50 grams of protein, and 10 to 30 grams of fat (table 16.5).

Lighter clients, mostly females, and those wishing to lose weight tend to use the lower ranges of the guidelines provided. Heavier clients, mostly males and those wishing to gain weight, tend to use the higher ranges of the guidelines. Those of average weight are often in the middle. If people eat significantly less than the amount suggested, they are likely to run out of energy during a hard workout. If people eat significantly more than this amount, they are likely to be full and feel stuffed when the workout begins, which does not promote maximal performance.

If your clients ask for more specific guidelines, you might suggest that they try to eat some of the foods outlined in table 16.6 before they work out and avoid some of the others listed.

CARBOHYDRATE LOADING

Athletes sometimes employ a more advanced method of nutritional eating that involves carbohydrate loading. The goal of carbohydrate

Table 16.5   Macronutrient Composition for a Small, Medium, and Large Meal

Small meal	Medium meal	Large meal
50 g carbohydrate	125 g carbohydrate	200 g carbohydrate
20 g protein	35 g protein	50 g protein
10 g fat	20 g fat	30 g fat
360 total calories	820 total calories	1,270 total calories

Table 16.6   Suggested Foods to Consume and to Avoid Before a Workout

Foods to eat	Foods to avoid
Skinless chicken breast	Cold cereal
Skinless turkey breast	Doughnuts
Fish (salmon, tuna, trout, and so on)	Pastries
Potato (baked, mashed)	Pop Tarts
Oatmeal	Large amounts of milk (may upset the stomach)
Sweet potato	Soda or equivalent (including diet)
Rice	Large amounts of fruit
Lean red meat	Fast food
Piece of fruit or a glass of fruit juice	Junk food
Bagel or wrap	Fried food
Olive oil	Any desserts
Any veggie (peas, corn, carrots, green beans, broccoli, and so on)	Protein bars*
	Protein shakes*
Salad (will likely need some starch with it)	Chinese food**
	Mexican food**

*Note: Protein bars and shakes are often hard to digest. Protein should not be the primary nutrient before a workout. These foods can be OK as part of a whole meal, but they are rarely ideal when eaten alone as a preworkout meal.

**Note: Foods from these cultures are not necessarily bad, but the Americanized version of them found in restaurants is often not ideal before a workout.

loading is to maximize glycogen stores and, in essence, trick the body into storing more glycogen than it normally does. This method is useful for two groups of people. Aerobic endurance athletes commonly perform it before they participate in long events during which total glycogen storage is key to performance. Glycogen, being a high-intensity fuel, is important in events like a marathon or triathlon (12). The second group that uses this method is bodybuilders. Glycogen is stored inside the muscles. When the muscles are full of glycogen, they tend to take on a more desirable appearance; they look more full, round, and hard. When the muscles are low on glycogen, they look flatter and smaller. Bodybuilders need glycogen not for performance, but for looks. Bodybuilding diets may look different from what is presented here, but the ultimate goal is the same—to have as much glycogen inside the muscles as possible at the start of the event (150).

Two methods are used for carbohydrate loading. The first is simple. Eat a meal particularly high in carbohydrate as the preworkout meal or the night before the event. For example, a runner might have a pasta meal the night before a marathon. The second method, a seven-day process, is significantly more involved. Because it is long and harder to follow, athletes should use this method only a few times a year. The process starts one week before the event date:

Days 1 through 3: Eat half of normal carbohydrate consumption, maintain normal protein and fat intake, and exercise intensely during this time.

Example: A runner eats 200 grams of carbohydrate per day instead of 400 grams and exercises hard.

Days 4 through 6: Eat 150 percent of normal carbohydrate consumption, maintain normal protein and fat intake, and perform little to no exercise during this time.

Example: A runner eats 600 grams of carbohydrate per day instead of 400 grams and performs no exercise to rest and taper before the race.

Day 7, Event: Consume the recommended preworkout meal and compete in the event.

The goal of this method is first to deplete the body of glycogen. By the end of day 3 in this process, the person should feel tired, low on energy, and a bit run down. The body tends to do a good job of absorbing the nutrients that it needs. If you are low on vitamin C and eat an orange, your body will try to grab as much of that vitamin C as possible. But if you have eaten two oranges a day for 10 days straight, your body is less likely to need vitamin C and thus will absorb less of it. In the carbohydrate-loading example, the body becomes depleted of glycogen by day 3. When carbohydrate is introduced back into the diet, the body supercompensates and stores a large amount of glycogen. If the runner usually has 400 grams of glycogen total, he or she might now have 430 grams of glycogen. That extra 30 grams is an extra 120 calories of fuel. At 15 calories per minute, the runner can do an additional 8 minutes of hard pushing, which might be just enough to set a personal record (PR) or place in the race (31).

POSTWORKOUT MEAL

The goal of the postworkout meal is to replenish the nutrients lost from exercise. The more intense the exercise is, the more important the postworkout meal becomes. The body acts like a sponge after exercise, and it seems to do a particularly good job of absorbing the needed nutrients and sending them to the proper spot. Theories differ about the timing of the postworkout meal. Some believe that eating should occur within 30 minutes of completing the activity, whereas others believe that there is a 2-hour window where the body is more receptive to nutrients. Still others think that the timing is not really important as long as the total amount of food taken in is correct. Consuming food shortly after a workout certainly cannot hurt, and doing so might make a significant difference in the uptake of nutrients, so people should eat as soon as possible after the workout is complete, particularly if the goal is to build muscle.

For the postworkout meal, the most important nutrient to eat is protein, although people don't need to consume more protein than carbohydrate and fat in this meal. Protein works to repair the damage caused to the muscle from the activity. The more intense the workout is, the more important protein consumption becomes. Carbohydrate is also important to consume after a workout to replenish the glycogen that was used up to fuel the workout. Some research shows that at this time it is better to consume, at least in part, some simple-to-digest carbohydrate because it can be converted to glycogen better than more complex carbohydrate can (41). Most likely a combination of some simple and some complex carbohydrate is best. Fat is also useful to provide taste, supply essential nutrients, and help build hormones.

People who are going to be less strict with their diets will do better by being less strict postworkout than preworkout. A person who overeats a bit or consumes some ice cream or other treat after a workout would not experience a negative effect on performance because the performance is already completed. Those who want to be very lean will have to be strict with both pre- and postworkout meals, but people who simply want to be fit and healthy can be strict with the preworkout meal but occasionally less strict with the postworkout meal.

In general, a personal trainer can suggest that a client consume 50 or more grams of carbohydrate (some simple carbohydrate is OK), 20 or more grams of protein, and 10 or more grams of fat.

SAMPLE DIETS

Personal trainers will find that they are frequently recommending a certain number of calories to clients to gain and lose weight. For example, 1,250-, 1,500-, and 1,750-calorie diets are commonly recommended for females who are trying to lose weight. Diets of 1,500, 1,750, and 2,000 calories (table 16.7) are commonly suggested for males who are trying to lose weight. Diets of 3,000, 3,500, and 4,000 calories (table 16.8) are often recommended for males who are trying to gain weight. To provide you with an idea of what that amount of food might look like and how a sample day might go, each of those diets is provided here. Keep in mind that the sample days are only examples. Clients should not eat the food outlined here, day after day, to accomplish

Table 16.7 Sample Weight-Loss Daily Food Plans for Varying Caloric Levels

1,250 calories	1,500 calories	1,750 calories	2,000 calories
1 small bagel (1 oz, or 28 g) 2 whole eggs 1 oz (28 g) of american cheese	1 small bagel (1 oz, or 28 g) 2 whole eggs 1 oz (28 g) of american cheese	1 small bagel (1 oz, or 28 g) 2 whole eggs 1 oz (28 g) of american cheese	2 small bagels (2 oz, or 57 g) 4 whole eggs 2 oz (57 g) of american cheese
3 oz (85 g) of chicken 1/2 cup of wild rice, cooked 3 cups of salad 1/2 serving of salad dressing	4 oz (113 g) of chicken 1 cup of wild rice, cooked 3 cups of salad 1/2 serving of salad dressing	5 oz (142 g) of chicken 1 cup of wild rice, cooked 3 cups of salad 1/2 serving of salad dressing	5 oz (142 g) of chicken 1 cup of wild rice, cooked 3 cups of salad 1/2 serving of salad dressing
3 oz (85 g) of salmon 1 small whole sweet potato 1 pat of butter or 1 tbsp of olive oil 2 whole tomatoes	4 oz (113 g) of salmon 1 cup of sweet potato 1 pat of butter or 1 tbsp of olive oil 2 whole tomatoes	5 oz (142 g) of salmon 1 1/2 cups of sweet potato 2 pats of butter or 2 tbsp of olive oil 2 whole tomatoes	5 oz (142 g) of salmon 1 1/2 cups of sweet potato 2 pats of butter or 2 tbsp of olive oil 2 whole tomatoes
2 oz (57 g) of chicken Tortilla 1/2 tomato 1/2 tsp of mayo 1 cup of carrots 1 small cucumber	2 oz (57 g) of chicken Tortilla 1/2 tomato 1/2 tsp of mayo 1 cup of carrots 1 small cucumber	2 oz (57 g) of chicken Tortilla 1/2 tomato 1/2 tsp of mayo 2 cups of carrots 1 small cucumber	2 oz (57 g) of chicken Tortilla 1/2 tomato 1/2 tsp of mayo 2 cups of carrots 2 small cucumbers

Table 16.8 Sample Weight-Gain Daily Food Plans for Different Caloric Levels

3,000 calories	3,500 calories	4,000 calories
2 packets of steel-cut oatmeal 8 oz (237 ml) of whole milk	3 packets of steel-cut oatmeal 12 oz (355 ml) of whole milk	3 packets of steel-cut oatmeal 12 oz (355 ml) of whole milk 1 1/2 cups blueberries
4 oz (113 g) of chicken 6 oz (170 g) of orzo 1 serving of peas (4 oz, or 113 g) Large apple 1 tbsp of olive oil	4 oz (113 g) of chicken 8 oz (227 g) of orzo 1 serving of peas (4 oz, or 113 g) Large apple 1 tbsp of olive oil	8 oz (227 g) of chicken 10 oz (283 g) of orzo 1 serving of peas (4 oz, or 113 g) Large apple 1 1/2 tbsp of olive oil
4 oz (113 g) of salmon 6 oz (170 g) of sweet potato 3 cups of garden salad 1 oz (28 g) of italian dressing Banana	4 oz (113 g) of salmon 8 oz (227 g) of sweet potato 3 cups of garden salad 1 oz (28 g) of italian dressing Banana	4 oz (113 g) of salmon 8 oz (227 g) of sweet potato 3 cups of garden salad 1 oz (28 g) of italian dressing Banana
Orange 1 protein bar 8 oz (237 ml) of whole milk	Orange 1 protein bar 8 oz (237 ml) of whole milk	Orange 2 protein bars 12 oz (355 ml) of whole milk
2 scoops of protein powder 8 oz (237 ml) of whole milk	2 scoops of protein powder 12 oz (355 ml) of whole milk Banana	2 scoops of protein powder 12 oz (355 ml) of whole milk

their goals. When it comes to nutrition, variety is important. No one single day can be ideal forever. You will also notice the foods are similar on each day. This choice was made intentionally to highlight how small changes in the diet can add up to significant caloric changes over time, which will yield results if followed consistently.

CARBOHYDRATE CYCLING

The idea behind carbohydrate cycling is that altering the amount of carbohydrate consumed per day may help stimulate the metabolism, increase fat burning, and provide adequate glycogen levels (table 16.9). In general, a person will choose to follow a certain number of lower-carbohydrate days (less than 100 grams per day) and a certain number of higher-carbohydrate days (more than 400 grams per day).

Weight-loss guidelines: four to six low-carbohydrate days (start with five)

One to three high-carbohydrate days (start with two)

Weight-gain guidelines: two to five high-carbohydrate days (start with three)

Two to five low-carbohydrate days (start with four)

Nutrition at the deep, chemical level can be complicated. Nutrition on the broader level of health does not have to be difficult. Clients, and all people, have the power to change their weight and body composition. Nutrition is a huge contributor to that process. Learning what types of food are healthy and beneficial to the body does not take years of study. Whenever possible, choose natural, unprocessed complex carbohydrate to provide energy. Those who are extremely active need a fair amount of energy; those who are not as active need significantly less energy. Choose natural, organic, healthy sources of protein and don't have too much concern about the amount of fat that will naturally come from those foods.

Table 16.9 Sample Daily Food Plans Using the Carbohydrate Cycling Method

Low-carbohydrate day	High-carbohydrate day
(No intake)	Banana or tea with sugar upon waking
3 hard-boiled eggs 1/2 serving of shredded carrots 1/2 serving of peas 1/2 serving of cauliflower 1/2 serving of sliced peppers 1 serving of shredded cheese 8 oz (237 ml) of whole organic milk	4 scrambled eggs 1 baked potato with butter and sour cream 1 serving of peas 1 serving of shredded cheese 1 yogurt smoothie
6 oz (170 g) of chicken breast 1 serving of snow peas 1 serving of sliced peppers 1/4 serving of orzo 3 cherry tomatoes 1 tbsp of olive oil Water	1 plain bagel 4 oz (113 g) of tuna fish 2 tomato slices 2 slices of cheese 1 low-fat raspberry yogurt
(No intake)	2 servings of Surge Workout Fuel during training**
Turkey wrap: 1 high-fiber thin wrap or tortilla 4 oz (113 g) of roasted turkey 2 servings of cheese Lettuce, tomato slices Water	Chicken burrito with rice and vinaigrette sauce Toppings as desired Water
2 servings of beef jerky Water	1 Met-Rx Big 100 Bar 8 oz (237 ml) of whole organic milk 2 servings of roasted nuts

**For the Surge drink, consume that before, during, and immediately after lifting.

Attempt to eat a variety of variously colored fruits and vegetables; one serving per meal is a good goal to shoot for. Consume in moderation or abstain from foods that are heavily processed and preserved, not closely related to their natural state, have ingredients that you are unable to pronounce, or are foods that would commonly be considered junk food. Learn to listen to the signals that your body gives you. If you are feeling energetic, alert, mentally sharp, and fit, you are likely making positive choices. If you are not feeling like that most of the time, try a new approach. Pay more attention to results than theories when it comes to nutrition. In general, listen to people who have achieved the results you seek more than those who just have theories about how to go about getting those results. Food should be a source of moderate enjoyment to complement life; it should not take over life.

CONCLUSION

Many clients need guidance from their personal trainer about key practical aspects of nutrition. Overweight is defined as having a BMI of 25; obesity is having a BMI of 30. Clients often resort to extreme practices and fad diets to lose weight. Some clients may have a history of eating disorders such as anorexia and bulimia. NPTI presents the metabolism formula that it uses to calculate a person's total metabolism. Energy balance can then be manipulated by helping clients gain weight by consuming additional calories or helping clients lose weight by creating a caloric deficit. This knowledge can help clients affect their body composition, which is one of the fundamental components of fitness and a topic that personal trainers need to be well versed in to meet their scope of practice.

Study Questions

1. What is the estimated BMR of a male client who weighs 182 pounds (82.6 kg)?

   a. 1,787 kilocalories per day

   b. 1,986 kilocalories per day

   c. 4,368 kilocalories per day

   d. 9,610 kilocalories per day

2. What is the total metabolism of a female client who weighs 145 pounds (65.8 kg), is lightly active, and consumes 1,700 calories a day?

   a. 1,878 kilocalories per day

   b. 1,916 kilocalories per day

   c. 2,021 kilocalories per day

   d. 2,226 kilocalories per day

3. To gain 1 pound (.45 kg) of a muscle per week, how many kilocalories should a client add to his or her maintenance level (if exercising hard)?

   a. + 157 kilocalories per day

   b. + 250 kilocalories per day

   c. + 315 kilocalories per day

   d. + 500 kilocalories per day

4. Which of the following postworkout food information matches the guidelines presented in this chapter?

   a. 150 grams of carbohydrate, 50 grams of protein, 25 grams of fat

   b. 150 grams of protein, 50 grams of fat, 25 grams of carbohydrate

   c. 100 grams of protein, 100 grams of fat, 30 grams of carbohydrate

   d. 100 grams of carbohydrate, 50 grams of fat, 10 grams of protein

5. A client is 70 inches (177.8 cm) tall and weighs 215 pounds (97.5 kg). What is his or her BMI? Is the client considered obese?

   a. 14.0 BMI, not obese

   b. 26.5 BMI, not obese

   c. 30.8 BMI, obese

   d. 38.3 BMI, obese

Resistance Training Program Design

Developing resistance training programs can be challenging, especially when you have to navigate nearly 20 steps to create a comprehensive program tailored to your client's goals. But the steps are logical and sequential, which helps you address the variables and components of an effective training plan.

WARM-UP

All workouts should start with a warm-up. The purpose of the warm-up is literally to warm up the body by sending blood to the areas involved. The first part of the warm-up prepares the body for the work it is about to do, helps muscles and joints become more limber, and reduces your client's chance of injury. The second part of the warm-up prepares the nervous system. The nerves start firing in the sequence that will help your client perform the activity that you are preparing him or her to do. You have likely seen this process in all sorts of events: the golfer practicing a swing before taking the actual one, the football kicker kicking the ball on the sidelines before he tries

a field goal, and the sprinter sprinting a few yards before a big race. This component of the warm-up is at least as important as being physiologically warmed up, and it is too often misunderstood and undervalued.

These two types of warm-ups are known as the general warm-up and the specific warm-up (table 17.1). The general warm-up is always performed first; as noted, it serves the purpose of literally warming up the body. Five to 10 minutes of some total-body movement is sufficient for the general warm-up. The most common warm-up is a brisk five-minute walk on the treadmill, but you can have your clients perform all sorts of warm-ups. Any cardio machine will suffice, and the rower is particularly good for the upper body. If a machine isn't available, the client can walk outside, walk or jog in place, walk or jog in small circles, walk up and down a flight of stairs, perform jumping jacks, jump rope, and so forth.

The most important thing to remember about the warm-up is that the workout hasn't started yet. The warm-up activity should be relatively easy, something that your clients

Table 17.1 Purposes of the General and Specific Warm-Ups

General warm-up	Specific warm-up
Increase body temperature	Practice the specific motor pattern
Promote blood flow	Increase the rate of muscular contraction
Increase heart and breathing rate	Enhance neuromuscular coordination by increasing the frequency of activation and motor unit recruitment
May increase performance	Allows the person to prepare mentally for the activity
May reduce risk of injury	May reduce the risk of injury

could maintain for 30 minutes if they had to. Many people make the warm-up too challenging, which defeats its purpose. You want your client's heart rate to increase gradually over the 5-minute span, not to spike up and double in 1 minute. The intensity of the warm-up should be about 60 percent of your client's maximum heart rate. Most people accomplish this by a brisk (3.5 to 4.5 mph, or 5.6 to 7.2 km/h) walk. Some coaches and athletes like to include dynamic stretches, mobility drills, foam rollers, and other flexibility exercises as part of the general warm-up. See chapter 25 for more details about this option.

The second part of the warm-up is the specific warm-up, which is always performed after the general warm-up. The purpose of this warm-up is to warm up the specific area that is going to be trained that day. This part of the warm-up prepares the nervous system for action. Often the best specific warm-up is to perform the exercise itself, just with lighter weights. For example, if your client is going to bench press and you plan to have him work out with 200 pounds (90.7 kg) for 10 reps, perhaps you can have him lift just 95 pounds (43.1 kg) for 12 reps, then 155 pounds (70.3 kg) for 8 reps, and then 200 pounds (90.7 kg). In that example, your client performed two warm-up sets before the work set.

In general, you should have your clients perform one to three warm-up sets per exercise. They will perform a greater number of warm-up sets on the first exercise and then fewer, maybe one or two warm-up sets, on subsequent exercises. Sometimes, by the middle of the workout, no warm-up sets are necessary, and you can go right into the work set with them. The higher the level of skill is in the exercise, the more neuromuscular coordination it requires and the more warm-up sets you want to include. In addition, the more weight your client is going to lift, the more warm-up sets you want him or her to perform. The older the client is, the longer and more thorough the warm-up should be, both the general warm-up and the specific warm-up. Older adults should warm up for at least 10 minutes instead of the usual 5. If your clients are trying a new exercise or an exercise that

they are not familiar with, always start with a warm-up set.

Many people take the attitude that a warm-up set is a waste of time, but that is not true. Clearly, a warm-up is beneficial not only for your clients' health and safety but also for their performance. Remember that neuromuscular coordination is the most important factor in performance, and a warm-up set gives your client a chance to practice perfect technique and visualize how he or she will perform on that exercise. As the weight gets heavier, form often begins to break down, and the warm-up provides a fresh memory of what perfect form feels like.

People often use too much weight in the warm-up. Here are a few guidelines. The weight that you start with should be very easy for the client. If the client needs a spot, the weight is too heavy. Clients should be able to double the number of reps that they performed with the warm-up. If you like your clients to warm up with 135 pounds (61.2 kg) for 12 reps on the bench, they should be able to lift 135 pounds (61.2 kg) for 24 reps. Generally, if your clients are using just one warm-up set, the warm-up weight should be approximately 50 to 75 percent (60 percent works well) of the weight of their first work set (not their 1RM). If you are going to have a client bench press 200 pounds (90.7 kg) on the first work set, you should have him or her warm up with somewhere between 100 and 150 pounds (45.4 to 68.0 kg); 135 pounds (61.2 kg) works nicely here. But if you are going to start a client with 150 pounds (68.0 kg) for the first work set, then you should have him or her warm up with 75 to 115 pounds (34.0 to 52.2 kg); 95 or 105 pounds (43.1 or 47.6 kg) works well here. In this instance, 135 pounds (61.2 kg) is too heavy for a warm-up because it is too close to the work set.

Table 17.2 provides common exercises and the number of warm-up sets that are usually performed for these exercises (sets are always written "weight × reps").

Generally, if your clients are lifting less than 20 pounds (9.1 kg), they do not need to perform a specific warm-up for that activity. They simply complete the general warm-up and then go at it. In addition, if your clients are performing fewer than 20 reps on most body-

Table 17.2 Sample Specific Warm-Up Sets for Example Work Sets

Work set	Warm-up sets
Squat 315 lb (142.9 kg) × 5 (5 sets)	45 lb (20.4 kg) × 12 135 lb (61.2 kg) × 8 185 lb (83.9 kg) × 5 235 lb (106.6 kg) × 5 275 lb (124.7 kg) × 3
Squat 150 lb (68.0 kg) × 8 (2 sets)	75 lb (34.0 kg) × 12 115 lb (52.2 kg) × 6
Bench press 275 lb (124.7 kg) × 5 (4 sets)	45 lb (20.4 kg) × 12 135 lb (61.2 kg) × 8 185 lb (83.9 kg) × 5 235 lb (106.6 kg) × 4
Bench press 200 lb (90.7 kg) × 10 (3 sets)	45 lb (20.4 kg) × 12 135 lb (61.2 kg) × 8 135 lb (61.2 kg) × 8
Bench press 185 lb (83.9 kg) × 8 (2 sets)	45 lb (20.4 kg) × 12 135 lb (61.2 kg) × 10
Bench press 60 lb (27.2 kg) × 12 (1 set)	35 lb (15.9 kg) × 12
Lat pull-down 150 lb (68.0 kg) × 10 (1 set)	100 lb (45.4 kg) × 10
DB military press 60 lb (27.2 kg) × 8 (2 sets)	20 lb (9.1 kg) × 12 40 lb (18.1 kg) × 8
DB lateral raise 25 lb (11.3 kg) × 12 (1 set)	15 lb (6.8 kg) × 12
Deadlift 315 lb (142.9 kg) × 8 (2 sets)	135 lb (61.2 kg) × 12 225 lb (102.1 kg) × 8
Leg press 720 lb (326.6 kg) × 6 (3 sets)	180 lb (81.6 kg) × 12 360 lb (163.3 kg) × 10 540 lb (244.9 kg) × 8
Leg press 100 lb (45.4 kg) × 15 (1 set)	60 lb (27.2 kg) × 12
Bicep curl 75 lb (34.0 kg) × 10 (1 set)	50 lb (22.7 kg) × 10
Tricep extension 50 lb (22.7 kg) × 12 (1 set)	30 lb (13.6 kg) × 12

weight exercises, you may not need a specific warm-up for them. If your clients are performing challenging body-weight exercises such as pull-ups or dips, you can have them warm up by using a machine. For example, if you want your client to complete eight pull-ups, he or she can perform one or two sets on a lat pull-down machine first. Use body weight to determine the warm-up weight. If the person weighs 170 pounds (77.1 kg), put 100 to 120 pounds (45.4 to 54.4 kg) on the machine. The client performs the set, rests, and then tries for the pull-ups.

PROGRAM DESIGN

Developing resistance training programs for your clients can be fun, but the process can also be confusing and perhaps a little intimidating. Because you can manipulate so many options and variables, the development process can seem overwhelming at first. The National Personal Training Institute's system of exercise program design is a series of steps that you can use to create effective and results-oriented training programs.

The core of this system is based on improving the client's primary resistance training goal. Reflect back to the beginning of this text. What is it that you, as a personal trainer, are trained to do? Personal trainers should be experts at improving the components of fitness. You want to relate a client's goal to one of the components of fitness and then build a program around that goal. Remember that a client who is new to exercise or has little training experience should follow the beginner workout outlined in chapter 18.

Clients often have goals related to the components of fitness: to increase strength, increase muscle size, increase muscular endurance, and lose weight (improve body composition). These goals are covered in this chapter. Other goals, such as to increase power, increase cardiovascular endurance, and tone up, are covered in their respective chapters.

NPTI's System of Exercise Program Design

- Establish the primary resistance training goal for that time period (mesocycle).
- Define and clarify the goal.
- List the expected outcomes.
- List the expected physiological adaptations.
- Analyze the program setup.
- Select the specific routine.
- Select the specific number of resistance training exercises per workout.
- Select the specific number of resistance training exercises per body part or movement.
- Select the specific exercises.
- Put the exercises in their proper order.
- Select the number of reps per work set.
- Select the load per set.
- Select the number of work sets per exercise.
- Select the number of warm-up sets per exercise.
- Choose the desired weight progression.
- Confirm that the selected number of reps per set matches the goal time under tension.
- Select the appropriate rest time between sets.
- Implement any tricks of the trade to elicit faster adaptations.
- Program an appropriate progressive overload.

The next several sections focus on a specific primary training goal and follow the NPTI's system of exercise program design to create a program. The client should have completed a minimum of two months of a beginning program (such as that described in chapter 18) before following the sample one-month programs for strength, hypertrophy, muscular endurance, or fat loss.

Define and Clarify the Goal: Increase Maximal Strength

The purpose of this program is to improve the client's ability to exert maximal strength in one all-out effort, that is, to improve the client's 1RM in the desired exercises.

List the Expected Outcomes

After following a strength-based program, clients should be able to lift more weight in the exercises that they were training on. In general, as strength increases, activities of daily living should become easier to perform, work capacity on related exercises should increase, sporting performance may increase, muscles may grow in size, resistance to injury should increase, and self-confidence should grow (20).

List the Expected Physiological Adaptations

Specific changes take place in the body when a client follows a muscular strength training program:

- Actin, myosin, and related filaments thicken and increase strength.
- Neuromuscular coordination increases, which can result from the following changes:
  - Increased frequency of activation
  - Improved ability to recruit motor units
  - Improved firing ability of motor nerves
- Motor units may begin to switch over to Type II motor units.
- Bone, tendons, and ligaments generally increase in strength along with the muscle.

- Increased power comes from the phosphagen system.

Analyze the Program Setup

Programming for strength requires a good balance of frequency versus intensity. The intensity must be high enough to elicit the adaptations that the client is seeking, but the frequency must also be high enough to improve the neuromuscular coordination of the person. A large part of strength can be viewed simply as skill, and building any skill, strength included, requires practice. Strength-based programs usually train a movement or area of the body one to three times per week, and two times per week is the most common option.

Select the Specific Routine

Strength can be increased in many ways. The goal of this section is to provide the personal trainer with a template of proven, time-tested methods that will build muscular strength. If a personal trainer chooses to emphasize intensity over frequency, the client will be lifting heavy weights one or two times a week for each area of the body. If a personal trainer chooses to emphasize frequency over intensity, the client will be lifting slightly lighter (but still heavy) weights two or three times per week for each area of the body. The specific routine chosen will be heavily dependent on the total number of training sessions per week. Table 17.3 describes several common routines to increase strength.

Select the Number of Resistance Training Exercises per Workout

Training for maximal strength can be time consuming and draining. In general, a moderate number of exercises is selected per workout. The number can be as few as 2 exercises or as many as 10, but 4 to 7 resistance training exercises per workout is the most common for a 60-minute personal training session.

Select the Number of Resistance Training Exercises per Body Part or Movement

In general, training for muscular strength consists of two to five exercises per muscle group. Larger muscles usually use more exercises than smaller ones.

Select the Specific Exercises

Exercise selection is important when it comes to training for strength. This point relates back to the principle of specificity—the body adapts specifically to the demand imposed on it. Generally, when training for strength, the goal is not to get better at a specific exercise just to lift more weight in that one exercise (unless the person is a competitive lifter). The hope is that by getting stronger at one exercise, the client will then be stronger in a variety of similar exercises and activities. This important

Table 17.3   Specific Strength Routines and Their Corresponding Frequency

Total training sessions per week	Frequency of each area per week	Specific routine
4	2	Upper–lower* repeated or push–pull** repeated
3	3	Total body***
3	1	Push, legs, pull routine
2****	2	Total body

*Upper refers to training the muscles of the upper body (chest, back, shoulders, and arms); lower refers to training the muscles of the lower body (glutes, quads, hamstrings, calves) and the core (abs and lower back).

**Push refers to training the pushing muscles of the upper body (chest, shoulders, and triceps); pull refers to training the pulling muscles of the upper body (back and biceps). Legs are usually included in a pull day because it is shorter than a push day, but that practice is not mandatory.

***Total body classically refers to performing an upper-body pushing movement, an upper-body pulling movement, and a compound exercise for the lower body. A specific area of the body can still be emphasized in a total-body routine.

****Training just twice a week for strength is likely not ideal, but that frequency may be all that the client can commit to at that time.

concept is called the transfer of skill, which expresses the idea that improved performance in one movement will translate to improved performance in another movement even if that second movement is not regularly practiced. For example, improvement in the bench press often yields improvement in push-ups even if push-ups are not practiced regularly. Improvement in the squat commonly results in an increased leg press even if the leg press is not used regularly. Those improvements result from the transfer of skill.

Most personal trainers and clients are aware of the idea of the transfer of skill, but they believe that it applies broadly, not specifically, which is incorrect. For example, performing a one leg exercise does not automatically improve every other leg exercise. To be clearer, the transfer of skill flows downhill. That means that the skill of a high-skill exercise will likely transfer to a lower-skill exercise but the transfer is unlikely to occur in the opposite direction. To expand on the examples given earlier, if a client trains hard on squats for a year, even if that is the only exercise the person does, when he or she attempts a leg press, his or her performance on the leg press will be significantly improved compared with what an untrained person could do. But if a client trains hard on the leg press for a year but never does anything else, that strength built in the leg press is unlikely to transfer immediately to yield an impressive squat. The client will need time, likely months, to learn how to use the strength developed in the leg press and apply it to the squat.

High-skill exercises are usually compound, free-weight exercises that require the ability to move in three dimensions and that stimulate large-muscle groups. Lower-skill exercises are usually isolation, machine-based exercises that require movement in only two dimensions. Note that lifting more weight is a component of skill. For example, more skill is needed to lift 800 pounds (362.9 kg) on the leg press than 200 pounds (90.7 kg). Note as well that although some exercises performed in the gym require higher skill than other exercises, some sports and activities (gymnastics, for example) involve movements that require significantly higher skill to complete than movements found in the gym. A relatively strong person in the gym will struggle to perform certain gymnastic moves if he or she has not regularly practiced those moves.

To take advantage of the transfer of skill in developing maximal strength, exercise selection should be guided by the following information. Select an exercise that allows the most weight to be lifted and requires the most skill. Both aspects need to be followed to elicit the best gains in strength; weights lifted must be heavy (for the client), and the exercises need to require a reasonable level of skill or technique. Table 17.4 contains five exercises for each area of the body that do a good job of building strength.

People are not expected to train only on these exercises or to perform all the exercises in every session. Most strength-based workout programs consist of four to seven total resistance training exercises per workout.

Put the Exercises in Their Proper Order

Exercise order is important in building strength. The traditional guidelines of starting the workout with high-skill, compound, free-weight exercises and then moving to lower-skill, isolation machine exercises (if even necessary) still apply. Advanced clients might perform doubles in which they return to a key, compound exercise at the end of the training session after already having trained on it at the beginning of the workout.

Select the Number of Reps per Work Set

When training for strength, the number of reps performed is generally low. This approach allows the person to lift more weight, and strength is traditionally tested by performing just a few reps, often just 1 rep. The number of reps per set will usually be 10 or fewer, and 1 to 6 reps per set is the standard recommendation (49).

Select the Load per Set

Strength-based programs almost always involve an intensity greater than 50 percent

Table 17.4 Ideal Exercises for Each Body Area to Build Strength

Chest	Back	Shoulders	Total body
Bench press	Pull-ups	Push press	Clean and press
Incline press	Chin-ups	Barbell military press	Farmer's walk
Decline press	Bent-over row	DB military press	Yolk walk
DB press	DB row	Power DB lateral raise	Sled drag
Dips	Cable row	Leaning lateral raise	Muscle-ups

Biceps	Triceps	Legs	Abs
EZ-bar curl	Close-grip bench	Squats	Hanging leg raise
Power curl	Board press	C deadlifts	Inverted sit-up
DB curl	Skull crushers	Sumo deadlifts	Cable crunch
DB hammer curl	DB overhead tricep extension	Good mornings	Dragon flags
Strict curl	V-grip tricep push-down	Leg press	Standing ab wheel

of the 1RM. An amount significantly higher than that is often recommended, particularly for advanced clients, and 85 percent or more of the 1RM is the standard.

Select the Number of Work Sets per Exercise

Strength programs usually are based on multiple sets per exercise. The standard is 2 to 6 working sets per exercise, although anywhere from 1 to 20 working sets can be employed. The classic strength-building set and rep program is 5 sets of five reps.

Select the Number of Warm-Up Sets per Exercise

Warm-up sets are important when training for strength. The purpose is to prepare the body and mind to perform at a high level. Warming up for the first exercise of the day usually involves two to six warm-up sets when training for strength; three warm-up sets works well. On subsequent exercises, zero to two warm-up sets are usually performed, and one warm-up set works well.

Choose the Desired Weight Progression

Multiple-set strength-based programs commonly involve ascending-set patterns, meaning that the weight lifted increases with each set. This pattern helps build neuromuscular coordination, and each set helps the client prepare for heavier weight. Straight sets, or sets across (same weight for all sets), can also work, as can a pyramid progression (weight increasing to a peak and then decreasing). Descending sets (weight decreasing each set) are rarely used when training for strength (189).

Confirm That the Selected Number of Reps per Set Matches the Goal Time Under Tension

Strength routines typically do not involve a long time spent under tension. Strength programs are most closely related with the phosphagen energy system, which yields high power but only for a short duration. The time under tension for each set is generally 15 seconds or less.

Select the Appropriate Rest Time Between Sets

The final key to a strength program is the rest between sets. Most texts recommend a longer rest, and this break is crucial for success. Some anecdotal evidence suggests that when the sets are intense, rest is the most important variable in determining whether strength or size is improved, especially for intermediate lifters. A client who is training for strength needs relatively long rests. The standard recommendation is 2 to 5 minutes. On a few extratough sets, you can let the client rest longer than that. The client should not rest for more than 15 minutes between sets, and 10 minutes is usually too long. A client who seems to need more than 5 minutes to recover fully probably needs to improve his or her general conditioning.

Implement Any Tricks of the Trade to Elicit Faster Adaptations

Some tricks or specific tools can be used to help reach each training goal. When training for strength, people should avoid doing some things and ought to do others to increase performance. When following a strength-building workout, they should avoid or use sparingly the following exercises and equipment:

- Smith machine
- Leg extension
- Chest machine
- Shoulder press machine
- Stability balls
- Anything using light dumbbells (less than 20 pounds, or 9.1 kg, for men; less than 10 pounds, or 4.5 kg, for women)
- Regularly training until failure
- The big four contraindicated exercises

"Sparingly" doesn't mean that the client should never perform those exercises—except that the big four contraindicated exercises should definitely be eliminated—it just means that unless an exercise is improving a specific weakness, it will not be as beneficial as other exercises and will not be a good use of the client's time and energy.

Not as many tricks apply to building strength as to building size, but here are some techniques to incorporate periodically for strength building:

- Cluster sets
- Negatives
- Partials
- Accommodating resistance
- Compensatory acceleration

Remember that a strength-based program should, of course, build strength. This goal is specific and measurable. Periodically, normally every two to three months, test your clients and see what kind of progress they have made.

If they are making progress, great, you are doing your job. If they are not making progress, evaluate their consistency and effort in the gym, the workout program, and your methods for elements that could be improved. Make sure that you are following the guidelines outlined earlier.

Program an Appropriate Progressive Overload

Implementing progressive overload is crucial when the goal is increased strength. The most common form of overload is simply increasing the weight, usually by 5 pounds (2.3 kg) but 2.5 to 20 pounds (1.1 to 9.1 kg) or 2 to 5 percent works well. The number of reps can also be increased up to a point after which the number of reps is dropped and the weight is increased. The number of work sets per exercise can be increased to build volume and provide the client with additional practice on the key exercises. Personal trainers looking to increase a client's strength should also look to progress the client to free-weight, barbell exercises. When the client is working with those exercises, proper technique should be constantly reinforced and reaffirmed. Linear progression works well for beginners and intermediates. After a client plateaus with that type of progression, more advanced methods can be used to induce further strength gains (180).

Sample One-Month Strength Training Workout Program

The application of the program design variables to design a resistance training program to increase muscular strength can create many different programs. Table 17.5 provides an example of a one-month program.

Upper- and lower-body workouts three days per week

Client—170-pound (77.1 kg) male, intermediate level

Starting 1RMs—185-pound (83.9 kg) bench, 250-pound (113.4 kg) squat, 330-pound (149.7 kg) deadlift

The compound exercises for this workout follow a 10, 5, 3 protocol, which means that on the first week 10 reps are used (usually

Table 17.5 Sample One-Month Strength Program for an Intermediate-Level Male Client

Upper body

Exercise	Workout 1	Workout 3	Workout 5	Workout 7	Workout 9	Workout 11
Bench press	45 lb (20.4 kg) × 8 95 lb (43.1 kg) × 6 120 lb (54.4 kg) × 10 135 lb (61.2 kg) × 10	45 lb (20.4 kg) × 8 95 lb (43.1 kg) × 6 115 lb (52.2 kg) × 5 135 lb (61.2 kg) × 5 155 lb (70.3 kg) × 5	45 lb (20.4 kg) × 8 95 lb (43.1 kg) × 6 125 lb (56.7 kg) × 3 140 lb (63.5 kg) × 3 155 lb (70.3 kg) × 3 170 lb (77.1 kg) × 3	45 lb (20.4 kg) × 8 95 lb (43.1 kg) × 6 125 lb (56.7 kg) × 10 140 lb (63.5 kg) × 10	45 lb (20.4 kg) × 8 95 lb (43.1 kg) × 6 120 lb (54.4 kg) × 5 140 lb (63.5 kg) × 5 160 lb (72.6 kg) × 5	45 lb (20.4 kg) × 8 95 lb (43.1 kg) × 6 130 lb (59.0 kg) × 3 145 lb (65.8 kg) × 3 160 lb (72.6 kg) × 3 175 lb (79.4 kg) × 3
DB incline press	35 lb (15.9 kg) × 6 55 lb (24.9 kg) × 6 55 lb (24.9 kg) × 6 55 lb (24.9 kg) × 6	35 lb (15.9 kg) × 6 55 lb (24.9 kg) × 8 55 lb (24.9 kg) × 8 55 lb (24.9 kg) × 8	35 lb (15.9 kg) × 6 55 lb (24.9 kg) × 10 55 lb (24.9 kg) × 10 55 lb (24.9 kg) × 10	40 lb (18.1 kg) × 6 60 lb (27.2 kg) × 6 60 lb (27.2 kg) × 6 60 lb (27.2 kg) × 6	40 lb (18.1 kg) × 6 60 lb (27.2 kg) × 8 60 lb (27.2 kg) × 8 60 lb (27.2 kg) × 8	40 lb (18.1 kg) × 6 60 lb (27.2 kg) × 10 60 lb (27.2 kg) × 10 60 lb (27.2 kg) × 10
Pull-ups	BW × 8 BW × 8	BW × 5 BW + 15 lb (6.8 kg) × 5 BW × 5	BW × 3 BW + 15 lb (6.8 kg) × 3 BW + 25 lb (11.3 kg) × 3 BW × × 3	BW × 10 BW × 10	BW × 6 BW + 20 lb (9.1 kg) × 5 BW × 6	BW + 10 lb (4.5 kg) × 3 BW + 20 lb (9.1 kg) × 3 BW + 30 lb (13.6 kg) × 3 BW × 3
45-degree bent-over row	95 lb (43.1 kg) × 8 135 lb (61.2 kg) × 10 155 (70.3 kg) × 10	95 lb (43.1 kg) × 8 145 lb (65.8 kg) × 5 165 lb (74.8 kg) × 5 185 lb (83.9 kg) × 5	135 lb (61.2 kg) × 3 165 lb (74.8 kg) × 3 185 lb (83.9 kg) × 3 205 lb (93.0 kg) × 3	95 lb (43.1 kg) × 8 140 lb (63.5 kg) × 10 160 lb (72.6 kg) × 10	95 lb (43.1 kg) × 8 150 lb (68.0 kg) × 5 170 lb (77.1 kg) × 5 190 lb (86.2 kg) × 5	140 lb (63.5 kg) × 3 170 lb (77.1 kg) × 3 190 lb (86.2 kg) × × 3 210 lb (95.3 kg) × 3
Overhead press	45 lb (20.4 kg) × 8 65 lb (29.5 kg) × 10 80 lb (36.3 kg) × 10	45 lb (20.4 kg) × 8 65 lb (29.5 kg) × 5 85 lb (38.6 kg) × 5 95 lb (43.1 kg) × 5	45 lb (20.4 kg) × 8 60 lb (27.2 kg) × 3 75 lb (34.0 kg) × 3 90 lb (40.8 kg) × 3 105 lb (47.6 kg) × 3	45 lb (20.4 kg) × 8 70 lb (31.8 kg) × 10 85 lb (38.6 kg) × 10	45 lb (20.4 kg) × 8 70 lb (31.8 kg) × 5 90 lb (40.8 kg) × 5 100 lb (45.4 kg) × 5	45 lb (20.4 kg) × 8 65 lb (29.5 kg) × 3 80 lb (36.3 kg) × 3 95 lb (43.1 kg) × 3 110 lb (49.9 kg) × 3
EZ-bar curl	45 (20.4 kg) × 8 70 lb (31.8 kg) × 8 70 lb (31.8 kg) × 8 70 lb (31.8 kg) × 8	45 (20.4 kg) × 8 70 lb (31.8 kg) × 10 70 lb (31.8 kg) × 10 70 lb (31.8 kg) × 10	45 (20.4 kg) × 8 70 lb (31.8 kg) × 12 70 lb (31.8 kg) × 12 70 lb (31.8 kg) × 12	45 (20.4 kg) × 8 75 lb (34.0 kg) × 8 75 lb (34.0 kg) × 8 75 lb (34.0 kg) × 8	45 (20.4 kg) × 8 75 lb (34.0 kg) × 10 75 lb (34.0 kg) × 10 75 lb (34.0 kg) × 10	45 (20.4 kg) × 8 75 lb (34.0 kg) × 12 75 lb (34.0 kg) × 12 75 lb (34.0 kg) × 12
Skull crushers	35 lb (15.9 kg) × 8 60 lb (27.2 kg) × 8 60 lb (27.2 kg) × 8 60 lb (27.2 kg) × 8	35 lb (15.9 kg) × 8 60 lb (27.2 kg) × 10 60 lb (27.2 kg) × 10 60 lb (27.2 kg) × 10	35 lb (15.9 kg) × 8 60 lb (27.2 kg) × 12 60 lb (27.2 kg) × 12 60 lb (27.2 kg) × 12	35 lb (15.9 kg) × 8 65 lb (29.5 kg) × 8 65 lb (29.5 kg) × 8 65 lb (29.5 kg) × 8	35 lb (15.9 kg) × 8 65 lb (29.5 kg) × 10 65 lb (29.5 kg) × 10 65 lb (29.5 kg) × 10	35 lb (15.9 kg) × 8 65 lb (29.5 kg) × 12 65 lb (29.5 kg) × 12 65 lb (29.5 kg) × 12

Lower body

Exercise	Workout 2	Workout 4	Workout 6	Workout 8	Workout 10	Workout 12
Squat	45 lb (20.4 kg) × 8 95 lb (43.1 kg) × 6 135 lb (61.2 kg) × 6 155 lb (70.3 kg) × 10 175 lb (79.4 kg) × 10	45 lb (20.4 kg) × 8 95 lb (43.1 kg) × 6 135 lb (61.2 kg) × 6 165 lb (74.8) × 5 185 lb (83.9 kg) × 5 205 lb (93.0 kg) × 5	45 lb (20.4 kg) × 8 95 lb (43.1 kg) × 6 135 lb (61.2 kg) × 6 165 lb (74.8) × 3 185 lb (83.9 kg) × 3 205 lb (93.0 kg) × 5 225 lb (102.1 kg) × 5	45 lb (20.4 kg) × 8 95 lb (43.1 kg) × 6 135 lb (61.2 kg) × 6 160 lb (72.6 kg) × 10 180 lb (81.6 kg) × 10	45 lb (20.4 kg) × 8 95 lb (43.1 kg) × 6 135 lb (61.2 kg) × 6 170 lb (77.1 kg) × 5 190 lb (86.2 kg) × 5 210 lb (95.3 kg) × 5	45 lb (20.4 kg) × 8 95 lb (43.1 kg) × 6 135 lb (61.2 kg) × 6 170 lb (77.1 kg) × 3 190 lb (86.2 kg) × 3 210 lb (95.3 kg) × 3 230 lb (104.3 kg) × 3
Deadlift	135 lb (61.2 kg) × 6 205 lb (93.0 kg) × 10 235 lb (106.6 kg) × 10	135 lb (61.2 kg) × 6 215 lb (97.5 kg) × 5 245 lb (111.1 kg) × 5 275 lb (124.7 kg) × 5	135 lb (61.2 kg) × 6 210 lb (95.3 kg) × 3 240 lb (108.9 kg) × 3 270 lb (122.5 kg) × 3 300 lb (136.1 kg) × 3	135 lb (61.2 kg) × 6 210 lb (95.3 kg) × 10 240 lb (108.9 kg) × 10	135 lb (61.2 kg) × 6 220 lb (99.8 kg) × 5 250 lb (113.4 kg) × 5 280 lb (127.0 kg) × 5	135 lb (61.2 kg) × 6 215 lb (97.5 kg) × 3 245 lb (111.1 kg) × 3 275 lb (124.7 kg) × 3 305 lb (138.3 kg) × 3
Leg press	180 lb (81.6 kg) × 8 290 lb (131.5 kg) × 10 335 lb (152.0 kg) × 10	180 lb (81.6 kg) × 8 315 lb (142.9 kg) × 5 360 lb (163.3 kg) × 5 405 lb (183.7 kg) × 5	180 lb (81.6 kg) × 8 295 lb (133.8 kg) × 3 340 lb (154.2 kg) × 3 385 lb (174.6 kg) × 3 430 lb (195.0 kg) × 3	180 lb (81.6 kg) × 8 300 lb (136.1 kg) × 10 345 lb (156.5 kg) × 10	180 lb (81.6 kg) × 8 325 lb (147.4 kg) × 5 370 lb (167.8 kg) × 5 415 lb (188.2 kg) × 5	180 lb (81.6 kg) × 8 305 lb (138.3 kg) × 3 350 lb (158.8 kg) × 3 395 lb (179.2 kg) × 3 440 lb (199.6 kg) × 3

(continued)

Table 17.5 *(continued)*

Exercise	Workout 2	Workout 4	Workout 6	Workout 8	Workout 10	Workout 12
Lower body *(continued)*						
Multi-directional lunges	BW 6 *6* *6*	BW 8 *8* *8*	BW 10 *10* *10*	BW + 10 lb (4.5 kg) 6 *6* *6*	BW + 10 lb (4.5 kg) 8 *8* *8*	BW + 10 lb (4.5 kg) 10 *10* *10*
Glute–ham raise	BW 8 *8* *8*	BW 10 *10* *10*	BW 12 *12* *12*	BW + 10 lb (4.5 kg) 8 *8* *8*	BW + 10 lb (4.5 kg) 10 *10* *10*	BW + 10 lb (4.5 kg) 12 *12* *12*
Cable crunch	100 lb (45.4 kg) × 10 100 lb (45.4 kg) × 10	100 lb (45.4 kg) × 10 100 lb (45.4 kg) × 10 100 lb (45.4 kg) × 10	100 lb (45.4 kg) × 10 100 lb (45.4 kg) × 10 100 lb (45.4 kg) × 10 100 lb (45.4 kg) × 10	110 lb (49.9 kg) × 10 110 lb (49.9 kg) × 10	110 lb (49.9 kg) × 10 110 lb (49.9 kg) × 10 110 lb (49.9 kg) × 10	110 lb (49.9 kg) × 10 110 lb (49.9 kg) × 10 110 lb (49.9 kg) × 10 110 lb (49.9 kg) × 10
Hanging leg raise	8 8	8 8 8	8 8 8 8	10 10	10 10 10	10 10 10 10

Italicized sets are warm-up sets.

for two sets), on the second week 5 reps are used (usually for three sets), and on the third week 3 reps are used (usually for four sets). The sets for the compound exercises are generally ascending when training for strength. The assistance exercises consist of a rep range progression by selecting a range of reps (6 to 12 is most common for assistance work) and progressing within that range of reps at the same weight. When the top end of the reps is reached, the weight is increased, the number of reps is reduced, and the process repeats.

It is not uncommon when training for strength to follow a percentage-based plan, particularly for the key exercises in the routine. Table 17.6 shows a sample six-week percentage-based plan that is effective for increasing strength in the key barbell exercises. This information applies to work sets only; it is assumed the person will perform the proper warm-up sets necessary to prepare for the work sets listed.

Define and Clarify the Goal: Increase Muscle Hypertrophy

The purpose of this program is to increase the size of the client's skeletal muscles. The muscles will grow larger as measured by their cross-section, and the proportions and muscularity of the person will change.

List the Expected Outcomes

After following a size-based program, clients should see an increase in muscle size of the trained areas. The client's percent body fat

Table 17.6 Sample Six-Week Percentage-Based Program to Build Strength

Week	Work set 1	Work set 2	Work set 3	Work set 4
1	80% × 2	86% × 2	92.5% × 2	NA
2	80% × 4	87.5% × 3	95% × 2	NA
3	80% × 2	86% × 2	92% × 2	97.5% × 2
4	80% × 5	87.5% × 4	95% × 3	NA
5	80% × 2	86% × 2	92.5% × 2	100% × 2
6	80% × 2	86% × 1	92.5% × AMRAP*	NA

*AMRAP = as many reps as possible.

should decrease, assuming that body weight stays the same. The client may experience an increase in muscle strength and related outcomes, the added muscle may help protect other areas of the client's body, and the client may think that he or she looks better because muscularity is more visible, which in turn may increase self-confidence.

List the Expected Physiological Adaptations

Specific changes take place in the body when a client follows a hypotrophy training program:

- Hypertrophy of the muscle occurs (muscle cross-sectional area increases).
- Contractile protein hypertrophy occurs.
- Noncontractile protein hypertrophy occurs.
- Hyperplasia may possibly occur.
- Type II muscle fibers increase in size.
- Bones, tendons, and ligaments generally increase in size and strength along with the muscle.

Analyze the Program Setup

Sized-based programs differ from strength-based programs in that the volume is usually increased, the frequency for each area is usually decreased, and the time under tension is longer. Size-based programs usually stimulate each area of the body one or two times per week, and clients typically follow a split routine in which the body is split up for training on different days.

Select the Specific Routine

The actual routine that a client follows to build muscular size can vary considerably. It will be heavily influenced by the number of weekly sessions performed. Most clients training for size work out two to four times per week. Some common examples of hypertro-

phy-based workouts are outlined in table 17.7.

Select the Number of Resistance Training Exercises per Workout

The volume is slightly higher in a size-based workout compared with a strength-based one. Most personal trainers therefore use five to eight exercises per workout when going for increased muscle size.

Select the Number of Resistance Training Exercises per Body Part or Movement

To fatigue and stimulate a muscle fully, three to five exercises per muscle are used. Smaller muscles may receive equal or slightly fewer exercises than larger muscles.

Select the Specific Exercises

Exercise selection is also important when training for size. The guideline is to select an exercise that allows the most weight to be lifted and the most isolation of the muscle. If the goal is to build size, a reasonable weight must be used and preference should be given to exercises that allow clients to lift more weight in the same movement, all else being equal. In addition, when training for size, the goal is to isolate, feel, and fatigue a specific muscle group. Muscles

Table 17.7 Specific Hypertrophy Routines and Their Corresponding Frequency

Total training sessions per week	Frequency of each area per week	Specific routine
4	2	Push–pull repeated or upper–lower repeated
4	1	Day 1: chest and biceps Day 2: legs and lower back Day 3: back and abs Day 4: shoulders and triceps
3	1	Day 1: chest and back Day 2: legs, lower back, and abs Day 3: shoulders and arms
2	2	Total body
2	1	Push–pull or upper–lower

don't work in true isolation, which would mean that one muscle contracts while the rest of the body is relaxed, but it is certainly possible to place significant emphasis on one muscle over another with exercise selection. Clients should feel the muscle that they are trying to grow during the set. If they don't, the exercise is likely to be less effective. Remember that stabilization increases muscle activation. One benefit of machines is that they add to stability and are generally more effective for increasing muscle size versus muscular strength. Table 17.8 lists five exercises per muscle group that are effective choices if the goal to increase muscle size.

Put the Exercises in Their Proper Order

The general guidelines presented in the beginner workout chapter still apply when training for size, but the personal trainer has more freedom to rearrange the order of exercises if hypertrophy is the goal. As a client progresses, using preexhaustion, supersets, and compound sets can all be useful to build size.

Select the Number of Reps per Work Set

When training for size, a client should usually lift a moderate number of reps per set, traditionally defined at 6 to 12 reps per set. But personal trainers usually have a lot of freedom when it comes to improving size because many rep selections can work. Lifting fewer than 6 reps of heavy weight is sometimes appropriate in an attempt to recruit more of the large Type IIb motor units. Lifting more than 12 reps of light weight can fully fatigue the muscle and hit as many motor units as possible. A good guideline is to vary the rep ranges over time. Approximately 50 percent of the time use 6 to 12 reps per set, 25 percent of the time use 1 to 5 reps per set, and 25 percent of the time use more than 12 reps per set, usually in the range of 15 to 25 reps. This method ensures that all muscle fibers are being stimulated, and the variation in training can help prevent plateaus and burnout.

Select the Load per Set

Because a client is traditionally lifting a moderate number of reps per set, the weight is also moderate. The weight needs to be heavy enough to stimulate and fatigue the muscle; otherwise, the muscle will not respond. But the weight needs to be light enough that the client can complete a number of reps that is sufficient to tax the muscle fully so that it has to respond to the stimulus. When using 6 to 12 reps per set, the standard is to lift 67 to 85 percent of the 1RM. On the sets in which the client uses fewer reps, the weight will go up to 85 percent or more of the 1RM. When the client performs a high-rep set, the weight will decrease, but it should not go below 50 percent of 1RM.

Select the Number of Work Sets per Exercise

High-volume work has been associated with muscular growth, so the most common recommendation to increase muscular size is to perform a reasonably large number of work

Table 17.8 Ideal Exercises for Each Body Area to Increase Hypertrophy

Chest	Back	Shoulders	Total body
Bench press	Bent-over row	Smith mx mil press	Clean and press
Smith mx bench	Mx row	Power DB lat raise	Squat
Machine press	DB row	Leaning DB lat raise	
DB press	Mx pull-down	Power DB rear delt raise	
Power DB fly	Pullover machine	Rear delt machine	

Biceps	Triceps	Legs	Abs
EZ-curl	Skull crushers	Leg press	Cable crunch
DB curl	Push-downs	Smith mx squat	RC leg raise
Cable curl	Close-grip bench	Squat	Decline sit-up
Power curl	Dips	Deadlift (any)	Mx crunch
DB hammer curl	DB overhead triceps	Leg extension, leg curl	Dumbbell side bend

sets per exercise. The standard is three to six work sets per exercise. In general, the smaller the number of reps performed, the larger the number of work sets completed and vice versa.

Select the Number of Warm-Up Sets per Exercise

Hypertrophy work also requires the use of warm-up sets, although the number of warm-up sets is generally fewer than what is incorporated when training for strength. To prepare for the first exercise of the day, two to four warm-up sets are typically performed before the first work set. For all subsequent exercises, zero to two warm-up sets are usually performed.

Choose the Desired Weight Progression

Size training can be associated with any type of weight progression, but descending sets are commonly used. Straight sets are also common, as are pyramids. Ascending sets are more commonly used for strength programs than for size programs.

Confirm That the Selected Number of Reps per Set Matches the Goal Time Under Tension

Time spent under tension is a more important variable when training for size than it is when training for strength. Hypertrophy is best achieved when muscles are under tension for a moderate time, defined as 15 to 45 seconds and an average of 30 seconds. This goal can be accomplished using a moderate number of reps and a relatively slow tempo (the 2:4 count works well for size) or with a larger number of reps at a fast tempo. The muscle should remain under tension throughout the set, so personal trainers should encourage clients to work on both the eccentric and concentric ranges of motion in each exercise.

Select the Appropriate Rest Time Between Sets

Another key variable in a size program is rest time between sets. Unlike the rest used in training for strength, the rest time is relatively short—30 to 90 seconds after each set. On large exercises, you can let your clients take 2 or even 3 minutes after the set before they go again, but 1 to 2 minutes is a good guideline. You do not want to allow near or full recovery; you want the client to begin each set in a slightly fatigued state. The client thus has to recruit more muscle fibers and release more hormones such as testosterone and growth hormone, both of which are important in improving muscle size. Because of the relatively short rest, the most common practice is to reduce the weight for each set or keep the weight the same. Increasing the weight for each set is difficult when full recovery does not take place between sets.

Implement Any Tricks of the Trade to Elicit Faster Adaptations

When training for size, many tricks can be employed to make the muscle work harder and elicit size gains. Here are some exercises and equipment to avoid. The list is not as long as it is for strength:

- Stability balls
- Anything using light dumbbells (less than 20 pounds, or 9.1 kg, for men; less than 10 pounds, or 4.5 kg, for women)
- The big four contraindicated exercises
- Lack of strength

Lack of strength is mentioned because some clients are interested in building size but they are not very strong. Therefore, they have to use light weight on most exercises that, when combined with shorter rests, may not be enough stimulus to force the muscles to grow. In this case the client would benefit by following a strength-based program for a while to build strength before switching over to a size-based program. Although no hard and fast rules define what is strong enough, males should likely be able to squat their body weight or 200 pounds (90.7 kg), whichever is less, bench press their body weight or 200 pounds, whichever is less, and deadlift 150 percent of their body weight or 300 pounds (136.1 kg), whichever is less, before they begin a size-specialization routine. Females should likely be able to squat 75 percent of their body weight or 100 pounds (45.4 kg), whichever is less, bench 50 percent of their body weight or 65 pounds (29.5 kg), whichever is less, and deadlift their body weight or 135 pounds (61.2 kg), whichever is less, before they begin a size-specialization routine. See the summary in table 17.9.

Here are some things to try periodically when training for size:

- Preexhaustion
- Compound sets
- Supersets
- Timed sets
- Drop sets
- Varying the angle of the stimulus
- Lifting slower to put more tension on the muscle
- Mentally trying to squeeze the muscle as it contracts during the exercise
- Developing a mind–muscle connection
- Getting a pump during the workout
- Feeling the lactate and unbuffered hydrogen ions in the muscles during a workout

Program an Appropriate Progressive Overload

Progression must be following in size-building routines to create the muscular adaptation that the client is looking for. Increasing the weight and increasing the number of reps per set are the most commonly used methods. Personal trainers can also increase the time under tension, decrease rest time, and use other intensity techniques to create progression. If a client plateaus in a certain exercise, the personal trainer should switch the client to a new exercise. Strength does not have to increase to see an increase in size.

Sample One-Month Hypertrophy Training Workout Program

Resistance training programs to increase muscular hypertrophy come in many forms. Table 17.10 shows an example of a one-month program.

Three-day split of push, pull, and legs and core

Client—170-pound (77.1 kg) male, intermediate level

Starting 1RMs—250-pound (113.4 kg) bench, 350-pound (158.8 kg) squat, 425-pound (192.8 kg) deadlift

This hypertrophy workout program is based on using slightly heavier weights and fewer reps for weeks 1 and 2 and then more reps and lighter weights for weeks 3 and 4. The first two weeks generally follow ascending sets, and the last two weeks of the month follow descending sets. After the month is complete, the routine can be repeated if desired with a focus on increasing each set 5 to 10 pounds (2.3 to 4.5 kg) or one to two reps.

Define and Clarify the Goal: Increase Muscular Endurance

The purpose of a muscular endurance program is to improve the client's ability to complete a repetitive physical task, that is, to improve the ability of the muscles to contract repeatedly. The client is also working on improving his or her ability to recover after challenging sets to reduce recovery time (20).

Table 17.9   Theoretical Strength Standard to Achieve Before Specializing in a Hypertrophy Training Program

Exercise	Male standard	Female standard
Squat	Body weight or 200 lb (90.7 kg), whichever is less	75% of body weight or 100 lb (45.4 kg), whichever is less
Bench	Body weight or 200 lb (90.7 kg), whichever is less	50% of body weight or 65 lb (29.5 kg), whichever is less
Deadlift	150% of body weight or 300 lb (136.1 kg), whichever is less	Body weight or 135 lb (61.2 kg), whichever is less

Table 17.10 Sample One-Month Hypertrophy Program for an Intermediate-Level Male Client

Day 1—push day			

Exercise	Week 1	Week 2	Week 3	Week 4
Bench press	*45 lb (20.4 kg) x 8* *95 lb (43.1 kg) x 5* *135 lb (61.2 kg) x 5* 175 lb (79.4 kg) x 8 195 lb (88.5 kg) x 6 205 lb (93.0 kg) x 5 215 lb (97.5 kg) x 5	*45 lb (20.4 kg) x 8* *95 lb (43.1 kg) x 5* *135 lb (61.2 kg) x 5* 180 lb (81.6 kg) x 8 200 lb (90.7 kg) x 6 210 lb (95.3 kg) x 5 220 lb (99.8 kg) x 5	*45 lb (20.4 kg) x 8* *95 lb (43.1 kg) x 5* *135 lb (61.2 kg) x 5* 185 lb (83.9 kg) x 10 170 lb (77.1 kg) x 12 155 lb (70.3 kg) x 15	45 lb (20.4 kg) x 8 95 lb (43.1 kg) x 5 135 lb (61.2 kg) x 5 190 lb (86.2 kg) x 10 175 lb (79.4 kg) x 12 160 lb (72.6 kg) x 15
Incline bench press	*95 lb (43.1 kg) x 6* 135 lb (61.2 kg) x 10 150 lb (68.0 kg) x 8 165 lb (74.8 kg) x 6	*95 lb (43.1 kg) x 6* 140 lb (63.5 kg) x 10 155 lb (70.3 kg) x 8 170 lb (77.1 kg) x 6	*115 lb (52.2 kg) x 6* 165 lb (74.8 kg) x 8 145 lb (65.8 kg) x 12 125 lb (56.7 kg) x 15	*115 lb (52.2 kg) x 6* 170 lb (77.1 kg) x 8 150 lb (68.0 kg) x 12 130 lb (59.0 kg) x 15
Cable crossover	30 lb (13.6 kg) x 10 30 lb (13.6 kg) x 10 30 lb (13.6 kg) x 10	30 lb (13.6 kg) x 12 30 lb (13.6 kg) x 12 30 lb (13.6 kg) x 12	20 lb (9.1 kg) x 20 20 lb (9.1 kg) x 20 20 lb (9.1 kg) x 20	20 lb (9.1 kg) x 22 20 lb (9.1 kg) x 22 20 lb (9.1 kg) x 22
Seated DB military press	*25 lb (11.3 kg) x 8* 40 lb (18.1 kg) x 10 50 lb (22.7 kg) x 8 60 lb (27.2 kg) x 6	*25 lb (11.3 kg) x 8* 40 lb (18.1 kg) x 12 50 lb (22.7 kg) x 10 60 lb (27.2 kg) x 8	*30 lb (13.6 kg) x 6* 55 lb (24.9 kg) x 10 45 lb (20.4 kg) x 12 35 lb (15.9 kg) x 15	*30 lb (13.6 kg) x 6* 60 lb (27.2 kg) x 10 50 lb (22.7 kg) x 12 40 lb (18.1 kg) x 15
Leaning DB lateral raise	25 lb (11.3 kg) x 10 25 lb (11.3 kg) x 10 25 lb (11.3 kg) x 10	25 lb (11.3 kg) x 12 25 lb (11.3 kg) x 12 25 lb (11.3 kg) x 12	20 lb (9.1 kg) x 15 20 lb (9.1 kg) x 15 20 lb (9.1 kg) x 15	20 lb (9.1 kg) x 18 20 lb (9.1 kg) x 18 20 lb (9.1 kg) x 18
Dips	*BW x 6* BW + 45 lb (20.4 kg) x 5 BW + 25 lb (11.3 kg) x 8 BW + 10 lb (4.5 kg) x 10	*BW x 6* BW + 55 lb (24.9 kg) x 5 BW + 35 lb (15.9 kg) x 8 BW + 15 lb (6.8 kg) x 10	AMRAP of BW 3 sets	AMRAP of BW 3 sets
Skull crusher	*65 lb (29.5 kg) x 6* 80 lb (36.3 kg) x 10 90 lb (40.8 kg) x 8 100 lb (45.4 kg) x 6	*65 lb (29.5 kg) x 6* 85 lb (38.6 kg) x 10 95 lb (43.1 kg) x 8 105 lb (47.6 kg) x 6	*65 lb (29.5 kg) x 8* 90 lb (40.8 kg) x 10 80 lb (36.3 kg) x 12 70 lb (31.8 kg) x 15	*65 lb (29.5 kg) x 8* 95 lb (43.1 kg) x 10 85 lb (38.6 kg) x 12 75 lb (34.0 kg) x 15
V-grip tricep push-down	90 lb (40.8 kg) x 10 90 lb (40.8 kg) x 10 90 lb (40.8 kg) x 10	95 lb (43.1 kg) x 10 95 lb (43.1 kg) x 10 95 lb (43.1 kg) x 10	100 lb (45.4 kg) x 10 90 lb (40.8 kg) x 12 80 lb (36.3 kg) x 15	105 lb (47.6 kg) x 10 95 lb (43.1 kg) x 12 85 lb (38.6 kg) x 15

Day 2—pull day			

Exercise	Week 1	Week 2	Week 3	Week 4
Pull-up	*BW x 6* BW + 10 lb (4.5 kg) x 8 BW + 20 lb (9.1 kg) x 6 BW + 30 lb (13.6 kg) x 6	*BW x 6* BW + 15 lb (6.8 kg) x 8 BW + 25 lb (11.3 kg) x 6 BW + 35 lb (15.9 kg) x 6	AMRAP of BW 3 sets	AMRAP of BW 3 sets
45-degree bent-over row	*135 lb (61.2 kg) x 6* 185 lb (83.9 kg) x 10 205 lb (93.0 kg) x 8 225 lb (102.1 kg) x 6	*135 lb (61.2 kg) x 6* 190 lb (86.2 kg) x 10 210 lb (95.3 kg) x 8 230 lb (104.3 kg) x 6	*135 lb (61.2 kg) x 6* *185 lb (83.9 kg) x 5* 205 lb (93.0 kg) x 10 185 lb (83.9 kg) x 12 155 lb (70.3 kg) x 15	*135 lb (61.2 kg) x 6* *185 lb (83.9 kg) x 5* 210 lb (95.3 kg) x 10 190 lb (86.2 kg) x 12 160 lb (72.6 kg) x 15
Hammer strength row	*140 lb (63.5 kg) x 6* 210 lb (95.3 kg) x 10 240 lb (108.9 kg) x 8 270 lb (122.5 kg) x 6	*140 lb (63.5 kg) x 6* 215 lb (97.5 kg) x 10, 245 lb (111.1 kg) x 8 275 lb (124.7 kg) x 6	*160 lb (72.6 kg) x 6* 230 lb (104.3 kg) x 10 210 lb (95.3 kg) x 12 180 lb (81.6 kg) x 15	*160 lb (72.6 kg) x 6* 235 lb (106.6 kg) x 10, 215 lb (97.5 kg) x 12 185 lb (83.9 kg) x 15

(continued)

Table 17.10 (continued)

Day 2—pull day (continued)			
Exercise	**Week 1**	**Week 2**	**Week 3**	**Week 4**
Power DB rear delt raise	30 lb (13.6 kg) x 10 30 lb (13.6 kg) x 10 30 lb (13.6 kg) x 10	30 lb (13.6 kg) x 12 30 lb (13.6 kg) x 12 30 lb (13.6 kg) x 12	20 lb (9.1 kg) x 20 20 lb (9.1 kg) x 20 20 lb (9.1 kg) x 20	20 lb (9.1 kg) x 22 20 lb (9.1 kg) x 22 20 lb (9.1 kg) x 22
EZ curl	*65 lb (29.5 kg) x 8* 85 lb (38.6 kg) x 10 100 lb (45.4 kg) x 8 115 lb (52.2 kg) x 6	*65 lb (29.5 kg) x 8* 90 lb (40.8 kg) x 10 105 lb (47.6 kg) x 8 120 lb (54.4 kg) x 6	*65 lb (29.5 kg) x 8* 100 lb (45.4 kg) x 10 85 lb (38.6 kg) x 12 65 lb (29.5 kg) x 15	*65 lb (29.5 kg) x 8* 105 lb (47.6 kg) x 10 90 lb (40.8 kg) x 12 70 lb (31.8 kg) x 15
DB hammer curl	35 lb (15.9 kg) x 10 35 lb (15.9 kg) x 10 35 lb (15.9 kg) x 10	35 lb (15.9 kg) x 12 35 lb (15.9 kg) x 12 35 lb (15.9 kg) x 12	25 lb (11.3 kg) x 20 25 lb (11.3 kg) x 20 25 lb (11.3 kg) x 20	25 lb (11.3 kg) x 22 25 lb (11.3 kg) x 22 25 lb (11.3 kg) x 22
Cable curl	70 lb (31.8 kg) x 10 90 lb (40.8 kg) x 8 110 lb (49.9 kg) x 6	75 lb (34.0 kg) x 10 95 lb (43.1 kg) x 8 115 lb (52.2 kg) x 6	*65 lb (29.5 kg) x 8* 105 lb (47.6 kg) x 10 90 lb (40.8 kg) x 12 70 lb (31.8 kg) x 15	*65 lb (29.5 kg) x 8* 110 lb (49.9 kg) x 10 95 lb (43.1 kg) x 12 75 lb (34.0 kg) x 15

Day 3—legs and core			
Exercise	**Week 1**	**Week 2**	**Week 3**	**Week 4**
Squat	*135 lb (61.2 kg) x 8* *185 lb (83.9 kg) x 6* 235 lb (106.6 kg) x 10 255 lb (115.7 kg) x 8 275 lb (124.7 kg) x 6 295 lb (133.8 kg) x 5	*135 lb (61.2 kg) x 8* *185 lb (83.9 kg) x 6* 240 lb (108.9 kg) x 10 260 lb (117.9 kg) x 8 280 lb (127.0 kg) x 6 300 lb (136.1 kg) x 5	*135 lb (61.2 kg) x 8* *205 lb (93.0 kg) x 6* 255 lb (115.7 kg) x 10 235 lb (106.6 kg) x 12 215 lb (97.5 kg) x 15	*135 lb (61.2 kg) x 8* *205 lb (93.0 kg) x 6* 260 lb (117.9 kg) x 10 240 lb (108.9 kg) x 12 220 lb (99.8 kg) x 15
Deadlift	*135 lb (61.2 kg) x 8* *205 lb (93.0 kg) x 6* 275 lb (124.7 kg) x 10 305 lb (138.3 kg) x 8 335 lb (152.0 kg) x 6	*135 lb (61.2 kg) x 8* *205 lb (93.0 kg) x 6* 280 lb (127.0 kg) x 10 310 lb (140.6 kg) x 8 340 lb (154.2 kg) x 6	*135 lb (61.2 kg) x 8* *225 lb (102.1 kg) x 6* 295 lb (133.8 kg) x 10 265 lb (120.2 kg) x 12 235 lb (106.6 kg) x 15	*135 lb (61.2 kg) x 8* *225 lb (102.1 kg) x 6* 300 lb (136.1 kg) x 10 270 lb (122.5 kg) x 12 240 lb (108.9 kg) x 15
Leg press	*180 lb (81.6 kg) x 8* *360 lb (163.3 kg) x 6* 540 lb (244.9 kg) x 5 585 lb (265.4 kg) x 5 405 lb (183.7 kg) x 15	*180 lb (81.6 kg) x 8* *360 lb (163.3 kg) x 6* 550 lb (249.5 kg) x 5 595 lb (269.9) x 5 415 lb (188.2 kg) x 15	*270 lb (122.5 kg) x 8* *405 lb (183.7 kg) x 5* 500 lb (226.8 kg) x 10 455 lb (206.4 kg) x 12 410 lb (186.0 kg) x 15	*270 lb (122.5 kg) x 8* *405 lb (183.7 kg) x 5* 510 lb (231.3 kg) x 10 465 lb (210.9 kg) x 12 420 lb (190.5 kg) x 15
Seated leg curl	*105 lb (47.6 kg) x 8* 135 lb (61.2 kg) x 12 157 lb (71.2 kg) x 10 180 lb (81.6 kg) x 8	*105 lb (47.6 kg) x 8* 142 lb (64.4 kg) x 12 165 lb (74.8 kg) x 10 187 lb (84.8 kg) x 8	*120 lb (54.4 kg) x 8* 172 lb (78.0 kg) x 10 150 lb (68.0 kg) x 12 127 lb (57.6 kg) x 15	*120 lb (54.4 kg) x 8* 180 lb (81.6 kg) x 10 157 lb (71.2 kg) x 10 135 lb (61.2 kg) x 15
Standing calf raise	200 lb (90.7 kg) x 15 230 lb (104.3 kg) x 12 260 lb (117.9 kg) x 10	205 lb (93.0 kg) x 15 235 lb (106.6 kg) x 12 265 lb (120.2 kg) x 10	180 lb (81.6 kg) x 20 180 lb (81.6 kg) x 20 180 lb (81.6 kg) x 20	185 lb (83.9 kg) x 20 185 lb (83.9 kg) x 20 185 lb (83.9 kg) x 20
Hyperextension	BW x 12 BW + 15 lb (6.8 kg) x 10 BW + 25 lb (11.3 kg) x 8	BW x 12 BW + 20 lb (9.1 kg) x 10 BW + 30 lb (13.6 kg) x 8	BW x 20 BW x 20 BW x 20	BW x 22 BW x 22 BW x 22
Hanging leg raise	10 10 10	11 11 11	Knees: 20 20 20	Knees: 22 22 22
Decline sit-up	40 lb (18.1 kg) x 12 50 lb (22.7 kg) x 10 60 lb (27.2 kg) x 8	45 lb (20.4 kg) x 12 55 lb (24.9 kg) x 10 65 lb (29.5 kg) x 8	30 lb (13.6 kg) x 20 30 lb (13.6 kg) x 20 30 lb (13.6 kg) x 20	30 lb (13.6 kg) x 22 30 lb (13.6 kg) x 22 30 lb (13.6 kg) x 22

Italicized sets are warm-up sets. AMRAP = as many reps as possible.

List the Expected Outcomes

After following a program based on muscular endurance, clients should be able to perform more repetitions at a given weight with the exercises that they have been training on. In general, activities of daily living should become easier as muscular endurance increases, work capacity on related exercises should increase significantly, the ability to recover between work sets and exercises should improve, and the muscle may increase in strength and possibly size. The client should be more resistant to injury and may have more self-confidence as his or her muscular endurance increases.

List the Expected Physiological Adaptations

Specific changes take place in the body when a client follows a muscular endurance training program:

- Stimulation of Type I and Type IIa motor units
- Increase in capillaries
- Increase in mitochondria
- Increase in myoglobin
- Increase in storage of glycogen in the muscles
- Ability to tolerate increased pH levels in the muscles
- Increase in red blood cells
- Increase in stroke volume (72)

Analyze the Program Setup

Programming for muscular endurance generally favors frequency over intensity. Because the number of reps is high and the load is low, the demand on the neuromuscular system is also low. Therefore, the body can recover relatively quickly from traditional muscular endurance exercises. Most muscular endurance programs follow a frequency of training each area two to four times per week.

Select the Specific Routine

Muscular endurance programs are usually designed around higher frequencies, so once-a-week routines that might be used for muscular size are less commonly followed. Table 17.11 provides common examples of sample muscular endurance workout programs.

Select the Number of Resistance Training Exercises per Workout

Generally, 5 to 10 resistance training exercises are used per workout session when working to improve muscular endurance.

Select the Number of Resistance Training Exercises per Body Part or Movement

The large number of reps and fast pace will fatigue a muscle rapidly. One to three exercises per muscle group are usually recommended to increase muscular endurance.

Select the Specific Exercises

Exercise selection is important for developing muscular endurance. Personal trainers should select the most challenging functional exercises that the client can complete for 20 or more reps to build muscular endurance. Functional exercise in this instance is an exercise that moves in three dimensions and has high probability of transferring to common, everyday activities. Challenging exercises require more skill and more stabilization. Don't forget that simply using more weight significantly increases the challenge. Table 17.12 lists

Table 17.11 Specific Muscular Endurance Routines and Their Corresponding Frequency

Total training sessions per week	Frequency of training each area per week	Specific routine
4	4	Total body
4	2	Upper and lower
3	3	Total body
2	2	Total body

three to five exercises for each area of the body that do a good job of increasing muscular endurance.

Put the Exercises in Their Proper Order

The order of the exercises performed for muscular endurance is significant. Because of the nature of training for muscular endurance, fatigue builds quickly. If one area of the body is extremely fatigued before the person moves on to another exercise, that fatigued area will significantly limit performance. Thus, exercise order should be large, key, compound, high-skill exercises first followed by smaller, isolation, and lower-skill exercises if necessary (44).

Select the Number of Reps per Work Set

When training for muscular endurance, the number of reps per work set is generally high. Most sets consist of 12 or more reps; 15 to 20 reps is the norm. Occasionally, ultrahigh rep sets can be performed, particularly if the client will be tested on something in which a large number of reps is the goal.

Select the Load per Set

The number of reps performed in an exercise has an inverse relationship with the load. When the number of reps is high, the load invariably must be reduced. Relatively light loads, usually defined as less than 67 percent of 1RM, are most commonly used to build muscular endurance.

Select the Number of Work Sets per Exercise

Training for muscular endurance involves a large number of reps per set, which results in a high volume per set. For that reason, the number of work sets per exercise can be relatively low compared with other training methods. Traditionally, two or three work sets are performed for each exercise.

Select the Number of Warm-Up Sets per Exercise

Fewer warm-up sets are employed when training for muscular endurance as compared with training for strength and size because the weight being used is lighter and the number of reps is higher. In general, zero to two warm-up sets are used to prepare for the first exercise in the session, and zero or one warm-up set is used for all exercises after that.

Choose the Desired Weight Progression

Weight progression during an exercise is usually static in muscular endurance programs. The high level of fatigue generated by the first work set makes it hard to increase the load significantly without reducing the number of reps; either straight sets or descending sets are usually used.

Table 17.12 Ideal Exercises for Each Body Area to Increase Muscular Endurance

Chest	Back	Shoulders	Total body
Bench press	Pull-up	Handstand push-up	Burpees
Push-up	Chin-up	Barbell military press	Bear crawl
Dip	Inverted row	DB military press	Thrusters
Ring push-up	DB row	DB lateral raise	
One-arm push-up	Flexed arm hang	DB rear delt raise	
Biceps	**Triceps**	**Legs**	**Abs**
EZ-bar curl	Close grip push-up	Squat	Plank
Suspension curl	Bench dips	Lunge	Sit-up
DB curl	Band push-down	Leg Press	Crunch
			Bicycle
			Wood chop

Confirm That the Selected Number of Reps per Set Matches the Goal Time Under Tension

Time under tension is usually quite long when training for muscular endurance, because the goal is prolonged effort. Most work sets are at least 30 seconds long, and 45 to 60 seconds is the norm. After a client can perform an exercise for longer than 2 minutes straight, greater results are likely to be achieved by making the exercise harder to perform for 45 to 60 seconds than by increasing the duration of the set.

Select the Appropriate Rest Time Between Sets

The rest time between work sets for muscular endurance is generally low, particularly when the goal is to build multiple-set endurance. The body must learn to adapt and recover even with minimal recovery time. Rest times are usually 1 minute or less, and 30 seconds or less is the most common recommendation.

Implement Any Tricks of the Trade to Elicit Faster Adaptations

Training for muscular endurance is generally straightforward, but a few tricks can be used in workout programs to help clients achieve the goal of building muscular endurance. These tricks include the following:

- Drop sets combined with a high number of reps per set
- Compound sets combined with a high number of reps pet set
- Body-weight exercises
- Timed sets
- Timed rests
- Stretching or light active recovery between sets to promote recovery

Program an Appropriate Progressive Overload

Progressive overload is still important when it comes to building muscular endurance. The most obvious choice is to increase the number of reps. Decreasing the rest time, increasing the load, and moving toward more challenging exercises are all valuable tools to build positive adaptations in a client.

Sample One-Month Muscular Endurance Training Workout Program

Applying the program design variables to design a muscular endurance training program can result in a variety of programs. Table 17.13 provides an example of a one-month program.

Two-day split of upper body and lower body

Client—155-pound (70.3 kg) female, early intermediate or late beginner level

Starting level—20 modified push-ups, 0 pull-ups

Define and Clarify the Goal: Weight Loss

The purpose of a weight-loss program is to create a caloric deficit while engaging in resistance training. Note that weight loss can be achieved in many ways—by controlling food intake, performing regular cardiovascular exercise, manipulating water intake—but the purpose of this program is to promote weight loss through resistance training. At the end of the program, clients should weigh less on a scale and should have reduced the amount of fat mass on their bodies as compared with the start of the program.

List the Expected Outcomes

After following a weight-loss program, clients should weigh less at the end of the program than when they started; their percent body fat should decrease or at least not increase; they might improve their muscle strength, muscle size, and muscle endurance; their activities of daily living should seem easier because they weigh less; cardiovascular endurance should improve; risk factors may improve if the weight loss is significant; health may improve and lifespan may increase if the weight loss is maintained; and clients may have greater confidence in themselves because they weigh less.

Table 17.13 Sample One-Month Muscular Endurance Program for an Early Intermediate or Late Beginner Female Client

	Upper body					
Exercise	**Day 1**	**Day 3**	**Day 5**	**Day 7**	**Day 9**	**Day 11**
Assisted pull-up	3 x 8	3 x 9	3 x 10	4 x 5 1 leg	4 x 6 1 leg	4 x 7 1 leg
Push-up	3 x 8	10, 8, 8	12, 10, 8	14, 11, 8	16, 12, 8	18, 14, 10
Body-weight rows at 5	8, 8, 6	10, 8, 6	12, 10, 8	Lower bar 3 x 6	Lower bar 3 x 7	Lower bar 3 x 8
Body-weight slide fly	8 out 8 up 8 out	8 out 8 up 8 out	8 out 8 up 8 out	10 out 10 up 10 out	10 out 10 up 10 out	10 out 10 up 10 out
Standing DB military press	10 lb (4.5 kg) x 12 10 lb (4.5 kg) x 12 12 lb (5.4 kg) x 12	10 lb (4.5 kg) x 14 10 lb (4.5 kg) x 14 12 lb (5.4 kg) x 14	10 lb (4.5 kg) x 16 10 lb (4.5 kg) x 16 12 lb (5.4 kg) x 16	12 lb (5.4 kg) x 8 12 lb (5.4 kg) x 8 15 lb (6.8 kg) x 8	12 lb (5.4 kg) x 10 12 lb (5.4 kg) x 10 15 lb (6.8 kg) x 10	12 lb (5.4 kg) x 12 12 lb (5.4 kg) x 12 15 lb (6.8 kg) x 12
Tube lateral raise	Power 12, 12 Strict 20, 20	Power 12, 12 Strict 20, 20	Power 12, 12 Strict 20, 20	Power 15, 15 Strict 25, 25	Power 15, 15 Strict 25, 25	Power 15, 15 Strict 25, 25
Assisted dips plus isometric hold	3 x 6 :10	3 x 7 :10	3 x 8 :10	3 x 9 :15	3 x 10 :15	3 x 11 :15
Flexed arm hang with band	:20 :15	:20 :15	:25 :20	:25 :20	:30 :25	:30 :25
Push-ups negative plus modified positive	3 x 8	3 x 10	3 x 12	3 x 6 military	3 x 8 military	3 x 10 military

	Lower body					
Exercise	**Day 2**	**Day 4**	**Day 6**	**Day 8**	**Day 10**	**Day 12**
Goblet squats	25 lb (11.3 kg) x 12 35 lb (15.9 kg) x 12 45 lb (20.4 kg) x 12	25 lb (11.3 kg) x 15 35 lb (15.9 kg) x 15 45 lb (20.4 kg) x 15	35 lb (15.9 kg) x 8 45 lb (20.4 kg) x 8 55 lb (24.9 kg) x 8	35 lb (15.9 kg) x 10 45 lb (20.4 kg) x 10 55 lb (24.9 kg) x 10	35 lb (15.9 kg) x 12 45 lb (20.4 kg) x 12 55 lb (24.9 kg) x 12	35 lb (15.9 kg) x 15 45 lb (20.4 kg) x 15 55 lb (24.9 kg) x 15
DB squats wide stance	25 lb (11.3 kg) x 12 35 lb (15.9 kg) x 12 45 lb (20.4 kg) x 12	25 lb (11.3 kg) x 15 35 lb (15.9 kg) x 15 45 lb (20.4 kg) x 15	35 lb (15.9 kg) x 8 45 lb (20.4 kg) x 8 55 lb (24.9 kg) x 8	35 lb (15.9 kg) x 10 45 lb (20.4 kg) x 10 55 lb (24.9 kg) x 10	35 lb (15.9 kg) x 12 45 lb (20.4 kg) x 12 55 lb (24.9 kg) x 12	35 lb (15.9 kg) x 15 45 lb (20.4 kg) x 15 55 lb (24.9 kg) x 15
Walking lunge (2 = one time up and back)	BW x 2 25 lb (11.3 kg) x 2	BW x 2 25 lb (11.3 kg) x 2	BW x 2 35 lb (15.9 kg) x 2	BW x 2 35 lb (15.9 kg) x 2	15 lb (6.8 kg) x 2 45 lb (20.4 kg) x 2	15 lb (6.8 kg) x 2 45 lb (20.4 kg) x 2
Glute–ham raise	16	18	20	22	24	26
Romanian deadlift	45 lb (20.4 kg) x 12 65 lb (29.5 kg) x 12 65 lb (29.5 kg) x 12	45 lb (20.4 kg) x 15 65 lb (29.5 kg) x 15 65 lb (29.5 kg) x 15	45 lb (20.4 kg) x 18 65 lb (29.5 kg) x 18 65 lb (29.5 kg) x 18	45 lb (20.4 kg) x 20 65 lb (29.5 kg) x 20 65 lb (29.5 kg) x 20	55 lb (24.9 kg) x 8 75 lb (34.0 kg) x 8 75 lb (34.0 kg) x 8	55 lb (24.9 kg) x 10 75 lb (34.0 kg) x 10 75 lb (34.0 kg) x 10
Donkey calf raise, one leg	12 x 3	14 x 3	16 x 3	18 x 3	20 x 3	22 x 3
Ab wheel	3 x 8	3 x 9	3 x 10	4 x 6	4 x 7	4 x 8
Rotations	5 x 30 3 sets	5 x 30 3 sets	5 x 35 3 sets	5 x 35 3 sets	5 x 40 3 sets	5 x 40 3 sets
Plank	1:30	2:00	2:30	3:00	3:30	4:00
Hyperextension	3 x 12	3 x 14	3 x 16	3 x 18	3 x 20	3 x 22
Body-weight squats to box	2 x 20	2 x 24	2 x 28	2 x 32	2 x 36	2 x 40

List the Expected Physiological Adaptations

Specific changes take place in the body when a client follows a program to lose body fat:

- Reduced total fat mass
- Reduced blood pressure
- Possible loss of lean mass if weight loss is rapid
- Increased insulin receptor sensitivity
- Decreased risk of cancers if weight loss brings about a healthy BMI and is maintained

Analyze the Program Setup

Weight-loss programs tend to be most similar in setup to muscular endurance programs. Generally, personal trainers choose to emphasize frequency over intensity. Most weight-loss programs are performed two to four times per week.

Select the Specific Routine

Weight-loss programs traditionally follow a total-body routine. Using total-body exercises and training large-muscle groups in each session allows a maximal number of calories to be burned. Some common examples of weight-loss workouts are outlined in table 17.14.

Select the Number of Resistance Training Exercises per Workout

Generally, 6 to 12 resistance training exercises are used per workout session when the goal is weight loss. This higher volume helps keep the client moving and exercising during the entire session.

Select the Number of Resistance Training Exercises per Body Part or Movement

Weight-loss programs use a good number of exercises per workout and a higher frequency of training for each area of the body. The total number of exercises per muscle group is therefore limited to one or two when training for weight loss.

Select the Specific Exercises

Inducing weight loss through resistance training is best achieved by selecting exercises that burn the most calories minute per minute and create the greatest excess postexercise oxygen consumption (EPOC). Personal trainers therefore generally want to select exercises that require standing rather than sitting, require some coordination and balance rather than rely on a machine to do that, and are challenging enough to disrupt homeostasis so that the body adapts to them. Listed in table 17.15 are several exercises for each area of the body that are effective at generating weight loss. Note that although all the exercises listed can burn many calories and create EPOC, not all clients, particularly those with a large amount of weight to lose, will be able to complete these exercises. Exercises should be regressed and modified to meet the client's needs and abilities (123). Table 17.15 lists several exercises per muscle group that are effective choices for weight loss.

Put the Exercises in Their Proper Order

If the goal is to produce weight loss, effort is more important than actual performance during a training session. When effort becomes the focus, the general rules of exercise order such as performing exercises with large-muscle groups first no longer apply. When in doubt the rules should still be followed, but a more common approach when training for weight loss is to mix up the order, to alternate between upper and lower body, to jump from one exercise to the next and then back again. To lose weight, the client should be huffing and puffing during the training session. The personal trainer is in essence mimicking a cardiovascular workout with resistance training, which ideally will produce positive changes in body composition and may end up being more enjoyable for the client.

Table 17.14 Specific Weight-Loss Routines and Their Corresponding Frequency

Total training sessions per week	Frequency of each area per week	Specific routine
4	4	Total body
3	3	Total body
2	2	Total body

Table 17.15   Ideal Exercises for Each Body Area to Promote Weight Loss

Chest	Back	Shoulders	Total body
Bench press Alt medicine ball push-up Walking sled press	Jumping pull-ups Renegade row Standing sled row	Handstand push-up Standing alt DB military press Lunging lateral raise	Battling ropes Medicine ball slam Bear crawl Sprinting Thruster
Biceps	**Triceps**	**Legs**	**Abs**
Power curl Biceps and triceps are generally not isolated when it comes to training for weight loss.	Close-grip push-up	Squat Jumping squats Frog jump Deadlift Walking lunge	Wood chop Sword swing Hanging leg raise

Select the Number of Reps per Work Set

The number of reps per work set can vary greatly when training for weight loss. High weight and a low number of reps can be used to stimulate the Type IIb fibers and create EPOC, but in general lower weight and a higher number of reps are chosen to increase heart rate and burn more calories per minute. The most common recommendation is 8 to 20 reps per set.

Select the Load per Set

Load can also vary greatly for weight-loss programs. The weight usually isn't heavy, but if it is too light, it may not promote positive adaptations. Thus, a weight between 50 and 70 percent of the 1RM is generally suggested.

Select the Number of Work Sets per Exercise

Multiple work sets per exercise are usually chosen to produce weight loss simply because multiple sets usually yield a greater workload. If too many sets are used, however, fatigue will become excessive and effort will suffer. A better course is to switch over to another exercise so that the client is fresher and can work harder rather than continue with an exercise after becoming exhausted doing it. Two to four work sets per exercise are traditionally used.

Select the Number of Warm-Up Sets per Exercise

Warming up for weight loss will be similar to warming up for muscular endurance. The weight used is often light, the number of reps is high, and performance is not as prioritized as it might be for the other goals. Zero to two warm-up sets are used for the first exercise, and zero or one warm-up set is used after that.

Choose the Desired Weight Progression

The client is likely to be lifting in a fatigued state for most of the training session. Straight sets or descending sets are therefore more desirable than ascending sets after the client is warmed up.

Confirm That the Selected Number of Reps per Set Matches the Goal Time Under Tension

Time under tension per set can vary considerably when training clients for weight loss. The time under tension is rarely short (less than 15 seconds), but if it is too long, the client may be intentionally moving slowly or even recovering during the set. The usual recommendation is 15 to 45 seconds under tension per set.

Select the Appropriate Rest Time Between Sets

Typically, a fat-loss program includes or allows little if any rest between exercises. To maximize EPOC, a client typically moves from exercise to exercise in a continuous manner rather than resting for a specific duration between exercises.

Implement Any Tricks of the Trade to Elicit Faster Adaptations

Personal trainers can use many tricks of the trade to help clients focus on weight loss during a workout session without reverting to classic cardiovascular work. Some of those tricks include the following:

- Supersets
- Combination exercises
- Active rest
- Circuit training
- Compound sets
- Timed rest
- Timed sets
- Drop sets
- Rest–pause reps
- Peripheral heart action training

Program an Appropriate Progressive Overload

Progressive overload for weight loss comes primarily by trying to increase work capacity. Achieving this means increasing the number of reps performed, increasing the weight lifted, and decreasing down time (time spent not being active). Over time the client should be able to perform more work and burn more calories in the same period (the personal training session).

Sample One-Month Fat-Loss Workout Program

A personal trainer can design many programs that will decrease a client's body fat. Tables 17.16 through 17.18 provide an example of a one-month program.

Total body training with cardio training and a strict diet

Client—132-pound (59.9 kg) female with 24 percent body fat, late intermediate level

Starting level—resistance training three times a week (total-body training)

A complex consists of the following exercises performed consecutively without rest:

- Romanian deadlift
- Hang clean
- Thruster
- Squat
- Good morning
- 90-degree bent-over row

Also, the jumping pull-ups and the burpees are supersetted, and the front squat and 400-meter run are supersetted. For an illustration of the burpee and the thruster exercises, refer to figures 17.1 and 17.2, respectively.

The shoulder series consists of performing one set of lateral raises, one set of front raises, and one set of rear delt raises consecutively. The push-up and kettlebell or dumbbell row exercises (figure 17.3) are supersetted with the goblet squat exercise (figure 17.4). Also, the deadlift and sled drag (figure 17.5) exercises are supersetted. The tabata routine consists of performing 20 seconds of the exercise followed by 10 seconds of rest; the number indicated is how many intervals of that is performed.

The frog jump exercise involves jumping forward, backward, to one side, and to the other side for the number indicated. The 4-1 routine means starting with four jumps in each direction, then immediately doing three jumps in each direction, then two jumps in each direction, and finally just one jump in each direction. The overhead farmer's walk exercise consists of holding one or two kettlebells with the arms overhead and walking for

Table 17.16 Sample One-Month Fat-Loss Program for a Late Intermediate Female Client (Day 1)

Exercise	Day 1	Day 4	Day 7	Day 10
Complex, 5 rounds	55 lb (24.9 kg) x 8	55 lb (24.9 kg) x 10	60 lb (27.2 kg) x 8	60 lb (27.2 kg) x 10
Jumping pull-up, 4 rounds	6	7	8	9
Burpee, 4 rounds	6	7	8	9
Front squat	95 lb (43.1 kg) x 12 2 sets	95 lb (43.1 kg) x 12 2 sets	95 lb (43.1 kg) x 12 3 sets	95 lb (43.1 kg) x 12 3 sets
400-meter run	2 sets	2 sets	3 sets	3 sets

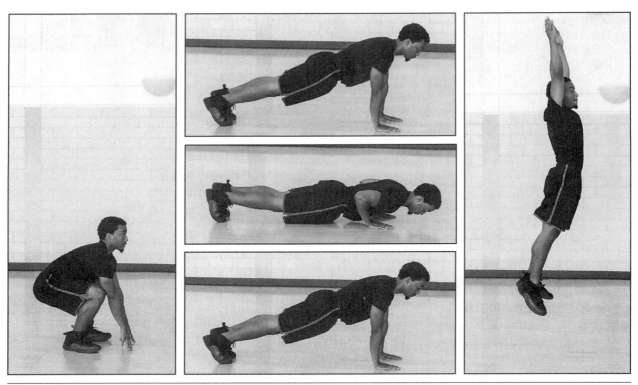

Figure 17.1 Five stages of the burpee exercise.

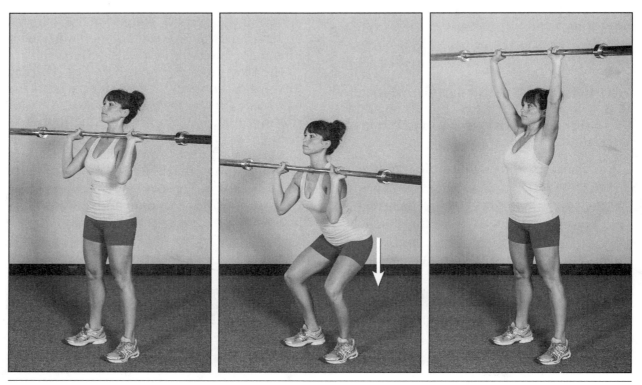

Figure 17.2 Three stages of the thruster exercise.

Table 17.17 Sample One-Month Fat-Loss Program for a Late Intermediate Female Client (Day 2)

Exercise	Day 2	Day 5	Day 8	Day 11
Shoulder series, 3 sets	8 lb (3.6 kg) x 10	8 lb (3.6 kg) x 12	10 lb (4.5 kg) x 8	10 lb (4.5 kg) x 10
Push-up plus DB row, 4 sets	12 25 lb (11.3 kg) x 6	14 25 lb (11.3 kg) x 7	16 25 lb (11.3 kg) x 8	18 25 lb (11.3 kg) x 9
Goblet squat, 4 sets	55 lb (24.9 kg) x 10	55 lb (24.9 kg) x 12	60 lb (27.2 kg) x 10	60 lb (27.2 kg) x 12
Deadlift, 5 sets	145 lb (65.8 kg) x 5	145 lb (65.8 kg) x 5	150 lb (68.0 kg) x 5	150 lb (68.0 kg) x 5
Sled drag, 5 sets	135 lb (61.2 kg)	135 lb (61.2 kg)	145 lb (65.8 kg)	145 lb (65.8 kg)
Tabata front squat	55 lb (24.9 kg) 5 intervals	55 lb (24.9 kg) 6 intervals	55 lb (24.9 kg) 7 intervals	55 lb (24.9 kg) 8 intervals

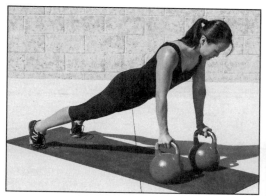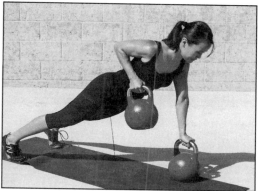

Figure 17.3 Pushup with kettlebell row.

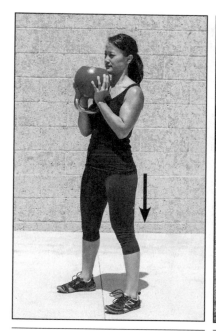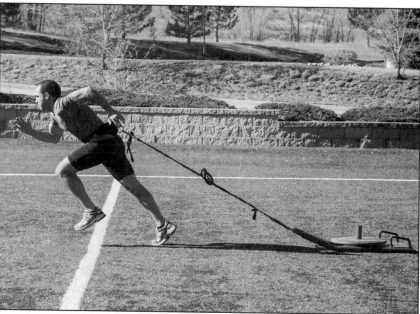

Figure 17.4 Goblet squat.

Figure 17.5 Sled drag.

Table 17.18 Sample One-Month Fat-Loss Program for a Late Intermediate Female Client (Day 3)

Exercise	Day 3	Day 6	Day 9	Day 12
Complex	55 lb (24.9 kg) x 9	55 lb (24.9 kg) x 12	60 lb (27.2 kg) x 9	60 lb (27.2 kg) x 12
Frog jump, 4 sets	4-1 each way	4-1 each way	5-1 each way	5-1 each way
Overhead farmer's walk with a kettle-bell, 4 sets	25 lb (11.3 kg)	25 lb (11.3 kg)	30 lb (13.6 kg)	30 lb (13.6 kg)
Prowler push alternating high and low, 6 total trips	50 lb (22.7 kg)	50 lb (22.7 kg)	60 lb (27.2 kg)	60 lb (27.2 kg)

a distance. Note that the frog jump and overhead farmer's walk are supersetted. Refer to figure 17.6 for an illustration of the prowler push exercise.

For a fat-loss program, an ideal approach is to combine the workouts in tables 17.16 through 17.18 with brisk walking at 4.0 miles per hour (6.4 km/h) or faster three or more times per week for 45 to 120 minutes. The client's heart rate should fall in the range of 60 to 70 percent of his or her maximum heart rate.

PROGRAMS BASED ON A CLIENT'S ONE-REPETITION MAXIMUM

Many of the one-month sample programs call for a client to lift a certain percentage of his or her one-rep max (1RM). A logical question that follows is, "What is my client's one-rep max?" There are two main ways to find a client's 1RM. The most accurate method is to have a client max out, although that approach is not appropriate or necessary for all clients. A personal trainer can estimate a client's maximum by analyzing a challenging set that a client has completed and using a conversion chart to predict the one-rep max. That prediction is easier and quicker to do, but it is less accurate than having the client max out. Both methods are outlined in the following sections.

Warm Up for a 1RM Test

When your clients are ready to attempt a maximum effort in an exercise, follow the procedure outlined here to help achieve maximal results. The ideal amount of warm-up undoubtedly varies from person to person;

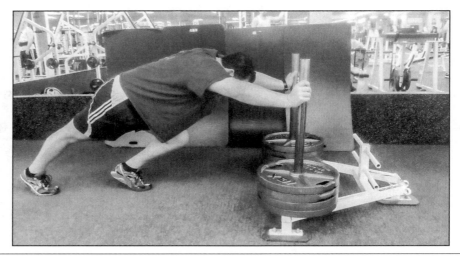

Figure 17.6 Prowler push.

some people find that they prefer to be fully warmed up, sweating, and almost slightly fatigued when they go for a max. Others find that just a few warm-up sets are enough to get them ready. Customizing and individualizing the warm-up routine is OK, but until you are familiar with how the person responds, start with the routine presented here.

Before you test a client's 1RM, a few words of caution are needed. First, clients should not max out on an exercise they are unfamiliar with. Although you might want to know the client's true starting point, too much risk is involved in asking an untrained person to lift maximal weights, particularly for any free-weight exercise. The client should practice with the exercise for four to eight weeks at a minimum before attempting to max out. Second, the client's form should be good. Minimal movement compensations should occur with normal work weight. If the client has a preexisting injury, even more caution should be used. The safety of the client is paramount, so the personal trainer should take every precaution necessary. You should feel comfortable spotting the weight that the client is going to lift, and recruiting additional spotters is rarely a bad idea on the particularly challenging sets. Equipment should be inspected, and safety pins or other apparatus should be properly installed at the correct height. Squats and bench press pose the most risk, so you must be particularly careful with those exercises. If a client wishes to max out at home on the bench, which is not recommended, using weightlifting collars is not recommended in case the lifter has to dump the bar. Any lifting attempts in the gym with a barbell should use the weightlifting collars to keep the weight locked on the bar.

To prepare for the max attempt, the client should perform both a general warm-up and a specific warm-up. The more intensely a client is training and the more weight he or she will be lifting, the more important the warm-up becomes. Therefore, a proper warm-up procedure is paramount when preparing for a max lift. The general warm-up can be just the basic 5 to 10 minutes of activity to get the client warm, improve blood flow, and prepare the body for general physical activity. A brisk walk, five minutes on the bike, 500 to 1,000 meters on the rower, and a sled drag are all good choices. Dynamic stretches and foam rolling can be included as part of the warm-up as well, after any cardio that is performed. The more inflexible or stiff an area is, the more important this warm-up will be. Most people comment that the warm-up and particularly some sort of stretching are more important for the lower-body exercises than for the upper body, but each client is different.

After your client has completed the general warm-up, you then have them perform a specific warm-up, which is the focus of this section. The purpose of the specific warm-up is to prepare the body for the specific activity that is to follow. Jogging 3 miles (4.8 km) is different from benching 315 pounds (142.9 kg), so the warm-up for each activity will be different. With resistance training, the best way to warm up for a heavy weight is to perform the same exercise with a lighter weight. Push-ups are an acceptable way to warm up for the bench, but performing some lighter weight bench presses is better. You are literally warming up the client's neuromuscular system, so you want to have the person practice the movement with light weight before he or she lifts the heavy weight.

To do this percentage-based warm-up, you need to know your client's max. You may not know the exact max (which may be why you want your client to max out), but you should have an idea of what it is. A conversion chart can be helpful here. If that doesn't work, use 5 or 10 pounds (2.2 or 4.5 kg) more than your client's best 3RM load. Pick a conservative number that you are confident the client can lift for one rep and use that number. When in doubt, go light and remember that what counts is not what the client starts with but what he or she ends up with. You are going to try to have your client hit his or her max in anywhere from 5 to 12 sets. The more weight the person can lift and the more skill needed to complete the lift, the more warm-ups you want the client to do.

Table 17.19 provides the basic outline of what the specific warm-up routine looks like. Some common examples with exact numbers follow so that you can see what the setup will look like when it is fleshed out.

The following tables specify how to warm up for some common maxes. At the end of each example, a suggestion is provided about how much to go up if your client is successful with the max attempt. Your client should perform a general warm-up (as described earlier) before each specific warm-up.

As mentioned earlier, people seem to need different levels of warm-ups. To account for this, three possible warm-up scenarios are offered for each example: a normal warm-up, a high-volume warm-up, and a low-volume warm-up. The high-volume warm-up is for someone who likes to be very warm and almost fatigued, is feeling extra stiff that day, or is lifting in a cold environment. The normal warm-up is the most effective for the majority of people, and you should use that one with your clients. The normal warm-up is based on the preceding chart. A low-volume warm-up is good for people who just like to grab the bar and go or are worried about becoming excessively fatigued before they max out.

Here are some key points to consider when testing a client's 1RM:

- Using convenient weights like 135 pounds (61.2 kg), 225 pounds (102.1 kg), and so on is acceptable when progressing through the warm-up.

- Jumps in weight should stay the same size or decrease in size; they should not be erratic or get larger.

- The biggest difference between the high-volume warm-ups and the low-volume warm-ups occurs in the lighter sets. After

getting to around 80 to 90 percent of the max, stick to one or two reps.

- Do not have the client warm up with anything at or above 95 percent of his or her max. That weight is heavy enough to tire out the client and not heavy enough to prove anything.

If your client has already maxed out previously, add 5 pounds (2.3 kg), or 10 pounds (4.5 kg) at most, and use that as the max set even if you hope that he or she will ultimately be able to do more. If the client hits his or her max, use your best guess, increase the weight, and try again. Increasing the weight 2 to 5 percent is usually best after a successful max attempt. The increase should definitely not be more than 10 percent. If the client is successful on that set, he or she rests and simply goes again. The client should not get tired and instead will probably find the excitement of hitting new maxes to be highly motivating. The momentum will seem to build on itself. Hitting a max on the way up is much easier than it is on the way down. A failure is very defeating, so don't expect to take 10 pounds (4.5 kg) off and then automatically see a success at that lower weight. Repeating a max that the client has already completed doesn't make much sense unless you really want to know whether he or she can do it again. Otherwise, try a new weight.

You will see a warm-up routine for both a squat of 405 pounds (183.7 kg) and a deadlift of 405 pounds in table 17.20. The two routines are presented to highlight the differences between the exercises even though the goal weight is the same. The higher-skill, less natural movement of the squat usually requires a

Table 17.19　How to Warm Up for a 1RM

Warm-up set	%1RM	Reps	Rest after set
1	~30–50%	8	~2 minutes
2	~60%	5	~2 minutes
3	~70%	3	~3 minutes
4	~80%	1	~3 minutes
5	~90%	1	~5 minutes
6 (max out)	100%	1	5–15 minutes
7+ (max out)	+ ~2–5%	1	5–15 minutes

longer, more intensive warm-up than a deadlift of equal weight. Competitive powerlifters can use this information if they wish to do so. They should put their first attempt (the opener) in as their max on this formula; the second and third attempts follow (powerlifters should not try to set a new PR on their first attempt in a meet).

Finally, the table includes only one female-specific example. But if your client is attempting to lift a similar weight to that for another example, even if it is a different exercise, that weight can still be a starting point for the client. For example, if a female is going to try to squat 185 pounds (83.9 kg) for a max, she could use the recommendations for a male benching 185 pounds as a starting point. The same theme is true for the men. If a male could bench 405 pounds (183.7 kg), use the squat or deadlift warm-up with that weight as a starting point. You can use the percentage guidelines if your client can lift more than the examples given, but at that level most lifters would have a decent idea of how to warm up. Don't be afraid to add sets if you think that your clients need it. Rarely should people use fewer than three warm-up sets before trying a max. Repeating some of the earlier warm-up sets can be useful to add some volume without tiring out a client. For example, a client can perform two sets at 135 pounds (61.2 kg) to get loose.

Clients generally need and want a lot of positive motivation during a maximal attempt. Clients might be a little intimidated by the weight

Table 17.20 Sample Warm-ups for Specific 1RM Attempts

Female bench 105 lb (47.6 kg) 1RM			Male bench 185 lb (83.9 kg) 1RM		
Normal	High	Low	Normal	High	Low
45 lb (20.4 kg) x 8	45 lb (20.4 kg) x 12	45 lb (20.4 kg) x 5	95 lb (43.1 kg) x 8	95 lb (43.1 kg) x 12	95 lb (43.1 kg) x 5
60 lb (27.2 kg) x 5	55 lb (24.9 kg) x 8	65 lb (29.5 kg) x 3	115 lb (52.2 kg) x 5	115 lb (52.2 kg) x 8	125 lb (56.7 kg) x 3
75 lb (34.0 kg) x 3	65 lb (29.5 kg) x 5	85 lb (38.6 kg) x 1	135 lb (61.2 kg) x 3	135 lb (61.2 kg) x 5	125 lb (56.7 kg) x 3
85 lb (38.6 kg) x 1	75 lb (34.0 kg) x 3	105 lb (47.6 kg) x 1*	155 lb (70.3 kg) x 1	155 lb (70.3 kg) x 2	145 lb (65.8 kg) x 1
95 lb (43.1 kg) x 1	85 lb (38.6 kg) x 1		170 lb (77.1 kg) x 1	170 lb (77.1 kg) x 1	165 lb (74.8 kg) x 1
105 lb (47.6 kg) x 1*	95 lb (43.1 kg) x 1		185 lb (83.9 kg) x 1**	185 lb (83.9 kg) x 1**	185 lb (83.9 kg) x 1**
	105 lb (47.6 kg) x 1*				

Male bench 250 lb (113.4 kg) 1RM			Male bench 315 lb (142.9 kg) 1RM		
Normal	High	Low	Normal	High	Low
115 lb (52.2 kg) x 8	95 lb (43.1 kg) x 12	135 lb (61.2 kg) x 5	145 lb (65.8 kg) x 8	135 lb (61.2 kg) x 12	160 lb (72.6 kg) x 3
145 lb (65.8 kg) x 5	135 lb (61.2 kg) x 8	175 lb (79.4 kg) x 3	185 lb (83.9 kg) x 5	135 lb (61.2 kg) x 12	205 lb (93.0 kg) x 3
175 lb (79.4 kg) x 3	135 lb (61.2 kg) x 8	200 lb (90.7 kg) x 2	215 lb (97.5 kg) x 3	185 lb (83.9 kg) x 8	235 lb (106.6 kg) x 2
205 lb (93.0 kg) x 1	165 lb (74.8 kg) x 5	225 lb (102.1 kg) x 1	245 lb (111.1 kg) x 1	225 lb (102.1 kg) x 5	265 lb (120.2 kg) x 1
230 lb (104.3 kg) x 1	195 lb (88.5 kg) x 3	250 lb (113.4 kg) x 1***	275 lb (124.7 kg) x 1	245 lb (111.1 kg) x 3	295 lb (133.8 kg) x 1
250 lb (113.4 kg) x 1***	215 lb (97.5 kg) x 1		295 lb (133.8 kg) x 1	265 lb (120.2 kg) x 2	315 lb (142.9 kg) x 1****
	235 lb (106.6 kg) x 1		315 lb (142.9 kg) x 1****	285 lb (129.3 kg) x 1	
	250 lb (113.4 kg) x 1***			300 lb (136.1 kg) x 1	
				315 lb (142.9 kg) x 1****	

Male squat 405 lb (183.7 kg) 1RM			Male deadlift 405 lb (183.7 kg) 1RM		
Normal	High	Low	Normal	High	Low
135 lb (61.2 kg) x 8	135 lb (61.2 kg) x 12	135 lb (61.2 kg) x 5	135 lb (61.2 kg) x 8	135 lb (61.2 kg) x 12	205 lb (93.0 kg) x 3
185 lb (83.9 kg) x 5	135 lb (61.2 kg) x 12	225 lb (102.1 kg) x 3	225 lb (102.1 kg) x 5	185 lb (83.9 kg) x 12	275 lb (124.7 kg) x 3
235 lb (106.6 kg) x 3	185 lb (83.9 kg) x 8	275 lb (124.7 kg) x 2	275 lb (124.7 kg) x 3	225 lb (102.1 kg) x 8	325 lb (147.4 kg) x 1
285 lb (129.3 kg) x 3	235 lb (106.6 kg) x 8	325 lb (147.4 kg) x 1	325 lb (147.4 kg) x 1	275 lb (124.7 kg) x 5	365 lb (165.6 kg) x 1
325 lb (147.4 kg) x 1	275 lb (124.7 kg) x 5	365 lb (165.6 kg) x 1	365 lb (165.6 kg) x 1	325 lb (147.4 kg) x 3	405 lb (183.7 kg) x 1*****
365 lb (165.6 kg) x 1	315 lb (142.9 kg) x 3	405 lb (183.7 kg) x 1*****	405 lb (183.7 kg) x 1*****	365 lb (165.6 kg) x 1	
405 lb (183.7 kg) x 1*****	345 lb (156.5 kg) x 1			405 lb (183.7 kg) x 1*****	
	375 lb (170.1 kg) x 1				
	405 lb (183.7 kg) x 1*****				

(continued)

Table 17.20 (continued)

Male deadlift 500 lb (226.8 kg) 1RM		
Normal	**High**	**Low**
135 lb (61.2 kg) x 8	135 lb (61.2 kg) x 12	135 lb (61.2 kg) x 5
225 lb (102.1 kg) x 5	225 lb (102.1 kg) x 12	225 lb (102.1 kg) x 3
315 lb (142.9 kg) x 3	275 lb (124.7 kg) x 8	315 lb (142.9 kg) x 2
365 lb (165.6 kg) x 1	325 lb (147.4 kg) x 5	405 lb (183.7 kg) x 1
415 lb (188.2 kg) x 1	375 lb (170.1 kg) x 3	455 lb (206.4 kg) x 1
455 lb (206.4 kg) x 1	425 lb (192.8 kg) x 1	500 lb (226.8 kg) x 1******
500 lb (226.8 kg) x 1******	465 lb (210.9 kg) x 1	
	500 lb (226.8 kg) x 1******	

*Increase weight by 2.5 to 10 pounds (1.1 to 4.5 kg) on the next attempt.

**Increase weight by 5 to 10 pounds (2.3 to 4.5 kg) on the next attempt.

***Increase weight by 5 to 15 pounds (2.3 to 6.8 kg) on the next attempt.

****Increase weight by 5 to 20 pounds (2.3 to 9.1 kg) on the next attempt.

*****Increase weight 10 to 30 pounds (4.5 to 13.6 kg) on the next attempt.

******Increase weight 10 to 40 pounds (4.5 to 18.1 kg) on the next attempt.

that they are lifting because it is likely heavier and simply appears bigger than what they are used to lifting. Maxing out is often particularly foreign for female clients, but both males and females will enjoy the process if it is set up correctly (although the process can be deflating if it is set up incorrectly). Clients often take their cues from the personal trainer. Believing in clients and encouraging them to do their best will go a long way. Failing during a max attempt should cause no shame; the shame occurs in letting fear prevent someone from trying. Finding a max can be both fun and extremely useful in helping you design a more accurate program and in giving you feedback on how the program is actually working; you can't fake a new max. But at the same time, you do not need to use this method with all clients.

1RM Testing

Most personal trainers have a client complete a warm-up set, increase the weight, have the client complete the first work set, and then wonder, "How much weight should I put on now?" But the weight should be the last variable to be determined. After your client finishes one set, you want to ask yourself, "How many reps do I want the client to get on the next set?" After you determine how many reps you want the client to complete, you should ask yourself how long you are going to let the client rest until the next set. After you have answered both of those questions, select the amount of weight that you believe will allow the client to complete the specified number of reps. Here are several guidelines, assuming that the first set was challenging. If it was easy, of course, you can increase the weight (99).

- If you want the client to complete a higher number of reps than he or she did on the first set, you need to go down in weight.

- If you want the client to complete the same number of reps as he or she did on the first set and the client is resting a long time (two minutes or longer), try the same weight.

- If you want the client to complete the same number of reps as he or she did on the first set and the client is resting a short time, you need to reduce the weight.

- If you want the client to complete fewer reps than he or she did on the first set and the client is resting a long time, increase the weight.

- If you want the client to complete fewer reps than he or she did on the first set and the client is resting a short time, try the same weight.

- Generally, from one set to the next, do not change the weight up or down more than 10 percent of the working set weight.

The next question is, "After I know how many reps I want and how long I will let the client rest, how do I choose the appropriate weight? Do I go up 10 pounds (4.5 kg), 15 pounds (6.8 kg), or 50 pounds (22.7 kg)? What do I do?"

Some personal trainers prefer a percentage-based chart; see tables 17.21 and 17.22 as two examples. The first is one derived from watching lifters perform a maximum effort lift and then, after they rest for a reasonable period, watching them perform a repetitive effort lift, usually in a lifting competition. The second chart is provided by the NSCA. Common criticisms of the NSCA chart are that it tends either to overpredict the max if using reps to estimate max or to underpredict the reps that the lifter will get at a certain percentage if using the 1RM.

Conversion charts are useful in helping determine a client's 1RM, and that is their most common purpose, but they are an underutilized tool in helping personal trainers predict how much weight a client should lift for each set. If a personal trainer prefers to use the percentage-based chart, here is an example of how that would work:

A client can perform lat pull-downs at 130 pounds (59.0 kg) for 10 reps for a tough set. The personal trainer wants the client to perform a challenging set of 6 reps on the lat pull-down. Use the following method (based on the NPTI conversion chart):

$$130 \div 0.792 = 164.1 \text{ pounds}$$
(74.4 kg) is the estimated 1RM

$$164.1 \text{ pounds} \times 0.868 = 140 \text{ pounds}$$
(63.5 kg), rounded to use real weights

The personal trainer puts 140 pounds (63.5 kg) on the machine, and the client attempts to perform 6 reps. If he or she does more than 6 reps, either the chart underpredicted his or her ability (it is just an estimation) or he or she could really complete more than 10 reps at 130 pounds (59.0 kg). If the client performs fewer than 6 reps, either the chart overpredicted his or her ability or the client's form wasn't very good on that set of 10.

To be accurate with the weight selected, use the specific conversion charts. But at times a personal trainer may just want to make a quick estimate of how much weight a client might need on an exercise. If a client is lifting 100 pounds (45.4 kg) or more on an exercise, a simple yet reasonably accurate number can be obtained by figuring that each rep is worth about 5 pounds (2.3 kg). Weight at the lower end of the scale, below 150 pounds (68.0 kg), is likely to be worth less, and weight over 250 pounds (113.3 kg) is likely to be worth more, but 5 pounds per rep is a reasonable guess.

Table 17.21 NPTI Percentage-Based Conversion Chart

Reps performed	Estimated % of 1RM
1	100%
2	96.8%
3	93.7%
4	91.2%
5	88.8%
6	86.8%
7	84.9%
8	83.0%
9	81.0%
10	79.2%
11	77.5%
12	75.9%

Table 17.22 NSCA Percentage-Based Conversion Chart

Reps performed	Estimated % of 1RM
1	100%
2	95%
3	93%
4	90%
5	87%
6	85%
7	83%
8	80%
9	77%
10	75%
12	67%
15	65%

Adapted, by permission, from NSCA, 2008, Resistance training, by T. Baechle, R.W. Earle, and D. Wathen. In *Essentials of strength training and conditioning*, 3rd ed., edited by T. Baechle and R.W. Earle (Champaign, IL: Human Kinetics), 397.

Returning to the previous example, if a client lifts 130 pounds (59.0 kg) for 10 reps and wants to do a set of 6, using 5 pounds (2.3 kg) per rep, the calculation would look like this:

10 reps − 6 reps = 4 extra reps × 5 pounds (2.3 kg) per rep = 20 extra pounds (9.1 kg)

130 + 20 pounds (59.0 + 9.1 kg) = 150 pounds (68.0 kg) for 6 reps

The result is not exactly the same as the prediction from the previous formula (140 versus 150 pounds), but it's close enough to provide a good set for the client. Maybe the person will complete 5 reps, maybe 6, maybe 7, but that weight will cause whatever adaptation the personal trainer is looking for. Jumping up to 170 pounds (77.1 kg) or increasing to only 135 pounds (61.2 kg) may not produce the same effect.

Some personal trainers don't use conversion charts because the charts don't always work for all people. But even if exceptions are found, the idea should not be tossed out the window. You can calculate a client's personal conversion chart relatively simply. To do this, you must know two key sets that the client performed on the same exercise, preferably separated by at least two reps or 20 pounds (9.1 kg). You then calculate the weight-per-rep value for that exercise. Here is an example of how this process works:

A client can bench press 150 pounds (68.0 kg) for 10 reps.

The same client can bench press 180 pounds (81.6 kg) for 4 reps.

Calculate the weight difference between the two sets:

180 pounds − 150 pounds = 30-pound difference (81.6 kg − 68.0 kg = 13.6 kg difference)

Calculate the rep difference between the two sets:

10 reps − 4 reps = 6-rep difference

Divide the weight difference by the rep difference to find the weight-per-rep value:

30 pounds ÷ 6 reps = 5 pounds per rep (13.6 kg ÷ 6 reps = 2.3 kg per rep)

After determining the weight-per-rep value, you can estimate with reasonable accuracy the weight for a client to lift for a given number of reps. In the previous example, if you want the client to lift a tough set of 6 reps, you would choose 170 pounds (77.1 kg) (150 pounds + 5 pounds per rep × 4 reps, or 68.0 kg + 2.3 kg per rep × 4 reps). If you want a set of 12 reps, you would choose 140 pounds (63.5 kg) (150 pounds − 5 pounds per rep × 2 reps, or 68.0 kg − 2.3 kg per rep × 2 reps). This method is not foolproof, but it provides a solid starting point to selecting the appropriate weight for each set. It also helps predict the client's max as his or her ability to perform more reps improves. Continuing with the previous example, if that client could now lift 180 pounds (81.6 kg) for 6 reps instead of 4, the client's maximum bench probably increased about 10 pounds (4.5 kg) (2 extra reps × 5 pounds per rep = +10 pounds, or 2 extra reps × 2.3 kg per rep = +4.5 kg).

CONTRAINDICATED EXERCISES

For each goal, guidelines can help personal trainers choose the best exercises to help their clients achieve their goals. At the same time, you are encouraged to try new exercises and come up with your own list of exercises that can help clients reach certain goals. Some exercises might work well with one client but not another. Part of personal training is catering the workout to the specific client you are working with. When in doubt choose an exercise from the list. If you never use exercises on the list, analyze your results critically. If you are achieving great results for the client, you are doing something right; if you are not achieving those results, you are doing something wrong. You can't argue with results. Assess your clients before and after training to see what is really happening with them.

Although you can choose from a huge number of exercises, four exercises that are performed regularly today should be contraindicated for personal-training clients, according to the NPTI. These exercises are contraindicated not because they are ineffective for training the target muscles but because they carry an excessive risk-to-reward ratio; they are simply too likely to cause injury when used long term.

Behind-the-Neck Military Press

This exercise is similar to the shoulder or military press exercise in which you push a bar overhead. The contraindicated version has the bar coming down behind the head to touch the base of the neck (figure 17.7). This exercise is effective for training the delts, but it is hard on the shoulder joint and often causes

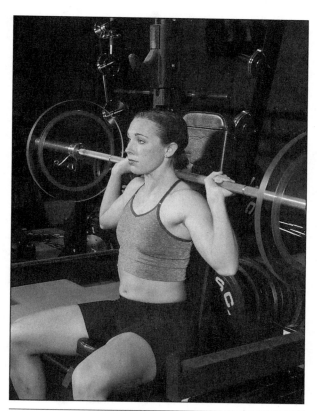

Figure 17.7 Behind-the-neck military press (contraindicated exercise).

problems with the rotator cuff, particularly the supraspinatus muscle. An excellent substitution for this exercise is simply to bring the bar down in front of the head and perform regular shoulder (military) press. This variation targets the delts just as effectively and does not place the same strain on the shoulder joint. Some people believe that doing a behind-the-neck military press stimulates the posterior deltoid, but that is not accurate. The posterior delt is the antagonistic muscle in this exercise and does not receive significant stimulus from performing a shoulder (military) press either in front of the head or behind the head. A shoulder (military) press is abduction of the shoulder while it is externally rotated, which is one of the prime actions of the anterior deltoid. The posterior deltoid performs the opposite action, adduction when externally rotated, as seen in a lat pull-down.

Behind-the-Neck Lat Pull-Down

To perform this exercise, the client sits in a lat pull-down machine and pulls the bar down behind the head so that it touches the base of the neck (figure 17.8). Again, this exercise is hard on the shoulder joint and the stabilizing muscles, although it does effectively target the lats. An effective substitution is to perform the regular lat pull-down exercise in which the bar comes down in front of the face. This variation targets the muscle equally well and does not place much strain on the shoulder joint. To mimic the muscular action of a behind-the-neck lat pull-down, the client simply maintains an upright position (instead of leaning back) while performing the exercise. Remember that pull-ups were around long before lat pull-down machines came on the scene, and the machines were designed to mimic pull-ups (and be easier). A pull-up with the bar in front of the head is much more natural than a pull-up with the bar behind the head. Behind-the-head pull-ups should also be avoided (102).

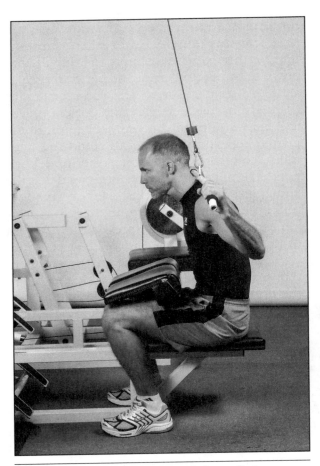

Figure 17.8 Behind-the-neck lat pull-down (contraindicated exercise).

Upright Row

To begin this exercise, the client holds a barbell while standing erect with the arms hanging straight in front. The movement is to lift the bar up to the chin and neck area with high-pointing elbows (figure 17.9). This exercise targets the middle delts and the traps, but it is rough on the shoulder joint. This exercise is common in the gym and even in aerobics classes. If the weight is very light, the exercise is not as bad for the joint, but the heavier the weight is, the worse it gets. Avoid including upright rows in your client's workout routines. This exercise is the only one that requires two exercises as substitutes; no single exercise safely mimics the upright row. The upright row can be performed with a limited range of motion (by pulling the bar up to the bottom of the chest instead of the neck or chin). This movement is not hard on

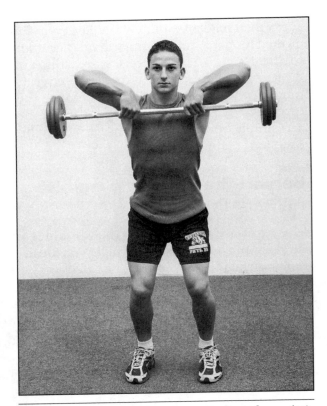

Figure 17.9 Upright row (contraindicated exercise).

the shoulder, but most people don't like how it feels. To train the same muscles, clients can perform a lateral raise for the middle delts and shrugs for the traps (not at the same time) (25).

The behind-the-neck military press, behind-the-neck lat pull-down, and upright row exercises cause impingement of the shoulder. In simple terms, the shoulder is put into a position where a muscle is pinched, normally the supraspinatus, between the acromion process of the scapula and the humerus (figure 17.10). The specific position to avoid is having the elbow above the shoulder and behind the body.

Barbell Bicep Curl

The final exercise on the contraindicated list is the barbell bicep curl (figure 17.11). A barbell refers to the straight, long bar that is used for the bench press exercise. A curl using a straight bar does target the biceps effectively, but it places a lot of stress on the wrist. If you compare the start position of the exercise to the finish position, at the finish position the wrists are significantly farther apart than the elbows.

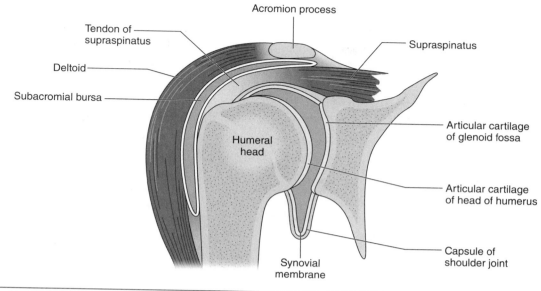

Figure 17.10   Shoulder impingement (contraindicated exercise).

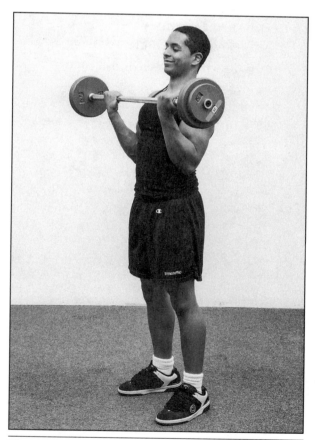

Figure 17.11   Barbell bicep curl (contraindicated exercise).

It is not natural for the wrists to stay straight and rigid as they curl upward.

The most effective substitute for this exercise is to use the EZ-bar instead. The EZ-bar was designed to be easier on the wrists, and the movement is more natural. Using dumbbells is fine as well because clients either shift the body slightly or do not totally supinate the dumbbell the same way they do a barbell. The heavier the weight that is used with the straight bar, the worse it is for the wrists (58).

CONCLUSION

NPTI suggests that personal trainers follow a step-by-step system to create effective workouts that cover the following points: establish a goal; list desired outcomes; select the routine; select the exercises for each workout; program training variables such as number of reps, load, number of sets, and rest time; incorporate any tricks of the trade deemed useful; and, finally, program progression to ensure that the goals are achieved. Following these steps will ensure that your workout programs are effective, time efficient, specific to the client and his or her goals, and fun to complete.

Study Questions

1. What is a good warm-up set for a client who is going to perform one warm-up set before performing a leg press set of 300 pounds (136.1 kg) × 10?

   a. 140 pounds (63.5 kg) × 8

   b. 180 pounds (81.6 kg) × 10

   c. 250 pounds (113.4 kg) × 12

   d. 270 pounds (122.5 kg) × 15

2. Resistance training using standard protocols is the least effective in improving which of the following characteristics?

   a. muscle strength

   b. muscle size

   c. $\dot{V}O_2max$

   d. muscle power

3. If a client is able to lift 180 pounds (81.6 kg) for 10 reps on the bench press, what is a logical guess for that client for a challenging set of 6 reps?

   a. 200 pounds (90.7 kg) × 6

   b. 220 pounds (99.8 kg) × 6

   c. 240 pounds (108.9 kg) × 6

   d. 260 pounds (117.9 kg) × 6

4. When training for size, which of the following programs matches the guidelines presented in this text?

   a. 8 to 10 reps, 75 percent of 1RM, four work sets per exercise, one-minute rest

   b. 3 to 8 reps, 80 percent of 1RM, one work set per exercise, two-minute rest

   c. 3 to 5 reps, 100 percent of 1RM, two work sets per exercise, three-minute rest

   d. 2 to 4 reps, 90 percent of 1RM, four work sets per exercise, four-minute rest

5. When training for multiple-set muscular endurance, what should the rest time be between sets?

   a. 2 to 5 minutes

   b. 1 to 2 minutes

   c. 30 to 60 seconds

   d. less than 30 seconds

Beginner Workout

This chapter details how to set up an appropriate beginner workout. A beginner is anyone who has never exercised before or a client who has taken extended time off from exercising. People new to exercises should follow a relatively specific program to help their bodies become accustomed to exercise without inducing significant muscle soreness and damage along the way. Imagine what would happen if a friend who had not exercised in years accompanied you to the gym and performed your workout, set for set, rep for rep. Would that be successful? Not likely. A more likely outcome is that your friend would fail during the workout, would be unable to do what you are doing, and would be extremely sore the next day and possibly injured. We do not want our untrained clients to feel that way.

A beginner is defined as anyone new to exercise, anyone who has not been working out consistently for three months straight, or anyone who has taken a prolonged layoff from regular activity (six months or more, even if that person was an advanced athlete). If your client played football in college but has not done any exercise in five years, you should definitely have him begin with the beginner workout. The beginner workout is a great place to start, and as you will see, *beginner* is not the same as *easy*.

GOALS OF THE BEGINNER WORKOUT

The beginner workout has three primary goals. First, the goal of the workout is to improve the components of fitness, all of them. This is a not a specialist workout. It is designed to strengthen your client's base level of fitness. Having a strong base is important to health and to performance of almost all athletic events. Second, the goal of the beginner workout is to prepare your client's body for more intense work to come. The client will not stay on the beginner workout forever, and the goal is to get the client off the beginner workout and on to intermediate workouts and beyond. Third, the purpose of the beginner workout is to teach your clients proper form and technique while exercising. Fully grasping the structure of the beginner workout will help you understand the setup of more complicated programs that you will come across.

DURATION OF THE BEGINNER WORKOUT PROGRAM

How long should clients follow the beginner workout? The answer depends on their goals and their fitness level, but most people should follow the beginner workout for two to three months. If a client used to have a high fitness level but has taken time off and is using the workout to get back in shape and learn how to do things right, he or she should follow this workout for one to two months. If you find that your client really likes this workout and is making good progress, you can have the person follow it for four or more months. Generally, though, after six months almost everybody should be ready to move on (10).

If you are worried that the beginner workout will be too mundane and boring for your clients or if you think that they hired you to give them a secret program designed for Olympic athletes, think again. Clients, especially new clients, are often intimidated by the idea of exercise. By definition, beginners are people who are not used to exercise. The bad news is that their fitness level is likely to be low. The good news is that any form of training will equate to progressive overload, and they will make positive adaptations to almost all forms of exercise. You don't have to apply the most advanced intensity techniques to a new client; that approach would not be wise. Instead, start with basic exercises and build the foundation. You can't rush fitness; if you try, the long-term results will be compromised. You don't plant a field of crops two days before the harvest. Instead, you develop a plan and stick with it.

PRINCIPLES OF THE BEGINNER WORKOUT

To follow this plan successfully, your clients need to work out consistently two, three, or four times per week. Generally, they perform a total-body routine. If they are training four times a week, they follow the beginner workout split outlined in this chapter. In each workout, clients lift weights and perform a cardiovascular workout to improve their $\dot{V}O_2$max and body composition. At the end of the workout, clients stretch to work on their flexibility.

The beginner workout consists of approximately 8 to 12 total resistance training exercises, usually one exercise per muscle group. The client performs one to three work sets per exercise following a warm-up set. Each set is 10 to 15 reps at moderate intensity. The set shouldn't be ridiculously easy, but the client should not be reaching failure on any set. The client rests 30 seconds to 1 minute after each set and each exercise. The weightlifting part of the workout takes approximately 30 minutes, although the first few days may take longer or you may not be able to get in all the suggested exercises because your client will not know what to do and will need a lot of instruction and demos. After the client gets the routine

down, you can move through it relatively quickly. Although the range of exercises is usually 8 to 12, personal trainers often use the lower end of that range simply because of time constraints. Generally, the exercises chosen for the beginner workout are considered relatively low-skill exercises that are easier to learn and don't require as much coordination. Often these exercises involve using machines, but not always. The selection of exercises depends on the client's fitness level and what equipment you have available. Normally, these exercises do not require a spotter (1).

When the weight training portion of the workout is over, you will have the client perform some cardiovascular exercise as prescribed in the following sections. The goal is to perform cardio training for 20 to 30 minutes, but if your client cannot continue that long in the beginning, don't worry; he or she can build up to that level.

DETERMINING LOADS FOR THE BEGINNER WORKOUT

How much weight should new clients lift when they begin? That question is difficult to answer because clients have varying levels of strength.

Warm-Up Loads

The loads listed in table 18.1 provide general guidelines for effective warm-up loads for many common exercises that apply to most beginning clients. If your client is significantly weaker than most people, you can lower this weight; if your client is stronger than most people, you can raise it a bit. Remember that this is a warm-up set, so the client should perceive it as easy to complete. After the set, you can ask the client how the weight felt. With that information and by judging how the client looked when he or she was performing the exercise, you can decide how much weight to add for the first work set (26).

Work Set Loads

After your client has completed the warm-up set, he or she is ready to perform the work sets.

Table 18.1 Sample Warm-Up Loads for Beginning Male and Female Clients

Exercise	Female	Male	
Chest press	10–20 lb (4.5–9.1 kg)	20–40 lb (9.1–18.1 kg)	
Bench press	25 lb (11.3 kg)*	45 lb (20.4 kg)	
Lat pull-down	30–40 lb (13.6–18.1 kg)	40–60 lb (18.1–27.2 kg)	
Cable row	30–40 lb (13.6–18.1 kg)	40–60 lb (18.1–27.2 kg)	
Military (shoulder) press machine	10–20 lb (4.5–9.1 kg)	20–30 lb (9.1–13.6 kg)	
DB military press	5–8 lb (2.3–3.6 kg)	10–15 lb (4.5–6.8 kg)	
EZ-bar curl	15–20 lb (6.8–9.1 kg)	25–35 lb (11.3–15.9 kg)	
DB curl	5–8 lb (2.3–3.6 kg)	10–15 lb (4.5–6.8 kg)	
Curl machine	10–20 lb (4.5–9.1 kg)	20–30 lb (9.1–13.6 kg)	
Tricep push-down	30–40 lb (13.6–18.1 kg)**	50–60 lb (22.7–27.2 kg)**	
Leg press	0–50 lb (0–22.7 kg)	50–90 lb (22.7–40.8 kg)	
Leg extension	20–30 lb (9.1–13.6 kg)	30–40 lb (13.6–18.1 kg)	
Leg curl	20–30 lb (9.1–13.6 kg)***	30–50 lb (13.6–22.7 kg)***	
Standing calf raise	60–80 lb (27.2–36.3 kg)	60–100 lb (27.2–45.4 kg)	
Seated calf raise	5–10 lb (2.3–4.5 kg)	10–25 lb (4.5–11.3 kg)	

*The bar is 45 pounds (20.4 kg), so you need to use a smaller, lighter bar to get this weight.

**Pulleys can vary greatly in resistance. If no pulley is set up at the bottom of the machine, divide this weight in half.

***The leg curl starting weight is higher than the leg extension because the leg is falling down (in a seated leg curl), so some weight is needed to balance that out.

Here the client uses a weight that is somewhat challenging but at this stage should not be unbearable. In all workouts, particularly in the beginner workout, form is important. When your clients are first learning how to perform the exercises, their form should be extra strict, almost textbook perfect. The client should lift using a 2:4 count, which means using a 2 count on the concentric portion of the exercise (the hard part) and a 4 count on the eccentric portion of the exercise (the easy part). You don't have to be super controlling about this by counting the speed on every single rep, but the client should be lifting relatively slowly and stay in control in the beginner phase of the program. The client should exhale when working (concentric phase) and inhale during the easy part, taking one breath per rep. The client should not reach failure at any point during this workout, meaning that the client should not get to a point where he or she can't lift the weight the desired number of repetitions. Even if the client enjoys training hard, remind the client that he or she will train the same muscle group two or three times a week. Until the client is used to working out, high-intensity training at high frequency is not recommended because he or she will become very sore. Extreme soreness causes many clients to quit working out; in addition, getting that sore is not necessary to see results (7, 16, 21).

When determining the weight for work sets for beginners, three methods are appropriate.

Method 1

Instruct the client to stay with the same weight and reps for each set (after the warm-up set). For example, if you are using the chest press, the client warms up with 60 pounds (27.3 kg) for 10 reps and then lifts 100 pounds (45.4 kg) for 10 reps. You repeat that two more times so that all the sets are the same:

Chest press 60 lb (27.2 kg) × 10; 100 lb (45.4 kg) × 10; 100 lb (45.4 kg) × 10; 100 lb (45.4 kg) × 10

This method is best if you want to increase muscular endurance because the client lifts the same load for each set even when tired. After the client can complete all three sets with the same weight, the next week you increase the weight by about 5 pounds (2.3 kg) to make it progressively more difficult. This weight and set arrangement is called straight sets or sets across.

Method 2

Direct the client to increase the weight with each set and either decrease the number of reps or use the same number of reps. With beginners, the latter choice is the most common. For example, if the client is using the chest press, the sets might look like this:

Chest press 60 lb (27.2 kg) × 10; 90 lb (40.8 kg) × 10; 100 lb (45.4 kg) × 10; 110 lb (49.9 kg) × 10

This method is best if your main goal is to increase the client's maximum strength because you are building intensity as each work set goes along. This format is also best for increasing neuromuscular coordination because you let the client practice with something and then make it progressively harder. This format works well with beginners because most beginners do not know exactly how much weight they should lift. They can pick a number, find that it is a little easy, and then work their way up. The disadvantages of this method are that the rest periods are short in the beginner workout and making the heaviest set at the end when they might be the most tired can limit their performance. This method is called ascending sets because the weight gets heavier with each set (7).

Method 3

Instruct the client to decrease the weight with each progressive work set after the warm-up set. In this method, your client starts with the heaviest weight that he or she can lift for the goal number of reps. Each set then becomes progressively easier. You can either increase the number of reps or keep the number of reps the same; the latter choice is the most common when using the beginner workout. If you were to use the chest press, the sets might look like this:

Chest press 60 lb (27.2 kg) × 10; 110 lb (49.9 kg) × 10; 100 lb (45.4 kg) × 10; 90 lb (40.8 kg) × 10

This method is the best if your client's main goal is to increase muscle size because the client is performing each set in a fatigued state, which is ideal for hypertrophy. This format also works well with the shortened rest periods that are prescribed in the beginner workout, because as the client gets more tired the sets become easier. The problem with this method is that most beginners are not comfortable launching into their heaviest set after just one warm-up. Going heavy on an exercise that they may not be familiar with is difficult. In addition, the personal trainer may be unable to predict accurately how much weight a beginner should lift for the hardest set; getting the weight right is a key component of this method. This method is referred to as descending sets, because the weight gets lighter after the first work set (29–30).

Because most beginners are not intimately familiar with the exercises and because of the importance of motor learning, particularly in the early stages of training, most personal trainers tend to use ascending sets. But all the methods can be effective. In addition, the primary resistance training goal has been highlighted to serve an educational viewpoint, but it is really splitting hairs. First, remember that the beginner workout is not a specialist workout, so the goal is not to focus on just one aspect of fitness. Second, the volume and work performed by each method is the same, so the results will likely be relatively similar. Finally, muscle strength, muscle endurance, and muscle size are related to each other, so it is logical to expect that all these qualities will improve on each of the programs. Factoring in your personal preference when choosing what to do is OK, if for no other reason than you will more effectively sell a program that you believe in. Second, think about what kind of goal you want to focus on for the client (strength, size, or endurance) and then go with that one. The bottom line is to get your clients to the gym, give them a great workout, have fun, and make some progress!

ADDING CARDIO TO THE BEGINNER WORKOUT

In the beginner workout, most clients perform traditional forms of cardio. This format is not mandatory; it is a guideline. After clients complete the resistance training portion of the workout, starting them on a simple piece of cardio such as the bike or treadmill works well. Then, over the course of a few weeks, progressing them to the elliptical machine, stair climber, and rowing machine is logical. Clients may want to break up the cardio on different pieces of equipment (for example, 12 minutes on the elliptical and 8 minutes on the rower), particularly after they are performing cardio for 20 minutes or more (19).

The intensity of cardio in the beginning should be relatively easy but still challenging enough to elicit adaptations. Training at 60 to 70 percent of MHR works well. Clients should be able to talk at this intensity. Many clients dislike cardio and are intimidated by it. If you force them to gut through a challenging cardio session, they may complete it that one time because you stood next to them and didn't let them quit, but that approach often reinforces their poor opinion of cardio. Instead, by prescribing a lower intensity, the workout experience can be more pleasant, which leads to greater buy-in from clients and builds confidence. As their enjoyment of exercise grows, then it is appropriate to throw more challenging modalities their way (13, 25).

You should be cautious about incorporating other forms of cardio into a beginning client's workout routine. Conditioning tools such as a jump rope, sled, prowler, sandbags, tire, and boxing all have their place, but an overzealous personal trainer can easily push a new client over the edge, especially if proper monitoring is not taking place. Those tools are more suitable for an intermediate level or advanced client. The classic cardio machines, although perhaps slightly boring, do a great job of building a base of cardiovascular fitness and help to ensure a positive experience.

CHANGING OR UPDATING THE BEGINNER WORKOUT

With all workouts, you need to introduce change at the proper points so that the client's body adjusts maximally. This point applies to the beginner workout as well, but you should change the workouts less frequently for those who are less experienced. The opposite is also true. The more advanced a client is, the more frequently you should change the workouts.

As you can see in table 18.2, the beginner workout should be changed every one to two months. This change depends on a few factors. Part of it is whether your client likes to change things up or prefers to do the same thing repeatedly. The other part of the equation is how much change is built into the existing program. For example, if your client is starting the beginner workout and working out two times a week, you can design a total-body program in one of two ways. First, you can create one workout plan and have the client perform that workout on both days of the week, usually for a month at a time before you modify it and have the client follow it for another month. Eventually, the client can progress to an intermediate-level workout. A second option is to design two workouts in the beginning. For example, if your client is training on Monday and Thursday, you could have the client perform workout A on Monday and workout B on Thursday to create more variation (the exercises for each muscle group are different from one workout to the next). For example, you might have the client use the chest press machine in workout A and perform push-ups in workout B. Because of the added variation, a client can follow this pattern for two months. In both examples, the number of times that a client completes each workout is the same (eight). Remember that beginners need to practice and learn the basic movements, so switching it up frequently is not a good idea. Clients need time to learn how to perform a new movement, and repetition is the only way to get that practice.

Table 18.2 Suggested Frequency for Implementing Change in a Workout

Level	How frequently to change the workout
Beginner	4–8 weeks
Intermediate	3–6 weeks
Advanced	1–3 weeks

SAMPLE BEGINNER WORKOUTS

This section includes two beginner workouts—a total-body routine performed twice a week and a split routine performed four times a week. You can choose to follow one of these routines with your beginning clients, or you can create your own using them as a template.

Most clients will be ready to move on from the beginner workout after two or three months, sooner if the client used to be in decent shape. A client who is older or is training less frequently (once or twice a week) can follow the beginner workout for a longer time. Ultimately, the client can follow the beginner workout as long as he or she enjoys it and, in your view, is continuing to benefit from it.

Two Times a Week Total-Body Routine

This type of beginner workout has the client performing exercises that train the upper body and the lower body—all in one workout session—and repeating that workout on two nonconsecutive days in a week.

For the first month (table 18.3), the client performs one warm-up set of 10 to 15 reps followed by one to three work sets of 10 to 15 reps. Rest is 30 to 60 seconds between sets. See table 18.4 for guidelines on the number of work sets and time spent on cardio. When

Table 18.3 Sample Beginner Workout: Two Times a Week Total-Body Routine (First Month)

Workout A	Optional workout B
Warm-up: 5 minutes treadmill or bike	Warm-up: 5 minutes treadmill or bike
Chest press machine	Incline press machine
Wide-grip lat pull-down	V-grip cable row
Shoulder press machine	DB front raise*
DB lateral raise*	Lateral raise machine*
Curl machine*	DB curl*
V-grip tricep push-down*	Machine tricep extension*
Leg press	Horizontal leg press
Leg extension*	Leg extension*
Seated leg curl*	Prone leg curl*
Standing calf raise*	Seated calf raise*
Abdominal crunch	Reverse abdominal crunch
Cardio (12–30 minutes)	Cardio (12–30 minutes)
Cool-down (3–5 minutes)	Cool-down (3–5 minutes)
Stretch (5–10 minutes)	Stretch (5–10 minutes)

*An exercise that is ideal to include but optional if time or other constraints exist.

Table 18.4 Sample Beginner Resistance Training Volume

	Beginner at lower fitness level, work sets and cardio time	Beginner at moderate fitness level, work sets and cardio time
Week 1	1 work set, 12 minutes cardio	2 work sets, 15 minutes cardio
Week 2	1 work set, 16 minutes cardio	2 work sets, 20 minutes cardio
Week 3	2 work sets, 20 minutes cardio	3 work sets, 25 minutes cardio
Week 4	2 work sets, 24 minutes cardio	3 work sets, 30 minutes cardio
Week 5 and beyond	3 work sets, ≥25 minutes cardio	3 work sets, ≥30 minutes cardio

in doubt, assume that the client is a beginner because starting too easy is always better than starting too hard.

For the second month, the client performs one warm-up set of 10 to 15 reps and then three work sets of 10 to 15 reps. The client should perform cardio for at least 20 minutes and probably closer to 25 to 30 minutes or more, but no more than 35 minutes. The client rests 30 to 60 seconds between sets. The personal trainer may find it necessary to complete the resistance training portion with the client, move the client to the cardio, and get him or her set up on that to finish the cardio, if the client is willing to do that. This approach saves time and is a good method to use if the client wants to perform a reasonable amount of cardio but also is performing a reasonable number of resistance training exercises during the personal training session. The asterisk in this list indicates exercises that are ideal to include but optional if time or other constraints exist.

Sample Beginner Workout A2: Two Times a Week Total-Body Routine (Second Month)

- Warm-up: 5 minutes treadmill or bike
- Bench press
- Hammer strength row
- DB military press
- Cable lateral raise*
- EZ-bar curl*
- Reverse grip tricep pull-down*
- Squat
- Leg extension*
- Seated leg curl*
- Rotary calf*
- Sit-up
- Cardio (20–35 minutes)
- Cool-down (5 minutes)
- Stretch (5–10 minutes)

Four Times a Week Split Routine

If you have a client who is enthusiastic about getting into shape, you can train him or her four times a week. This schedule poses a problem, however, because generally the goal is to take a day off after a workout, especially when following a total-body routine. To solve this problem, the client follows a split routine in which he or she works out four times a week but targets each muscle group only twice a week. The easiest and most practical split for beginners is an upper-body and lower-body split routine:

Upper-Body and Lower-Body Split Routine

Day 1: Upper body (chest, back, shoulders, biceps, triceps)

Day 2: Lower body (legs, abs, lower back)

Day 3: Repeat day 1

Day 4: Repeat day 2

Technically, the abs and lower back reside on the upper body, but that day is already relatively full and the muscles of the core tend to work closely with the muscles of the lower body. For those reasons, the abs and lower back are placed on the lower-body day. The benefit of this method compared with a total-body routine is that each day is a bit shorter, particularly during the first couple of weeks because the number of exercises is not as great.

Table 18.5 shows a sample program with upper-body exercises (without abs and lower back) on one day and lower-body exercises (including abs and lower back) on a second day. The first day tends to be a bit longer than the second day and a little more intensive on the upper body, but the client gets a more complete rest between workouts on this program.

In the first week, your clients perform one warm-up set of 10 to 15 reps and then two work sets of 10 to 15 reps. They rest 30 to 60 seconds between sets. They perform cardio for 12 minutes, cool down for 3 minutes, and then stretch for 5 to 10 minutes. In the second week, your clients perform one warm-up set and three work sets of 10 to 15 reps, so you are adding one work set per exercise in the second week. They perform cardio for 16 minutes, cool down for 4 minutes, and then stretch for 5 to 10 minutes.

Table 18.6 shows the next two weeks of the split routine. For week 3 you add a second exercise to each muscle group. Generally, you want the client to perform the exercises in the order listed here. The client is doing one warm-up set and dropping back to two work sets per exercise. The total volume is four work sets per muscle group (two plus two), which is up one set from the week before and helps create overload. The client performs cardio for 20 minutes, does a 5-minute cool-down, and then stretches for 5 to 10 minutes. For week 4, you repeat week 3 but add a work set so that the client performs three work sets per exercise instead of two. The client completes cardio for 24 minutes, does a 5-minute cool-down, and then stretches for 5 to 10 minutes.

Table 18.7 shows the second month of the split routine, a challenging and effective pro-gram. For the entire month the client should be performing one warm-up set and three work sets. The warm-up set on the second exercise for that muscle group is optional but still rec-ommended. The biggest thing is to continue to use a short rest period to keep this workout from taking too much time. These workouts should take the client somewhere between 75 and 90 minutes including everything, so you have to make an effort to move fast. Keeping the rest period short is more important than using heavier weight, so use a lighter weight if necessary to get through the workout in the recommended time (19, 33). The client will have plenty of time to lift heavy later; the goal of this workout is to build the foundation. With

Table 18.5 Sample Beginner Workout: Four Times a Week Upper-Body and Lower-Body Split Routine (First Two Weeks)

Day 1	Day 2
Warm-up: 5 minutes on treadmill or bike	Warm-up: 5 minutes on treadmill or bike
Chest press machine	Leg press
Wide-grip lat pull-down	Leg extension
Hammer strength military press	Leg curl
DB lateral raise	Standing calf raise
V-grip tricep push-down	Lower-back machine
EZ-bar cable curl	Crunches
Cardio	Cardio
Cool-down	Cool-down
Stretch	Stretch
Day 3	**Day 4**
Repeat day 1	Repeat day 2

Table 18.6 Sample Beginner Workout: Four Times a Week Upper-Body and Lower-Body Split Routine (Weeks 3 and 4)

Day 1	Day 2
Warm-up: 5 minutes on treadmill or bike	Warm-up: 5 minutes on treadmill or bike
Chest press machine	Leg press
Chest fly machine	Horizontal leg press
Wide-grip lat pull-down	Leg extension
V-grip cable row	Leg curl
Hammer strength military press	Standing calf raise
DB lateral raise	Seated calf raise
Rear delt machine	Crunches
V-grip tricep push-down	Reverse crunch
DB tricep kickback	Lower-back machine
EZ-bar cable curl	Cardio
DB curl	Cool-down
Cardio	Stretch
Cool-down	
Stretch	

Table 18.7 Sample Beginner Workout: Four Times a Week Upper-Body and Lower-Body Split Routine (Month 2)

Day 1	Day 2
Warm-up: 5 minutes	Warm-up: 5 minutes
Bench press	Smith machine squat
Incline press machine	Leg press
Reverse-grip lat pull-down	Leg extension
DB row	Leg curl
DB military press	Abductor machine
Lateral raise machine	Adductor machine
DB rear delt raise	Rotary calf
Skull crusher	Seated calf raise
Rope tricep push-down	Crunches
EZ-bar curl	Reverse crunch
Machine curl	Hyperextensions
Cardio	Cardio
Cool-down	Cool-down
Stretch	Stretch
Day 3	**Day 4**
Repeat day 1	Repeat day 2

this method, personal trainers often take their clients through the resistance training portion and then set them up on the cardio. Clients can then complete the cardio, cool-down, and stretch on their own time. If that doesn't work, some of these exercises may need to be eliminated to fit the workout into the usual 60-minute time frame. Generally, you can eliminate the second exercise per muscle group or the isolation exercises. If the client is sufficiently fit, the exercises can be supersetted to save significant time.

ANALYSIS OF THE BEGINNER WORKOUT

The beginner workout has been outlined in detail because a large number of clients are beginners and personal trainers need to understand the ins and outs of the program and the rationale for the setup. The beginner workout can be analyzed with NPTI's system of exercise program design presented in chapter 17.

Define and Clarify the Goal

The purpose of this program is to enhance the components of fitness including muscular strength, muscular endurance, body composition, and cardiovascular endurance to improve a client's fitness level, health status, and ability to accomplish activities of daily living.

List the Expected Outcomes

After following a program designed for beginners, the client should express greater maximal strength, greater muscular endurance, reduced body fat, and improved $\dot{V}O_2max$. The client should have fewer risk factors for coronary artery disease and should find activities of daily living easier to complete.

List the Expected Physiological Adaptations

Specific changes take place in the body when a client follows a beginner workout program:

- Actin and myosin and related filaments thicken and increase strength.
- Neuromuscular coordination improves.
- Bone, tendons, and ligaments generally increase in strength along with the muscle.
- Myoglobin and capillary density increases.
- Blood volume, aerobic capacity, and anaerobic capacity increase.

Analyze the Program Setup

Create a program for beginners that has the client working out two to four times a week. Three times a week is best.

Select the Specific Routine

The most common routines designed for beginners include total-body routines. Occasionally, an upper–lower routine is used if the client is training four times per week. Table 18.8 describes several common routines.

Select the Number of Resistance Training Exercises per Workout

The beginner workout consists of 8 to 12 resistance training exercises per workout.

Select the Number of Resistance Training Exercises per Body Part or Movement

Commonly, one or two exercises per muscle group or movement are selected.

Select the Specific Exercises

Beginners usually start exercising on lower-skill exercises (table 18.9). Machines, cables, and more stable free-weight or body-weight exercises are often chosen as a starting point.

Clients are not expected to train only on these exercises or to perform all the exercises in every session.

Put the Exercises in Their Proper Order

Exercise order is somewhat important in working with beginners. The traditional guidelines of starting the workout with high-skill, compound, free-weight exercises and then moving to lower-skill, isolation, machine exercises still apply. Personal trainers might incorporate supersets to save time if the client can handle the increased workload.

Select the Number of Reps per Work Set

Beginners should perform 10 to 15 reps per work set.

Table 18.8 Specific Beginner Routines and Their Corresponding Frequency

Total training sessions per week	Frequency of each area per week	Specific routine
4	2	Upper–lower* repeated
3	3	Total body
2	2	Total body

*Upper refers to training the muscles of the upper body (chest, back, shoulders, and arms); lower refers to training the muscles of the lower body (glutes, quads, hamstrings, calves) and the core (abs and lower back).

Table 18.9 Ideal Exercises per Body Area for Beginners

Chest	Back	Shoulders
Chest press mx	Wide-grip lat pull-down	Military press mx
Push-ups	Band assisted pull-up	Seated DB military press
Bench press	Cable row	Lateral raise
DB press	DB row	Rear delt raise
Flys	Straight-arm lat pull-down	Overhead press

Biceps	Triceps	Legs	Abs
EZ-bar curl	V-grip tricep push-down	Leg press	Crunch
Machine curl	Tricep extension mx	Leg extension	Reverse crunch
DB curl	Skull crusher	Leg curl	Clam
DB hammer curl	DB tricep extension	Lunge	Plank
Cable curl	Close-grip bench press	Squat	Ball crunch

Select the Load per Set

The load is usually defined as being light to moderate when working with beginners. The 1RM in the various exercises may not be known; therefore, have the client start light and incorporate progressive overload. If the 1RM is known, the client usually lifts between 40 and 65 percent of the 1RM on the work sets.

Select the Number of Work Sets per Exercise

One to three work sets per exercise is suggested for beginners.

Select the Number of Warm-Up Sets per Exercise

Warm-up sets are useful for beginners because they are new to exercising. The warm-up sets serve as a learning tool and a refresher of proper form. One or two warm-up sets are usually performed on the first exercise in the session, and zero or one warm-up set is used on the subsequent exercises.

Choose the Desired Weight Progression

Personal trainers can choose the weight progression they wish to use with beginners, but ascending sets are standard to facilitate neuromuscular coordination and preparedness.

Confirm That the Selected Number of Reps per Set Matches the Goal Time Under Tension

Beginners should experience some time under tension. Performing 10 to 15 reps and using a 2:4 tempo usually leads to 20 to 40 seconds of time under tension.

Select the Appropriate Rest Time Between Sets

Beginners should rest 30 to 60 seconds between work sets.

Implement Any Tricks of the Trade to Elicit Faster Adaptations

Beginners are new to exercise, so using numerous intensity techniques with them is neither necessary nor desirable. The most common intensity techniques to be used with beginners would be supersets to save time and preexhaustion if a beginner has a hard time feeling a muscle contracting during an exercise.

Program an Appropriate Progressive Overload

Progressive overload is important for beginners. Generally, they experience rapid strength increases. Many beginners can add 5 pounds (2.3 kg) or increase the load by 2 percent every week for several consecutive months, so linear progression is usually considered ideal for them. Increasing the number of reps per set, increasing the number of sets per exercise, increasing the number of exercises per muscle group, and progressing to more challenging exercises are commonly used forms of overload for beginners.

CONCLUSION

The goals of the beginner workout are to increase the components of fitness, teach the client proper form and technique, prevent injury, and prepare the body for more intense activity in subsequent programs. Beginners should generally follow a total-body routine of 8 to 12 resistance training exercises consisting of one or two exercises per muscle, one to three work sets per exercise, 10 to 15 reps per set, and 30 to 60 seconds of rest between sets. Beginners should warm up appropriately, perform resistance training, do cardiovascular work at 60 to 70 percent of MHR, cool down, and complete the workout with a flexibility program. They should follow this program two or three times a week for two or three months, or longer if necessary.

Study Questions

1. True or false: If an advanced client takes three weeks off from regular training, that client must return to the beginner workout.

   a. true

   b. false

2. What is one of the goals of the beginner workout?

   a. Create intense soreness so that the client becomes immune to that feeling in the future.

   b. Employ intensity techniques to achieve quick results.

   c. Specialize in whatever fitness goal the client is aiming toward.

   d. Prepare the body for a more intense workout to follow the beginner phase.

3. How many strength training exercises does the beginner workout use for a total-body routine?

   a. 1 to 3 exercises

   b. 3 to 5 exercises

   c. 8 to 12 exercises

   d. 10 to 15 exercises

4. What is the standard sequence for a beginner workout?

   a. warm-up, resistance training, cardio, cool-down, stretch

   b. warm-up, cardio, resistance training, cool-down, stretch

   c. warm-up, cardio, resistance training, stretch, cool-down

   d. stretch, cool-down, cardio, resistance training, warm-up

5. Which sequence of exercises is the correct order of performance for the beginner workout?

   a. military press, chest press, lat pull-down, tricep push-down, bicep curl

   b. chest press, lat pull-down, military press, bicep curl, tricep push-down

   c. lat pull-down, tricep push-down, bicep curl, chest press, military press

   d. chest press, lat pull-down, bicep curl, tricep push-down, military press

Squat

Some people say that the squat is the king of all exercises. It is grueling, demanding, and difficult to perform correctly, but it gives great results. Few people squat regularly, and fewer still squat properly, so knowing how to squat and performing it well puts you in an exclusive club.

TRAINING GOALS

Aside from the Olympic lifts, the squat is probably the highest skill exercise in the program of most clients. Learning and mastering the technique takes time. At first, most people feel and look awkward, but if they stick with it, the squat can yield impressive results. Improving the technique for the squat will aid in reaching three goals: to improve health, performance, and the 1RM.

Improve Health

If the goal is to improve overall health by improving the components of fitness, the squat exercise provides many benefits. It increases balance and coordination because performing it requires moderately high skills; it is considered highly functional because it mimics a natural movement for humans and because improvements in squatting ability transfer well to many activities and sports; it is a structural exercise that places a positive load on the bones, muscles, tendons, and ligaments; it releases anabolic hormones; it can increase EPOC to assist in fat loss and increased $\dot{V}O_2max$; and it is the most useful and specific exercise that people can do to increase muscular strength in the lower body.

Clients who include the squat exercise in a program to improve health and other components of fitness need to follow several general technique guidelines to get set up to perform the exercise:

- Set the safety racks (sometimes called cross bars) in the squat rack (if they can be moved) at a height just below the shoulders.
- Stand in front of the bar and place the pinky fingers on the "rings" on the bar where there is no knurling (the rough texture of the Olympic bar); if the shoulders are inflexible, place the hands farther apart. Clients who are more flexible can often grasp the bar with a narrower grip.
- Put the feet under the bar and squat down and under the bar.
- Position the bar just below the base of the neck on top of the traps, not on the bones of the neck (avoid C7 in particular).
- With the feet directly under the body and the bar, inhale and stand up; in that position, the bar should clear the rack with the client fully supporting it.
- Take two to four steps backward to get into position in the middle of the squat rack.
- Stand tall with the feet a little wider than shoulder-width apart and point the toes slightly out or straight ahead, whichever is more natural.
- Exhale and then inhale again before beginning the descent.

To begin a squat, the first thing that moves is the hips. Instruct clients to push their hips backward as if they were trying to stick their butt out. As their hips move backward behind the body, allow the knees to bend and then drop down in a controlled fashion into the squat (figure 19.1). Ideally, they should go down so that the middle of their thighs is parallel to the ground or just below. Their knees can move forward, but they should focus on keeping their heels and feet flat on the ground. As clients descend, they will end up leaning forward, so be sure to instruct them to lean from the hips, not by rounding the back. Have them keep the chest up and look straight ahead. After clients are down low enough, instruct them to reverse direction and head back up. Have them return to the starting position with their legs straight and body upright. That movement is one rep.

During the squat, most clients find that looking straight ahead is the most comfortable position for the head, but it is OK to look slightly up or down to a maximum of 45 degrees in either direction. Do not allow clients to look up or down excessively; looking at the ceiling or looking at the feet would be excessive (16). Make sure that clients are keeping the chest up and the lower back slightly arched. In rising from a squat, clients maintain the body position and don't allow the torso to lean forward or the upper back to round.

Clients should avoid several techniques or movements:

- Looking up or down excessively
- Rounding the back
- Letting the bar roll down the back
- Setting up unevenly
- Going only halfway down
- Bending the knees first
- Letting the knees move significantly in front of the toes
- Rising up on the toes

Improve Performance

Regardless of the goal, clients always need to use good form when performing the squat exercise. Not much can be changed when squatting to improve performance, but some modifications can make the exercise easier.

The formal name of the squat is the back squat because the bar sits on the back, as opposed to a front squat exercise in which the bar is held at the front of the shoulders at the base of the neck (figure 19.2). There are two

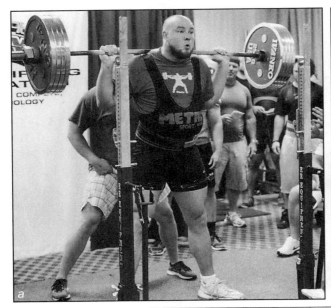
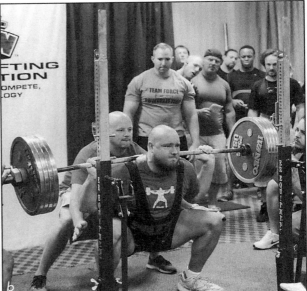

Figure 19.1 The proper *(a)* starting and *(b)* ending positions of the squat.

types of back squats. Most people perform the high-bar back squat (figure 19.3) in which the bar is placed right at the top of the upper back, just below C7, but not directly on the neck. This placement works well because it helps people maintain good form. But clients can lift more weight with the low-bar back squat (figure 19.4) in which the bar is placed farther down the back, about 2 to 3 inches (5.1 to 7.6 cm) lower than the high-bar position. The bar is on the middle of the traps and rhomboids, just above the rear delts. Low-bar squats force clients to lean forward more, thereby placing more stress on the lower back and hips. But in this position the bar is closer to the center of gravity, and clients are less likely to fall forward during the exercise. Depending how a person is built and trained, a low-bar squat can often allow the client to lift 50 to 100 pounds (22.7 to 45.4 kg) more than he or she can using a high-bar squat (20).

Using a wider stance can also help to improve your clients' squatting performance. Instead of the standard hip-width position, have your clients move each foot out about 2 to 4 inches (5.1 to 10.2 cm). This position will feel more natural in combination with a low-bar position. A wider stance involves the hip muscles (glutes) more, and because they are the strongest muscles in the body, trying to use them as much as possible makes sense. A wider stance also results in a shorter range of motion, which in turn makes the exercise easier. A wider stance places more stress on the hips, so be sure to move clients to a wider stance gradually. Be careful not to go too low with a wide stance, because doing this can place additional stress on the hip joints.

Increase the 1RM

Squatting with a heavy weight is an intense activity. Remember that clients should max out only on exercises that they have been practicing for a while (at least a month or two) and that they can complete in good form.

The setup and positioning of your client's body is important when attempting a 1RM. The client starts with the grip in the normal position and then moves the hands closer by

a few finger widths on each side. This action will cause the back muscles to tighten up, thereby creating a more solid base for the bar. Again, you will probably want clients to use a low-bar position if they are familiar with it. Moving the grip in can bother the shoulders and elbows if used too frequently, so save this for the extra heavy, low-rep sets. A tight grip combined with the low-bar position often feels

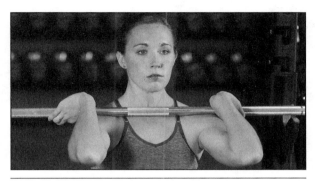

Figure 19.2 Bar position for the front squat.

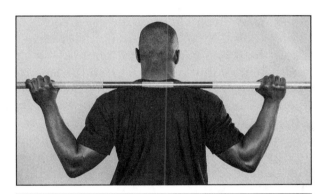

Figure 19.3 Bar position for the high-bar back squat.

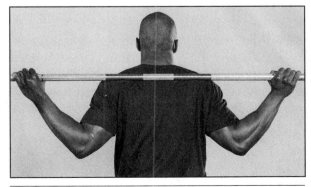

Figure 19.4 Bar position for the low-bar back squat.

best when the client uses an open grip, which has the thumb on the same side as the fingers. This grip reduces pressure on the wrist.

Make sure that the chest is up high and that the client's head is back. To get set properly, after the client grabs the bar and gets underneath it, have him or her try to stand up without moving the bar as if trying to scratch the middle of the back with the bar. Because the hands are still on the bar, this position causes the back to arch and tightens the muscles. Instruct the client to maintain that position while lowering him- or herself back under the bar so that the person begins the exercise without being hunched over. After the client is in position, have him or her drive the base of the neck back into the bar as if trying to push it off the back; this action is called packing the neck. This setup will help keep the center of gravity back and the bar stable. The client should maintain that position throughout the exercise.

After the body is set, the client places the feet underneath the body. The feet should be right under the body so that the client will have a strong walk out (the act of lifting the bar up and walking it out of the racks). If the feet are too far in front or behind, lifting the bar off the racks will be tough. Some people stagger their feet for the lift off, but when a person begins to lift heavy weights (more than 400 lb or 181.4 kg), this movement is not advisable. Get the client's feet under the body and then have the person take a big breath in, achieve proper position, tighten everything up, and lift the bar off the racks. This movement should be forceful; you are trying to get the client's first thought to be "This isn't that bad" as opposed to "Wow, this is heavy." Almost any weight feels heavy when it is sitting on a person's relaxed back, but if everything is tight and the person launches into it, the weight will not feel as heavy. The goal of the walk out is to build confidence, not ruin it.

After the bar is up and off the racks, the client needs to walk it back into position. Have the client take controlled steps and try to get into a pattern of always taking the same number of steps each time he or she walks the bar out. Practice this with every set, even with light weight, so that it becomes natural. Make sure that the client does not lose good position while walking the bar out. Try to minimize the number of steps taken; some people can get set in two steps, which is the minimum necessary. Most people take two steps and then a slight shuffle on each foot to get in the right position. Your client should not take more than four steps. The more steps the person takes, the more energy he or she expends. This is not a big deal when the client is not lifting heavy weight, but if the client is going heavy and hopes to get good at squats, he or she will want to refine the walkout.

After the walkout is completed and the client is standing straight, have him or her exhale but keep the body tight. The person should then inhale again and while doing so attempt to lift the chest even higher and again pack the neck. After he or she inhales and is set, instruct the client to hold his or her breath. The client is now ready to begin the descent, so have him or her break with the hips and then the knees. Cue the client to keep the chest up and keep looking straight ahead. Have the client go lower than he or she thinks necessary—the top of the acetabulum (where the femur meets the pelvis to compose the hip joint) should be below the top of the knee. A simple visualization is that a marble placed at the top of the knee while the client is at the bottom of the squat would roll down toward the hips. If it would, the client is low enough for the squat to be considered full and proper. If the marble would not roll down toward the hips, the client is performing a partial squat. After the client is down at the proper position, tell him or her to blast into the bar as if trying to launch it up in the air with the legs. Tell the client to think of the force coming from the lower back, as if a pulley were attached to the lower back and lifting him or her up to the ceiling. Have the client keep a tight grip on the bar, brace the core so that the trunk is like a strong column for support, and keep the chest up and neck back while driving upward. Instruct the client to exhale while completing the lift or when the client knows that he or she will be able to do it. Again, your client should not hold his or her breath on the normal sets, but it is OK to hold the breath and produce the Valsalva maneuver for a 1RM, especially during competition. At the completion of the exercise, the client should stand up straight with the legs straight, take a strong step forward, and place the bar on the racks. The client needs to watch the fingers when returning the bar to the racks to keep them from being crushed, particularly if the client has a wide grip.

FLAWS IN SQUAT TECHNIQUE

When people perform poorly in a squat, they normally have a problem with some aspect of their technique. The following sections discuss some of the common flaws and ways in which you can attempt to correct them.

Insufficient Squat Depth

The most common problem in the squat is not squatting deep enough (figure 19.5). If clients want to improve their health or the appearance of their legs, they need to squat so that their

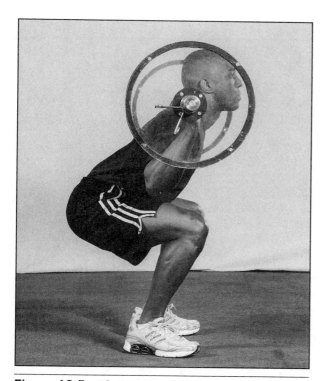

Figure 19.5 Three-quarter squat through a partial range of motion.

thighs are parallel to the floor or a bit lower. Most people go down only about half that far because they don't take enough time to learn how to squat properly. By squatting only halfway down, people can use much more weight, often double, than they can use if they are using good form. Everyone wants to go heavy as soon as possible, so they load up the weight. People have to be patient enough to use light weight while they are learning (31).

To learn how to squat to a proper depth, the first thing to do is to have clients use just the bar or a very light weight—10-pound (4.5 kg) dumbbells work best—and have them squat all the way down. Now instruct them to look at themselves in the mirror, both to the front and to the side if they can, to see their movements and notice what it feels like to be in the lowest position. The goal is to do the same thing with the training weight. People often use proper depth when they warm up, but when the weight is heavier they start cutting the depth, which is cheating. People are not really squatting if they don't go all the way down.

One of the benefits that clients gain by working with a personal trainer is that you can tell them how far they are going down. Show them what proper depth is first so that they know what it looks like. Then, while they are lifting, you can tell them whether each rep was deep enough. After a while, clients will learn what a good rep feels like, but you may want to review the form periodically to make sure that it is still correct.

A third technique to help clients learn how to squat deeply is to place a band behind them at the depth that you are trying to get them to. Now when clients go down low enough, their butts will touch the band. You and they will know that they performed the squat correctly. Of course, the band has to be set up at the right depth. For most people, this is 10 to 18 inches (25.4 to 45.7 cm) off the ground, depending on how tall the person is, how long the legs are, and how thick the person is in the hip and butt region (thin people need a higher band). Almost no one should have a band higher than 18 inches (45.7 cm), so if the bottom of your client's butt is not within 18 inches (45.7 cm) of the floor on each squat, he or she is not going down deep enough. After using the band for a while, remove it but have clients keep their form the same. Use the band to help your clients learn how to squat, but don't let it become a crutch. A simple exercise band will work just fine for this. Be sure that the client doesn't trip on it going in and out with the weight on his or her back.

A box squat, similar to squatting to a band, is another technique that you can use to help your clients learn proper squat depth. A box squat is a regular squat in which the client squats down to a box, sits on it for a second, and then stands back up. Set up the box so that it allows the client to go down to the proper depth; a box 10 to 18 inches (25.4 to 45.7 cm) high works well. Normally, the client straddles the box, so don't make it too wide, and make sure that the box is sturdy enough to support the client and the weight. Instruct the client not to drop onto the box or try to bounce off it because doing so can be jarring to the spine. The client should sit gently on the box, pause, and then stand back up. You might want to put a thin cushion or pad on the box for a little support. Aerobic steps work well to make a box. Adjusting the height by changing the number of risers under the box is easy. Four risers normally work well, and a thin yoga pad adds some comfort. Set the aerobic step long ways in the squat rack and then just have the client straddle the box while he or she is squatting. Aerobic steps work well because you find them in almost any gym, but any type of sturdy box will work. See figure 19.6 for an example of this exercise.

Finally, the client needs to have the right stance to go deep in a squat. Most people, particularly beginners, place their feet too close together, so they feel awkward and unstable at the bottom of a squat. The narrow stance makes them more comfortable at the top of the squat, but that is the easy part. When learning to squat with proper depth, clients will likely want to put their feet wider than shoulder-width apart and have their toes pointed out. With a narrow stance, most people cannot go deep enough without letting the knees go too far forward or without bending too far forward. If you are finding it difficult to get your clients

to go low enough, spread their feet apart. As clients become more used to squatting and more flexible in that movement, they may find that they are more comfortable bringing their feet in a bit, but most people are strongest in a wider stance. But if people choose to go extra wide, as in a stance similar to that used in a sumo deadlift, they will likely not be able to get their hips low enough for the squat to be fully effective.

Rolled-Forward Bar Position

Often during a heavy squat, the bar will roll forward on your client's neck on the ascent, making the squat much more difficult. As the bar rolls forward, the center of gravity moves forward. This shift in weight causes the client to lean extra far forward, as in the good morning exercise. The client may even fall forward so that the bar actually falls over his or her head.

You can do several things to prevent this bar roll.

- Put the barbell in a low-bar position on the back to help prevent the client from falling forward.

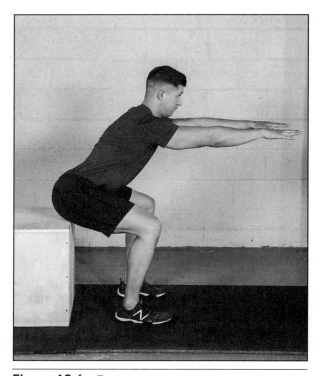

Figure 19.6 Box squat.

- Make sure that the client keeps the upper back tight during the squat.

- Instruct the client to hold the bar on the back, not just let it rest on the back. Tell the client to pull the bar down onto the back as if performing a lat pull-down with the bar on the back. The pulling motion helps keep the bar in place. The client should grip the bar with a slightly narrower grip. This grip makes the upper body extra tight, and the tight muscles help prevent the bar from rolling forward.

- Instruct the client to keep the chest up and drive the base of the neck into the bar. Sometimes, looking up too much can incline the upper back forward, allowing the bar to roll forward. Have the client keep his or her gaze in the midrange.

- Use a good squat bar that allows the sleeves of the bar to swivel without moving the bar. The sleeves are the thicker sections of the barbell where the weight goes. The sleeves should be well greased, and if you spin them they should turn for a while on their own without moving the bar. Some older bars or bars that haven't been taken care of have rusty or sticky sleeves. When you spin the sleeves on these bars, either they stop spinning almost immediately or the entire bar moves with the sleeve. Neither situation is desirable. When a person squats and moves backward, the weights on the bar tend to roll forward a bit. If the bar is not in good condition, it will roll with the weights. A bar rolling around, even a quarter of an inch (.6 cm), does not feel good on the back and it can throw a person out of his or her groove, especially on a heavy squat, so make sure that you have a good squat bar for your clients.

- Make sure that your clients keep a good setup position during the walkout. Clients may have a great setup under the bar, but after lifting it off the racks and walking it back, they are hunched over and in a terrible starting position. Remember, how people lift the bar off the racks is not as important as their position immediately before beginning the actual squat, so make sure that your clients keep or improve their body positioning during the walkout. You want your clients to start a squat standing up straight (not leaning forward). The legs should be straight, the feet should be in the position they want them in for squatting, the chest should be up, the neck should be driven back into the bar, the elbows should be almost under the bar (some people like to drive their elbows up), and the upper back should be tight. Have them look straight ahead and take a deep breath. Now they are ready to squat.

MUSCLES INVOLVED IN THE SQUAT

Many muscles are trained during the squat, which is one of the reasons that it is an outstanding exercise. The squat is clearly the best exercise to test leg strength. During the concentric part of the exercise, the hips, knees, and, to a lesser extent, the trunk are extending, so the muscles that perform those movements are all working.

The squat, along with most other compound leg exercises, has a double agonist. Both the glutes and the quads are working extremely hard in a squat. Both movements are crucial to achieving a squat, so both muscles are agonists. If we had to pick just one muscle as the agonist, it would be the glutes, but the quads are working too much to be considered just a synergist in this exercise (59). Working with the glutes and the quads as synergists are the hamstrings (minus the short head of biceps femoris), which are helping to extend the hip. In addition, the erectors and the quadratus lumborum are working to help keep the trunk stable and help extend the trunk during the ascent.

The squat uses many important stabilizers. The abductors and adductors are working to keep the thigh and knee stable; in fact, the adductor magnus is a synergist during hip extension. If your client's knee buckles or shakes during a squat, then his or her abductors and adductors might be weak. Remember, people are likely to go to where they are strong, so if the knees buckle in, the abductors may be weak; if they buckle out, which is rarer, the adductors may be weak. If the knees just shake, then the client is probably not used to the weight, and both abductors and adductors could be strengthened.

The obliques and abs are working as stabilizers to keep the trunk stable. Think of the trunk as a column that is supporting the weight, the bar, on the back. You want your client's column (the trunk) to be thick and strong, so have him or her squeeze the abs isometrically during the squat. If your client is wearing a belt, he or she can push the abs against the belt to generate good thoracic pressure.

Having well-developed upper-body musculature is helpful in carrying and bracing the bar; the traps, rhomboids, lats, and rear delts all contribute to supporting the bar. Keep in mind that these muscles are only useful stabilizers and will not receive enough stimuli to grow in size and strength just from a squat.

NAUSEA DURING THE SQUAT

The squat is a demanding exercise. It taxes many muscles in the body, most of which are large muscles that require a good deal of blood. After performing a squat, people often have high blood pressure, are gasping for breath, and may feel a bit lightheaded. Of course, breathing properly and using sensible intensity can help with this.

In addition to being exhausting, the squat also creates pressure on the fluid ball in the abdominal region. The weight is exerting pressure on the body in a downward position, while the legs are exerting pressure in an upward direction into the body. When the abdominal muscles and diaphragm are kept tight, the most unstable thing in that area is the stomach. All that pressure makes the body want to empty

the contents of the stomach, and clients may vomit while they squat (rare) or, more commonly, after they finish squatting several tough sets. In addition, during any demanding set, the body sends blood out to the muscles and away from the core of the body—the stomach and intestines. If your client has a lot of undigested food in the stomach when beginning intense exercise, the body may want to get rid of that food, which it does by vomiting (15).

Squatting is a brutal exercise, but the goal is certainly not to make your clients vomit. Like all things, the body adapts to doing squats, and the more a person squats, the more he or she becomes used to this sensation. In addition, although you or your clients may want to train at high intensity, the goal is not to vomit or faint. If your client throws up when you train the legs with him or her, it means that the person is likely not eating properly before lifting. You should talk about eating proper preworkout foods, setting aside more time to digest the food, and eating less before working out. Alternatively, you might be training your client too hard. People can feel exhausted and have a good workout without throwing up.

EXERCISES THAT ASSIST THE SQUAT

Like the bench press, the squat is a high-skill movement. In fact, it is a higher skill movement than the bench press, and it takes longer to learn and master. In addition, when you don't squat, your ability to do so will go away faster than your ability to bench press if you stop doing that exercise. The key to successful leg training is consistency. If you can get your clients to train their legs at least once a week for a year, they will make major progress. People like to skip their legs in favor of minor exercises, but the core of a person's strength comes from the hips, so the legs should not be neglected.

The best exercise to help the squat is, of course, the squat itself. First, clients must take the time to learn how to squat properly with light weight. Get your client's form down solidly and then begin to increase the weight. Ultimately, clients will be able to squat a lot of weight compared with what they do on other exercises, but rushing to lift heavy weights will compromise their overall potential.

Primary Exercises

Here are some exercises that have a strong correlation with the barbell back squat.

- High-bar squat
- Low-bar squat
- Full squat
- Three-quarter squat
- Half squat
- Bottom quarter squat
- Box squat
- Band squat
- Rack squat
- Front squat
- Safety bar squat

Supplemental Exercises

Here is a list a good exercises that can benefit the squat, assuming that the client is continuing to squat while incorporating these exercises. These supplemental exercises should not be considered good substitutions for the squat.

- Leg press
- Lunge
- Smith machine squat
- Hack squat
- Horizontal leg press
- Step-up
- One-legged squat
- Conventional deadlift
- Sumo deadlift
- Glute–ham raise
- Romanian deadlift
- Good morning
- Reverse hyperextension

Isolation Exercises

Isolation exercises do not have a large positive effect on the squat because the transfer of skill for those exercises is low. But if you think that your clients have a weak point, you can use isolation exercises with them to help increase the strength of that muscle. Again, if you have your clients perform these exercises and squat at the same time, the gains in these exercises might transfer over to improving their squatting ability.

- Leg curl
- Leg extension
- Abductor exercises
- Adductor exercises

SPOTTING THE SQUAT

The squat requires a competent spot because of the potential for serious injury. Anytime a weight is over a client's head or face, or the weight can crush the person, that exercise needs to be spotted. To start, the personal trainer should ensure that optimal safety is practiced by having the client squat inside a squat rack or a power rack. The benefit of this is twofold; it separates the client from other people in the gym, and the safety racks prevent a catastrophic injury. Set up the safety racks just below where the bar is at the bottom of the squat and make sure that they are installed correctly. That way, if a client falls or collapses or something strange happens, the worst that will happen is that the bar will crash down to the safety racks. The client will be embarrassed and shaken but likely unhurt.

To spot a squat, you should stand behind the client. You may wish to assist the client when the walkout is performed, and you can either grab the bar (between the hands and the shoulders of the client) or spot the client's upper chest, but a spot on a walkout is rarely needed. If a client struggles to walk out the weight, what will happen when he or she attempts to squat it? When the client is in position to begin the squat, you will be behind the client, have your knees slightly bent, and have the palms supinated about 6 to 12 inches (15.2 to 30.5 cm) under the client's front delts. You will not be in direct contact with the client at this time. As the client squats down, you must mimic the client and squat down with him or her. Maintain that 6- to 12-inch distance under the front delts with your hands. As the client rises from the bottom of the squat, you again mimic the motion. The proper position to spot a squat is shown in figure 19.7.

If a client is going to fail during a squat, he or she will usually do one of two things. First, the client might just drop straight down, so you must be prepared for that. Second, the client may fall forward. The most common technique mistake, even with experienced squatters, is to let the bar shift forward so that it is no longer in a straight line with the center of the foot. That will tilt the client forward. The bar may roll up on the client's back, tilting the person farther forward, and suddenly the client is trying to do the good morning exercise with a heavy squat weight, a movement that rarely works. You must be able to prevent this from happening. If a client needs a spot, you put your hands on the client's upper-chest and front deltoid region (the latter is preferred when spotting a female). You place your hands firmly in that area and hug the client to you so that the client's upper back is in contact with your chest. Together

the client and you complete the squat. Placing the hands on the lower back or obliques is not effective when trying to spot someone squatting heavy, particularly if the person starts to fall forward, because grabbing someone's sides does nothing to prevent the upper body from rounding forward (5).

You must use common sense when spotting a client. If the client is just warming up or is going relatively light, you do not need to mimic their actions so closely because doing so can feel a little invasive and looks a little odd. Having the safety racks set up is still a good idea, even with the lighter sets. If the client is squatting a very light weight that you can curl, then you can choose to spot the bar and not the body. This method is sometimes preferable when a male is spotting a beginning female client. But clients will quickly be able to squat more weight than you are comfortable holding, so you need to spot the upper body of the client as described earlier. You should use your own legs to help spot the client, not just your arms, which is why you are squatting down and up with the client at the same

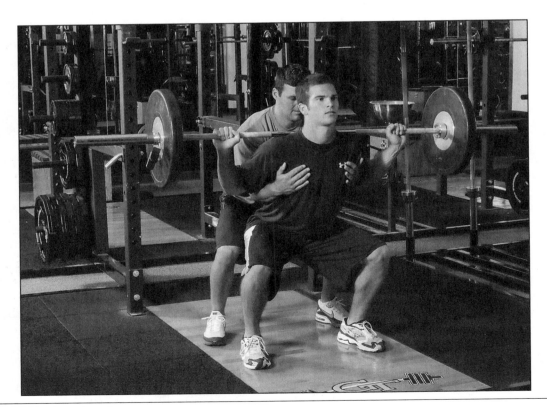

Figure 19.7 Spotting the squat.

time. But if the client is able to lift the weight, you should not overspot the client by assisting when it is unnecessary, thus reducing the workload that the client completes. You might choose to overspot brand new clients for the first few reps to make sure that they don't fail or fall, but after clients are familiar with the movement, overspotting is unnecessary and generally counterproductive.

EQUIPMENT AND APPAREL FOR THE SQUAT

When squatting, clients need to be appropriately dressed and ready for a good workout. In addition, some clients might wonder about the pros and cons of wearing a weight belt or knee wraps.

Shoes

Wearing the proper type of shoes is important for the squat. You want your clients to wear a shoe with a firm sole and some ankle support. Running shoes are not ideal for a squat, and a heavy squat can pop the bubble in air-filled shoes. A flat-soled high top is good, but deadlifting shoes (they look like wrestling shoes) are better if you prefer the feet to be flat. Further, special shoes are designed just for the squat; they can be expensive ($60 or more), are not comfortable to walk around in, and look somewhat weird, but they feel good for heavy squatting. Also, Olympic weightlifting shoes work well (figure 19.8). Some people want to emulate the barefoot experience when squatting; the Vibram Five Finger shoes work well for this. Most clients find that regular cross-training shoes with a solid support base work well.

Weightlifting Belt

Clients can wear a weightlifting belt when they squat (figure 19.9). Generally, they should save the belt for a heavier set with low reps, maybe a challenging set of five or fewer reps. Some personal trainers set a weight guideline. For instance, if your clients will be lifting over 400 pounds (181.4 kg), you will have them wear

a belt. But you do not need to require clients to wear a belt. In any case, do not have them wear a belt for the warm-up sets or sets with lighter weight unless they are protecting an injured area (43, 90).

Wrist Wraps

Heavy squats, particularly in the low-bar position, can place strain on the wrist. If your clients want to wear wrist wraps to add support, that is fine.

Knee Wraps

People often wrap their knees when they squat or when they train heavy with the legs. Knee wraps serve two purposes. The first is to help the person lift more weight. When the knee is wrapped with the legs straight, the joint is locked in that angle. Then when the leg is

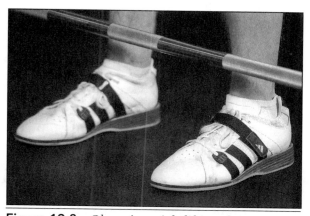

Figure 19.8 Olympic weightlifting shoes.

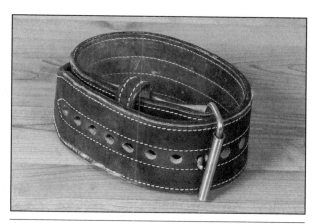

Figure 19.9 Weightlifting belt.

bent, the knee wants to spring back in position. This helps the person lift more weight. The amount of assistance varies greatly depending on the type of wrap used and how tightly it is wrapped, but tight power-lifting knee wraps add 20 to 50 pounds (9.1 to 22.7 kg) to the lift, in some cases even more, with an average of about 30 pounds (13.6 kg).

The second function of a knee wrap is to help protect the knee by keeping everything tight and in place. Research to support the efficacy of knee wraps is lacking, although some people swear by them. If your client is using a knee wrap for support, it does not need to be very tight; a knee brace or knee sleeve is probably adequate. In fact, some evidence indicates that extremely tight wraps are detrimental to the knees because they restrict the natural range of motion and do not allow good blood flow to the knee and calf. If your clients want to use tight knee wraps and you decide to allow that, they should take them off after each set. In addition, try to time it so that when the wraps are on, the client is ready to lift.

BEGINNING SQUAT TRAINING PROGRAMS

A simple five-week beginning training program for the squat involves starting at low resistance so that the person can learn the proper technique and perform the exercise through the proper range of motion. If a client wants to perform the squat exercise more than once a week, the workouts can simply be repeated for added practice.

For a Healthy Male

- Week 1: 45 lb (20.4 kg) × 12, 95 lb (43.1 kg) × 10, 95 lb (43.1 kg) × 10, 95 lb (43.1 kg) × 10
- Week 2: 45 lb (20.4 kg) × 12, 95 lb (43.1 kg) × 10, 95 lb (43.1 kg) × 10, 105 lb (47.6 kg) × 10
- Week 3: 45 lb (20.4 kg) × 12, 95 lb (43.1 kg) × 10, 105 lb (47.6 kg) × 10, 115 lb (52.2 kg) × 10

- Week 4: 45 lb (20.4 kg) × 12, 95 lb (43.1 kg) × 10, 115 lb (52.2 kg) × 10, 125 lb (56.7 kg) × 10
- Week 5: 45 lb (20.4 kg) × 12, 95 lb (43.1 kg) × 10, 115 lb (52.2 kg) × 10, 135 lb (61.2 kg) × 10

For a Healthy Female

- Week 1: 25 lb (11.3 kg) × 12, 45 lb (20.4 kg) × 10, 45 lb (20.4 kg) × 10, 45 lb (20.4 kg) × 10
- Week 2: 25 lb (11.3 kg) × 12, 45 lb (20.4 kg) × 10, 50 lb (22.7 kg) × 10, 55 lb (24.9 kg) × 10
- Week 3: 25 lb (11.3 kg) × 12, 45 lb (20.4 kg) × 10, 55 lb (24.9 kg) × 10, 65 lb (29.5 kg) × 10
- Week 4: 25 lb (11.3 kg) × 12, 45 lb (20.4 kg) × 10, 60 lb (27.2 kg) × 10, 70 lb (31.8 kg) × 10
- Week 5: 25 lb (11.3 kg) × 12, 45 lb (20.4 kg) × 1 0, 65 lb (29.5 kg) × 10, 75 lb (34.0 kg) × 10

CONCLUSION

The squat is an important exercise because it helps improve strength, bone density, mobility, balance, and coordination, and it has a positive transfer to other movements and exercises. The proper form for the squat involves keeping the feet flat, the knees in line with the toes, the trunk rigid, and descending as low as possible without expressing compensations. A personal trainer might modify a client's form on a squat depending on the client's goals such as improved health, improved performance, or squatting with a maximal weight.

Common flaws in the squat include not going deep enough, letting the bar roll forward, letting the heels come up, and allowing the knees to move inward. The agonists for the squat are the glutes and quads; the hamstrings, erectors, and adductors are strong synergists. The primary movement is hip, trunk, and knee extension, which takes place in the sagittal plane.

Various exercises can help improve the squat, but exercises that more closely resemble some aspect of it have a better transfer to squatting ability. Personal trainers need to know how to spot a squat exercise, which involves standing behind the client, squatting down with him or her, and, if assistance is needed, placing the hands on the client's upper chest and helping him or her stand up. Equipment is available to help with squatting mechanics and performance, such as hard-soled shoes, lifting belts, wrist wraps, and knee wraps, should a client choose to use them.

The squat is a valuable exercise, but learning the proper form takes time. All exercises carry risks, and squatting improperly carries great risks. The rewards of squatting with proper form over the long term can be high, and the squat is a great tool for a personal trainer to use when it is appropriate for the client.

Study Questions

1. What two muscles are usually considered agonists in a squat?
   a. quads and hamstrings
   b. glutes and erectors
   c. soleus and gastrocnemius
   d. glutes and quads

2. What are the primary movements that occur in a squat?
   a. hip extension, trunk extension, and knee extension
   b. hip flexion, trunk extension, and knee extension
   c. hip flexion, trunk flexion, and knee extension
   d. hip flexion, trunk flexion, and knee flexion

3. According to most authorities, where should a lifter look when squatting?
   a. up at the ceiling
   b. directly ahead
   c. down at the feet
   d. eyes closed on all attempts to feel the weight

4. What position should a personal trainer take to spot the squat?
   a. standing behind the client with the hands on the client's obliques
   b. standing in front of the client, facing the client, with the hands on the barbell
   c. standing behind the client with the hands coming under and around the trunk to support the client's front deltoids and upper-chest area
   d. sitting in a chair 15 feet (4.6 m) to the side of the client to judge depth

5. What is the proper depth for a client to reach during a squat assuming that he or she does not express any contraindication?
   a. The top of acetabulum should be lower than the top of the knee.
   b. The knee must make a 90-degree angle.
   c. The femur must be parallel to the floor.
   d. The bottom of the ischium must be below the patella.

Bench Press

If you're involved in fitness or have spent any time working out, at one point or another you have been asked the question, "How much do you bench?" The answer to that question is the most common way of measuring a person's strength. Honestly, the bench press may not deserve its position of supremacy above all other exercises, and a huge bench press does not necessarily indicate fantastic athleticism, but it is still the go-to representation of strength.

TRAINING GOALS

Many people are interested in improving their bench press, sometimes for no other reason than having an impressive answer to that common question. Some people want to improve their bench to improve their health, others because a big bench generally means a bigger chest, others because it will help their performance in sport, and still others because it is their sport itself. The purpose of this chapter is to help you better understand the bench press and ultimately help you improve your clients' bench-pressing ability.

In some sense, a bench press is a simple exercise. Lie down on a bench, hold a bar with your arms straight, bring it down to your chest, and then push it back up until your arms are straight again. Of course, when analyzed, the exercise is more complex than that. The level of analysis will depend on your goals. Improving the technique for the bench press will aid in reaching three goals: to improve health, performance, and the 1RM.

Improve Health

Increasing your client's bench press means increasing his or her muscular strength, one component of fitness. To perform a bench press properly for health, clients need to follow these procedures:

- Have your clients lie down on a bench so that their eyes are underneath the bar.
- Have your clients place their feet flat on the floor about 2 feet (61 cm) apart.
- Clients should keep the spine in a neutral position. The back should be basically flat with just a tiny arch.
- Instruct your clients to tuck their shoulder blades slightly together before they begin the exercise.
- Provide them with a spot to help them unrack the weight, known as getting a liftoff, if they are lifting heavy, but they can probably handle it themselves at this stage.
- Have your clients lift the bar off the racks and bring it over the chest. The bar should be straight above the chest, in line with the nipples.
- Direct your clients to bring the bar down with their elbows slightly tucked in and not flared out to the sides (figure 20.1). The elbows should not be in line with the shoulders; they should stick out from the body at about a 45- to 60-degree angle (a 90-degree angle would be in a straight line with the shoulders). The elbows should stay under the bar.

- Have your clients touch the bar to the chest with their forearms perpendicular to the bar; if this position is achieved, the grip is the correct width. If the grip is too wide or too narrow, clients will not be able to lift as much weight and their results will be compromised.
- After the bar touches the chest, instruct clients to press it straight up to the ceiling, continuing to press until their arms are straight. Their arms should extend evenly, keeping the bar level.
- As they press upward do not allow them to round their shoulders. You want them to know that they are trying to press the bar up without excessively moving their shoulder blades.
- Clients should keep the head and neck in line with the body, keep the head back on the bench, and look straight ahead.

Clients should avoid several techniques or movements:

- Lifting the butt off the bench
- Dancing with the feet (should be stable)
- Slamming the bar on the chest
- Cutting the range of motion short (failing to touch the bar to the chest)

- Flaring the elbows out to the side
- Letting the head come off the bench
- Looking to either side or watching one arm
- Letting one side of the bar go up faster than the other
- Using an open grip (not closing the thumbs around the bar on the side opposite the fingers)
- Excessively arching the back
- Letting the wrists bend backward

Improve Performance

The technique for your clients to use when you are trying to increase their bench press performance is similar to the form they use for improving their health, with just a few differences. When your clients are lifting heavy loads, you need to make sure that the upper body is stable. Have them accomplish this by pulling their shoulder blades very tightly together before they begin, even before they lie down on the bench. They can accomplish this by pulling their arms back as though performing a row. Have them squeeze the rhomboids, traps, and rear delts together, trying to make the back hard and firm. This

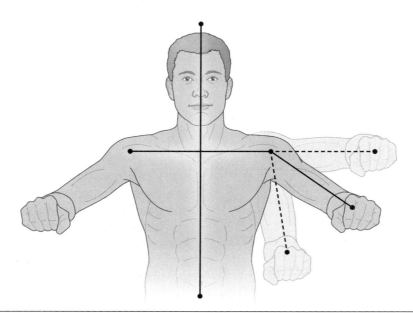

Figure 20.1 Correct and incorrect positions of the humerus in relation to the body during the bench press.

From Starting Strength: Basic Barbell Training. Copyright 2007 The Aasgaard Company. Used by permission.

action will lift the chest, which decreases the range of motion and makes the bench press easier. They need to maintain this position as they lift off the bar. To help them keep this position, either give them a liftoff or make sure that they are far enough under the bar that they can easily press it up.

Right before clients receive the liftoff, have them take a deep breath and hold it during the liftoff. After the bar is set over the chest, instruct them to exhale and then inhale again. Inhaling with a deep breath also serves to raise the chest slightly. Clients should hold their breath as they lower the weight to the chest and then exhale as they push it back up. Normally, you want them to exhale through the sticking point, or the difficult part of the range of motion for that particular client. For most people this point is about halfway up. If clients are performing multiple reps, tell them to inhale on the way back down and then repeat. They don't have to hold the bar straight to inhale each time, just on the first rep (16).

You will want clients to arch the back slightly during the exercise. There should be no tension in the lower back, nor should the back cramp up during the exercise. By having them pull the shoulder blades back and down and then lift the chest, they can usually produce an acceptable arch. To increase their stability, clients should keep their feet flat on the floor and relatively far apart.

As clients are pressing the bar up, they may find that they have greater strength if they press the bar up and back slightly so that the bar travels in an arc going back up over the head. If the bar begins at the middle of the chest, as you watch them press it up and slightly back, the bar should end up over the upper chest or clavicle (figure 20.2). This arc should not be excessive; it should follow a natural range of motion. The main problem with arcing the bar is that a person might lower the bar to touch the chest at the wrong point. If you choose to tell your clients to arc the bar, make sure that each rep is the same and that the bar touches the chest in exactly the same place each time. Do not let the elbows flare out too much (more than 90 degrees) as the bar is pressed up and arced back, and instruct clients to keep their elbows tucked in at the bottom of the movement. Make sure that their wrists are straight and not bent backward, because that will cause them to lose power (20).

Increase the 1RM

If your goal when showing clients how to bench press is to have them lift the most weight possible, follow these guidelines. Powerlifters

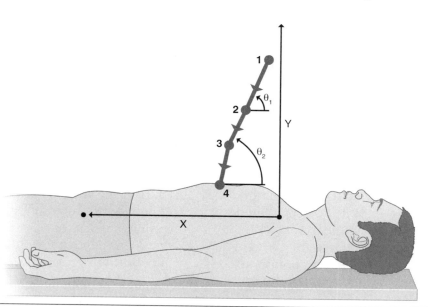

Figure 20.2 Proper bar path during a bench press.

compete only by performing a 1RM in competition, and performing a 1RM is the truest way of testing strength.

When people perform a 1RM bench press, the same general rules apply. They can do a few things to squeeze out some extra pounds. Your client's body position should be similar to a bench press for performance, but in this case it is acceptable to arch the back. Some benefits and some disadvantages are associated with doing this. When people arch the back, they raise the chest, which decreases the range of motion of a natural bench press and therefore makes it easier. It is similar to performing a decline bench press. The disadvantages of allowing your clients to arch the back are that they are more likely to injure the lower back. Some people are more flexible than others in this area. Although arching the back is legal in powerlifting competitions, do not confuse that with raising the butt off the bench, which is not legal. The upper back and butt must remain on the bench, but the lower back can be off the bench.

Long-term training is more important than lifting a bit of extra weight and getting hurt. If you want your clients who are focused on improving their 1RM to arch their backs, you should not have them use that technique on most of their training sets. Have them arch their backs just for heavy sets of five or fewer reps; three or fewer is even better. They should perform the arch enough so that it feels comfortable, but they should not use it all the time because the risk of injury is too significant.

When clients are maxing out, you want them to change their breathing slightly as well. Instruct them to inhale before the liftoff and then hold their breath as they get the bar in position over the middle chest. They exhale and then take a big inhale again. Have clients hold their breath as they bring the bar down to the chest and continue to hold their breath as they press the weight upward. Tell them to exhale either at the end of the rep or when they know that they can complete the rep. If you choose to tell them to hold their breath, make sure that you use this technique only on sets of three or fewer reps. Tell clients to breathe in after each rep; do not have them hold their breath for the entire set. Any set that includes more than three reps requires clients to breathe normally as described in the section "Improve Performance." If clients don't breathe, they will run out of oxygen and subsequently energy on their longer sets. Remember that this technique is appropriate only for strength athletes, not most personal-training clients. When in doubt, be conservative and safety conscious (22).

When telling clients how to grip the bar, the same general rules apply to maxing out as to regular training. Most people are stronger with a wider grip but not always; you should have them experiment with different grips to find what is best for them. Keep in mind that occasionally a grip that feels good with a light weight will not feel good with a heavy weight. Wider is better because a wide grip requires a smaller range of motion, but if you have them go too wide, they will be weak at the bottom of the bench (115). Going too wide can also be rough on the shoulders. The widest legal grip in a competition is 81 cm (about 32 inches), which is the width that is attained by putting a pointer finger on the ring on a standard bar. The best starting point is to have the forearms perpendicular to the bar at the bottom of the movement or at the sticking point, whichever feels better (42, 55).

Again, make sure that your clients are using a closed grip that has the thumb on the side of the bar opposite the fingers, enabling them to close the hand around the bar. This grip is important for safety, because the bar is much less likely to fall out of their hands and crush the chest or face. In many competitions, benching with an open grip is illegal, although federations have different rules.

As clients drive the bar upward, instruct them to keep their upper back muscles tight, which tightens the whole upper body. Clients may want to imagine that the bar is immovable and that they are trying to press their back into the bench as far as they can. When they are pressing, you can have your clients attempt to drive with their hips. Doing this is fine as long as the butt does not come off the bench. They are trying to channel the energy from their hips into the bar to make it go up (31). The sequence of photos in figure 20.3 shows the stages of the bench press exercise.

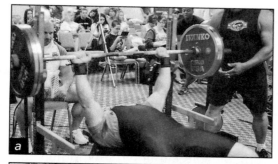

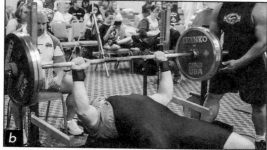

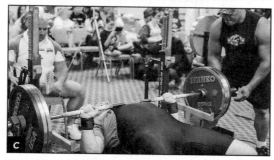

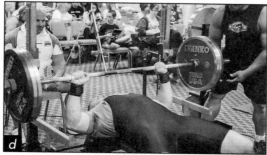

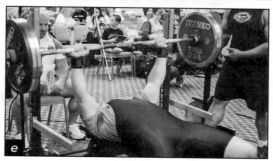

Figure 20.3 Stages of the bench press: *(a)* start, *(b)* descent, *(c)* touch, *(d)* ascent, *(e)* lock out.

For a 1RM, you normally want your clients to arc the bar up and back (toward the face) as described earlier. Gripping the bar tightly can help the muscles in the arm contract, particularly the triceps. You want to encourage your clients to keep their wrists in line with their forearms as they press up. Some clients find that allowing the wrists to relax slightly and roll backward, or extend, on the way down and then roll slightly forward, or flex, on the way up helps get the bar through the sticking point. Tell clients to keep their shoulder blades locked together, and do not let them protract their shoulders as they press the bar up. Have clients bring the bar down with their elbows tucked, keep them tucked for the beginning of the press, and then start to flare their elbows out as they press, never flaring more than 90 degrees. A flare to approximately 70 degrees in the middle of the range of motion usually works best.

BENCH PRESS PAUSE

When people participate in a bench press competition, they must bring the bar down, rest it on the chest, and keep it motionless. Then, after the bar is visibly still, they can press it back up. In some organizations, the referee yells, "Press!" as a signal that the lifter can then push it up. Pausing the bar on the chest makes it harder to push up because it dilutes the stretch reflex, which weakens the involved muscles. Most people can expect to lose 5 percent or about 10 to 20 pounds (4.5 to 9.1 kg) off their max because of the pause. If your clients lose strength because of the pause even after they get used to it, their form during a regular bench press without a pause may not be as good as it should be, and they may be bouncing the weight off the chest. The pause is necessary in competition because without the pause, it would be difficult to distinguish a light touch of the chest (called a touch-and-go rep) from a moderate bounce and from a full slam on the chest that uses it as a springboard to bounce the weight back up (62).

If you decide to have your clients rest the bar on the chest or have the bar just touch the chest, make sure that the bar does not sink into the chest. Some people relax as the bar hits the chest, making the lift much more difficult for them. Tell your clients to keep the upper body very tight so that the bar is just lightly resting on the chest. Then, when it is time to press, they explode upward and drive the bar to the lockout.

You do not need to have all clients, or even those interested in increasing their 1RM, pause a bench press. The pause can teach clients to react a bit more slowly. Clients who are training for power or for a fast reaction time might want to train to reverse the weight as quickly as possible after the bar hits the chest. If clients want to try their hand in a powerlifting competition, they will have to get used to a pause. If clients are weak at the bottom of the movement or comment that they don't often feel the chest working in a bench press, making them pause their reps (on all sets or at least on a back down set) can be a useful technique to fix both problems.

MUSCLES INVOLVED IN THE BENCH PRESS

Most people know that the pecs are the agonist in a bench press and the front delts and triceps are the main synergists, but that is not the complete picture. The most important muscle left out of that understanding is the lats. The lats are involved in a bench press, as explained in detail in chapter 11. The lats insert on the front of the humerus, so when the humerus goes behind the body, the lats help pull the humerus forward. They are working particularly hard during the first couple of inches of the bench press. Table 20.1 lists the muscles involved in a bench press and the way in which they contribute to the movement.

FAILURE DURING THE BENCH PRESS

When clients are performing the bench press, you need to know their sticking point, the point in the range of motion that is the most challenging, and the position of the bar when they fail.

Some people fail down low; others fail up high. Knowing where this occurs is important because that tells you the location of their weak link. To analyze the bench press, we divide the ascent of the bar into the bottom, middle, transition, and top portions of the movement.

Bottom Portion of the Ascent

The bottom part of the bench press is the beginning of the exercise, normally the first 2 to 4 inches (5.1 to 10.2 cm) of the range of motion. The two most important muscles in this part of the range of motion are the lats and the pecs, in that order. The lats help drive the bar off the chest, and the pecs continue that movement upward. Clients who fail in the bottom range of motion probably have one of three problems. First, they might be bringing the bar down in the wrong spot. Make sure that the bar hits the middle of the chest. If clients bring the bar too high, toward the head, or too low, on the belly, they will not be able to generate much force at the bottom. To correct this, make sure that in performing every rep, clients have the bar hitting the chest in the same place. In addition, you can use negatives by having them take a heavy weight and practice bringing it down in the right spot (109).

The second problem could be that your client's hands are too far apart. A wide grip

Table 20.1   Muscles Involved in the Bench Press

Agonist	Major synergists	Minor synergists	Stabilizers
Pecs	Front delt Triceps Lats Subscapularis	Middle delt Coracobrachialis Teres major	Rotator cuff Elbow flexors Rhomboids Middle traps Forearm extensors Forearm flexors Serratus anterior

is helpful because it offers a smaller range of motion, but the drawback of a wide grip is that getting the bar going in the beginning is tough (115). Any grip that involves a finger going beyond the ring on the bar is a wide grip. That doesn't mean the grip is too wide, but it might be, so if a client is using a wide grip and getting no power at the bottom, that might be the issue. If all the fingers are outside the knurled rings, then the grip is almost assuredly too wide, as well as being illegal in competition. Try narrowing the client's grip a finger or two to see how that feels at the bottom.

The third problem could be that the client's muscles are simply weaker at that point in the range of motion. Again, the muscles in question are the lats and the pecs. To strengthen those muscles for the bench press, the client can perform the following exercises:

- Lats—bent-over row, pull-up, dumbbell row, cable row, lat pull-down
- Chest—wide bench press, low incline bench press, pause bench press, low incline DB press, neutral grip dumbbell press, neutral grip chest press machine

Middle Portion of the Ascent

The middle of the bench press is where most people fail. If a normal bench press has a range of motion of about 18 inches (45.7 cm), the middle portion of the ascent is from the 4th inch (10.2 cm) to the 10th (25.4 cm) or 12th inch (30.5 cm). The primary muscle working here is the pecs.

If your client fails in the middle range of motion, one of three problems is the likely cause. The most common reason is poor form, most likely allowing the elbows to flare out too quickly. This problem is particularly common among beginner and intermediate clients. When the elbows flare out to the side, more emphasis is placed on the shoulders, particularly the front delt. The front delt is not as strong as the pecs, or at least it shouldn't be, so this is not advantageous for a heavy bench press. In addition, elbow flare normally signals weaker lats. To fix elbow flare, train the lats using the exercises listed previously and have the client practice each rep with good form.

Stop the set as soon as you see the elbows flare out. Four to eight weeks might be needed to fix this problem, and during that time the client's bench might even go down, but ultimately it will move up significantly after the client learns how to bench press properly. In addition, practicing dumbbell presses with a neutral grip can help the client learn the proper elbows-tucked position (34).

A second problem is speed. A client who lifts the bar slowly off the chest is more likely to stall in the middle range of motion. When lifting heavy, the goal is to blast the bar off the chest, moving it as fast as possible. To work on improving your client's speed, you can incorporate plyometrics into the routine (75, 87). The two best chest plyometric exercises are clap push-ups and drop catch push-ups, described in chapter 24. In addition, lifting a lighter weight as fast as possible can improve speed.

The third problem might just be that the chest is weak at that point compared with the other muscles. To improve the strength of the chest for the middle range of motion of the bench press, clients can perform bottom three-quarter (range-of-motion) bench press, incline bench press, dumbbell press, dumbbell incline press, push-up (preferably weighted or on rings), floor press, two-board press, dip, decline bench press, or a combination of those exercises.

Transition Portion of the Ascent

If your clients fail in the transition, in the middle-upper range of motion, their shoulders are probably weak (8). The transition part of a bench press is a small range where the chest stops contributing as much force to the exercise and the triceps are getting ready to take over. In an 18-inch (45.7 cm) range-of-motion press, this phase likely starts somewhere between 10 and 12 inches (25.4 and 30.5 cm) and goes for about 2 inches (5.1 cm).

To fix this issue, have clients try arching the bar up and back slightly. This often helps drive the bar through the higher sticking points. In addition, clients can allow their elbows to flare out ever so slightly to increase their mechanical advantage, but they should not do this too soon. They should maintain good speed through the middle of the range of motion and work on the shoulders. Good exercises for the shoulders include the barbell military (shoulder) press, dumbbell military press, Smith machine military press, military rack lockout, and three-board press.

Top Portion of the Ascent

Finally, if your clients fail in the upper range of motion, if they can't lock out the weight (i.e., fully extend the elbows), their triceps are probably weak, at least in that movement pattern. To help correct this problem, instruct your clients to try arching the bar as they press and allowing their elbows to flare out slightly.

People normally don't fail in the upper part of the range of motion because mechanically they have the advantage at that point. Generally, people can lock out significantly more than they can bench press. Failure in this part of the movement indicates that some neuromuscular issue is present. Probably what is happening is that the body is learning to decelerate the lighter weight near the lockout to prevent injury, and this is causing the muscles to shut down as the client presses heavier weight. This problem seems to occur more often in people whose arms are longer than average. To correct this, have the client try the following exercises: band press, three-to five-board press, rack lockout, reverse grip tricep pull-down, skull crusher, military lockout, band lockout, close-grip bench press, JM press, and triceps isolation exercises with the shoulder girdle in bench press position (for better transfer).

EXERCISES THAT ASSIST THE BENCH PRESS

When training to increase the bench press, performing the exercise all the time is not recommended. Clients need to work on various supplemental exercises to help strengthen the muscles that perform the bench press. But simply selecting random exercises for the chest, lats, shoulders, and triceps is a poor approach. The principle of specificity and skill transfer applies here. Remember that if you want your clients to improve in a high-skill exercise like the bench press, you need to have them practice mainly high-skill movements. Choose a maximum of 25 percent low-skill movements (see table 20.2); the rest should be high-skill movements.

One of the great things about a bench press is that it is a relatively high-skill exercise, at least when compared with other resistance training exercises. Remember that the transfer of skill flows downward, so clients who become more proficient at a high-skill exercise will become more proficient at a low-skill exercise. If you have them practice the bench press exclusively for six months and their bench goes up 50 pounds (22.7 kg), their performance on a chest press machine will also improve significantly. Getting better at the bench press has a positive effect on all the exercises listed in table 20.2, not just the ones with a high relationship. It has the most powerful effect on the compound exercises, but any exercise that involves the chest will be improved by improving the bench press. That result is what makes the bench press one of the most valuable exercises for the upper body.

Table 20.2 Relationship of Assistance Exercises to the Bench Press

Highest relationship	High relationship	Moderate relationship	Low relationship
Bench press	Wide bench press Close-grip bench press Incline bench press Decline bench press Floor bench press Two- or three-board press Pause bench press Bench press with chains or bands	Dip Push-up DB press (any angle) Ball DB press Smith machine bench press Partial bench press Negatives	Chest press machine (any angle) Hammer strength machine (any angle) DB fly (any angle) Chest fly Cable crossover Pec deck

SPOTTING THE BENCH PRESS

Like the squat, the bench press is an exercise that the personal trainer needs to know how to spot. You should stand behind the client, near his or her head, when the client is lying on the bench (figure 20.4). You should take an alternated grip on the bar and place your hands inside the grip of the client, unless the client is performing a close-grip bench press, in which case your hands will be outside his or her grip. You can provide a liftoff for the client. If this happens, you and client should set up some sort of system to ensure that the client is ready to receive the full weight of the bar. Remember that it is more important that the client is ready to lift the weight than the personal trainer.

When spotting the bench press, you should bend your knees and keep your back arched; do not try to use just your arms when you spot somebody. The weight will likely be out in front of you, so your leverage will be poor. Also, remember that you are in charge. If you are worried about your ability to spot the client if he or she performs another rep, then the set ends there, even if the client wants to keep going. You decide when the set stops (5).

EQUIPMENT FOR THE BENCH PRESS

When competing in the bench press, some powerlifters wear a special superthick, tight shirt that provides stability to their shoulders and gives them great rebound at the bottom of the movement. With current bench shirt technology, bench shirts usually add 20 percent to 50 percent to what a person is able to lift. That effect is one reason why the best bench press ever recorded is just over 700 pounds (317.5 kg), and the best bench press with a bench shirt is over 1,100 pounds (499.0 kg). The two situations are different, and we cannot compare a bench press performed without a shirt, often called a raw bench press, to a bench press performed while wearing a bench press shirt, often called an equipped bench press.

BEGINNING BENCH PRESS TRAINING PROGRAMS

A simple five-week beginning training program for the bench press involves starting at low resistance so that the person can learn the proper technique and perform the exercise through the proper range of motion. If a client wants to perform the bench press exercise more than once a week, the workouts can simply be repeated for added practice.

For a Healthy Male

- Week 1: 45 lb (20.4 kg) × 12, 75 lb (34.0 kg) × 10, 75 lb (34.0 kg) × 10, 75 lb (34.0 kg) × 10
- Week 2: 45 lb (20.4 kg) × 12, 75 lb (34.0 kg) × 10, 75 lb (34.0 kg) × 10, 85 lb (38.6 kg) × 10
- Week 3: 45 lb (20.4 kg) × 12, 75 lb (34.0 kg) × 10, 85 lb (38.6 kg) × 10, 95 lb (43.1 kg) × 10
- Week 4: 45 lb (20.4 kg) × 12, 75 lb (34.0 kg) × 10, 95 lb (43.1 kg) × 10, 105 lb (47.6 kg) × 10

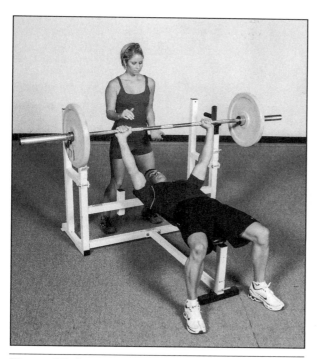

Figure 20.4 Spotting the bench press.

- Week 5: 45 lb (20.4 kg) × 12, 75 lb (34.0 kg) × 10, 95 lb (43.1 kg) × 10, 115 lb (52.2 kg) × 10

For a Healthy Female

- Week 1: 25 lb (11.3 kg) × 12, 35 lb (15.9 kg) × 10, 35 lb (15.9 kg) × 10, 35 lb (15.9 kg) × 10
- Week 2: 25 lb (11.3 kg) × 12, 35 lb (15.9 kg) × 10, 35 lb (15.9 kg) × 10, 45 lb (20.4 kg) × 10
- Week 3: 25 lb (11.3 kg) × 12, 35 lb (15.9 kg) × 10, 45 lb (20.4 kg) × 10, 50 lb (22.7 kg) × 10
- Week 4: 25 lb (11.3 kg) × 12, 35 lb (15.9 kg) × 10, 45 lb (20.4 kg) × 10, 55 lb (24.9 kg) × 8
- Week 5: 25 lb (11.3 kg) × 12, 35 lb (15.9 kg) × 10, 45 lb (20.4 kg) × 10, 55 lb (24.9 kg) × 10

Note: The standard barbell in a gym is 45 pounds (20.4 kg). Often gyms will have pre-loaded smaller barbells of 15 pounds (6.8 kg), 25 pounds (11.3 kg), and 35 pounds (15.9 kg) that can be used if the standard barbell is too heavy for that workout.

CONCLUSION

The bench press involves lying on a bench in a supine position, bringing a bar down to the chest, and then pressing it back up until the arms are straight. A personal trainer might modify the form on the bench press for a client depending on whether the goal is simply to improve health, to increase performance, or to perform the highest bench press possible. A bench press can be performed in touch-and-go style, or it can be paused on the chest. Pausing the bench press reduces momentum, which makes the lift harder. The agonists for the bench press are the pec major. Strong synergists include the front delts, triceps, lats, and subscapularis. The movement is closest to horizontal shoulder adduction and elbow extension, taking place in the transverse plane.

To help improve a client's bench press, the personal trainer should know where the person fails during the exercise. Failure might be a result of poor neuromuscular coordination or might indicate that certain muscles are weak. Various exercises can help improve the bench press. Generally, the exercises that more closely resemble the bench press involving a barbell have the most powerful effect. A personal trainer should spot the bench press with an alternated grip, hands inside the client's hands, bent knees, and a flat back.

The bench press may be the most popular exercise. It has a positive transfer to other upper-body pressing exercises. The bench press can be a higher risk exercise given the nature of the shoulder joint, so care should be exercised to ensure that proper form is used. Ultimately, a client is likely to lift a large amount of weight on the bench press compared with other upper-body exercises.

Study Questions

1. What is the agonist in a bench press?
   a. latissimus dorsi
   b. anterior deltoid
   c. biceps brachii
   d. pectoralis major

2. What are the main synergists in a bench press?
   a. pectoralis minor and biceps brachii
   b. triceps brachii and anterior deltoid
   c. rhomboids and posterior deltoid
   d. pectoralis major and rectus abdominis

3. What primary movements occur in a bench press?
   a. horizontal shoulder adduction and elbow extension
   b. horizontal shoulder abduction and elbow extension
   c. shoulder extension and elbow flexion
   d. shoulder abduction and elbow flexion

4. What is the proper angle for the humerus in relation to the torso at the bottom of the lift?

    a. 0- to 15-degree angle

    b. 45- to 60-degree angle

    c. 90- to 100-degree angle

    d. 125- to 140-degree angle

5. Which of the following exercises would most likely improve the 1RM on a bench press?

    a. push-ups with body weight

    b. one-arm ball dumbbell press

    c. one-arm dumbbell row

    d. barbell incline press

Deadlift

The deadlift is simple: You just bend down to the weight, pick it up, and stand up straight with it. Yet the deadlift is grueling. It is the simplest of the big three exercises in that it requires the least skill. In addition, a person's ability to perform the deadlift remains for a relatively long time after he or she stops deadlifting because the neuromuscular coordination required for the deadlift is the least specific of the three exercises. The basic motor pattern remains intact even after someone stops deadlifting. In contrast, if a person stops squatting, that motor pattern degrades relatively quickly.

TRAINING GOALS

Although the deadlift has the lowest skill level of the three exercises, it is not easy to learn. As with the squat, extra time should be taken to learn the proper form with the deadlift. Spend time with light weights building your client's foundation before you move on to heavier weights. This advice can be tough to follow. Most people can deadlift a good amount of weight right from the start, and lifting two or three plates on each side of a bar in a short time is fun. But then the form can break down as your clients try to go heavier, and they either hurt themselves or get frustrated by the lack of progress and quit the exercise. If you make them take time in the beginning to learn how to perform the exercise properly, performing the exercise will be much safer and ultimately they will be able to lift much more weight. Improving the technique for the deadlift will help clients achieve three different goals: to improve health, performance, and the 1RM.

Improve Health

The deadlift, much like the squat, is likely to benefit a large majority of clients. The deadlift is the most functional of the big three barbell lifts because it directly mimics what people do in real life—a person bends down, picks something up, and then stands with it. The deadlift is a structural exercise so it is beneficial to bone health. It targets a large number of muscle groups and teaches them to work together in a synergistic fashion. It can cause a positive hormonal release, it is effective for eliciting hypertrophy, and it can create EPOC, which helps burn fat and can build $\dot{V}O_2$max and work capacity.

For clients who include the deadlift exercise in a program to improve health and other components of fitness, proper technique starts with the lower back. During the entire deadlift movement, you want the client's lower back to be slightly arched. Ideally, it should be flat, but slightly arched is better. You do not want the lower back to round, as would happen if they were to bend forward to touch their toes. This posture would put them in a weak position that is more likely to cause injury to the spine.

To get into the starting position to perform the exercise, clients should follow several general technique guidelines:

- Arch the back by lifting the chest up toward the ceiling and pulling the shoulder blades back together.

- Tilt the butt backward and upward so that the top of the butt goes toward the lower back.

- Imagine a pencil rolling down the lower back and then push the butt out to try to catch it with the top of the butt. This motion will cause the lower back to arch, which is also called an anterior pelvic tilt (2, 32).

To start a deadlift, have the client walk up to the bar where it rests on the ground and get the feet set. The feet should be about shoulder-width apart. Most people have their toes pointing out slightly. Make sure that the client is standing close to the bar; it should almost be touching the shins when the person is standing up straight. The stance for the deadlift will be narrower than it is for the squat.

After the feet are set, instruct the client to lift the chest and pull the butt back, thus arching the back. Tell the client to maintain that position and bend forward, starting with the hips, as he or she reaches down and grabs the bar with a pronated grip. When the hands get lower than the knees, the client flexes the knees to get low enough to grasp the bar with the hands just outside the legs while maintaining an arched back. The wider the hands are, the higher the client will have to lift the bar, which increases the difficulty of performing the exercise (26).

After the client grabs the bar, tell him or her to use the bar to stabilize him- or herself, lift the chest, and push the butt back again to make sure that the lower back has a slight arch. At the bottom position, the client should be able to see his or her chest fully in the mirror. The hips should be higher than the knees but lower than the chest. As you look at the client from the side, the goal is to have the bar under the spine of the scapula. If the hips are too low, the spine of the scapula will be behind the bar. If the hips are too high, the spine of the scapula will be in front of the bar. When the client is set, tell him or her to take a deep breath, brace the core, and then lift up the bar. The client should be looking straight ahead or up slightly (37).

As the client lifts the bar, tell him or her to drive with the legs but maintain stability in the upper body. The person should visualize lifting the bar with the upper body first. While lifting the bar, he or she is pulling up with the upper body and driving with the legs. The client can visualize a pulley attached to his or her upper back (where the squat bar would be) heading up toward the ceiling. The pulley would be pulling the person up; it would lead with the upper body. The goal is for the legs and trunk to straighten out all at once. If one area (joint) is locked out before the other, the momentum is often killed and the rep may not be completed.

After your client has completed one rep, the descent is important because you want him or her to end in the proper starting position and be able to complete another rep. After the client is at the top and locked out, you want him or her to begin lowering the bar by first bending at the hips, as if bowing to an audience. Instruct the client to keep the chest up and to keep looking straight ahead. After the bar clears the knees, the client should bend the knees and allow the knees to move forward. Cue the client to maintain the arched position of the back the whole time. The client should lower the bar until it lightly touches the floor, reverse direction, and lift it up again. Instruct him or her to avoid rounding the back while setting the weight down. The client should not pause with the weight on the floor to reposition him- or herself unless necessary.

The client should avoid these techniques or movements:

- Rounding the lower or upper back
- Starting with the bar in front of the middle of the foot
- Dropping the hips too low
- Bending the arms
- Shrugging the weight at the top of the movement
- Leaning back excessively at the top of the movement
- Using a supinated or open grip
- Practicing the exercise with the bar resting on the ground (the bar should begin 8 inches [20.3 cm] off the ground because that is the radius of a 45-pound [20.4 kg] plate)

Improve Performance

Deadlift technique will not change too much from the basic form, but you can have clients do several things to boost performance. When people are first learning the lift, they tend to feel more comfortable with a slightly wider stance, but after clients have practiced the movement and gained the necessary flexibility, they should try to bring their feet in a little closer.

A good way for clients to find the proper foot position in the deadlift is to take one step and then perform a maximum vertical jump. One step means that each foot can move once, but they have to start the jump with both feet on the ground. Wherever your clients naturally put their feet when they jump is their natural power position, so it is a good starting point for their feet during the deadlift.

The easiest way for your clients to boost deadlift performance is to use an alternated grip, which involves one hand being supinated and the other pronated. It doesn't matter which one they chose to be up. They simply pick the most comfortable position and stick with it. Most often clients choose to place their nondominant hand up (supinated). Having an alternated grip will help them hold on to the bar. Amazingly, just reversing one hand can increase grip strength by 100 pounds (45.4 kg) or more (or 20 to 30 percent). The drawback of using an alternated grip is that it

can cause uneven development of the back muscles, particularly the erectors and traps. Clients should save the alternated grip for heavy training sets and use a regular pronated grip for all other sets. You could have your clients try alternating the hand that faces up to even out their muscular development, but don't do anything that will negatively affect the motor pattern of a proper deadlift. In addition, don't expect clients to be able to switch the supinated hand and deadlift the same amount without any practice. If they have a hard time holding on to the bar even with an alternated grip, use chalk, which is discussed in more detail later in the chapter (8).

Hip movement is important in a deadlift, especially as the weight gets heavier. At the start of the deadlift, the hips are in an anterior pelvic tilt position. But after the bar clears the knees and heads toward lockout, clients should drive their hips forward. At the completion of the ascent, the hips should not be in an anterior pelvic tilt position; rather, they should be in a neutral position right under the torso. The body should make a straight line, and clients should not have their butts sticking out at the top of the movement. The start and finish position of a conventional (standard) deadlift is seen in figure 21.1.

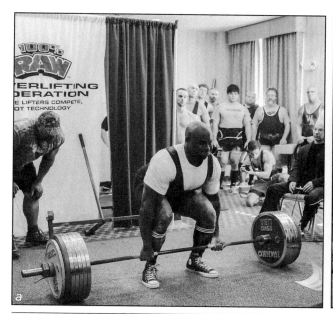 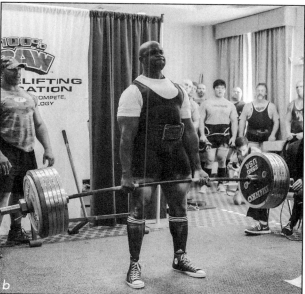

Figure 21.1   Conventional deadlift: *(a)* starting position; *(b)* ending position.

Increase the 1RM

The deadlift is likely the best test of total-body strength of the three powerlifting exercises. The technique to lift the most weight possible is similar to what was described in the previous section with a few modifications.

Try bringing the client's stance in even more and experiment with various foot angles. If your client's adductors are strong, try pointing the toes more. Also, bring the grip in tightly; the hands should be close to the legs.

As with any version of a deadlift, clients should try to start with and maintain an arched back, particularly the lower back, during the movement. A trick to do this is to have clients approach the bar and raise the arms above the head, arching the entire back as they do this. People can get a better arch with their arms over the head than held down at their sides. Attempting to keep that new arch involves bending slowly at the hips and reaching for the bar. After they grab the bar, they should reset the arch as much as possible.

In terms of grip, an alternated grip is again preferred. Some clients will choose to use a hook grip, which is similar to a closed grip except that the thumb goes under the first two fingers. This type of grip is common in Olympic weightlifting, but it also can be used for the deadlift exercise. A hook grip allows clients to keep both hands pronated, which provides more symmetrical stimulus and places less stress on the biceps. The disadvantage is that it takes a while to develop a tolerance for this grip because it is uncomfortable at first (17).

After lifting the bar off the floor, clients will want to drag the bar along their legs, particularly the thighs. Holding a heavy deadlift away from the legs is impossible anyway, so the bar will literally drag up the shins and thighs. This is normal and expected. The bar may even cut the shins slightly or leave red marks on the thighs. Using sports tape or wearing track pants can alleviate this problem.

Some advanced clients allow the upper back to round slightly during a deadlift. At no point should the lower back round, but a round upper back allows the hands to be held lower, which means that the bar doesn't have to be lifted as high. But if the upper back rounds too much, pulling a heavy weight back into position can be difficult, resulting in a failed lockout. When the upper back rounds, the lower back tends to follow, so use this method with caution.

Clients should attempt to look up during the exercise. Doing so will help prevent the upper back from rounding excessively, enhance the contraction of the back musculature, and help the client achieve the lockout position.

FLAWS IN DEADLIFT TECHNIQUE

Beginners make several common mistakes when performing the deadlift. Here are some of them explained in detail.

Rounding the Back

Your clients must keep the lower back slightly arched. Focus on that as you watch your clients from the side while they perform the deadlift with very light weight. Make sure that the lower back is not rounding. You can even have clients watch themselves in the mirror from the side when they are lifting light weights, but don't have them watch themselves from the side when they go heavy because they might strain their necks. Tell clients to memorize what it feels like to be in the proper position and stick with the light weight until they can do that naturally. A rounded back is shown in figure 21.2.

Bending the Arms

Some people try to pull the bar up with their arms as if they were performing a row. This method is not effective, and when clients get strong, they will not able to lift the same weight with the arms that they will be able to lift with the body. Have your clients keep their arms totally straight and relaxed. Tell them to think of the arms as hooks that are holding on to the weight and attaching it to the body. The only part of the arms that they need to focus on is the grip, which should hold tightly to the bar.

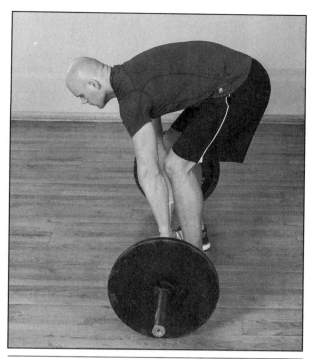

Figure 21.2 Example of a rounded back during the deadlift (a contraindicated position).

Starting Too Far From the Bar

When your clients get into position for the deadlift, make sure that they are standing close to the bar. Their shins should be touching or almost touching the bar. If they start with the bar far away, their first motion will be to pull or roll the bar back to them, which wastes energy. In addition, a bar position too far from the shins places undue stress on the lower back. Instruct clients to keep the bar close to them at all times.

Beginning With a Dip to Gain Momentum

Some people drop down, grab the bar, and get into position. When they are ready to go, they drop down another inch or two (about 2 to 5 cm), often bending their arms in the process, and then pull up hard as if they are trying to lift the bar off the floor as quickly as possible. The dip before the deadlift is not ideal for three reasons. First, preloading is an important factor in force development. Clients preload when they bend down, grab the bar, and pull on it slightly to get set. If they dip right before that,

they are eliminating the preloading, which has been shown to decrease force production, sometimes significantly. The second problem with this method is that they can really do this only on the first rep, because you do not want them to pause significantly after each rep. Generally, you want your clients' reps to look the same, each a mirror image of the others. A significant alteration of form on one rep is not desirable. A third reason that this method is not effective is that the dip and subsequent pull often seem to get people out of proper position, especially as the weight becomes heavy.

Using the Back Muscles Too Much

When people first learn how to do the deadlift, they are often pleasantly surprised at how much weight they can lift. Most people can lift more on the deadlift than they can on any other barbell exercise. As they begin to go heavier, they rely more on their back and less on their legs. This method is a mistake because the legs are strong and you want your clients to use them as much as they can. Many people begin the exercise in the proper position but straighten out their legs first to get the bar moving. Now they are significantly bent over, their legs are almost straight, and the weight is only three inches (7.6 cm) off the floor. To complete the rep, they have to use almost all back and hamstrings, as they would for a stiff-legged or romanian deadlift, which is harder than a conventional deadlift. Therefore, tell your clients that they need to be patient and not rush to lift heavy loads. In addition, tell them to be patient during the rep. If they let their form break during the rep just to get the weight going, then later during the range of motion when they need to lock out the weight, they may not be able to do so because they are not in the proper position.

MUSCLES INVOLVED IN THE DEADLIFT

The deadlift trains many muscles of the body, which is one reason that it is an effective and grueling exercise. The main movement is trunk extension, so the agonist in the deadlift is the erectors, which are focused in the lower back and run the length of the spine. Keep in mind that trunk extension is not necessarily the same thing as spine extension. In a deadlift we want to keep the spine extended during the whole lift; the muscles will contract primarily isometrically to do this. But to straighten out the trunk (the spine can be extended while bending forward), people must produce trunk extension, which is the main action in a deadlift. In addition, the hips are performing hip extension, so the glute maximus and hamstrings, all heads except the short head of the biceps femoris, are contributing significantly to this lift. The legs are performing knee extension as well, so the quads are working, but they are in a strong position with limited range of motion and don't get a huge stimulus. That said, if a person's quads are weak compared with other muscles, they will negatively contribute to the strength of the pull, particularly with the power off the floor (21).

Other muscles working in a deadlift are the quadratus lumborum, which almost always works as a synergist with the erectors. The traps are receiving a lot of stimulus during a deadlift because the weight wants to round the shoulders forward and people have to fight that movement by isometrically holding the shoulders back. The upper and middle traps get the most stimuli. But your clients do not need to perform a shrug during the deadlift; those two exercises are different. The simple act of deadlifting places enough stimuli on the traps to get them to respond. Finally, the forearm flexors receive a lot of stimulus. Ultimately, your clients will be able to use a lot of weight when they deadlift so their grip will get a good workout. Their forearms will respond by getting bigger and, more important, stronger, especially in isometric grip strength.

FAILURE DURING THE DEADLIFT

If your clients fail when performing a deadlift or if they are unable to complete the lift, you need to know where in the range of motion they failed. You want to identify their weakness so that they can focus on improving it.

Bar Liftoff From the Ground

If clients fail because they can't lift the bar off the ground or can lift it off the ground only a few inches, they have a weak start. They are not developing enough power at the beginning of the exercise. You can do several things to help them improve the start.

First, you can add deficit deadlifts to the client's program. This exercise involves performing a deadlift while standing on a platform or starting with the bar closer to the ground than normal. The proper starting bar height for a deadlift is 8 inches (20.3 cm) off the ground, which is the radius of a 45-pound (20.4 kg) weight plate. For a deficit deadlift, the bar is lower than 8 inches off the ground, but not so low that it negatively affects form. The most common recommendation is to adjust the height by 1 to 4 inches (2.5 to 10.2 cm). For a 1-inch (2.5 cm) adjustment, you can have the client stand on one or two extra rubber mats or use 35-pound (15.9 kg) weight plates instead of 45-pound weight plates. The smaller plates will put the bar lower to the ground, making the exercise harder and allowing the client to work on the weak point. For a more significant height change, you can have the client stand on an aerobic step. Steps fit nicely inside the weights on a barbell, and they are 4 inches (10.2 cm) high, enough to make the exercise significantly harder but not enough to alter technique. Don't put any risers (the plastic squares) under the step; just use the step itself. Another option is to use 25-pound (11.3 kg) plates on the deadlift, but doing this can be annoying if your client is lifting heavy loads (41). An example of a deficit deadlift is provided in figure 21.3. Make sure that the client doesn't round his or her back to achieve the additional range of motion required by this exercise.

Clients may use a stance that limits the power they can generate to lift the bar off the ground. If they are using a sumo deadlift, bring the stance in a few inches and see whether that

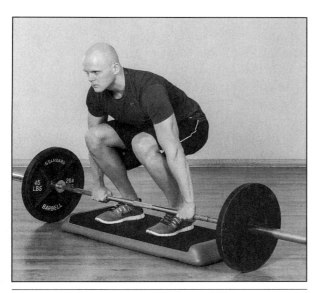

Figure 21.3 Deficit deadlift.

helps. If they are using a conventional deadlift, try widening or narrowing the stance. Try both positions and see which one feels better.

You can work on developing your clients' beginning power by having them squat and jump. When people jump, they need to produce power immediately, so practicing that will help your clients develop the speed necessary to get the weight moving. Olympic lifting is also a good method to develop speed and power.

The last thing to do to improve the bar liftoff from the ground is to tell your clients to get mad. The deadlift is not a complex activity. After your clients know how to do it, you want them to channel all their energy into lifting the weight. People have more energy when they are angry. Most people can't walk up to a heavy weight and crack a joke or have a big smile on their face and then lift it. Instruct them to focus and attack the weight. This approach will get their adrenaline flowing and improve the function of the entire body. They will be amazed at what a difference this attitude can make.

Lockout

Some people can lift the weight off the ground but then struggle to lock out the weight. If a client can get the weight above the knees but cannot finish it, then you need to work on his or her lockout ability. There are several ways to do this.

First, have your client perform deadlifts with two resistance bands that are anchored under a squat rack or power rack and looped over the bar. Position the bands just inside the sleeves on the bar but wider than where the client will grip the bar. As a side note, make sure that you have additional weight on the rack to which the bands are hooked or use a rack that is bolted to the floor. This is important because when the client lifts the bar, the rack may tip over if it is not sufficiently anchored. The bands will be slack in the beginning, but when the bar reaches the knees, tension develops and builds significantly during the lockout. The bands can add 100 to 200 pounds (45.4 to 90.7 kg) of resistance at the top of the deadlift. The bands match the strength curve of the deadlift because the lockout is the easiest and strongest part for the client. Make sure that the client fully locks out the weight with each rep and does not just lift the bar partially up and then back down. Many clients note that using bands combined with heavy weight is draining on the central nervous system, so use this technique for just one to three weeks and then take a break for a while (38).

Another exercise to help the lockout is the rack pull. Clients perform a regular deadlift with the bar at a higher than normal starting position. To do this, you need to use a squat rack. A good starting bar height for this exercise is somewhere between 11 and 14 inches (27.9 and 35.6 cm), which is 3 to 6 inches (7.6 to 15.2 cm) higher than usual (but it should still be below the knees). Rack pulls are easier than a regular deadlift, so your clients should be able to use more weight than usual. Do not overemphasize exercises to improve the lockout at the expense of training with the regular deadlift exercise because the client is likely to develop a different weak point.

A final problem with the lockout is grip strength. Clients who have a weak or slipping grip on something cannot apply the maximum pressure to it. As their grip slips, their back pulls with less force. If they are maxing out, they may not be able to lift the weight. Working on grip strength is a big factor.

To make sure that your clients have a strong grip during the deadlift, you can do several things. First, they should use an alternate grip on the heavy weight. This technique will make a huge difference. Second, they should use chalk when performing deadlifts of any significant weight, which is anything heavier than a warm-up. Chalk makes a huge difference because it increases friction and dries up any moisture on the hands. Third, they should rarely use straps. Fourth, they can use a bar slightly thicker than normal, which is a great way to fix any grip issues (31). The bar does not need to be super thick. Most bars are 28 millimeters. A 29- or 30-millimeter bar is enough of a difference to have a big effect. Have your clients perform all their regular deadlifting on the thicker bar. When they switch over to the regular bar, they will be amazed at how much easier it feels. Note that you do not have to use an actual thick bar in which the bar is as thick as the sleeve is. These are OK, but the weight used will be so limiting that undertraining the other muscles is likely.

Fifth, you can work your clients' forearms and grip to improve their grip strength. For the deadlift, your clients do not need a tremendous amount of crushing, concentric strength. Instead, they need the ability to keep their fingers closed, so you want to improve their isometric and eccentric strength. You can develop this through regular forearm work and by just having them practice holding on to something for as long as possible.

Finally, when your clients perform a deadlift, make sure that you always have them use a closed, not open, grip. Having clients lift with a closed grip is a good approach whenever they are lifting something that is hard to grip, as occurs during most back exercises. When clients are performing a deadlift, instruct them to keep their grip tight on all sets, even the warm-ups.

Back Position

The last significant reason why clients may fail when performing a deadlift is the tendency to allow the back to round over. This position is dangerous; avoiding it is so important that you should stop a client who rounds over the back even in the middle of a set. Although you do not spot the deadlift, you should tell a client to set the bar down if he or she is starting to round over the back during a deadlift. The client can readjust the form and try again, or just end the set.

People round their backs for a number of reasons, and here are some ways to prevent that. First, make sure that clients start in an arched back position. They should get the butt relatively low and keep the chest up. Clients should look as if they are a quarter to halfway down in a squat. Then, when they pull the weight up, have them pull first with the upper body; don't allow them to move their legs first. They should keep the chest high and the shoulders pulled back the whole time. If your clients do all this and still can't keep their shoulders from rounding, then the muscles holding the shoulders back are weak. They need to strengthen the middle traps (perform the shrug exercise but in a 30-degree forward-flexed position), rhomboids (add more back exercises), and, to a lesser extent, the rear delts (add more shoulder exercises). Just having the client perform deadlifts more often with a weight that they can lift with consistently perfect form will help. Remember that in almost every exercise in the gym, you want your clients to have their shoulders retracted, so over time this position should become strong (29).

EXERCISES THAT ASSIST THE DEADLIFT

Table 21.1 lists primary and secondary exercises that will help clients become stronger and more proficient at performing the deadlift. Of course, the best thing to do is to practice the deadlift exercise itself with good form. The conventional deadlift is the traditional, standard deadlift exercise, so obviously it is listed as the primary exercise to improve clients' overall ability to deadlift. For this version, clients position their hands outside their legs. Most people are strongest using this form. The conventional deadlift places the most emphasis on the lower back and then somewhat evenly distributes the load among the glutes, hams, traps, forearms, and quads. People who are taller and thinner

Table 21.1   Exercises and Their Relationship to the Deadlift

Primary assistance	Possible secondary assistance
Conventional deadlift	Glute–ham raise
Sumo deadlift	Hyperextension (weighted)
Squat	Leg curl
Good morning	Barbell bent-over row
Romanian deadlift	Bicep curl
Stiff-legged deadlift	Lower-back machine hyperextension
Deficit deadlift	Shrug (with a slight forward lean)
Rack pull	Farmer's walk
Deadlift with bands	Power clean
Snatch grip deadlift	Reverse hyperextension
	Leg press
	Grip-related exercises

with long arms and a stronger back tend to favor the conventional deadlift.

The deadlift has several variations, and each has a slightly different emphasis. For the sumo-style deadlift (or just sumo deadlift), clients position their hands inside their legs. The stance is very wide, approximately double shoulder-width apart. The rationale is that with a wide stance and a close grip, people have a shorter range of motion to lift the bar. Although that is true, the downside is that a wide stance can make it hard to generate much power at the bottom of the exercise. Sumo deadlifts place a lot of emphasis on the erectors and glutes and require the leg muscles to be more involved than they are in the conventional deadlift. The exercise also emphasizes the adductors, quads (particularly the inner part, the vastus medialis), traps, and forearm flexors. Clients who are shorter and stockier with stronger legs tend to favor the sumo deadlift (15, 16). The start and finish position of a sumo deadlift is shown in figure 21.4.

Another variation of the deadlift is the stiff-legged deadlift (sometimes called the straight-leg deadlift). The movement is similar to the conventional deadlift, but clients keep their legs straight through the exercise. Therefore, the movement is at the trunk, not the knee. The stiff-legged deadlift trains the erectors and the hamstrings, and some contribution comes from the glutes, traps, and forearm flexors. Your clients will use less weight on the stiff-legged deadlift than the conventional deadlift with the knees straight but not locked out. Clients who are flexible may need to stand on

a raised surface to get a full range of motion if the weight plates hit the ground on the way down before they feel a stretch.

When performing a stiff-legged deadlift, clients need to bend their knees on the first rep as if it were a conventional deadlift, pick up the weight but not count that rep, and start at the top. The stiff-legged deadlift is a good hamstring and lower-back exercise, but the drawback is that it puts more stress on the lower back. Tell clients that you are having them do this exercise as a way of focusing on specific muscles (hamstrings and erectors) but you do not want them to pick up something from the floor with this form; instead, they should use the conventional deadlift movement. The stiff-legged deadlift is shown in figure 21.5.

A third version of the deadlift is the romanian deadlift (RDL for short). This exercise is a hybrid between the stiff-legged deadlift and the conventional deadlift. In an RDL, your clients may bend their knees, but the knees should not push forward. An RDL looks a lot like the good morning exercise, but the weight is in the hands instead of on the back. A simple instruction for clients is to tell them to create as much distance between the chin and the butt as possible; this approach usually results in good RDL form. The RDL trains the hamstrings, erectors, glutes, traps, and forearms, much like the stiff-legged deadlift does. It is an easier version of the stiff-legged deadlift, but it is still harder than a conventional deadlift. It is a good variation because it is somewhat safer than the stiff-legged deadlift, and it is better

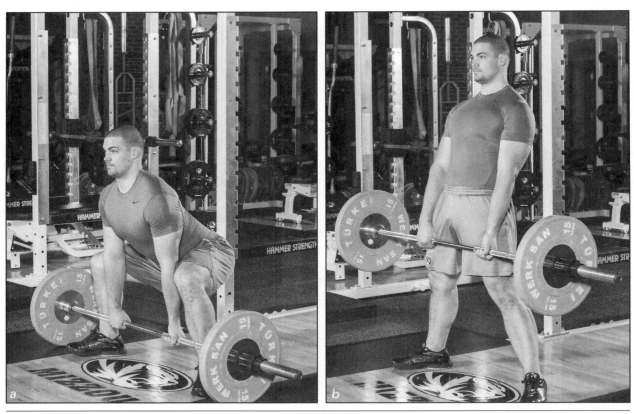

Figure 21.4 Sumo deadlift: *(a)* starting position and *(b)* ending position.

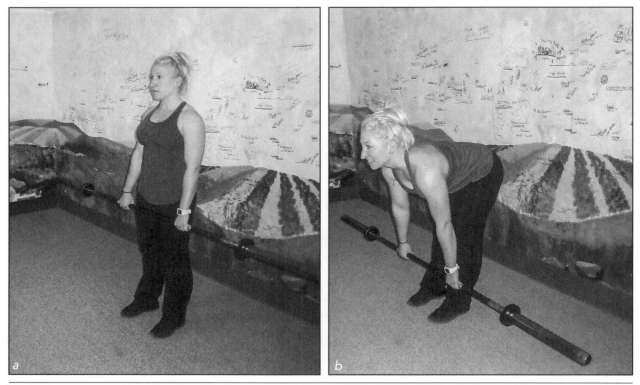

Figure 21.5 Stiff-legged deadlift: *(a)* starting position and *(b)* ending position.

for people who are not flexible. The ending position of the RDL is shown in figure 21.6 (the starting position is the same as shown in figure 21.5a). Note that the knees are bent compared with the stiff-legged deadlift shown in figure 21.5b.

EQUIPMENT AND APPAREL FOR THE DEADLIFT

Your clients do not need fancy equipment to deadlift well, but a couple things are useful. The two most common tools, aside from chalk, are deadlifting shoes and a belt.

Shoes

The first key piece of equipment is good deadlifting shoes. A good shoe for deadlifting has a thin sole, because the thicker the sole of the shoe is, the higher the person has to lift the weight. A half inch (about 1 cm) may not seem like much, but when someone is lifting very heavy weights, it can make a noticeable differ-

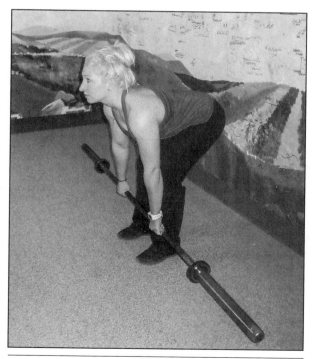

Figure 21.6 Romanian deadlift (RDL) ending position.

ence. The most common deadlifting shoe is a wrestling shoe. Wrestling shoes are available at almost any store that sells sport shoes. Some people deadlift in slippers or just their socks, but that does not give the foot much support and is more likely to slip. If your clients like the option of going barefoot but train in a gym, you might suggest the Vibram five-finger shoes, which can be a good compromise.

Weightlifting Belt

Clients may also choose to wear a weightlifting belt while performing deadlifts. The belt may increase intra-abdominal pressure, which creates a more stable trunk and allows greater transfer of power. The belt may also provide a measure of safety to the lower back and spine, and it can serve as a cue not to flex the lower back. Overreliance on the belt, however, may weaken the abdominal muscles over time. As with wearing a belt for the back squat exercise, your clients should wear a belt only on their heavy work sets (46).

BEGINNING DEADLIFT TRAINING PROGRAMS

The deadlift, like the other two key exercises, takes a while to master, but after your clients become skilled at it, they can often lift very heavy weights. Here are sample beginning workouts for a male and female of average strength who have never trained using the deadlift exercise.

For a Healthy Male

- Week 1: 45 lb (20.4 kg) × 12, 95 lb (43.1 kg) × 8, 95 lb (43.1 kg) × 8, 95 lb (43.1 kg) × 8
- Week 2: 45 lb (20.4 kg) × 12, 95 lb (43.1 kg) × 8, 95 lb (43.1 kg) × 8, 115 lb (52.2 kg) × 8
- Week 3: 45 lb (20.4 kg) × 12, 95 lb (43.1 kg) × 8, 115 lb (52.2 kg) × 8, 135 lb (61.2 kg) × 8
- Week 4: 95 lb (43.1 kg) × 8, 115 lb (52.2 kg) × 8, 135 lb (61.2 kg) × 8, 155 lb (70.3 kg) × 8

- Week 5: 95 lb (43.1 kg) × 8, 135 lb (61.2 kg) × 8, 150 lb (68.0 kg) × 8, 165 lb (74.8 kg) × 8

- Week 6: 95 lb (43.1 kg) × 8, 135 lb (61.2 kg) × 8, 155 lb (70.3 kg) × 8, 175 lb (79.4 kg) × 8

- Week 7: 95 lb (43.1 kg) × 8, 145 lb (65.8 kg) × 8, 165 lb (74.8 kg) × 8, 185 lb (83.9 kg) × 8

For a Healthy Female

- Week 1: 25 lb (11.3 kg) × 12, 45 lb (20.4 kg) × 8, 45 lb (20.4 kg) × 8, 45 lb (20.4 kg) × 8

- Week 2: 25 lb (11.3 kg) × 12, 45 lb (20.4 kg) × 8, 45 lb (20.4 kg) × 8, 55 lb (24.9 kg) × 8

- Week 3: 25 lb (11.3 kg) × 12, 45 lb (20.4 kg) × 8, 55 lb (24.9 kg) × 8, 65 lb (29.5 kg) × 8

- Week 4: 25 lb (11.3 kg) × 12, 55 lb (24.9 kg) × 8, 65 lb (29.5 kg) × 8, 75 lb (34.0 kg) × 8

- Week 5: 25 lb (11.3 kg) × 12, 55 lb (24.9 kg) × 8, 70 lb (31.8 kg) × 8, 80 lb (36.3 kg) × 8

- Week 6: 25 lb (11.3 kg) × 12, 55 lb (24.9 kg) × 8, 70 lb (31.8 kg) × 8, 85 lb (38.6 kg) × 8

- Week 7: 25 lb (11.3 kg) × 12, 55 lb (24.9 kg) × 8, 75 lb (34.0 kg) × 8, 90 lb (40.8 kg) × 8

CONCLUSION

The deadlift exercise involves approaching a loaded bar on the ground, squatting down, and standing up with the weight while keeping the arms straight. A personal trainer might modify a client's form based on a goal of increasing health, improving performance, or simply being able to deadlift the most weight possible. Several flaws can occur while deadlifting, including rounding over, bending the elbows, starting too far from the bar, trying to dip and jerk the bar, and not using the legs to help move the weight.

Four variations of the deadlift are widely used. A conventional deadlift is the standard deadlift; it involves placing the hands outside the legs and bending the knees. During a sumo deadlift, the client places the hands inside the legs and uses a very wide stance. This variation targets the legs and inner thighs more and the back less. A stiff-legged deadlift removes the assistance of the quads and places more emphasis on the hamstrings. It is more useful for flexible clients. A romanian deadlift also emphasizes the hamstrings, and it tends to be slightly safer than a stiff-legged deadlift. It is more useful for inflexible clients.

Many types of exercises can help improve the deadlift. Generally, the exercises that use a barbell and mimic the movements performed in a deadlift are the most useful. Some equipment is available to assist with the performance of a deadlift including chalk to help with grip, flat-soled shoes to reduce the range of motion of the barbell, and a belt to add support to the back. Personal trainers do not actively spot the deadlift, but they are attentive with cues and feedback to the client who is performing it.

The deadlift exercise can be rewarding for clients because of the loads being lifted, the muscles being trained, and the transference that occurs to other activities. It carries risk if proper form is not used. Personal trainers should ensure that clients take time to learn proper form before they begin to lift heavy weights.

Study Questions

1. What are the primary movements in a deadlift?
   a. trunk flexion, hip flexion, knee flexion
   b. trunk extension, hip flexion, knee flexion
   c. trunk extension, hip extension, knee flexion
   d. trunk extension, hip extension, knee extension

2. Which of the following synergistic muscles would be contracting primarily isometrically in a deadlift?

    a. quads

    b. hamstrings

    c. traps

    d. triceps

3. When contrasting a stiff-legged deadlift versus a conventional deadlift of equal weight, which of the following muscles works harder in the stiff-legged deadlift?

    a. quads

    b. hamstrings

    c. forearm extensors

    d. biceps brachii

4. If a client has trouble locking out the deadlift, which of the following choices would be least likely to improve that sticking point?

    a. rack deadlifts from 14 inches (36 cm) high

    b. deadlifts with weight and resistance bands

    c. deficit deadlifts

    d. romanian deadlifts

5. If a client wants to improve performance in a deadlift but can no longer grip the bar with a pronated grip, what grip can the personal trainer suggest to improve the client's grip strength during a deadlift?

    a. alternated grip

    b. open grip

    c. closed grip

    d. supinated grip

Aerobic Training Program Design

Cardiovascular endurance—the ability of the heart, blood, blood vessels, and lungs to work together to provide oxygen to the body—is one of the five components of fitness. Personal trainers must understand how these four structures function to be able to develop an effective cardiovascular endurance training program.

Cardiovascular exercise is any rhythmic, continuous motion that involves large-muscle groups and is performed without stopping for five or more minutes. For a simple illustration, just think of any exercise that raises and maintains the heart rate for an extended period. True cardiovascular exercise, often shortened to "cardio," does not involve any stops until the person is finished, whereas aerobic exercise, as it is typically practiced, can include short rest periods.

HEART

The heart is a complex organ. It is a muscle composed of cardiac muscle cells that are not under voluntary control. The heart is divided into four chambers. The top two chambers are called the right and left atriums; they receive blood from the body. You can remember that term because an atrium in a building has high ceilings, and it may serve as a lobby or entrance hall where you would meet or receive someone. Your heart receives the blood in the atrium. The bottom two chambers are called the right and left ventricles. The word *ventral* normally refers to something that is lower in the body. These chambers hold the blood and then send it back out into the body.

The heart works by pumping blood through blood vessels. The two major types of blood vessels are arteries and veins. Arteries always carry blood away from the heart, and that blood is usually highly oxygenated. You can remember this by thinking of AAA, which stands for arteries always away. Veins always carry blood back to the heart, and that blood is usually low in oxygen. Blood that has a lot of oxygen will be bright red, whereas blood that is low in oxygen is more bluish. Veins tend to be closer to the surface and more visible than arteries, and because they are carrying oxygen-depleted blood, they look blue under the skin. When you bleed, your blood looks red because the oxygen in the air turns it red.

Figure 22.1 is a diagram that outlines the flow of blood in the body. The chart is purposefully simplistic to help you understand how blood flows throughout the body; it is not designed to be anatomically correct. After you understand this diagram, we can move on to something that more closely resembles a real heart, as opposed to a floor plan.

Let's use an example to illustrate the course of blood through the body. In the following example, the client is performing a bicep curl. A drop of blood starts in the biceps during the curl and travels from there.

- In the biceps, the blood drops off the "good" stuff, nutrients and oxygen (O_2), and picks up the "bad" stuff, waste products and carbon dioxide (CO_2).
- The blood then enters a vein and begins its journey back to the heart.
- The blood is low on O_2 as it enters the right atrium (RA). The RA receives blood from the body.

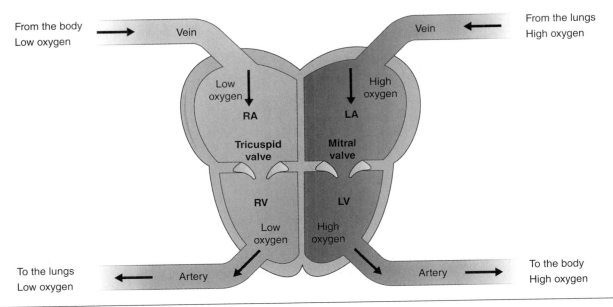

Figure 22.1 Blood flow through the heart and body.

- The blood then moves down from the RA into the right ventricle, passing through the tricuspid valve.
- The right ventricle (RV) pumps and sends the blood out to the lungs. The purpose of this trip is to pick up O_2.
- The blood, still low in O_2, travels through an artery to the lungs.
- In the lungs, gas exchange occurs. O_2 is picked up, and CO_2 is dropped off.
- The blood leaves the lungs through veins and returns back to the heart with a high amount of O_2.
- The blood enters the heart in the left atrium (LA).
- The blood moves down into the left ventricle (LV), passing through the bicuspid, or mitral, valve.
- The LV pumps and sends the blood out to the body. The purpose of this trip is to supply the muscles and organs with oxygen.
- The blood travels through arteries to reach its destination, in this case the biceps.
- In the biceps, the blood again drops off the good stuff and picks up the bad stuff. The cycle continues.

- The blood normally makes a full circuit through the body once every minute or so at rest.

Now that you have the general pattern of blood flow, we can examine the structure of the heart. Your heart is about the size of your fist—or a little larger, especially if you are well trained—and it is mostly hollow, because it functions as a container that holds blood. Figure 22.2 provides a picture of an anatomically correct heart.

When looking at figure 22.2, note a couple of things. First, two veins lead into the RA. The top one drains the upper body; the bottom one drains the lower body. The artery that goes from the RV to the lungs heads upward first. That makes sense because if you have to pump something, you want to perform the hard part (making blood go uphill) first. Then that artery, the pulmonary artery, branches off to the right and left lungs. In this instance, the blood in an artery is low on oxygen.

From the lungs, the blood goes back to the heart through the pulmonary veins, one from each lung. In this instance, the blood in a vein has a high amount of oxygen. It enters the LA and then goes to the LV. The LV is the biggest and strongest part of the heart because it has to send blood out the farthest. The lungs are only a short distance away, but the

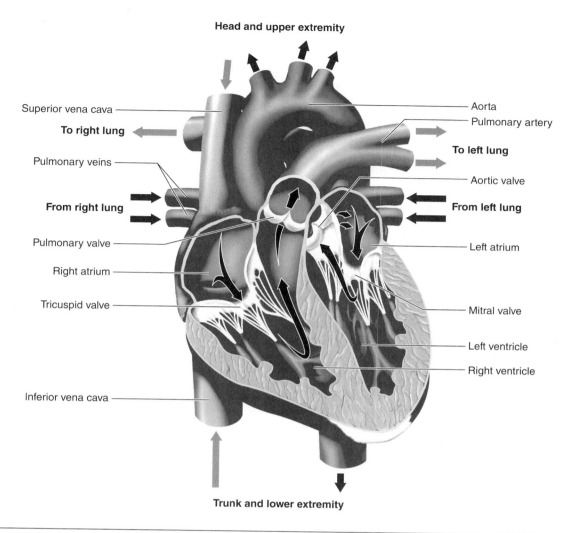

Figure 22.2 Structure of the human heart.

journey up to the head or down to the feet is tougher.

The artery leading out of the LV is called the aorta; it is a big tube that heads upward first. It then loops around the top of the heart and heads downward. At the top of the loop, three main arteries branch off it. These three arteries supply the right arm, the head, and the left arm, respectively. As the aorta heads downward, it supplies the lower body with blood. The tubes leading into the heart from the body (the inferior and superior vena cava) and the tube heading out from the heart (the aorta) are large, about the size of a garden hose. You could easily fit your finger inside one of those tubes, and they can carry a lot of blood.

A discussion of the heart usually includes information about what happens during a heart attack (a myocardial infarction). The purpose of this summary is not to make you an expert on heart attacks, but to provide a general description. The heart is both a big container that holds blood and a muscle that needs blood itself for oxygen and nutrients. The heart is unable to use the blood that is inside it, so it must pump its own blood. Imagine water in a water bottle. If your goal is to get the outside of the water bottle wet, you need to get the water out of the bottle (say by squeezing it). It is ironic that in a heart attack all this good blood is sitting in the heart but the heart cannot use any of it.

The coronary artery is a special artery that carries blood to the heart. Because this artery is relatively small, about the size of a straw, it can become blocked or restricted. When this happens, blood flow to the heart decreases. That reduction weakens the heart and impairs the pumping action, so less blood is supplied to the body. The body needs more blood, the already weakened heart works harder, and a vicious cycle is created. After a while, the heart stops beating altogether, which is a heart attack. For that reason, CPR can be effective. The heart still has some good blood (assuming that it can get oxygen), so artificially pumping the blood for a heart that has stopped will make the system work.

The coronary artery divides into several smaller arteries. If these become blocked, another route needs to be created. This procedure is called a bypass, and the number of arteries treated is usually included in the description. Thus, a double bypass means that two arteries were rerouted, a quadruple bypass means that four were rerouted, and so on. Bypass surgery is performed to prevent a heart attack or to repair the heart after a cardiac incident. Heart disease is the number one killer of North Americans; more than 33 percent of Americans will die from heart disease. Often, the first sign of heart disease is a heart attack. Luckily, regular exercise and weight management help control the risk of heart disease.

Here are some important terms to understand in our discussion of the heart.

Pulse

Pulse, or heart rate (HR), is the number of heartbeats per minute (bpm). An average pulse is 60 to 80 beats per minute. Resting pulse drops as fitness increases. A person's resting pulse may drop as much as 10 beats per minute after he or she works out for six months. Elite aerobic endurance athletes often have a pulse below 60 beats per minute, and it can be 50 beats per minute or even lower. A slow heart rate is good because it indicates that at rest the body is hardly working. Maximal heart rate (MHR) changes little as fitness increases. In fact, if it does anything it tends to decrease a little bit (5 to 10 beats per minute). Keep in mind that the formula *MHR = 220 minus age* is an estimate that can be significantly off the

mark. The standard deviation for that formula is at least plus or minus 10 beats in either direction.

Stroke Volume (SV)

The amount of blood pumped out by the heart in one beat is called stroke volume (SV). An average SV is between 60 to 70 milliliters per beat at rest. As fitness increases, the SV at rest increases. When a person is in better shape, the heart is able to eject more blood with each pump, indicating that it is operating more efficiently. Stroke volume commonly increases 15 to 30 milliliters per beat as an adaptation to exercise, and it can increase even more in advanced aerobic endurance athletes. Maximal SV also increases as fitness increases. During exercise, the heart is able to pump out more blood with each beat, providing more blood to the body. Maximal SV is about 120 milliliters per beat in untrained people, and it can go up 15 to 30 milliliters per beat in trained subjects and even more in advanced aerobic endurance athletes.

Cardiac Output

The amount of blood pumped out by the heart in one minute is referred to as cardiac output (abbreviated as the letter Q). The average cardiac output while resting is about 4.5 liters per minute (196). If you think about it, you already know the formula for this. You need to know two bits of information—how often the heart is beating and how much blood is pumped out in each beat. So, the formula is

$$Pulse \times SV = Q$$

As fitness increases, cardiac output at rest stays about the same. Remember that cardiac output is a factor of HR and SV. Because resting HR decreases and SV increases as an adaption to training, the two essentially cancel each other out. What cardiac output is really describing is how much blood the body needs. At rest the body needs about the same amount of blood whether the person is fit or not (assuming that the person weighs the same). Stroke volume goes up because the heart is working more efficiently, and pulse then goes down because it doesn't need to be as fast to supply the same amount of blood to the body.

Maximal cardiac output is a different story. Maximal cardiac output is how much blood a person can pump in one minute at the highest intensity. This quantity increases significantly with training, often by three to four liters after several months of training. Again, this result should make sense. Maximal pulse is basically unchanged, but maximal stroke volume increases significantly. Because Q = SV × pulse, if one greatly increases and the other stays the same, Q will increase. Elite athletes can often pump more than 30 liters of blood in a single minute. Imagine trying to drink 15 2-liter bottles of soda in one minute.

Heart Volume

The size of the heart is its volume; because it is three dimensional, as its size increases so does its volume. Remember that the heart is a muscle, so its size can change. Heart volume varies significantly. A big factor is simply size; the bigger a person is, the bigger the heart is. Training can alter the size of the heart. It is a muscle, and muscles can grow. Average heart volume is about three-quarters of a liter for most adults, and training can increase that by 10 percent in several months. The heart volume of elite athletes can be more than one liter. The way that the heart responds to exercise is still being studied, but it is generally believed that this increase in heart size is beneficial to both health and performance.

Blood Pressure

The pressure that the blood exerts against the arterial walls is blood pressure (BP). Blood is like water in a hose; it is trying to get out of the hose but normally cannot break through the wall of the hose. If the pressure becomes too great for a hose and a leak occurs, you know about it because you see water shooting out. Blood in arteries and veins behaves in the same way. It is trying to get out, but as long as the blood pressure does not go too high, it cannot escape. Generally, the lower the blood pressure is, the better a person's health is, although

extremely low pressure can lead to problems such as fainting or blacking out.

Blood pressure has two components—systolic and diastolic. Systolic blood pressure is the pressure against the vessel walls when the heart is beating. It will always be higher than the other component, diastolic blood pressure. Diastolic blood pressure is the pressure against the vessel walls when the heart is relaxed, when it is between beats. You can remember the two components by thinking that *systolic* sounds like *system*. When the system is operating, the heart is beating, so that is the systolic blood pressure. But if the heart stays relaxed, what happens? The person dies. So *dia*stolic pressure occurs when the heart is not beating. Normal blood pressure is 120/80 mm Hg.

When a person exercises regularly, the heart, lungs, and corresponding vessels operate more efficiently. The arteries and veins become more elastic. With regular training, aerobic exercise causes a decrease in blood pressure. This is thought to occur because of the effect of the exercise itself and because an increase in aerobic exercise usually results in weight loss, which also helps lower blood pressure. As a person is exercising, blood pressure is elevated over resting levels, but regular exercise generally lowers resting blood pressure over time. Sometimes, a person with borderline or mild hypertension (diastolic blood pressure below 105 mm Hg) can lower blood pressure with just exercise. Suggest to your clients that they speak with their doctors for specific information about blood pressure, exercise, and medication.

Arteriovenous Oxygen Difference

This value, the difference between the amount of oxygen in the arteries and in the veins, is normally abbreviated *a-vO$_2$ difference*. Remember that arteries generally carry highly oxygenated blood and veins do not. As an artery feeds blood to a muscle, the muscle uses up the oxygen, and the blood returns to the vein without much oxygen. The more efficient the muscles are, the more oxygen they use up. Having a lot of oxygen in the veins is of little benefit because it is essentially wasted. The goal is to have a large a-vO$_2$ difference (23).

For example, let's say that 10 pKa (a unit of measure in chemistry) of oxygen were in your arteries and 4 pKa of oxygen were in your veins. You would have an a-vO$_2$ difference of 6 pKa. Someone else who had 10 pKa of oxygen in the arteries and 2 pKa of oxygen in the veins would have an a-vO$_2$ difference of 8 pKa. The 8 is better than the 6 because it indicates that the other person was using more oxygen than you were; his or her system was more efficient.

As you exercise, you teach your body to use oxygen more effectively. This in turn yields a lower a-vO$_2$ difference. Generally, the body has plenty of oxygen at rest, but an increase in the a-vO$_2$ difference is evident during exercise.

See table 22.1 for a summary of how the key cardiovascular components adapt to the long-term effect of regular aerobic exercise training.

BLOOD

Blood volume is the amount of blood in the body. Normal blood volume in the adult human body is between four and five liters. As fitness increases, the body literally makes more blood. The body can add about a half liter after several months of training, and fit people have a blood volume of five to six liters. The function of blood in the body is to deliver nutrients to the body and remove waste products. More blood means that more nutrients can be delivered. Think of how you feel after you donate blood and reduce your blood volume; having additional blood has the opposite effect.

The major cells in blood are red blood cells. They help bind with and carry oxygen and deliver it to the muscles and organs. As fitness increases, the body produces more red blood cells. The greater number of red blood cells increases the amount of oxygen that the blood can carry, which increases endurance. Anemia results from a low red blood cell count, possibly from a lack of iron in the diet. Anemia causes people to feel tired, weak, and exhausted, even if they aren't doing anything active.

BLOOD VESSELS

Capillaries are little baby arteries and veins. Think of a tree with its roots branching off into the ground. As the roots go deeper into the ground, they become smaller and thinner, finally branching into tiny roots that absorb water and nutrients. Capillaries are the ends of arteries and veins, where the blood is being dropped off and picked up. People have the ability to grow new capillaries, just as the tree can grow new roots. As fitness increases, the body grows new capillaries, allowing better blood delivery and an increased supply of oxygen to the body (171, 191, 210).

LUNGS

The lungs play a crucial role in the cardiovascular system by oxygenating the blood. The lungs also respond to exercise. Most people take 12 to

Table 22.1 Key Cardiovascular Components and How They Change Because of Regular Aerobic Exercise

	Before training		After training	
	At rest	Maximal	At rest	Maximal
Pulse	60–80 bpm	~180–200 bpm	Decreases	Stays the same
Stroke volume	60–70 ml/beat	~110–120 ml/beat	Increases	Increases
Cardiac output	~4.5 L/min	~20 L/min	Stays the same	Increases
Blood pressure	120/80 mm Hg	Increases	Decreases slightly	Stays the same
a-vO$_2$ difference	~6.0 ml	Increases	Increases slightly	Increases

15 breaths per minute at rest, but that number can decrease as fitness increases. In addition, as fitness improves, the maximal breathing rate, the breathing rate during intense exercise, can increase. Simply put, a person who gets in better shape learns to breathe faster and more regularly, thus providing the body with more oxygen.

Besides changing their breathing rate change, people can improve their ability to deliver oxygen to the blood. The pulmonary ventilation rate increases significantly during exercise (meaning that they can consume more oxygen per minute) as their fitness increases. When they can consume more oxygen, their $\dot{V}O_2$max goes up.

ADDITIONAL ADAPTATIONS

In addition to changes that occur in the heart, blood, blood vessels, and lungs, adaptations take place at the microscopic level to a client's muscle fibers and to overall body weight. See table 22.2 for a summary of the changes.

Cellular

When regular aerobic exercise is performed, the cells in the body undergo physiological changes. As you can probably guess, these changes correspond with the body's ability to use oxygen. One of the major changes is in the mitochondria within a cell. Mitochondria are an organelle. An organelle is a structure inside a cell that is visible only under a microscope. As you know, the body is a single entity containing a bunch of organs, each performing its own important task. Organs are made of up tissues, and tissues are made up of similar cells. Each cell can act as a single entity with a bunch of organelles (little tiny organs) inside of it that perform important tasks. Mitochondria are one of those organelles (191).

The function of mitochondria is to help provide energy to the cell. They are thought of as the powerhouse of the cell. In addition, the mitochondria have the ability to use oxygen to produce energy. After people perform aerobic training, the mitochondria grow in both size and number. People who have trained aerobically have more and larger powerhouses, so they can produce more energy. With more energy, they can go for longer without getting tired.

Muscle Fibers

The majority of aerobic training targets the slow-twitch Type I muscle fibers. These fibers are weak but have good endurance. Unless a person is performing a lot of sprinting or burst-of-energy activities, the Type II muscle fibers are not being trained. Type I muscle fibers generally do not get large when trained and may even shrink in response to training. Do not mistake a defined muscle for a large one. Marathon runners and the like are often highly defined because of their low body fat, but their muscles aren't big. In fact, their muscles are often smaller than those of untrained people.

Table 22.2 Additional Cardiovascular Components and How They Change Because of Regular Aerobic Exercise

	Before training		After training		
	At rest	**Maximal**	**At rest**		**Maximal**
Breathing rate	12–15 min	Increases	Decreases		Increases
Pulmonary ventilation	~7 L/min	Increases	Decreases slightly		Increases
Blood volume	~4.5 L	–	Increases		–
Heart volume	~750 ml	–	Increases		–
Capillaries	~250–300	–	Increases		–
% Type I fibers	~50–55%	–	Stays the same or increases		–

Genetics determines a person's starting point for the percentage of slow- and fast-twitch muscle fibers in each muscle. Most people have about 50 percent slow-twitch fibers and 50 percent fast-twitch fibers in most muscles. Whether training can alter those numbers is unclear, although recent studies are indicating that training can change the percentage long term. Short-term training does not seem to have a powerful effect on that ratio. In some studies, elite aerobic endurance athletes have an extremely high percentage of slow-twitch muscle fibers, often around 80 percent. That number is too high to be explained by genetic selection, so over a long period the muscle fibers may begin to change. But that hypothesis has not been clearly proved in the lab.

Body Weight

Most people know that regular aerobic exercise contributes to weight loss. Aerobic exercise is a good way to burn calories and create the caloric deficit necessary to lose weight.

Remember that body weight is an important component in a person's $\dot{V}O_2max$. The heavier a person is, the harder it is to have a high $\dot{V}O_2max$. Conversely, the lighter a person is, the easier it is to have a high $\dot{V}O_2max$. The heart and lungs do grow as a person grows, but those organs will not be able to maintain an increase in size that corresponds with a person's overall weight gain. A 300-pound (136.1 kg) person, even if muscular, will not have a heart and lungs in exact proportion as a fit 150-pound (68.0 kg) person. Elite aerobic endurance athletes are almost always small; their engines are large in proportion to their bodies. Most elite aerobic endurance male athletes weigh less than 150 pounds (68.0 kg), and many are closer to 135 pounds (61.2 kg). A small body coupled with a large heart and lungs is a potential powerhouse for endurance.

Besides being a good way to lose body weight, cardio is a good way to lose body fat. Generally, people who perform a lot of aerobic training have less body fat than those who do not. Elite male aerobic endurance athletes often have body-fat levels in the single digits (5

to 8 percent), whereas the average for a male is 15 percent or slightly higher (154).

Exercise, particularly moderate exercise, helps regulate the appetite, which in turns helps control cravings and leads to better weight management. Intense exercise can sometimes leave a person feeling very hungry, so this effect varies from person to person.

Cardiovascular exercise causes many beneficial adaptations in the body, for both health and physical performance:

- Decreased heart rate at rest
- Increased $\dot{V}O_2max$
- Increased stroke volume at rest and maximally
- Increased cardiac output maximally
- Increased lung capacity
- Increased arteriovenous difference
- Increased mitochondria in the cells
- Increased blood volume
- Increased number of capillaries
- Increased number of red blood cells
- Increased number of aerobic enzymes
- Increased number of myoglobin
- Increased ability to recover between sets or after exercise
- Decreased body weight
- Decreased body fat

AEROBIC TRAINING ZONES

Most of your clients know that they should train aerobically on a regular basis, but they may not follow that guideline. The goals for this chapter are to illustrate different ways to use cardiovascular exercise, provide a variety of aerobic training programs from beginner through more advanced, and demonstrate ways to keep it entertaining without sacrificing effectiveness. If your clients are aerobic endurance athletes, they will need specialized programs to train for their specific goals. If your clients primarily want to lose weight, they will require a different sort of aerobic program to reach that goal.

Cardiovascular endurance is powered primarily by the oxidative energy system. The oxidative system is the main power source behind any activity that lasts five or more minutes. Everyone reading this book is in the oxidative system right now, unless he or she is reading and sprinting at the same time. The oxidative system (described in detail in chapter 8) uses oxygen, hence the name, and the fuel sources of fatty acids, from fat, and glucose, from glycogen and protein. At lower-intensity cardio, as measured by heart rate, a greater percentage of fat is burned; at higher-intensity cardio, a greater percentage of glucose is burned.

When personal trainers suggest that their clients perform cardio, they often talk about performing that aerobic exercise in one of two zones. One zone is called the fat-burning zone, which is traditionally defined as aerobic exercise at an intensity of 60 to 70 percent of MHR (for a longer duration). The second zone is the cardiovascular training zone (also called the cardio training zone), which is traditionally defined as aerobic exercise at an intensity of 70 to 85 percent of MHR (for a shorter duration). Over the years, much discussion has occurred about which zone is the best to train in and why one is better than the other. Each zone has benefits and drawbacks (198).

Fat-Burning Zone

This zone is typically thought of as low-intensity cardio. Keeping the heart rate at 70 percent or less means that the workload is not too difficult. People can normally maintain this pace for a longer time—at least 30 minutes and often for 1 to 2 hours. Most authorities agree that this is a good zone for beginners to train in. It is intense enough to create a positive response in the body and hard enough to burn a decent number of calories. At the same time, it is easy enough that most people can complete the exercise without exhausting themselves. In addition, talking, socializing, or watching TV is possible at this intensity, and the time goes by relatively quickly. The talk test is useful here—if clients can talk comfortably while

exercising, their heart rate is probably below 70 percent of MHR and they pass the talk test. When performing cardio in the fat-burning zone, people should do it for a relatively long time—20 minutes at a minimum, up to 60 minutes for most people, and even more for aerobic endurance athletes. Untrained beginners might start with less; they should follow the beginner cardio program outlined in this book. Because of the length of time necessary to be effective and because this type of cardio is relatively easy to program and follow, clients do not usually perform low-intensity cardio with their personal trainers.

The fat-burning zone gets its name because exercise in this zone burns a higher *percentage* of fat. When a person is sitting around at home, watching TV, or relaxing, the body is considered to be at a state of rest. Most people burn approximately 1 to 1.5 calories per minute in this state, depending primarily on how much they weigh. At rest, people burn approximately 70 percent of their calories from fat and 30 percent of their calories from glucose. You may be surprised to learn that when you are sitting around, or even sleeping, you are in the best fat-burning zone; the downside is that you are burning so few calories that it doesn't matter where the energy is coming from.

We all know that to lose weight a person needs to increase the number of calories burned per minute, and that is accomplished by exercise. The intensity and type of exercise determine how many calories a person burns per minute, but when exercising at moderate intensity most people burn 4 to 20 calories per minute, with the vast majority expending 5 to 15 calories per minute. Let's say that a client gets on the treadmill and starts walking at 4 miles per hour (6.4 km/h) with no incline (about 5 METs). If the client is in reasonable shape, that should not raise the heart rate above 70 percent of MHR, so the person would be in the fat-burning zone. Let's say that a particular exercise burns 5 calories per minute. If the client performs that activity for one hour, he or she would burn 300 calories. Although the proportion varies depending on the person and the activity, exercising in the fat-burning zone uses approximately 60 percent fat and

40 percent glucose. Therefore, the amount of energy burned looks like this:

Total fat calories burned (60 percent) = 180 calories of fat

Total glucose calories burned (40 percent) = 120 calories from glucose

Total calories burned = 300 calories

Cardio Training Zone

This training zone gets its name because training at this intensity provides the most benefit to the heart and lungs. If your client's goal is to improve $\dot{V}O_2$max, he or she should train in this zone. People can improve their $\dot{V}O_2$max in the fat-burning zone, but not as rapidly. This zone involves exercising at higher intensity. The main benefit of exercising above 70 percent of MHR (other than $\dot{V}O_2$max improvement) is that the activity burns many more calories per minute. As the level of intensity increases, people burn more glucose to fuel that intense exercise; remember that carbohydrate is a high-intensity fuel source. The percentage of fat burned decreases progressively, and the percentage of glucose burned increases progressively. But the amount of fat that people burn doesn't go down; in fact, it tends to go up.

Imagine that the person from the previous example who was walking at 4 miles per hour (6.4 km/h) decides to run at 7 miles per hour (11.3 km/h). That person will now burn about 10 calories a minute (about 10 METs). To make everything equal, assume that the activity is performed for an hour. Again, without knowing a number of specific variables, a personal trainer cannot know exactly what percentages a client is burning, but a reasonable estimate is that the percentages have flipped. The client is now burning 40 percent fat and 60 percent glucose. To run the numbers now, the amount of fuel burned looks like this:

Total fat calories burned (40 percent) = 240 calories of fat

Total glucose calories burned (60 percent) = 360 calories from glucose

Total calories burned = 600 calories

If we compare the 240 calories of fat burned in this example to the 180 calories of fat burned in the previous example, we can see that this person burned more total fat by exercising in the cardiovascular training zone (see figure 22.3). Generally, the harder a person performs cardio, the more total fat he or she will burn. Although the percentage of fat goes down, it is a percentage of a much larger pie. If you were offered 40 percent of $600 or 60 percent of $300, which would you take?

Advantages and Disadvantages of the Aerobic Training Zones

Does the higher number of fat calories burned in the cardio training zone mean that everybody should always use that training zone? Not necessarily, although certainly more people should use it than should use the fat-burning zone. A client who is an aerobic endurance athlete such as a runner, cyclist, rower, swimmer, or triathlete client should be spending most of his or her training time in this zone. A client who is mostly concerned with total weight (fat) loss should spend most of his or her time in this zone. How many high-level aerobic endurance athletes do you see who are not lean? If you want to improve your client's $\dot{V}O_2$max and overall aerobic fitness, this is their zone (91).

The fat-burning zone offers two major benefits. First, performing in this zone is relatively easy. For some people, the idea of performing cardio is so intimidating that they just skip it all together. From a fitness point of view, performing 30 minutes of easy cardio is much better than doing nothing at all. The second benefit of the fat-burning zone is that it burns very little muscle. One of the problems of the cardio training zone is that when a person runs low on glucose, which could be a result of insufficient carbohydrate as part of the pre-workout meal or low glycogen stores because of being on a diet, the body will start using muscle to gets its glucose from amino acids. For people interested in preserving their muscle mass—bodybuilders, powerlifters, weightlifters, and so forth—burning muscle can be a nasty side effect of intense cardio. This effect

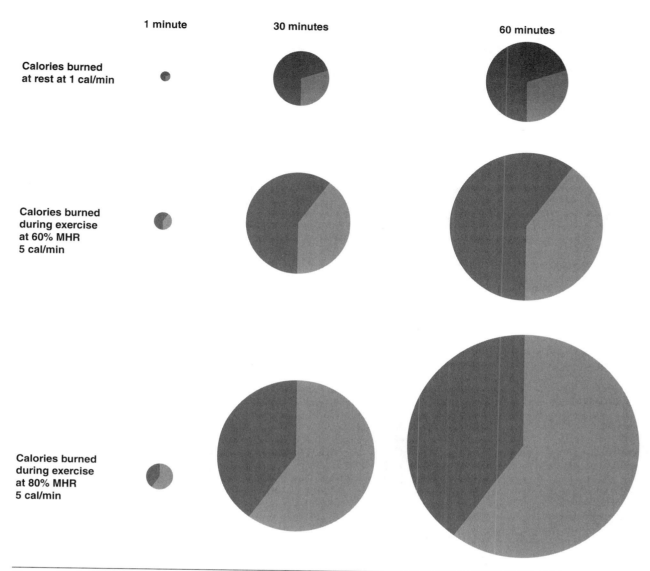

Figure 22.3   Percentage of fat and carbohydrate calories burned at rest and during exercise.

is further exacerbated if the client is already on a diet. The more muscle a person has, the more likely the person is to use that muscle as fuel. Intense cardio becomes a lot less desirable. The solution is to perform cardio in the fat-burning zone, but it has to be performed for a long time, 30 to 60 minutes or longer, to be effective.

Some clients like to perform their fat-burning cardio early in the morning before they eat anything. At that time, glycogen stores are low, so performing an intense workout is difficult. Exercising after a fasting period is not recommended for a cardio training zone

workout, but it is an ideal time to perform a fat-burning zone workout, especially if the goal is to lose body fat. Lifting weights and then performing cardio can provide a similar effect. The weightlifting will burn off some glycogen, thus priming the body to burn a bit more fat during the cardio session. But if this order is reversed and the body is low on glycogen from the cardio, the client will either perform poorly or the body will turn to amino acids (protein from muscles) to get its energy for weightlifting.

To summarize, here are the forms of cardio and the type of client best suited to each.

Cardio Training Zone

- Aerobic endurance athletes
- People who participate in events in which $\dot{V}O_2max$ is important to success
- People who are interested in improving aerobic performance

Fat-Burning Zone

- Bodybuilders
- Powerlifters
- Weightlifters
- People who are concerned about sacrificing muscle mass
- People who are already very lean
- Untrained beginners
- Seniors
- People on a strict, low-calorie diet who also lift weights
- People who perform cardio in the morning on an empty stomach

Either Zone

- People who are interested in improving overall health and fitness
- People who are interested in losing the most total body weight
- People who are interested in losing the most total body fat

Although the heart rate percentages are distinct for each zone, remember that the heart rate formulas themselves rely on estimations of the client's true MHR. Clients may have a MHR above or below what a formula predicts. Here is an easy way to assess a client's training zone. If the client can perform the cardio activity for 45 minutes or longer, is confident that he or she will not fail or have to stop during the exercise, and can carry on a conversation with you while exercising, then the client is most likely in the fat-burning zone. If the client struggles to perform the exercise for 30 minutes and cannot easily converse, the client is in the cardio training zone.

A caution here is that cardio machines are not always accurate in calculating how many calories a client is burning. When you enter the client's weight, the accuracy increases, but generally the machines overestimate how many calories are burned. The machines are consistent, so if a client burned 300 calories on a treadmill one day and 450 calories the next day, you know that the client burned more calories on the second day, even if it may not have been exactly 450.

If a machine requires the user's weight to be entered but you do not want to ask the client what he or she weighs or the client does not want other gym members to see what he or she weighs, you can just enter 111 as way to bypass that screen. Of course, the data will not be accurate if the client does not weigh 111 pounds (50.3 kg), but it can be a quick way to skip a potentially uncomfortable situation.

FACTORS THAT AFFECT CARDIOVASCULAR PERFORMANCE

Nine factors affect a client's cardiovascular performance. If a client has any interest in performing well in any type of aerobic endurance event, you need to be aware of these factors so that you can help the person improve his or her performance. In addition, an athlete can try to determine where he or she stands in relation to competitors on these factors. If the client is weak on one of them, you can help him or her improve in that area.

$\dot{V}O_2max$

The first factor, $\dot{V}O_2max$, is generally considered the most important. Remember, $\dot{V}O_2max$ refers to the ability of the heart and lungs to deliver oxygen to the body. Most people score between 20 and 80 milliliters per kilogram per minute. A score of 80 is world class, produced by an Olympic marathon runner, for example, and a score of 20 is very low, which would indicate difficulty climbing one or two flights of stairs. Most people have a $\dot{V}O_2max$ in the range of 30 to 40 milliliters per kilogram per minute. The number indicates how many milliliters of oxygen is being provided to each kilogram of body weight each minute, so a higher number indicates the ability to provide more oxygen to the body. If you begin to think of activities as requiring a certain amount of oxygen, then the importance of this number becomes obvious. For example, if walking at 4.0 miles per hour (6.4 km/h) requires 30 milliliters per kilogram per minute, running at 6.0 miles per hour (9.7 km/h) requires 40 milliliters per kilogram per minute, running at 8.0 miles per hour (12.9 km/h) requires 50 milliliters per kilogram per minute, and a person's $\dot{V}O_2$max is 45 milliliters per kilogram per minute, you can clearly see that the person should be able to jog at 6.0 miles per hour but running at 8.0 miles per hour might be too much. These numbers are not exact, but they illustrate the point. As a person's fitness improves, his or her $\dot{V}O_2$max goes up and so does the ability to perform more challenging cardio.

Three major variables are associated with $\dot{V}O_2$max. The first is the heart. The ability of the heart to pump blood determines how much blood can flow around the body and therefore how much oxygen can be delivered. The second is the lungs. Gas exchange occurs at the lungs where oxygen is brought in and carbon dioxide is released. The ability of the lungs to grab oxygen determines how oxygenated the blood will be. The third variable is body weight. As will be discussed later, body weight has a major effect on $\dot{V}O_2$max. For a high $\dot{V}O_2$max, a person needs to have a low body weight. Sex is also somewhat important to $\dot{V}O_2$max, mainly because a man's heart is larger than a woman's relative to body mass. On average, males' $\dot{V}O_2$max will be about 5 to 6 points higher than females' $\dot{V}O_2$max, which is one reason that men generally perform better than women in cardiovascular events.

Lactate Threshold

The second key factor in aerobic performance is lactate threshold. When a person exercises, particularly with intensity, lactate and unbuffered hydrogen ions build up in the muscles and blood. At first, this is no big deal, but as the lactate and other by-products accumulate, performance begins to decline. Ultimately, the person must either stop altogether or decrease intensity to keep going. This is not just a question of willpower; everybody has a point at which the lactate will build up so much that he or she has to stop exercising. If you put an elite bicyclist on a bike going up a 25-degree incline and told him to pedal at 25 miles per hour (40.2 km/h), even he would reach a point where he could no longer do it (15, 32, 233).

The good news is that lactate threshold can improve, just as $\dot{V}O_2$max can improve. As a client trains hard and experiences the buildup of lactate, his or her body becomes more efficient at handling that substance and buffering it. When a client starts exercising, he or she might last 10 minutes on the stair climber, but after two months of training, he or she might be able to stay on the stair climber for 30 minutes without the legs giving out. The key to building up lactate threshold is to experience lactate during training. Your client cannot exercise at low intensity all the time and then expect to have a high lactate threshold. Generally, a client will experience lactate accumulation at higher intensities during cardio, particularly at 80 percent of MHR or greater. Interval training (discussed later) involving the fast glycolysis energy system is a good way to improve this factor in aerobic performance (46, 127, 135).

Muscle Fiber and Motor Unit Type Composition

The third factor in aerobic performance is a person's individual muscle fiber and motor unit type in a specific muscle. The two main types of muscle fibers and motor units are Type I and Type II (see chapter 6). Type I is good for endurance, whereas Type II is better for power. A person's percentage of each type is determined by genetics, although long-term training may possibly cause a shift in these fiber types. In addition, each muscle has its own percentage of Type I and Type II muscle fibers. If the goal is to be a good marathon runner or long-distance cyclist, having a large number of Type I muscle fibers in the legs will be beneficial. Elite aerobic endurance athletes have been shown to have 75 percent or more slow-twitch muscle fibers, whereas most of the population has around 50 percent or slightly higher. Figure 22.4 shows

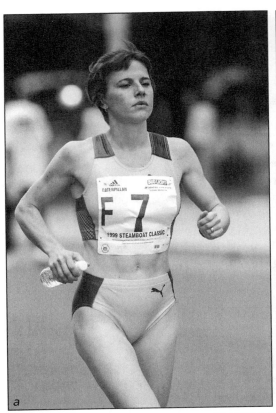 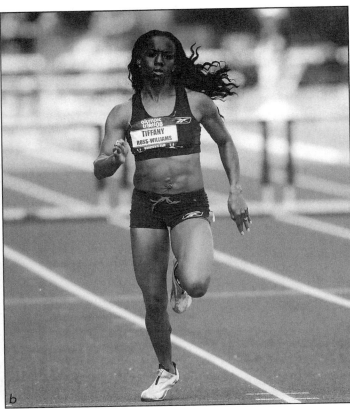

Figure 22.4 Physique differences between *(a)* a distance runner and *(b)* a sprinter.

the difference between the build of a distance runner and that of a sprinter.

Exercise Economy

Exercise economy refers to how efficient a person is during a specific exercise or activity. A client who is very efficient does not waste energy, will not become as tired during the workout, and will have more energy left after the workout is over. A person who is inefficient wastes energy, will become tired, and will not perform as well. Examples of ways to improve exercise efficiency include having proper running form, riding a lightweight bicycle, wearing an aerodynamically shaped helmet, running in lightweight running shoes, and wearing a bodysuit for swimming. Examples of things that negatively affect exercise economy are zigzagging while jogging, swinging the arms sideways while running, jumping too high with each running step, pounding the ground flat-footed with each step, pushing the bike pedal down but not pulling it up at the same time

with the opposite leg, and riding a mountain bike with flat tires on the pavement (76, 138).

If clients are interested in performance, you want to have them do everything they can to be as efficient as possible. Clients should have good shoes and good equipment, and they should master the form of movement that they are doing. But if they are using cardio for the sole purpose of burning calories, then exercise economy is no longer as important. Generally, you want your client's form on the exercise to be correct, but if a person is riding a bike just to lose weight, the weight or efficiency of the bike doesn't make any difference. In fact, slight inefficiencies will burn more calories per minute, which is acceptable if the inefficiency will not cause them to stop the exercise prematurely.

Fat as Fuel

During aerobic exercise, the two primary fuels are fatty acids and glucose (from glycogen). These two fuels each contribute a certain amount of energy to the exercise. But the supply of these two fuels is not equal. Even relatively lean people will have several pounds of fat on them. For example, almost all people have at least 5 pounds (2.3 kg) of fat; even this amount is incredibly low. Five pounds of fat represents 17,500 potential calories (3,500 × 5). That same person will likely have only 300 or 400 grams of glycogen stored in the body, which is at most 1,600 calories. Intense cardio can burn 1,000 calories per hour or more, so glycogen storage becomes a limiting factor in how long someone can maintain an intense pace during cardio. Because glycogen is limited and fat is not, the goal is to save the glycogen as much as possible (84, 107).

As a person's cardiovascular fitness increases, his or her body starts to burn more fat both at rest and during exercise. What happens is that the body learns to rely more on fat and fatty acids for fuel at higher intensities. In addition, as a person gets in better shape, he or she can exercise harder while maintaining a lower heart rate. The increased ability to burn fat means that the body is burning less glycogen. The person can then conserve glycogen, which means that he or she can go longer at the same speed or go slightly faster for the same period. Consider the following example of two marathon runners. Both are running at 10 miles per hour (16.1 km/h), and each has 350 grams of glycogen stored in the body.

- Person A runs at 10 miles per hour and burns 20 kilocalories per minute at 60 percent carbohydrate and 40 percent fat, which is 12 kilocalories of carbohydrate per minute and 3 grams of glycogen per minute, or 180 grams of glycogen per hour. After two hours person A will have burned 360 grams of glycogen, which exceeds the amount stored, so person A will have to decrease intensity after that. In other words, person A will have to slow down before reaching the 20-mile (32.2 km) point in the race.

- Person B runs at 10 miles per hour and burns 20 kilocalories per minute at 50 percent carbohydrate and 50 percent fat, which is 10 kilocalories of carbohydrate per minute and 2.5 grams of glycogen per minute, or 150 grams of glycogen per hour. After 2 hours person B will have burned 300 grams of glycogen and will still have 50 grams left. Therefore, person B can run 25 minutes longer than person A at the same pace and, as a result, be close to finishing the marathon at normal race pace.

The example shows that aerobic endurance athletes benefit by burning fat rather than burning carbohydrate. An increased ability to burn fat is also helpful for people interested in health, fitness, and weight loss because the body burns a higher percentage of fat at rest as well as during exercise. Over the course of days, weeks, or months, even a small difference adds up. Generally, to get this effect, people need to exercise at moderately high intensity, in the cardio training zone.

Body Weight

This factor is really a subset of $\dot{V}O_2max$ because $\dot{V}O_2max$ takes body weight into account. When performing a cardio event, having the lightest body weight possible is ideal. There are two main reasons for this. The first is simply effort. More effort or energy is required to move a larger body than a smaller one. Even if the body is mainly muscle, more energy is needed to move 150 pounds (68.0 kg) for 10 miles (16.1 km) than to move 120 pounds (54.4 kg) for the same distance. Because energy is precious in an aerobic event, the less energy a person spends, the better off he or she is.

The second reason is that although the heart and lungs can grow in response to training, they do not grow in proportion to the rest of the body. The heart and lungs of a 300-pound (136.1 kg) person will not be proportional to the heart and lungs of a 100-pound (45.4 kg) person. Another analogy that illustrates this point is a car and its engine. To make a car faster, you increase the size of its engine while trying to keep the weight of the car to a minimum. But if you put a really big engine in a really heavy car or truck, the vehicle will still be relatively slow. Most 18-wheelers you see on the road have big engines, but they are slow because their engines are not large in proportion to their size. The inverse is also true. Motorcycles generally have small engines that are weak compared with the engines in cars, but because motorcycles are relatively light, they are much faster than cars. In any major aerobic endurance event, the smaller people will generally perform better. Most elite endurance athletes weigh less than the average person because they have smaller muscles and low body fat. Rarely does a heavier person win an aerobic event.

Skill

Skill is closely related to exercise economy. A highly skilled person makes efficient movements and doesn't waste energy; an unskilled person wastes energy and therefore finds the exercise more difficult. This contrast can be seen when an aerobic endurance athlete with a high $\dot{V}O_2max$ tries a new or unfamiliar type of cardiovascular exercise. For example, if a skilled runner wants to complete a triathlon, he or she will have to learn how to bike and swim. The first attempt at swimming will leave the runner out of breath after just a few minutes because his or her movements will be inefficient. As time goes by, the person can dramatically improve his or her swimming ability.

Body Type

A person's body type affects how well he or she performs certain activities. Unfortunately, personal trainers cannot control this variable. A client who has short arms or legs will be at a disadvantage compared with someone who has longer arms or legs. Of course, clients can significantly improve their fitness whatever their body type. At the elite levels of sport, however, a genetic factor is clearly at play. Everyone can get better, even much better, but not everyone can be a world champion.

Mind-Set

The final key variable that affects aerobic performance is a person's mind-set (also called mind state). People who are highly motivated can achieve great things. In sport competition, lesser-skilled opponents often beat better-trained people because they have a stronger mind-set. Some evidence indicates that the power of belief can even affect physiology, so you should strive to instill in your clients a positive attitude and self-confidence (43).

FITT PRINCIPLE

The FITT principle—referring to frequency, intensity, time, and type—is important in helping you design and evaluate resistance and cardio training programs. Each variable needs to be set up correctly to maximize cardiovascular benefit.

Frequency

Clients commonly ask how often they should perform cardio; the answer depends on their training goals. Table 22.3 provides commonly recommended and ideal frequency guidelines (58, 176).

Intensity

Intensity for cardiovascular exercise can be measured in several ways. The primary way is to measure a person's heart rate while he

Table 22.3 Cardiovascular Goals and Training Frequency Guidelines

Goal	Sessions per week	
	Common guideline	Ideal recommendation
Improve cardiovascular fitness	3 or more	4–7
Decrease body fat	4 or more	4–9
Improve health	2–4 or more	3
Maintain cardiovascular fitness	1–3	2
Gain weight	0-2	1

or she is training and then determine the percentage of MHR. The heart rate formulas are a good starting point, but they are not absolute guidelines. A good training range is 60 to 85 percent of MHR; anything less than 60 percent is too easy and may not cause adaptations, and anything over 85 percent may be too challenging to perform for any length of time (179).

Another way to measure intensity is to use a rating of perceived exertion (RPE) scale. This subjective measure asks a person to rank how hard he or she is exercising. The two main scales are the Borg 6 to 20 scale, which spans from 6 to 20, and the Borg CR10 scale, which ranges from 1 to 10. The Borg 6 to 20 scale seems to be better suited for cardiovascular exercise, and the Borg CR10 scale seems to work well for weight training (42).

To use the RPE scale, you hold up a chart and ask your client, "How hard are you currently working?" The client ranks his or her effort on the scale provided. You may be thinking that the range of 6 to 20 is odd; why not just use 1 to 15? The genius behind the scale is that adding a zero to the end of the number provided by the client is a reasonable estimate of the client's heart rate. Normally, clients should be in the 13 to 15 range on the Borg scale when performing cardio, which translates to exercising in a heart rate range of 130 to 150 beats per minute.

If you do not want to take pulse and use scales, a simple way of monitoring the intensity of cardio is to see what level or speed your clients are working at and then gradually increase it. If a client is used to riding the bike at level 4, try level 5. If a client normally walks at 3.5 miles per hour (5.6 km/h), try 3.6 miles per hour (5.8 km/h). If the client is planning to do cardio for 25 minutes, have him or her try 30 minutes. Just as with lifting weights, following

progressive overload and gradually increasing the intensity of the cardio workout will improve cardiovascular fitness. This method works well because clients can start at an easy pace and achieve a high fitness level if they stick with it long enough. Table 22.4 provides suggested increases in intensity and the time frame in which they should occur.

Time (Duration)

The duration of a cardio workout depends on your philosophy and your client's goals. Cardio is usually performed for 20 minutes or longer, although if time is limited, nothing is wrong with occasionally doing cardio for 10 to 15 minutes. The most common recommendation for a cardio workout is 20 to 30 minutes. Anything longer than 45 minutes is considered long for cardio, but a workout of that duration is fine; a cardio workout can last 2 or more hours. If a client is training for an extended aerobic endurance event, some of his or her cardio workouts need to be about that long. If a client is trying to lose weight, you generally want him or her to perform cardio for as long as possible; a good initial goal is 30 to 60 minutes. If you are trying to maintain or increase your client's cardiovascular fitness, then 20 to 30 minutes of more intense cardio generally suffices (105, 219).

If a client is going to perform a cardio workout that would extend beyond the end time of the training session, you should get him or her started on the machine with the proper settings, level, and so forth. Then, when the session is over, you can leave him or her to finish the cardiovascular workout while you move to another client. This technique increases compliance, because clients are more likely to complete the cardio workout if you help them

Table 22.4 Optimal Progression for Standard Cardiovascular Training Machines

Mode of exercise	Overload	Time frame
Bike	Increase by one level or by 5 RPMs	Every 2–4 weeks
Treadmill	Increase speed by .1 mph (.16 km/h) or incline by 1%	Every 1–2 weeks
Elliptical	Increase by one level or increase speed by 5 strides	Every 2–4 weeks
Stair climber	Increase by one level	Every 2–4 weeks
Rowing machine	Increase kcal/h by 10 or decrease 500 m time by 1 s	Every 1–2 weeks

get started rather than rely on them to do it all on their own.

You may choose to break up the cardio workout time on different pieces of equipment or types of activities. If you want your clients to perform a cardio workout for 45 minutes, they could bike for 15 minutes, use the treadmill for 15 minutes, and then finish with the stair climber for 15 minutes. The rest after working on each machine should be relatively short, a minute or two maximum. Your goal is to keep the client's heart rate elevated. Again, the principle of specificity applies. If a client is training for a long event such as a marathon, dividing the cardio may not be a good idea because the effort will not mimic the race. But if your client is just trying to lose weight, get healthy, and improve endurance, breaking up the monotony a bit by using different machines may be a good approach.

If your client cannot initially complete a full 20 minutes, starting with less than that is acceptable. Refer to the beginner workout section for a specific cardio plan for your clients based on fitness level. Try to increase the time that your clients spend on cardio by 2 to 5 minutes every couple of weeks until they hit their goal time.

Type

The type of cardio that a client does will affect the results. In addition, each machine has pros and cons.

Treadmill

The treadmill is a functional piece of equipment because it trains an activity that we do regularly in everyday life—walk. A good goal for most clients is to be able to walk 4 miles (6.4 km) in an hour. If a client is unable to do this, his or her fitness level is likely not sufficient to meet the demands of daily life. The treadmill is easy to learn. Most people need only five minutes to feel comfortable on it, and when people run or walk briskly at an incline, they burn a relatively large number of calories.

Clients who have never used the treadmill should start at 2 miles per hour (3.2 km/h) until they get the feel of it. You can quickly move them up to about 3 miles per hour (4.8 km/h). From there, move up slowly.

People can either walk or run on the treadmill. If clients don't like to run, you can have them walk at an incline, which is a good way to burn extra calories. Running is great exercise, but it is not for everybody. It is high impact and can be rough on the feet, knees, and lower back, particularly if the person is heavy. For female clients who weigh over 160 pounds (72.6 kg) or male clients who weigh over 200 pounds (90.7 kg), you might want to work on building up their fitness level before they start jogging.

Do not start the incline too high. Most treadmills go up to a 15 percent incline; some go as high as 50 percent. Most clients should start at 2 or 3 percent. You can then increase the incline by 1 percent every one to two weeks as they improve. Any incline over 5 percent when running or over 10 percent when walking adds noticeably to the difficulty of the activity.

The muscles involved in walking or running on a treadmill are the glutes, quads, hamstrings, hip flexors, calves, and tibialis anterior. The adductors and abductors are stabilizers, as are the abs, lower back, and obliques. The upper-body muscles and bones receive little stimulus by walking or jogging.

One of the most common problems that people have with the treadmill is that it gives them shin splints. Shin splints can be related to overworking the tibialis anterior muscle. Doing too much too soon, going too fast, using too steep an incline, and wearing poor footwear all contribute to shin splints. The key is to start with a relatively easy amount of work and then gradually build up (224). See chapter 27 to learn about how to overcome shin splints.

Bike

The two main types of exercise bikes are recumbent and upright (figure 22.5). Recumbent bikes have the body reclined backward and the feet extended out in front. The upright bike resembles a traditional bicycle; the person sits on a seat, leans forward with the upper body, and positions the feet underneath the hips and knees.

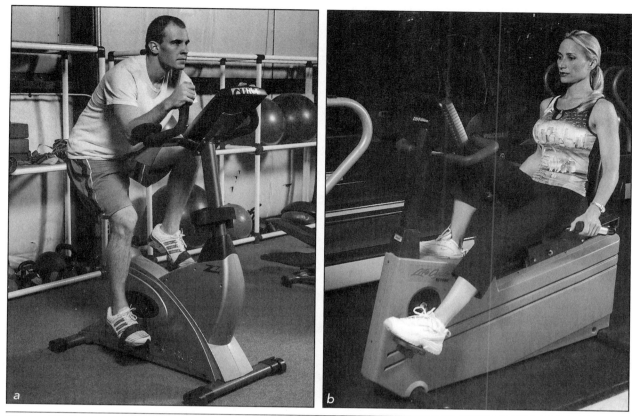

Figure 22.5   An *(a)* upright bike and a *(b)* recumbent bike.

The bicycle is an extremely efficient machine; some insist that it is the most efficient machine ever created. It allows us to take our power and apply it in such a way that we can travel much farther and faster without an increase in energy expenditure. This efficiency allows highly effective targeting of the heart and lungs. In simple terms, the bike is excellent at building up a person's $\dot{V}O_2max$. Few variables limit a person's performance on the bike, so it is the truest test of cardiovascular power. The bike is good at training the leg muscles, particularly for endurance. Finally, a stationary bicycle is easy to ride when a person has injuries or other complications that may prevent him or her from performing other types of exercise (180).

Unfortunately, riding a bike for a long time can be uncomfortable. Sometimes this discomfort is minor, but riding the bike for 20 minutes or longer nearly every day can be challenging if every minute of the activity feels uncomfortable. The degree of comfort is often a personal thing. Some people like the

way the bike fits them; others find it uncomfortable. If you have clients who find the bike uncomfortable, have them try different types of bikes or different kinds of seats. They can even try placing some padding or cushioning on the seat. The second big drawback of the bike is that it burns the fewest calories per minute of all the cardio equipment. Remember that the bike is extremely efficient. That efficiency is desirable in terms of travel and energy expenditure, but it is not desirable in terms of calorie burning. A more efficient activity requires less energy, so it burns fewer calories per minute. To be clear, a person can become lean just by riding a bike; look at any endurance cyclist. But minute per minute, most clients exercising at the same intensity will burn more calories on any other piece of cardio (with the exception of the upper-body ergometer). Because of this efficiency, the bike is not the best exercise mode for weight loss. A client will have to bike longer to achieve the same results. If the client doesn't mind that or enjoys cycling for long periods, that is fine. But if a person is pressed for time and is using cardio to lose weight, limit the use of the bike to once or twice a week at most.

The muscles involved when using the bicycle are the glutes, quads, hamstrings, and, to a lesser extent, the calves. If you instruct clients to pull up on the pedal as well as push down, they will also use their hip flexors and tibialis anterior. The recumbent bike places slightly more stress on the glutes, whereas the upright bike places slightly more stress on the quads. The bike is a good alternative if a client has shin splints. Most stationary bikes are designed to be pedaled at a speed of 80 RPMs (revolutions per minute). Instruct clients to stick to that recommendation. Going excessively slow will either shut the bike off or make the tension feel too hard, and going very fast will reduce the tension.

Elliptical Machine

This type of machine was designed to simulate the motion of running but with reduced impact. It gets its name because the platforms move in an ellipse, an elongated circle. There are two types of elliptical machines. Cross trainers have handles that move, so they work both the upper body and the lower body. Elliptical machines do not have moving handles, so they work just the lower body. Cross trainers are beneficial in that clients can either push or pull with their arms, using most of the muscles in the upper body. But the handles are often connected to the platforms and move as the user moves the feet, so many people just rest their hands on the handles and do not work their upper bodies. A drawback of the cross trainer is that it is difficult for people to reach the same speed as they can on a regular elliptical machine, limiting its application.

The elliptical machine has many advantages. First, it creates little impact. If you have clients who find it difficult to run, they should be able to use the elliptical machine with little problem. Second, it is effective at burning a large number of calories. Generally, people who use this machine will use at least as many calories as they will on the treadmill. Finally, people can reach high speeds and sprint on

an elliptical machine, an activity that can be uncomfortable on a treadmill and is generally challenging on indoor machines. Clients can get their feet moving very quickly on these machines for short periods, which make them ideal for interval training.

The two drawbacks of the elliptical machines are that they are somewhat unnatural and take a while to learn. For the first few minutes, many people find the machines uncomfortable, but they shouldn't give up because they are too beneficial to avoid altogether. Most people are comfortable using the bike and treadmill after just 5 minutes, but becoming comfortable on the elliptical machine takes much longer. Most people need about 20 minutes before they feel comfortable on the elliptical machine. The 20 minutes doesn't have to be continuous. If your client does a 5-minute warm-up on that machine four days a week, by the end of the first week, he or she should feel comfortable.

The second drawback of the elliptical machine is that it relies on a fixed movement. The stride length is predetermined, a circumstance not relevant to real life. In real life, when people run faster, they take longer strides, and when they run slower, they take shorter strides. On this machine, however, the only way to go faster is to make the feet move faster. In addition, this movement is not functional. The only time that a person produces an elliptical movement is in the gym on the elliptical machine. If your client wants to become an outstanding runner or cyclist, the principle of specificity is important, so he or she must run or bike to become accomplished at those activities. Doing only the elliptical will not make a person excel at other activities.

Because the movement of the elliptical machine is not natural (it is not walking, running, or stepping), you should focus on your clients' form while they are using this machine. Make sure that they keep their feet flat the entire time and do not go up on the toes during the movement. When the leg is at the bottom part of the movement, it should be straight. Many people keep their knees significantly flexed during the entire workout, which causes the lower back and quads to cramp up. You should instruct clients to stand up tall and look straight ahead with the chest up and shoulders back. Ideally, they should swing their arms as they glide, but if they need to hold on for balance, that is acceptable, especially when they are first learning the movement. If a client does need to hold on, see whether he or she can do that with just a couple of fingers. Do not let clients lean on or over the machine and do not let them lock their arms out to support themselves. Leaning on the machine makes the exercise easier and burns fewer calories, thus defeating the purpose of expending calories. For clients new to exercise, try building up their aerobic fitness on the bike and the treadmill for a week or two before you have them try the elliptical machine.

The muscles involved during an elliptical motion are the glutes, quads, hip flexors, hamstrings, and calves. By going backward on the machine, a person can place more emphasis on the hip flexor muscles and less on the glutes. On the cross trainer, pushing with the arms targets the pushing muscles, which are the chest, shoulders, and triceps. Pulling with the arms uses the pulling muscles of the lats, rhomboids, teres major, traps, rear delts, and biceps.

Stair Machine

The stair machine is a good, tough piece of cardio equipment, designed to mimic the action of walking up stairs. There are two main kinds of stair machines. The first is the traditional stair climber in which the feet go on the pedals (figure 22.6). The pedal then drops, and the feet are lifted. A second kind of stair machine is called the stepmill. A stepmill is a machine that has real stairs built into it, and clients must literally climb the stairs as they fall away. Stair climbers are more common than stepmills, but many gyms have both types of machines. Stepmills are generally considered more difficult, and you have to instruct clients to pay attention when they are on a stepmill because they could literally fall off the machine. In addition, clients are positioned higher when using a stepmill, so it is a somewhat more dangerous.

When using a stair machine, clients should place the balls or center of the feet on the pedals and keep them there. The feet should not come off the pedals at any time. Clients let

one foot drop the normal distance of a step, about 8 to 12 inches (20.3 to 30.5 cm), and then lift it and repeat the process on the other side. One of the most common mistakes that people make on the stair machine is taking tiny steps, not full normal-sized steps. If your clients need to hold on to the machine for balance, they can do so but should use just a few fingers. They should not lean forward on the machine or lock out their elbows for support. Swinging the arms is acceptable, particularly at faster speeds. Some old stair machines have the pedals connected to each other so that when one pedal goes down the other one comes up (like a bicycle). This setup is not ideal, so try to avoid those machines. In addition, any machine in which the knee shoots far out in front of the toes can harm the knees, so avoid those machines as well. Luckily, the machines that have the connected pedals are often the ones that allow the knees to go forward, so you

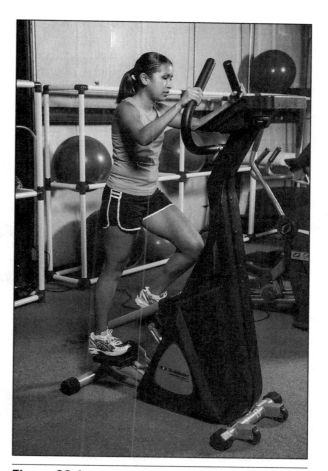

Figure 22.6 A stair climber.

can just avoid using that machine altogether. The stair machine can be a little rough on the knees, so if clients have sensitive knees, have them go easy the first few times to see how they feel. In addition, many people complain that their feet fall asleep while using the stair machine. The constant pressure of the foot against the pedal cuts off the circulation. To prevent this, instruct them to loosen their shoes so that they are not as snug. They should then alternately lift their feet off the pedals every few minutes and shake them out.

The stair machine is great for burning calories, building up $\dot{V}O_2max$, and strengthening the leg muscles. It is slightly more intense than riding a bike or performing the easier levels of the treadmill, so it is not recommended for untrained clients. Clients should perform cardio workouts for two to four weeks on other machines before they try the stair machine. In addition, heavy clients may feel the stair machine more in the legs than in the heart and lungs, sometimes to the point where their legs are burning and they have to stop the exercise, even though they are not out of breath. Let clients know that they will get used to this over time but prepare them for that sensation. If clients are experiencing this difficulty, start them with

five minutes on the stair machine and then gradually increase the time.

An interesting point about the stair machine is that it goes so slowly on its lowest levels that it can feel harder than going at a normal pace. Using the stair machine at level 1 may be so awkward that it gets tiring. Try level 2 or 3 with your clients so that they can get in a rhythm when they are first starting out.

The muscles that are involved when climbing stairs are the glutes, quads, hamstrings, hip flexors, and calves.

Rowing Machine

The rowing machine is a useful piece of cardio equipment because it is the only type of cardio that significantly builds strength, particularly in the upper body, aside from the upper-body ergometer (figure 22.7). The fancy name for the rowing machine is the ergometer, which is what people involved in crew, the sport of rowing, call a rowing machine.

To get started with the rowing machine, have clients sit in the seat facing the machine. You want their feet to be strapped to the foot boards. If they are too inflexible to grab the handle, you may have to hand it to them, because they may not be able to reach it after

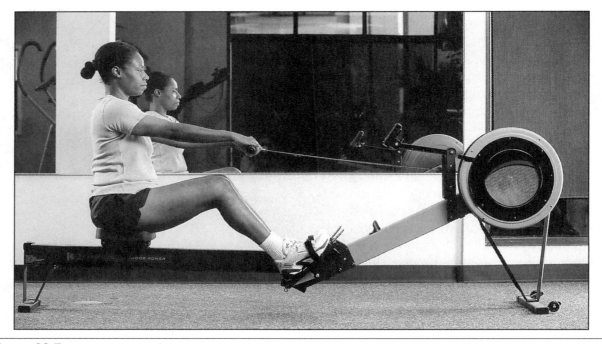

Figure 22.7 A rowing machine.

they are strapped in. If their feet are too low, they will lose power, so their feet should be as high as possible without the handle banging up against their knees. When they are ready, they lean slightly forward with arms straight and legs bent, as if they were trying to reach the fan on the machine. The most common grip to use is a pronated, or palms-down, grip with the hands held relatively far apart on the handles. To begin, clients straighten their legs, lean back slightly, and pull the handle into the belly. The cable should be straight and parallel to the floor when the handle touches the belly. The body position at the end of a row is similar to what it should be at the end of a cable row, leaning back about 15 degrees.

You may see people do different things with their wrists on the rowing machine. These people are usually rowers who are practicing for the actual act of rowing, which involve twisting the oars while rowing. If your clients are using the rowing machine for the sole purpose of getting a good workout, they do not need to do anything with their wrists. If clients complain that their forearms are getting tired, suggest that they loosen their grip on the handle or try a closed grip. In addition, they should not bend their wrists as they row. Many people bend their wrists for the last inch or two (about 2 to 5 cm) of the range of motion. That action is not good for their wrists and puts them in a weak position. In almost all exercises, the goal is to keep the wrist straight, essentially as an extension of the forearm.

The muscles that are trained when using a rowing machine are primarily the muscles in the legs and the back. They include the glutes, quads, hamstrings, tibialis anterior, hip flexor, lower back, lats, rear delts, rhomboids, traps (middle), biceps, brachialis, brachioradialis, and forearm flexors. The only main muscle groups neglected by this piece of equipment are the pushing muscles—the chest, shoulders, and triceps (75, 158).

The rowing machine is probably the hardest piece of cardio to use, mainly because most clients' upper-body muscles are not designed to be trained for 20 to 30 minutes continuously. Start clients with just 5 minutes on the rowing machine and increase that time as appropriate.

Rowing is also a good warm-up for an upper-body resistance training workout.

Some clients find the rowing machine boring, so be prepared for some grumbling if you regularly put them on that machine for more than 10 minutes. Clients who really enjoy rowing can enter ergometer machine competitions that involve all sorts of distances. A standard rowing race is 2,000 meters, which usually takes a decent rower between 6 1/2 and 7 1/2 minutes to complete. Typical clients need at least 8 minutes to complete the distance. Rowers measure their pace in 500-meter increments. Just as runners might talk about running a 6-minute mile, rowers might talk about rowing at a 1:35 500-meter pace.

The rowing machine is one piece of cardio where being heavier is an advantage because the larger body mass gives more power and momentum to the pull. Long arms and legs are also a distinct advantage. Rowing competitions are divided by gender and weight. The dividing line is 135 pounds (61.2 kg) for females and 165 pounds (74.8 kg) for males.

See table 22.5 for a summary of the pros, cons, recommended intensity progressions, and relative difficulty for common cardiovascular training machines.

TYPES OF CARDIOVASCULAR TRAINING

Each client should have a goal for the cardio part of the program. When clients lift weights, they do not lift weights simply to build muscle. Instead, they choose to emphasize strength, hypertrophy, or muscular endurance. The same is true for cardio training. In general, people want to focus on maximum speed, speed endurance, lactate threshold, muscular endurance, cardiovascular endurance, or weight loss. Different types of cardio training focus on each of these goals.

Steady-State Cardio

This type of cardio is the most common. For this type of training, clients get on a machine

Table 22.5 Description of Cardiovascular Training Machines

Type of cardio	Pros and cons	Progression	Difficulty
Treadmill	Pros: functional, mimics real life, easy to learn, can modify intensity, low impact when walking, burns a high number of kilocalories per minute, weight bearing Cons: has some impact, high impact when running, can aggravate or cause shin splints, can fall, hard to sprint on	+.1 mph (.16 km/h)/week +1% incline/week +2–5 min/week	Easy to advanced
Bike	Pros: easy to learn, low impact, doesn't bother shin splints, good way to increase V̇O₂max, good for interval training Cons: not weight bearing, burns the fewest number of kilocalories per minute, doesn't involve the upper body musculature, seat may be uncomfortable	+1 level every other week +.5–1 mile (.8–1.6 km)/week +2–5 min/week	Easy to advanced
Elliptical machine	Pros: low impact, emulates running, can train upper body on some machines, can work hard at low impact, good for nonjoggers, can go forward or backward, good for interval training Cons: not functional, doesn't mimic real life, can take a while to learn and feel comfortable with, fixed stride length	+1 level every other week +5 SPM/week (strides per minute) +2–5 min/week	Somewhat easy to advanced
Stair climber	Pros: low impact, can work hard, weight bearing, stimulates leg muscles, somewhat functional Cons: can hang on machine, can take minimal steps, might fatigue legs before arms, might bother knees, feet tend to fall asleep	+1 level every other week +2–5 min/week	Medium to advanced
Stepmill	Pros: functional, can work hard, weight bearing, stimulates leg muscles Cons: can hang on machine, can fall, hard to double step, tendency for users to look down and watch their feet, might be too hard for some clients, might fatigue legs before heart, might bother knees	+1 level every other week +2–5 min/week	Medium high to advanced
Rowing machine (ergometer)	Pros: can stimulate muscles, hits large number of muscles, trains upper body more than other cardio, can work hard, can burn a high number of kilocalories per minute Cons: takes a while to learn form, can be hard on the back and grip, hard to do for a long time, doesn't train upper-body pushing muscles, can aggravate shin splints	−1 to −3 sec/500 m every week +1–3 min/week	Advanced

Note: The progression listed is for a beginner; intermediate or advanced level clients may not be able to progress that fast. Level of difficulty is also given for a beginner. For example, the rowing machine is likely too advanced for a beginner to start on, but a client does not have to be advanced to use the rowing machine.

and go at a certain speed for a certain length of time. Normally, this form of cardio lasts at least 15 minutes and may go up to about 60 minutes. The key to this type of cardio is that the intensity does not change during the workout. People like this form of cardio because they can get in a zone and either focus on things such as TV or music or just relax and go with the exercise. This type of cardio is good for losing weight, building up low-force muscular endurance, and improving cardiovascular endurance (32).

Examples

Walk on treadmill at 4.0 miles per hour (6.4 km/h) at a 2 percent incline for 45 minutes

Jog outside at a 9:00-mile (5:35 km) pace for 4 miles (6.4 km)

Ride the bike at level 6, 80 RPMs, for 24 minutes

Use the elliptical machine at level 11, 140 strides, for 30 minutes

Long, Slow Distance Training

As the name implies, this form of cardio involves going longer than the person usually goes and at a slower pace. This type of training is sometimes abbreviated as *LSD*. The purpose of this form of cardio is to build up low force or cyclic muscular endurance so that the legs do not get tired when running a marathon, for example, and to build cardiovascular endurance. Because of the time spent performing this exercise, it is also effective for losing weight. LSD is similar to steady-state training, but the key element is that it lasts longer than usual. Clients should go at least 5 minutes longer than normal and often 15 to 30 minutes longer than normal. This form of cardio usually lasts 30 to 120 minutes. Because clients are going longer than normal, their speed is lower so that they can make it to the end. The volume of work performed can be stressful on the joints, so have clients build up to the longer duration, slightly increasing the work that they do each time. Normally, clients do only one or two LSD training sessions per week. Because this type of training takes longer than a traditional personal training session, personal trainers often suggest to clients that they perform this activity outside the regular training sessions.

Examples

- Walk on treadmill at 3.5 miles per hour (5.6 km/h) at a 2 percent incline for 75 minutes

- Jog outside at a 10:00-mile (6:12 km) pace for 6 miles (9.7 km)

- Ride the bike at level 4, 80 RPMs, for 45 minutes

- Use the elliptical machine at level 8, 130 strides, for 60 minutes

Pace, or Tempo, Training

This type of training is performed to get the body accustomed to a specific pace or speed. For example, let's say someone has a goal of running a 5K in 21 minutes. A 5K is about three miles long, so to complete three miles in 21 minutes, he or she needs to run at a 7-minute mile pace (4:20/km). A 5K is slightly longer than 3 miles, so the person would need to go slightly faster, but for our purposes we will focus on the 7-minute mile. Your client can run a 7-minute mile but cannot currently maintain that pace for 3 miles; he or she gets tired after the first mile. Your client needs to build up speed endurance, which is the ability to maintain a certain speed for a certain time. He or she should include pace or tempo training in the program to get accustomed to running at a 7-minute pace.

Because of the relatively high speed and intensity of this type of training, the length of time for this type of cardio is generally shorter than it would be for steady-state cardio. The duration depends on how long the person wants to be able to maintain a certain speed, but generally the length of time for this form of cardio is 15 to 45 minutes. This kind of training is relatively difficult, and your client's heart rate will be high (in the cardio training zone) when he or she is performing this form of exercise. Over time, you increase the time that the client spends at this speed to allow the body to get used to maintaining that speed. If a client will be spending a short amount of time at the goal pace, performing more than one round of this type of training is possible. For example, the client above could run 1.25 miles (2.0 km) at a 7-minute mile pace, walk for a mile (1.6 km) to recover, and then run another 1.25 miles at race pace. This plan allows more work to be performed. Pace or tempo training is most effective at building speed endurance, cardiovascular endurance, and lactate threshold, but it is also effective at promoting weight loss.

Examples

- Walk on treadmill at 4.5 miles per hour (7.2 km/h) at a 2 percent incline for 30 minutes

- Jog outside at a 7:30-mile (4:39 km) pace for 2 miles (3.2 km)

- Ride the bike at level 8, 80 RPMs, for 18 minutes

- Use the elliptical machine at level 11, 160 strides, for 20 minutes

Interval Training

The term *interval training* is used in fitness to describe many different forms of exercise. At its most basic level, it means doing something fast or hard for a short time, doing something slow or easy for a short time, and then repeating the sequence. The textbook definition of interval training is a period of high-intensity work followed by a period of low-intensity recovery with a work–rest ratio of 1:1. Thus, for every second your clients are training, they are resting for 1 second. If they sprint for 30 seconds, they then rest for 30 seconds.

When performing interval training, the time spent training varies, but each interval usually lasts between 30 seconds and 5 minutes. Anything over 5 minutes is probably too long, and the person will not be able to maintain the intensity for that duration. Anything under 30 seconds would require an increase in intensity that would have to be followed by a longer rest period, therefore resulting in work and rest periods that are uneven (138).

To select the proper intervals and intensity, you need to know the client's steady-state pace. If you do not know the steady state, you are likely to make the workout either too hard or too easy. For example, let's say that a person can run at 6 miles per hour (9.7 km/h) on the treadmill for 30 minutes. That pace is his or her steady state.

To design the interval program, you first decide how long the intervals are going to be. The longer they are (3 to 5 minutes), the more that program focuses on cardiovascular endurance; the shorter they are (30 seconds to 1 minute), the more that program focuses on speed and lactate threshold. You choose to go in the middle and decide that each interval will be 2 minutes long. You know that the steady state is 6 miles per hour (9.7 km/h), so you want to start from there. You want to maintain that average intensity, so at the end of the workout you want the average intensity to be 6 miles per hour (9.7 km/h). The easy way to do this is to remember that however much you go up from the steady state, you need to go down the same amount. Two good choices come to mind.

Choice 1

Fast: 7 miles per hour (11.3 km/h) for 2 minutes

Average speed: 6 miles per hour (9.7 km/h)

Slow: 5 miles per hour (8 km/h) for 2 minutes

Choice 2

8 miles per hour (12.9 km/h) for 2 minutes

4 miles per hour (6.4 km/h) for 2 minutes

Of course, other choices would work, such as 6.5 and 5.5, and 7.5 and 4.5, but you get the idea. The difference between choice 1 and choice 2 is that in choice 1, the person is running the whole time, whereas in choice 2 the person will probably be walking the slower interval (4.5 miles per hour [7.2 km/h] on the treadmill is usually the cutoff point between walking and running for most people). You need to decide whether you want the client to walk. If you want to work on endurance without rest, then you probably don't. If the goal is to make the work interval hard and the activity that the client is training for allows extra rest, that interval might be perfect.

After you have chosen an interval, you then decide how many intervals you want the client to complete. Currently one full interval takes 4 minutes (two fast and two slow), so five rounds would be a 20-minute workout, not including a warm-up and cool-down. Normally, interval training lasts 10 to 30 minutes. It can be an entire workout on its own, or it can be part of a longer workout, such as 10 minutes of interval training followed by 20 minutes of steady-state training.

The key to intervals is pace. If the difference between the steady state and the interval is too little, the workout won't seem much different, but if the difference is too great, the client will not be able to complete the workout. Certainly, going up in difficulty by 50 percent or more would be too much; a 10 to 30 percent increase is a good range, and 20 percent is ideal. Interval training is effective at building maximum speed, speed endurance, lactate threshold, and cardiovascular endurance. Depending on how the workout is set up, it can be effective at promoting weight loss as well. Interval training is an ideal form of cardio for people who participate in anaerobic sports—sports that require high bursts of energy followed by a quick rest period.

Examples (Based on Pace, or Tempo, Standards)

Run on the treadmill at 5.5 miles per hour (8.9 km/h) for 1 minute, walk at 3.5 miles per hour (5.6 km/h) for 1 minute, both speeds at a 2 percent incline, and repeat 15 times for a total of 30 minutes

Jog outside at a 7:00-mile (4:20 km) pace for 2 minutes, jog at an 8:00-mile (4:58 km) pace for 2 minutes, and repeat until a total distance of 2 miles (3.2 km) is covered

Ride the bike at level 10 for 1 minute, ride at level 6 for 1 minute, maintaining 80 RPMs throughout, and repeat 9 times for a total of 18 minutes

Use the elliptical at 180 SPM for 1 minute and then at 140 SPM for 1 minute; maintain level 11 throughout and repeat 10 times for a total of 20 minutes

Repetition Training

A type of interval training is called repetition training or sprint training. Like regular interval training, this kind of training also involves two parts, one fast and one slow, but unlike in interval training, the work–rest is ratio is not 1:1; instead, it is usually 1:3, 1:4, or 1:5. The work part of the interval for repetition training normally lasts 5 to 30 seconds; 10 to 15 seconds is the most common. The rest part of the interval normally lasts from 30 seconds to 2 minutes. Remember that the more intense the work is, the more rest the person needs to recover. Here are three common set-ups for repetition training:

- Work for 30 seconds, rest for 1:30 seconds (1:3 ratio)
- Work for 15 seconds, rest for 45 seconds (1:3 ratio)
- Work for 10 seconds, rest for 50 seconds (1:5 ratio)

Repetition training offers several benefits. During the work intervals, the person's heart rate skyrockets, often climbing to near maximal levels. This method helps the person become accustomed to working at high intensity. In addition, the high intensity required for this type of work normally produces lactate, which in turn builds the person's lactate threshold. Because the person is working as hard as possible, repetition training helps build maximum speed and some speed endurance. This type of training can help raise the metabolism even after the workout is over, and it can help build lean muscle, so it can have a positive effect on weight loss. This form of cardio is good for power athletes because it closely mimics their sport. And finally, many clients find it is simply more fun to do, and whenever we can make cardio fun, that is a good thing.

Examples (Based on Pace, or Tempo, Standards)

Run on the treadmill at 7.5 miles per hour (12.1 km/h) for 30 seconds, walk on the treadmill at 3.5 miles per hour (5.6 km/h) for 90 seconds, maintain a 2 percent incline throughout, and repeat 15 times for a total of 30 minutes

Run outside at a 6:00-mile (3:43 km) pace for 30 seconds, jog at an 8:00-mile (4:58 km) pace for 90 seconds, and repeat for a total distance of 2 miles (3.2 km)

Bike at 110 RPMs for 15 seconds and then at 70 RPMs for 45 seconds; maintain level 8 throughout and repeat 18 times for a total of 18 minutes

Use the elliptical at a speed of 220 SPM for 15 seconds and then at a speed of 140 SPM for 45 seconds; maintain level 11 throughout and repeat 20 times for a total of 20 minutes

Note: Performing as many repetitions as prescribed would be unusual; the examples were developed to be consistent with the previous ones. As noted earlier, the usual approach is to spend the last 5 to 15 minutes of cardio performing this type of activity.

Examples (Based on Pace, or Tempo, Standards)

When setting up a repetition cardio plan, you should know a person's steady-state ability and then design a plan that maintains that pace evenly throughout the repetition training. Unfortunately, the math is not as simple as it was for interval training because the work–rest ratio is uneven, but we can still figure it out.

> Walk on the treadmill at 4.5 miles per hour (7.2 km/h) at a 2 percent incline for 30 minutes
>
> Jog outside at a 7:30-mile pace (4:39 min/km) for 2 miles (3.2 km)
>
> Ride the bike at level 8, 80 RPMs, for 18 minutes
>
> Use the elliptical machine at level 11, 160 strides, for 20 minutes

In the first example, the client can walk on the treadmill at 4.5 miles per hour (7.2 km/h). If you are going to use repetition training as part of the program, this person must be able to run, at least a little bit. If someone has not done this type of training before, it is best to do interval training for a month or two and then bump up the intensity to repetition training.

To maintain the same steady-state average, you need to know what work–rest ratio you want to use. Remember, a 1:3 to 1:5 ratio is most common. Let's start with a 1:3 ratio. What that means is that for every second the person is working, he or she will rest for 3 seconds. Another way of saying that is that the person will be working for 1 out of every 4 seconds. If you want the person to work for 30 seconds straight and you use a 1:3 ratio, you have to let him or her rest for 90 seconds (30 × 3 = 90). So one set would be 2 minutes long—30 seconds of work followed by 90 seconds of rest.

Here is where the math gets a little tricky. To maintain the steady state, you have to increase the work intensity because the person is working at that level for only one-third of the time that he or she is resting. For example, if the person jogs at 5 miles per hour (8 km/h) for 30 seconds and then walks at 4 miles per hour (6.4 km/h) for 90 seconds, the average speed is not 4.5 miles per hour (7.2 km/h) because the person spends three times as long at the 4 miles per hour (6.4 km/h) level. The average is 4.25 miles per hour (6.8 km/h), which is an easier workout than the steady-state workout.

The way to figure out how to average repetition training is to take the rest level and multiply it by the rest ratio. For example, the person spent 30 seconds at 5 miles per hour (8 km/h) and performed three segments of 30 seconds at 4 miles per hour (6.4 km/h), so that really looks like 5 + 4 + 4 + 4 = 17. Divide that number by the total number of segments (4) to get the average. Therefore, you have 17 ÷ 4 = 4.25 miles per hour (6.8 km/h). If you wanted to have an average of 4.5 miles per hour (7.2 km/h), you would have to increase the work part of the exercise to 6.0. That would be 6 + 4 + 4 + 4 = 18 ÷ 4 = 4.5 miles per hour (7.2 km/h). A little trick to remember is that however much you go down from the steady state to determine the rest interval, you need to go up three to five times that amount (depending on the ratio) for the work level. You went down .5 miles per hour (.8 km/h) to get the rest interval, so you needed to go up 3 × .5, or 1.5 miles per hour (2.4 km/h), for the work interval. Therefore, 4.5 + 1.5 = 6 miles per hour (9.7 km/h). Here are some possible ways to set up 30 seconds of work and 90 seconds of rest to produce an average of 4.5 miles per hour.

- 30 seconds at 6 miles per hour (9.7 km/h), 90 seconds at 4 miles per hour (6.4 km/h)
- 30 seconds at 7.5 miles per hour (12.1 km/h), 90 seconds at 3.5 miles per hour (5.6 km/h)
- 30 seconds at 9 miles per hour (14.5 km/h), 90 seconds at 3 miles per hour (4.8 km/h)

If you want the client to sprint for 15 seconds and then rest for 45 seconds, the work–rest ratio is again 1:3. But the shorter work interval allows the person to go more intensely. You can use the same intensity listed earlier because the work–rest ratio is the same, but the first one is likely too easy unless the person is not used to running at all. So for this example you might do the following:

- 7.5 miles per hour (12.1 km/h) for 15 seconds, 3.5 miles per hour (5.6 km/h) for 45 seconds
- 9.0 miles per hour (14.5 km/h) for 15 seconds, 3.0 miles per hour (4.8 km/h) for 45 seconds
- 10.5 miles per hour (16.9 km/h) for 15 seconds, 2.5 miles per hour (4.0 km/h) for 45 seconds*

    *Not all treadmills go above 10 miles per hour.

If you want to use a 1:5 ratio so that the person exercises hard for 10 seconds and then rests for 50 seconds, use the same principle. Now the person is resting for five times as long as he or she is working, so the work interval should be even harder. Here are some examples:

- 7.0 miles per hour (11.3 km/h) for 10 seconds, 4.0 miles per hour (6.4 km/h) for 50 seconds
- 8.5 miles per hour (13.7 km/h) for 10 seconds, 3.7 miles per hour (6.0 km/h) for 50 seconds
- 10 miles per hour (16.1 km/h) for 10 seconds, 3.4 miles per hour (5.5 km/h) for 50 seconds

Getting the hang of planning repetition training and intervals just takes a little while. Sticking with the steady-state average intensity at first is recommended because interval and repetition training are generally harder than doing steady-state work. Just the fact that you are changing the intensity makes the workout more challenging. After a client adapts to that, you can bump up the intensity slightly.

Here is a list of other ways to program repetition training, again using the previous examples:

Jog outside at a 7:30-mile (4:39 km) pace for 2 miles (3.2 km) (8 miles per hour [12.9 km] for 15 minutes)

Work at a 6:00-mile (3:43 km) pace for 30 seconds

Rest at an 8:00-mile (4:58 km) pace for 90 seconds

or

Work at a 4:30-mile (2:47 km) pace for 15 seconds

Rest at an 8:30-mile (5:07 km) pace for 45 seconds

or

Work at a 3:45-mile (2:19 km) pace for 10 seconds

Rest at an 8:15-mile (5:07 km) pace for 50 seconds

Note: All these workouts would be brutal!

Ride the bike at level 8, 80 RPMs, for 18 minutes

Changing level, all at 80 RPMs

Work at level 11 for 30 seconds

Rest at level 7 for 90 seconds

or

Work at level 14 for 15 seconds

Rest at level 6 for 45 seconds

or

Work at level 18 for 10 seconds

Rest at level 6 for 50 seconds

Changing speed, all at level 8

Work at 110 RPMs for 30 seconds

Rest at 70 RPMs for 90 seconds

or

Work at 119 RPMS for 15 seconds

Rest at 67 RPMs for 45 seconds

or

Work at 130 RPMs for 10 seconds

Rest at 70 RPMs for 50 seconds

Elliptical machine, level 11, 160 strides, for 20 minutes

Changing level, all at 160 strides

Work at level 14 for 30 seconds

Rest at level 10 for 90 seconds

or

Work at level 14 for 15 seconds (level 17 is
probably too hard)

Rest at level 10 for 45 seconds

or

Work at level 16 for 10 seconds

Rest at level 10 for 50 seconds

Changing speed, all at level 11

Work at 190 strides for 30 seconds

Rest at 150 strides for 90 seconds

or

Work at 220 strides for 15 seconds

Rest at 140 strides for 45 seconds

or

Work at 260 strides for 10 seconds

Rest at 140 strides for 50 seconds

As you can see, repetition training generally
works better when speed is being manipulated
instead of the level of resistance. Changing
the level works well for interval training, but
the level is often either too easy or too hard
when it is changed enough for repetition
training.

Repetition training can be extremely intense,
so it is usually performed no more than once
or twice a week. Repetition training normally
lasts 5 to 20 minutes. It can be performed as
part of a longer cardio workout, such as during
the last 10 minutes of a 30-minute workout, or
as a stand-alone workout. Generally, if you are
using longer intervals (30 seconds of work, 90
seconds of rest), the session is 15 or 20 minutes
long. If the entire work and rest interval is a
minute or less, the session normally last 5 to
10 minutes.

The difficulty of this training is cumulative.
Even if the client has no problem with the first
one or two work sets, do not jump to increase
the intensity. After the 5th or 10th interval,
the client may be exhausted.

Repetition and interval training should not
be performed intensely until the client has
developed a base level of cardiovascular fitness.

Step Training

Step training is not about your basic aerobics
class. Instead, it refers to a way of setting up
a cardio program to hit different intensities
during the workout. Step training is similar to
interval training, but interval training always
consists of just two levels of difficulty. Step
training always includes three or more levels
of difficulty, normally three to five (see figure
22.8). It is called step training because a graph
of the workout intensity would look like a
series of steps.

To set up a step training workout, you need
to know a person's steady-state level on that
piece of equipment. You then set up a series of
steps or levels around that steady state. Normally, each step lasts 30 seconds to 5 minutes,
so the time frame is the same as that for interval
training. But because there are more than two
steps, completing one round of steps will take
longer than completing one round of interval
training (38).

To start, you want to decide how many
steps your client is going to do. Again, three is
the minimum, and using three to five steps is
common. When you are first doing this, pick
an odd number of steps, three or five, simply
because the math is much easier. If you choose

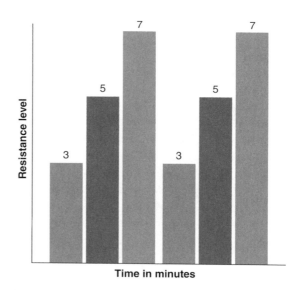

Figure 22.8 Step training with one minute being spent on levels 3, 5, and 7, respectively, and
then repeating those steps.

an odd number of steps, simply make the middle step the steady-state intensity and then work around that. So start with three steps.

Next, decide how long each step will be. Each step is the same length as one block in interval training, so they are 30 seconds to 5 minutes long. Normally, each step is the same length, so let's choose one minute per step. The shorter each step is, the more you can alter the difficulty; the longer each step is, the less you can alter the difficulty. Finally, you have to select the intensity for each step. Let's start with the examples listed earlier.

Walk on the Treadmill at 4.5 Miles per Hour (7.2 km/h) at a 2 Percent Incline

Changing speed

- Step 1: 4.3 miles per hour (6.9 km/h) at a 2 percent incline for 1 minute
- Step 2: 4.5 miles per hour (7.2 km/h) at a 2 percent incline for 1 minute
- Step 3: 4.7 miles per hour (7.6 km/h) at a 2 percent incline for 1 minute

Changing incline

- Step 1: 4.5 miles per hour (7.2 km/h) at a 0 percent incline for 1 minute
- Step 2: 4.5 miles per hour at a 2 percent incline for 1 minute
- Step 3: 4.5 miles per hour at a 4 percent incline for 1 minute

As you can see in the examples, the steady-state intensity was used in the middle step (step 2). Then the intensity was lowered slightly in step 1 and raised slightly in step 3. However much of the intensity was lowered in step 1, it was raised in step 3. This maintains the average intensity. In the first example, the speed couldn't be changed much because the person is walking and has almost topped out on walking speed, so small changes were made. Generally, step training involves smaller jumps in intensity than interval training does, and the jumps are definitely smaller than they are in repetition training. Keep in mind that it is best to alter just one variable at a time when you are learning how to do this. After you master it, feel free to change more than one variable but be careful that you do not make the workout too hard or too easy.

Examples (Based on Pace, or Tempo, Standards)

Treadmill 4.5 Miles per Hour (7.2 km/h) at a 2 Percent Incline for 30 Minutes, Five-Step Program

4.3 miles per hour (6.9 km/h) at a 2 percent incline for 1 minute

4.4 miles per hour (7.1 km/h) at a 2 percent incline for 1 minute

4.5 miles per hour (7.2 km/h) at a 2 percent incline for 1 minute

4.6 miles per hour (7.4 km/h) at a 2 percent incline for 1 minute

4.7 miles per hour (7.6 km/h) at a 2 percent incline for 1 minute

Repeat six times for a total of 30 minutes

Jog Outside at a 7:30-Mile (4:39 km) Pace for 2 Miles (3.2 km), Three-Step Program

Jog at an 8:00-mile (4:58 km) pace for 2 minutes

Jog at a 7:30-mile (4:39 km) pace for 2 minutes

Jog at a 7:00-mile (4:20 km) pace for 2 minutes

Repeat about three times or until 2 miles is covered

Bike at Level 8 at 80 RPMs for 18 Minutes (Four-Step Plan)

Level 5 at 80 RPMs for 90 seconds

Level 7 at 80 RPMs for 90 seconds

Level 9 at 80 RPMs for 90 seconds

Level 11 at 80 RPMs for 90 seconds

Repeat three times for a total of 18 minutes

Elliptical at Level 11 at 160 SPM for 21 Minutes

Level 9 at 160 SPM for 1 minute

Level 11 at 160 SPM for 1 minute

Level 13 at 160 SPM for 1 minute

Repeat seven times for a total of 21 minutes

Jog Outside at a 7:30-Mile (4:39 km) Pace

Three-step plan—changing pace
- Step 1: 8:00-mile (4:58 km) pace for 2 minutes
- Step 2: 7:30-mile (4:39 km) pace for 2 minutes
- Step 3: 7:00-mile (4:20 km) pace for 2 minutes

Four-step plan—changing pace
- Step 1: 8:15-mile (5:07 km) pace for 1 minute
- Step 2: 7:45-mile (4:48 km) pace for 1 minute
- Step 3: 7:15-mile (4:30 km) pace for 1 minute
- Step 4: 6:45-mile (4:11 km) pace for 1 minute

Five-step plan—changing pace
- Step 1: 8:00-mile (4:58 km) pace for 1 minute
- Step 2: 7:45-mile (4:48 km) pace for 1 minute
- Step 3: 7:30-mile (4:39 km) pace for 1 minute
- Step 4: 7:15-mile (4:30 km) pace for 1 minute
- Step 5: 7:00-mile (4:20 km) pace for 1 minute

Bike at Level 8 at 80 RPM

Three-step plan—changing level
- Step 1: level 7 for 2 minutes
- Step 2: level 8 for 2 minutes
- Step 3: level 9 for 2 minutes

Four-step plan—changing level
- Step 1: level 5 for 1 minute
- Step 2: level 7 for 1 minute
- Step 3: level 9 for 1 minute
- Step 4: level 11 for 1 minute

Five-step plan—changing level
- Step 1: level 6 for :30
- Step 2: level 7 for :30
- Step 3: level 8 for :30
- Step 4: level 9 for :30
- Step 5: level 10 for :30

Elliptical Machine, Level 11, 160 Strides

Three-step plan—changing strides
- Step 1: 150 strides at L11 for 1 minute
- Step 2: 160 strides at L11 for 1 minute
- Step 3: 170 strides at L11 for 1 minute

Four-step plan—changing strides
- Step 1: 130 strides at L11 for 1 minute
- Step 2: 150 strides at L11 for 1 minute
- Step 3: 170 strides at L11 for 1 minute
- Step 4: 190 strides at L11 for 1 minute

Five-step plan—changing strides
- Step 1: 100 strides at L11 for 30 seconds
- Step 2: 130 strides at L11 for 30 seconds
- Step 3: 160 strides at L11 for 30 seconds
- Step 4: 190 strides at L11 for 30 seconds
- Step 5: 220 strides at L11 for 30 seconds

Performing interval, repetition, and step training offers many benefits. A simple one is that these forms of training break up the time on cardio into chunks that seem to make the workout go by faster. They also allow clients to hit higher intensities, albeit for a short time, than they would if they did only steady-state training. They are also more fun, which alleviates the problem that cardio is not generally regarded as fun. But the best thing about these types of training is that they overload the body in a gradual fashion.

When clients are performing steady-state training, any increase in speed means that they perform the whole workout faster. That plan works well in the beginning, but after a while, clients plateau and can no longer increase their pace .1 miles per hour (.16 km/h) per week, week after week. But they can still improve. When clients are able to complete a routine of varying intensity such as the interval, reps, or steps, you can change just one block of their intensity. The change averages out to a small increase—big enough to be noticed by the person but not so big that the body cannot do it.

If you want to make the intense part of the activity harder, then increase the working level slightly or increase the working level of the last one or two steps by the smallest amount possible. If you want to improve your clients' recovery ability, then increase the resting level slightly. This approach allows you to increase the difficulty continually without automatically running into a plateau.

Here are examples of how to increase the overall average intensity of interval and step training.

Interval Training—Walk on the Treadmill at 4.5 Miles per Hour (7.2 km/h) at a 2 Percent Incline

Week 1

- Walk at 4.5 miles per hour (7.2 km/h) at a 0 percent incline for 2 minutes
- Walk at 4.5 miles per hour at a 4 percent incline for 2 minutes
- Average intensity is 4.5 miles per hour at a 2 percent incline

Week 2

- Walk at 4.5 miles per hour (7.2 km/h) at a 0 percent incline for 2 minutes
- Walk at 4.5 miles per hour at a 5 percent incline for 2 minutes
- Average intensity is 4.5 miles per hour at a 2.5 percent incline

Week 3

- Walk at 4.5 miles per hour (7.2 km/h) at a 1 percent incline for 2 minutes
- Walk at 4.5 miles per hour at a 5 percent incline for 2 minutes
- Average intensity is 4.5 miles per hour at a 3 percent incline

Week 4

- Walk at 4.5 miles per hour (7.2 km/h) at a 1 percent incline for 2 minutes
- Walk at 4.5 miles per hour at a 6 percent incline for 2 minutes
- Average intensity is 4.5 miles per hour at a 3.5 percent incline

Interval Training—Ride the Bike at Level 6 at 80 RPMs

Week 1

- Bike at level 4 for 1 minute
- Bike at level 8 for 1 minute
- Average intensity is level 6

Week 2

- Bike at level 5 for 1 minute
- Bike at level 8 for 1 minute
- Average intensity is level 6.5

Week 3

- Bike at level 6 for 1 minute
- Bike at level 8 for 1 minute
- Average intensity is level 7

Week 4

- Bike at level 6 for 1 minute
- Bike at level 9 for 1 minute
- Average intensity is level 7.5

Step Training—Run on the Treadmill at 7.0 Miles per Hour (11.3 km/h), Three Steps

Week 1

- Run at 6.7 miles per hour (10.8 km/h) for 1 minute
- Run at 7.0 miles per hour (11.3 km/h) for 1 minute
- Run at 7.3 miles per hour (11.7 km/h) for 1 minute
- Average intensity is 7.0 miles per hour (11.3 km/h) per hour

Week 2

- Run at 6.8 miles per hour (10.9 km/h) for 1 minute
- Run at 7.0 miles per hour (11.3 km/h) for 1 minute
- Run at 7.3 miles per hour (11.7 km/h) for 1 minute
- Average intensity is 7.03 miles per hour (11.3 km/h)

Week 3

- Run at 6.8 miles per hour (10.9 km/h) for 1 minute

- Run at 7.1 miles per hour (11.4 km/h) for 1 minute
- Run at 7.3 miles per hour (11.7 km/h) for 1 minute
- Average intensity is 7.067 miles per hour (11.4 km/h)

Week 4

- Run at 6.8 miles per hour (10.9 km/h) for 1 minute
- Run at 7.1 miles per hour (11.4 km/h) for 1 minute
- Run at 7.4 miles per hour (11.9 km/h) for 1 minute
- Average intensity is 7.1 miles per hour (11.4 km/h)

Step Training—Elliptical Machine at 150 Strides at Level 6

Week 1

- 130 strides for 1 minute
- 150 strides for 1 minute
- 170 strides for 1 minute
- Average intensity is 150 strides

Week 2

- 130 strides for 1 minute
- 150 strides for 1 minute
- 180 strides for 1 minute
- Average intensity is 153 strides

Week 3

- 130 strides for 1 minute
- 160 strides for 1 minute
- 180 strides for 1 minute
- Average intensity is 156 strides

Week 4

- 140 strides for 1 minute
- 160 strides for 1 minute
- 180 strides for 1 minute
- Average intensity is 160 strides

As you can see from the examples, making small changes to either the intervals or the steps leads to larger changes over time. Remember that the more advanced your clients get, the slower they will progress (unfortunately), so you have to set up ways to allow their bodies

to progress more slowly. Most machines do not have a resistance level of 6.5; it is either 6 or 7. A client may be at the stage where 6 is too easy but 7 is too hard. Setting up his or her training like this allows you to build up the intensity gradually to get the person used to level 7.

When clients are performing interval, repetition, or steady-state training, you need to decide how many cycles they are going to do. One complete cycle is performing all the work and rest periods for a certain interval or performing all the steps for step training. For example, walking at 4 miles per hour (6.4 km/h) for 2 minutes and then running at 7 miles per hour (11.3 km/h) for 2 minutes is one cycle that is 4 minutes in length. A five-step plan, where each step is 1 minute in duration, would consist of one cycle that is 5 minutes long. To figure out how many cycles to include in each cardio workout, simply take the time that you plan to have your client perform and then divide that by the duration of the cycle. If you have a 4-minute cycle and you want your client to train on cardio for 24 minutes, the client can do six cycles (24 ÷ 4 = 6) or six complete intervals. If you have a 5-minute cycle for a step program and you want your client to exercise for 20 minutes, the client could do four complete cycles of that step program.

Do not forget to include a warm-up and a cool-down in the cardio. The warm-up is normally 5 minutes at a steady state, and the cool-down is normally 3 to 5 minutes long. For the cool-down, you decrease the workload each minute to bring the heart rate gradually back to normal. Therefore, the warm-up could be 5 minutes of walking on the treadmill at 4 miles per hour (6.4 km/h). The client would then begin jogging using the interval routine, which takes 24 minutes, and then cool down by walking, each minute a bit slower than the one before, for 5 minutes. The total workout time would be 34 minutes.

After the client completes one full cycle of interval training or step training, he or she normally goes back to the beginning and repeats the process. The client who is doing levels 5, 7, and 9 on the bike, each for a minute, would return to level 5 and begin the second cycle immediately after completing the minute at level 9. This sequence works well because the easiest period follows the most difficult period, which is when the person needs the rest.

As clients get more advanced, they can do backward steps. They follow the regular step routine, but after finishing that cycle, they go back down in difficultly, reversing the cycle. So if a client does levels 5, 7, and 9, he or she would then do levels 9, 7, and 5, each for a minute. This sequence is much more challenging because now the person is doubling the time spent at the most difficult work level. The compensation occurs when the time at the easiest work level is doubled (2 minutes at level 5), but generally that is not enough to make up for the extra time at the tough one.

Fartlek Training

This type of cardio training is sometimes called random training because in essence that is what it is. Fartlek training involves performing some sort of intervals, that is, periods of work followed by periods of rest, but no set guideline dictates the length of the work or rest periods. When you hit the random button on the bike and the computer generates various levels, or hills, that is an example of Fartlek training. You do not know if you are going to get three blocks of the steepest hill or three blocks of the smallest hill or something in between.

The rationale behind Fartlek training is that in real life, activities are not always broken down into neat, specific intervals. When you are running a marathon you do not know that the next hill lasts exactly two minutes and then you get two minutes of rest. As you climb that hill, you might look up and see another hill right away. When you are playing football, the defense and offense generally play for the same length of time, so when you come off the field, you can expect a few minutes of rest. But what happens when your team turns the ball over on the first play? Although you just played against a 12-play drive, you get only 30 seconds of rest before you have to go in again. The idea behind Fartlek training is to prepare an athlete or fitness enthusiast for anything. Fartlek training is good at building $\dot{V}O_2$max, lactate threshold, mental toughness, and pos-

sibly maximum speed and speed endurance. The way that a Fartlek program is designed has a significant effect on the way the body adapts to it (59, 183).

You can set up Fartlek training in your client's program in many ways. As mentioned, many cardio machines have a random option that will do it for you. If several people are involved, you can give each person a turn in choosing how hard to go and how long to go. Coaches often use Fartlek training. For example, a football coach has his players shuffle their feet. Every time he blows the whistle, the players have to drop down and do a push-up. The coach can choose to blow the whistle five times in a row, or he can let them shuffle their feet for a minute straight. That training session is an example of Fartlek training.

EXCESS POSTEXERCISE OXYGEN CONSUMPTION

Excess postexercise oxygen consumption (EPOC) is a measure of the elevation of metabolism after a training session. In general, light to moderate activity creates little EPOC; 5 or 10 minutes after a workout is over, a client's metabolism returns to near resting levels (as indicated by pulse, breathing rate, and so on) (134). More intense exercise will leave the client's metabolism significantly elevated for an extended time, often 30 minutes or more but sometimes up to several hours after extremely intense routines. This effect can promote significant fat loss. EPOC can be created without performing incredibly long workouts; an intense 30-minute workout might create 2 hours' worth of elevated EPOC. If a client's normal resting metabolic rate is 1 kilocalorie per minute, or 60 kilocalories per hour, after performing that intense activity his or her metabolic rate might average 2.5 kilocalories per minute, or 150 kilocalories per hour. For the two hours following the activity, metabolism remained elevated. Besides burning calories during the 30 minutes of exercise, which might total 360 kilocalories at a rate of 12 kilocalories per minute, the client burns an additional 180 calories above normal (150 per hour × 2 = 300 kilocalories – basal rate of 120 = 180 extra calories). When repeated several times over the course of the week, the additional calories burned add up. An extra benefit is that the calories burned in the EPOC period are largely fat calories. This process can help explain why sprinters and bodybuilders, athletes who may not perform much traditional cardiovascular training, can still be lean.

Note that cardio is not the only form of activity that creates EPOC. Intense training of any type—such as body-weight exercises (if they are challenging enough), resistance training, conditioning modalities, and many sports—can create the same effect (160). The key is intensity; lower levels of intensity generate little EPOC. Note as well that a client cannot compound the effects of EPOC (5, 24, 63). For example, a personal trainer might read that an intense cardio workout creates two hours of EPOC and an intense resistance training workout creates two hours of EPOC. Those two activities performed back to back will not yield four hours of EPOC. The body does not know that it performed cardio or weights or sprints; it just perceives that it went through an intense activity. After the body is stimulated and the metabolism is elevated, it will respond accordingly. But if multiple separate sessions are planned in a day (as with athletes engaged in two- or three-a-days), EPOC can occur after each session.

The more well-trained a client becomes, the harder it is to create EPOC on a regular basis. In addition, constantly taking a client to that state, several times a week, might induce overtraining. As with most intensity techniques, there is a time and a place for generating EPOC. But for late beginning and early intermediate clients, creating EPOC can be an effective method to promote weight loss without asking the client to perform several additional hours of exercise per week.

CONCLUSION

The heart powers the cardio system. It is made up of four chambers: two atriums and two ventricles. Veins carry blood into the heart; arteries carry blood away from the heart. When the cardiovascular system is trained regularly, many positive adaptations occur, including increased stroke volume, decreased resting pulse, and increased maximal cardiac output. Additional specific physiological responses include increased number and size of mitochondria, increased number of capillaries, increased number of red blood cells, more efficient lungs, decreased body weight, and a preferential focus on the Type I muscle fibers.

Cardiovascular work can take place in one of two broad zones. The fat-burning zone is a name for lower-intensity cardiovascular exercise generally performed below 70 percent of MHR and so named because a higher percentage of the fuel is fat. The cardio training zone is the name of the zone above 70 percent MHR. Exercise in this zone tends to cause the most positive adaptations of the cardiovascular system. The key physiological factors that affect a person's ability to perform cardiovascular work include $\dot{V}O_2max$, lactate threshold, muscle fiber type, exercise economy, fuel utilization, body weight, skill, body type, and mind-set.

The FITT principle is a useful tool to help program cardiovascular work for clients. Several types of cardiovascular programs are available for personal trainers to use with clients, including steady-state work; long, slow distance training; step training; interval training; repetition training; pace, or tempo, training; and fartlek training.

Cardiovascular endurance is a key component of fitness, and many clients need guidance with it. Proper cardiovascular programming will help clients see and feel results, and the training doesn't need to be boring or tedious. Personal trainers should be able to program cardiovascular exercise for the proper frequency, intensity, type, and time for their clients all while factoring in their enjoyment of that activity.

Study Questions

1. Which of the following are common physiological adaptations to chronic cardiovascular exercise?

    a. decreased mitochondria, decreased blood volume, decreased myoglobin

    b. increased number of capillaries, increased blood volume, decreased body fat

    c. increased body fat, increased mitochondria, increased myoglobin

    d. decreased lactate threshold, increased $\dot{V}O_2max$, increased exercise economy

2. Which of the following exercise programs would most likely create EPOC?

    a. a two-hour long, slow distance walk at 55 percent of MHR

    b. a weightlifting session of five sets of two reps at 60 percent of MHR with four-minute rests between sets

    c. a 45-minute steady-state session on the treadmill at 70 percent of MHR

    d. a 15-minute repetition training program with a 1:3 work-to-rest ratio working at 90 percent of MHR for 15 seconds for each work period

3. If a client can maintain a steady-state average of 5.5 miles per hour (8.9 km/h) on the treadmill for 30 minutes, what is a logical interval training program to maintain the steady-state aver-

age for this client? The workout will last 30 minutes.

    a. 6.5 miles per hour (10.5 km/h) work for one minute, 4.5 miles per hour (7.2 km/h) rest for one minute, repeat 15 times

    b. 6.0 miles per hour (9.7 km/h) work for one minute, 4.0 miles per hour (6.4 km/h) rest for one minute, repeat 15 times

    c. 7.0 miles per hour (11.3 km/h) work for one minute, 5.0 miles per hour (8.0 km/h) rest for one minute, repeat 15 times

    d. 10.5 miles per hour (16.9 km/h) work for one minute, .5 miles per hour (.8 km/h) rest for one minute, repeat 15 times

4. Which type of aerobic training program would likely have the biggest positive effect on maximal speed?

    a. interval training program

    b. pace, or tempo, training program

    c. repetition training program

    d. steady-state training program

5. At which of the following intensities does a client burn a greater total amount of energy from fat?

    a. 50 percent of MHR for 30 minutes

    b. 60 percent of MHR for 30 minutes

    c. 70 percent of MHR for 30 minutes

    d. 80 percent of MHR for 30 minutes

Flexibility

Flexibility is defined as the range of motion (ROM) at a joint. A joint is defined as the point where two bones meet; anywhere two bones meet, movement is possible. The body has three main types of joints:

- Fibrous joints, such as the joints in the skull, are fused and allow little movement.

- Cartilaginous joints, such as the joints in the vertebral column, allow a small range of motion.

- Synovial joints, such as the joints at the knee and shoulder, allow a large range of motion.

As a personal trainer, you will be concerned primarily with the main joints in the body and the range of motion that they offer. The ability of a joint to move is controlled primarily by muscles, and the tightness of those muscles is usually the limiting factor in a person's flexibility. Those joints include the neck, shoulder (including the scapula), elbow, wrist, finger, trunk, hip, knee, and ankle.

COMMON TESTS OF FLEXIBILITY

Flexibility is one of the components of fitness, and several tests are designed to measure it. The most common test is the sit-and-reach test in which the subject sits with the legs straight out in front and tries to reach the toes (figure 23.1). How close to or how far beyond the toes the person can reach is the flexibility score. That test has been standardized, and scores can be compared with others in the relevant age group (see chapter 3). Keep in mind that all flexibility tests are measuring flexibility only in the tested muscles and joints. Someone could score well on a sit-and-reach test but then do poorly on a flexibility test for the ankles or shoulders.

A test to measure shoulder flexibility is the shoulder elevation test (figure 23.2). To perform this test, the subject lies on his or her belly with one or both arms straight out over the head, as if pretending to fly. The person grasps a yardstick with the hands (or one hand, if using only one arm for the test) about 12 inches (30.5 cm) apart. He or she then raises the yardstick as high off the ground as possible while keeping the arms straight and the rest of the body still. The height that the person can raise the yardstick is the score.

The wall test is designed to give a quick assessment of upper-body flexibility, particularly of the shoulder girdle. To perform this test, the subject places the heels, hips, upper back, and head against a wall. He or she then bends the elbows at 90 degrees and brings the elbows to shoulder height with the hands up (figure 23.3). A person with normal shoulder flexibility should be able to place the elbows and forearms against the wall without losing any of the previously established points of contact or excessively arching the back. From there, the person slides the arms up and down, maintaining a 90-degree bend in the elbow. The personal trainer is looking for points, if any, where the elbows and forearms come off the wall. This test does not identify people who have high levels of flexibility, but it does a good job of assessing those with poor flexibility. Clients who struggle with this test often

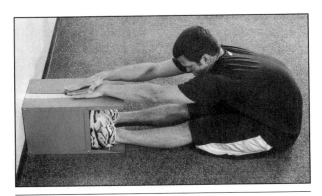

Figure 23.1 Sit-and-reach flexibility test.

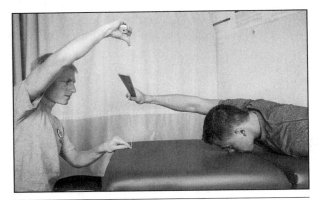

Figure 23.2 Shoulder elevation flexibility test.

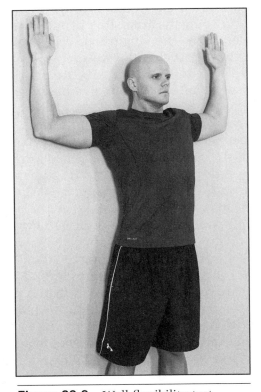

Figure 23.3 Wall flexibility test.

have tight internal rotators of the shoulder or a rounded upper back, which can lead to postural problems and potential shoulder problems in the future (1). Clients who have a hard time with this test also have a hard time completing military (shoulder) press exercises with proper technique.

The overhead squat is a good test to assess the flexibility of many muscles of the body at the same time. It requires clients to stand up, lift their arms over the head, and then squat down. The personal trainer is looking at the alignment and position of the thoracic region of the trunk, the lower back, and the legs. How the body compensates to get into the low squatting position can provide an idea of the muscles that are tight.

FACTORS THAT AFFECT FLEXIBILITY

Several factors affect a person's flexibility. Some of these factors can be changed and controlled, but others cannot. Normally, the goal of a flexibility program is to maintain or optimize the natural range of motion for that joint.

Joint Type

A joint is found anywhere two bones meet. As mentioned earlier, some joints are more flexible than others. The most flexible type of joint in the body is called a ball-and-socket joint. It has this name because the bone looks like a ball that is inserted into a socket. The bone can then swivel around in that socket to produce movement. Ball-and-socket joints can produce all the normal movements of the body and can function in any plane. The shoulder and hip are the two ball-and-socket joints in the body. Of those two, the shoulder joint is more flexible. The hip is also flexible, but it gives up some of its flexibility for stability. That tradeoff is common; more flexibility requires less stability and vice versa. For example, people have a larger ROM at the shoulder than they do at the hip, but the shoulder is more likely to be hurt or to be dislocated than the hip is (97).

Body Shape and Limb Length

The overall shape of the body has an effect on flexibility. A person with short arms will do poorly on a shoulder extension or sit-and-reach test. Someone who has extra-long arms will perform better on those types of tests. Generally, the shorter, stockier body types do not have the same level of flexibility as the thinner, wiry types. But all people can significantly improve their flexibility over time.

Activity Level

You may have heard the saying "Use it or lose it." This maxim is normally applied to muscle, because if you build up muscle but then stop exercising, most of the extra muscle will go away. The same is true of flexibility. People who practice flexibility frequently and perform activities such as yoga and regular stretching will increase their flexibility. But not being active or discontinuing a former activity will cause a decrease in flexibility. So the combination of getting older and becoming less active results in a reduction of flexibility. Staying active and regularly using the body in its natural range of motion will help improve, or at least maintain, a normal level of flexibility.

Age

Age has an effect on flexibility. Children, particularly young children, tend to be extremely flexible because their tissues are not as stiff as adults' tissues, they have less muscle than adults do, and some of their bones are not fused together as they are in adulthood, particularly the bones in the spine and hip (17). Their joints therefore have a greater ROM than the joints of adults do, thus giving them greater flexibility. As we age, our flexibility decreases. Normally, this decline does not significantly affect our health until our lack of flexibility causes us to have trouble getting up off the floor or tying our shoes. As we age, our muscle tissue atrophies. In its place, the body lays down connective tissue, which is a process called fibrosis. This connective tissue is much harder and less pliable than muscle tissue, so it is less flexible. Aging alone results in a usually manageable decrease in flexibility. Unfortunately, the effects of aging are often combined with a lack of physical activity, which can also result in a decrease in flexibility.

Weight Training

Clients often ask whether weight training will affect their flexibility. The answer is yes. Of course, the next question is about how weight training will affect their flexibility. Will it make them more flexible or less flexible? The answer is, "It depends." That answer may not be what they were looking for, but it is the truth.

If a client starts an exercise program being very inflexible, using a full range of motion on exercises will normally result in an increase in flexibility. For example, if a person has difficulty bringing the hands back to the chest, as in a bench press, regularly performing a bench press and attempting to reach a full range of motion will increase flexibility over time. One word of caution is needed here. Do not have your clients use heavy weights to force the body to stretch. The weight that people normally lift or even slightly less than that will be effective at increasing flexibility.

On the other hand, if a client starts an exercise program being very flexible, weight training will probably result in a decrease in flexibility. This decline can usually be offset with heavy stretching after the workout. Working out tends to tighten up loose muscles, which is an undesirable side effect for some people, such as martial artists, gymnasts, and ballet dancers. Reducing the intensity of the weight training can help combat this tightening, as can lifting through a full range of motion and aggressively and regularly stretching the trained muscles. Stretching between resistance training sets can be particularly effective.

Weight training can have some specific effects on flexibility if training is done in a certain way. For example, regularly or exclusively using partial reps and heavy weights can shorten the muscles' natural range of motion. For example, performing bicep curls in which the elbow does not extend more than 90 degrees can result in a shortening of the biceps muscle and tendon. The natural position of the arm will become bent, and straightening the arm, formerly a natural movement, will feel like a significant stretch (135).

Weight training builds muscle, and large muscles can sometimes interfere with the range of motion at a joint. This issue is most prevalent with the upper body. For instance, if your biceps are particularly large, they can prevent you from bending your elbow as much as someone who has smaller biceps because the biceps literally get in the way. For that reason, Olympic lifters do not train the biceps because they can interfere with the proper position when holding a bar in the clean and jerk.

TYPES OF STRETCHING

There are four main types of flexibility exercises. With all of them, the goal is to move the muscle's insertion away from the origin or vice versa. As with most aspects of fitness, each method of stretching has something positive about it.

Static Stretching

The most basic type of stretching is static stretching, a passive stretch that can be done with or without a partner. This type of stretching may be the safest because the movements are slow and gentle. Overstretching a muscle is possible, so care should be taken, particularly when recruiting a partner to help perform the exercises. In static stretching, clients get into a position that induces a mild stretch and then hold that position, normally for 15 to 30 seconds. If the stretch feels good and clients feel as if they are getting something out of the stretch, they can go longer, even up to several minutes. Breathing deeply during the stretch is important, and with each exhale, clients should try to get slightly more out of the stretch (9, 15). The stretch should go to the point of mild discomfort, but not severe pain. On an intensity scale of 1 to 10, with 1 being no stretch and 10 being extreme, something in the range of a 4 or 5 is the goal. The muscle held in position may possibly tighten up and make the stretch

uncomfortable. If that happens, decreasing the range of motion slightly is OK. A stretch for each muscle is usually performed one to three times. The goal is for the flexibility of that muscle and joint to increase over time (11). See figures 23.4 through 23.15 for the common static flexibility exercises.

If possible, clients should have some objective method of measuring how far they can stretch. It can be something simple such as noting that they can reach the top row of the shoelaces, then the third row, then the end of the shoes, then the ground, and finally the ground with all the fingertips. Having a point of reference for objective measurement will encourage clients to stretch intensely enough to increase their flexibility.

Dynamic Stretching

This type of stretching is active and involves movement on the part of the person doing it. Dynamic stretches are rarely done with a partner. Dynamic stretches are quick, controlled movements that do not involve bouncing at the end of the range of motion. A swimmer performing arm circles or a punter kicking his leg in the air are examples of dynamic stretches. Each dynamic stretch normally takes one or two seconds to perform, and as with lifting weights, clients normally perform a certain number of reps for each dynamic stretch. Eight to 12 reps is most common. After 20 reps the muscle gets tired and does not stretch as well. Dynamic stretches are most commonly used by athletes, but anyone can benefit from doing them (70, 95, 100).

Ballistic Stretching

A ballistic stretch is like a dynamic stretch that adds bouncing at the end of the range of motion. Leaning forward to touch the toes and then bouncing in that position is an example of a ballistic stretch. Ballistic stretching carries a higher risk of injury, which is why it is not often performed. Some clients enjoy ballistic stretches because they can feel the muscle being worked, although almost any form of stretching that is effective will be felt. A ballistic

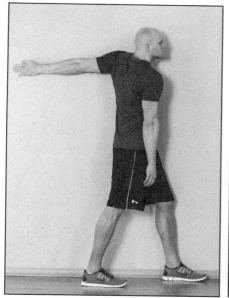

Figure 23.4   Chest stretch.

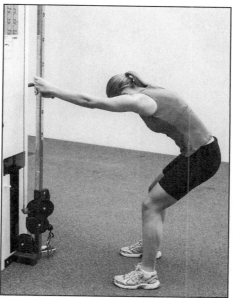

Figure 23.5   Lat stretch.

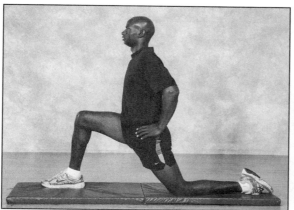

Figure 23.6   Hip flexor stretch.

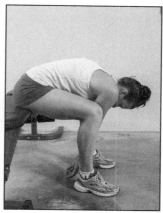

Figure 23.7   Erector spinae stretch.

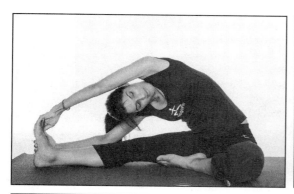

Figure 23.8   Quadratus lumborum stretch.

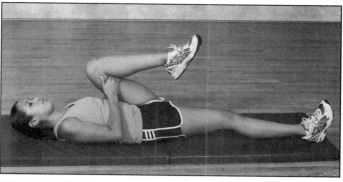

Figure 23.9   Glute stretch.

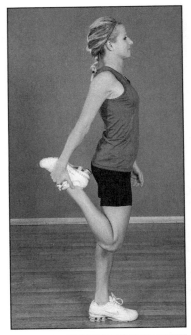
Figure 23.10   Quad stretch.

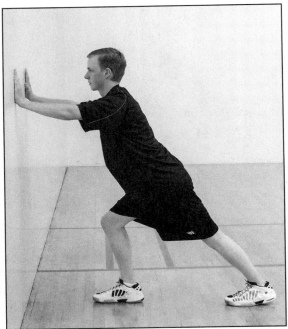
Figure 23.11   Gastroc stretch.

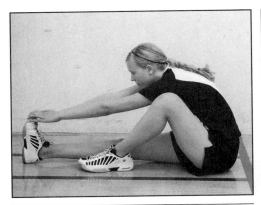
Figure 23.12   Hamstring stretch.

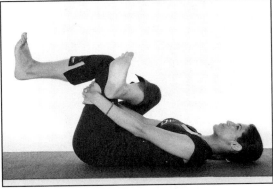
Figure 23.13   Piriformis stretch.

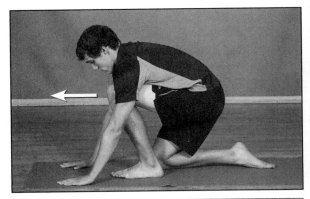
Figure 23.14   Soleus stretch.

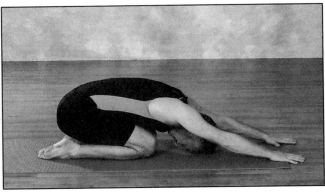
Figure 23.15   Child's pose stretch.

stretch causes the muscle spindle to activate, which might help prepare that muscle group for action, but a stretch that is performed too frequently might desensitize the muscle spindle and result in stretch reflex (118).

Proprioceptive Neuromuscular Facilitation Stretching

This type of stretching, typically abbreviated as PNF, involves sequentially contracting and relaxing a muscle. PNF stretching is effective at increasing flexibility, and anecdotal evidence suggests that it increases static flexibility faster than regular static or dynamic stretching does. The movements involve the contraction of a muscle, so they require more effort and burn more calories than a regular stretch does. PNF stretching is not considered a workout, but it is more active than static stretching. In addition, strength can be increased through PNF stretching, particularly in the ends of the range of motion and when the initial strength levels are low. This type of stretching can be particularly beneficial for older adults, although they must take care not to overexert during the stretches (8).

All PNF stretches have a similar pattern that includes three or more parts. The first part is a static stretch that is normally held for 10 to 15 seconds. The second part involves contracting the stretched muscle for about 6 seconds (as a general guideline). There is nothing magical about 6 seconds as opposed to 5 or 7 seconds, but 6 seconds is long enough to build significant tension in the muscle without tiring the muscle or promoting cramping. The third phase involves another static stretch of the muscle, normally lasting 10 to 30 seconds. This stretch is more intense than the first static stretch.

There are four main types of PNF stretches (132):

Hold–Relax

- Statically stretch the targeted muscle for 10 to 15 seconds.
- Contract the targeted muscle for 6 seconds with no movement (i.e., perform an isometric contraction).

- Statically stretch the targeted muscle for 10 to 30 seconds but at a greater intensity than before.

Contract–Relax

- Statically stretch the targeted muscle for 10 to 15 seconds.
- Contract the targeted muscle for 6 seconds with movement and then allow the limb to return to the starting point through a concentric contraction.
- Statically stretch the targeted muscle for 10 to 30 seconds but at a greater intensity than before.

Hold–Relax With Antagonist Contraction

- Statically stretch the targeted muscle for 10 to 15 seconds.
- Contract the targeted muscle for 6 seconds with no movement (perform an isometric contraction).
- Contract the muscle opposite the targeted muscle to pull the limb farther into the stretch and statically stretch the muscle for 10 to 30 seconds.

    Note: Some sources call this stretch a hold–relax with agonist contraction, but the agonist is the muscle being stretched and the one first being contracted. The antagonist is the muscle opposite the one being stretched (and focused on), so the name is hold–relax with antagonist contraction.

Hold–Relax Repeated

- Static stretch the muscle for 10 to 15 seconds.
- Contract the targeted muscle for 6 seconds with no movement (perform an isometric contraction).
- Statically stretch the targeted muscle for 10 seconds but at a greater intensity than before.
- Contract the targeted muscle for 6 seconds with no movement (perform an isometric contraction).

- Statically stretch the targeted muscle for 10 seconds but at a greater intensity than before.
- Contract the targeted muscle for 6 seconds with no movement (perform an isometric contraction).
- Statically stretch the targeted muscle for 10 to 30 seconds but at a greater intensity than before.

The hold–relax repeated flexibility exercise takes the longest to perform, but many clients comment that they enjoy it the most. It involves multiple muscle contractions, which in turn allows a greater stretch of the muscle. It is essentially the hold–relax stretch repeated two more times in the same sequence.

The principle behind PNF stretching is that a muscle is most flexible immediately after it contracts. This phenomenon is called autogenic inhibition. Autogenic inhibition occurs because muscle tension stimulates the Golgi tendon organ, which in turns increases the relaxation of that muscle after the contraction is stopped. Keep in mind this is an immediate effect. People will not get this effect if they contract their muscles, relax, get a drink of water, and then stretch. The instant that they stop contracting their muscles, they need to increase the stretch, within one second or less.

In the hold–relax with antagonist contraction stretching exercise, the body is taking advantage of a phenomenon called reciprocal inhibition, which occurs when the contraction of a muscle forces its antagonist to relax. Taking advantage of reciprocal inhibition is also useful when people have a muscle that is cramping. When that occurs, people want to contract the opposite muscle. Normally, the hamstrings cramp near the knee, so in that case people would want to contract the quads and straighten the knee. This contraction of the opposite muscle forces the cramped muscle to relax.

WHEN TO PERFORM FLEXIBILITY EXERCISES

Personal trainers are often asked, "When should I stretch out?" With a few exceptions, it is rarely a bad time to stretch, so people should stretch whenever they want to. The three main times to stretch in relation to exercise are before a workout, during a training or exercise session, and after a workout.

Before a Workout

Some clients like to stretch before they exercise. This order is common, and stretching can serve as part of the warm-up. General stretching is normally completed after a total body warm-up, such as walking on the treadmill for five minutes. If the workout is going to involve a challenging range of motion, then stretching before the workout is definitely a good idea. For example, if a client's shoulders are very stiff and he or she may not be able to bring the bar all the way down to the chest for the chest press, the client should stretch out before performing that exercise (80).

While stretching before exercising is acceptable, some people have the mistaken idea that it is mandatory. Warming up is certainly a good idea, but stretching does not need to be a part of the warm-up. If clients are training for strength or power, or plan on lifting very heavy weights, stretching before they work out is likely not a good idea. Numerous studies and anecdotal evidence have shown that stretching before lifting heavy weights decreases maximal strength. The effect is not huge, but even a 3 to 5 percent difference can be significant with large amounts of weight. Maximal strength declines because stretching, particularly static stretching, desensitizes the stretch reflex and loosens the muscles. When training for strength and power, people want a sensitive, active stretch reflex and tight muscles. The muscles should be flexible enough to perform the exercise properly but tight enough to provide a good rebound at the end of the range of motion. Dynamic stretches do not seem to cause the same reduction in strength and power as static stretches do, so if people wish to stretch before an event and want to achieve maximal performance, dynamic stretching exercises are the best choice (126).

A drawback of stretching before exercise is that the muscle is cold and likely to be stiff. In terms of flexibility performance, better results are attained after warming up. The chance of injury is also slightly greater when stretching cold (6). People are usually the coldest and the stiffest when they first get out of bed in the morning, so some flexibility experts advocate stretching first thing in the morning. Not all experts agree with this recommendation, because people are stiff for a reason. The synovial fluid in the joints might be low, and some evidence indicates that the disks in the vertebral column are also low on fluid when people first get up. These conditions will compromise the ability of the joints to withstand much bending and stretching.

During Exercise

Many people like to stretch while they are in the middle of exercising, and this approach can also be beneficial. The muscles tighten up during the exercise and produce waste products. Stretching can help counteract this tightness and, by promoting blood flow, can help remove the waste products. The muscles are usually warm at this point, so stretching them during exercise gives good results. Stretching during an exercise session can also be an efficient use of time. If people are going to spend 10 minutes stretching and they spread that out during the workout when they would just be passively resting, they will have 10 minutes at the end to spend on additional training.

Stretching while exercising is not advisable for strength and power athletes for the same reason that stretching before exercise is not a good idea (14). But after the core exercises are completed, stretching during the assistance exercises can be effective and saves time, and the minor loss of power is likely not noticeable. Personal trainers should note that stretching between intense resistance training sets is likely to reduce the pump in a muscle, which some experts believe is key to stretching out the fascia and promoting muscle growth.

After Exercise

Most experts believe that the best time to stretch is after exercise. The muscles are warmest at this time, and stretching cannot negatively affect performance because the performance part of the workout has ended. Stretching at the end of a workout can also function as part of the cool-down. Some research shows that stretching after working out can help reduce, but not eliminate, muscle soreness.

Guidelines for Stretching

- Try to stretch at the end of each workout.
- Stretch each muscle a minimum of two times per week.
- Stretching should normally last 5 to 15 minutes.
- Stretch to the point of mild discomfort.
- Try to have each side of the body be evenly flexible.
- Breathe deeply and try to relax when stretching.
- Focus on the shoulder girdle, trunk, and hip flexibility.
- Stretch on a stable surface.

EXTREME STRETCHING

Another type of stretching is called extreme stretching. Suggested by John Parillo and Dante Trudel, extreme stretching uses weights to produce a stretch on the area more intense than what is felt in a regular stretching routine. The hypothesis behind this idea is that extreme stretching, much like a pump, will expand and stretch the fascia (i.e., the endomysium, perimysium, and epimysium) surrounding the muscle tissue. The thought is that the space available inside the fascia can limit the total amount of muscle tissue that the body can add; after the available space is filled with muscle fibers, no new fibers or myofibrils can be added. Extreme stretching is put forth as a method to create more space. Studies of humans have produced little scientific evidence of this theory, but evidence from animal studies gives credence to the theory; for example, if weights are hung from a bird's wing, the chest muscle of the bird will grow new muscle fibers. Caution should be used if this method is used on clients.

STRETCHING TOOLS

A variety of tools are available to the personal trainer to aid in improving clients' flexibility and performance.

Yoga Strap

A simple and inexpensive strap (see figure 23.16) allows people to replicate the effects of having a partner while working alone. By folding or looping the strap over a limb, people can use the arms or legs to achieve a better stretch. People can attempt to simulate some of the PNF stretches this way.

Foam Roller

Foam rollers have experienced a surge in popularity in the last 10 years. The essential idea is that they loosely replicate soft-tissue massage, sometimes referred to as myofascial release. The rolling action over tight or knotted soft tissue can open it up and cause it to become more mobile. Most of the muscles in the body can be foam rolled. The general idea is to start at either the origin or insertion of the muscle and roll the full length of the muscle. People can apply more or less pressure as desired, and many kinds of foam rollers are available. The softer, less dense foam rollers are easier to use and better for beginners or for use on muscles with many adhesions and knots. The harder, denser foam rollers are better for more experienced clients or for use on healthier muscles that are no longer receptive to the softer foam rollers. A good recommendation is to roll the length of the muscle slowly, covering an inch (2.5 cm) per second. People should go slow and try to force the muscle to relax as much as possible. They should note the location of sensitive areas or trigger spots and return to them. They can sit on the sensitive spot for approximately 30 seconds, or until the pain diminishes, before moving on. If a muscle is sensitive, people should try to hit at least two trigger points before moving on to another muscle. Muscles usually have various angles of pennation or separate heads, so angling the foam roller to hit as much of the muscle as possible is a good technique (for example, when foam rolling the calf, people can point the toes in, out, and straight up) (149). See figure 23.17 for an example of a common type of foam roller.

Balls

In some areas of the body, the foam roller is too broad or not dense enough to apply enough pressure. To create the needed pressure, people can use a ball for a specific pressure point (see figure 23.18). The ball can be a racquetball, tennis ball, or a lacrosse ball; those balls are listed in order from low density to high density.

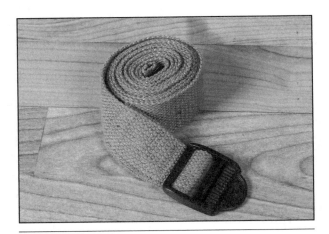

Figure 23.16 Yoga strap.

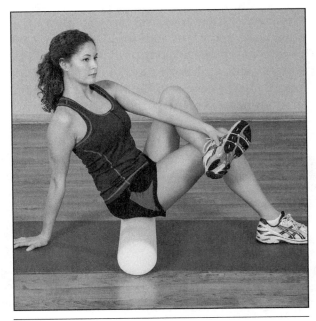

Figure 23.17 Foam roller.

Specific spots where balls tend to work well include but are not limited to the bottom of the feet, the calves, the distal portion of the quad, the piriformis and the abductors, the pec minor, and the rhomboids (88).

Bands

Some of the bands found in the gym, particularly jump stretch or flex bands, can be used to get a good stretch (figure 23.19). The band can be looped around an area such as the hand or foot and attached to a stable base like a power rack. The person can then use the band to stretch out the desired area. The more the band is stretched, the more tension or stretch it will apply to the targeted area.

STRETCHING ORDER

To prepare for an intense activity, people should first perform a general warm-up. They follow that up with some soft-tissue massage using the foam roller or a ball. They then stretch each area with a yoga strap or bands by performing static or PNF flexibility exercises,

attempting to activate the area by performing dynamic stretches and other muscular activation techniques. They can round out their preparation by performing a specific warm-up, such as doing three or four warm-up sets of squats to prepare for a squat workout, and then start the real workout. This process does not have to require a significant amount of time. The whole process, not including the specific warm-up sets, can be completed in 10 minutes or less. You can show clients how to do this on their own. After mastering the routine, they can arrive 10 or 15 minutes early to run through their preparation so that they do not use up their time with you. Of course, the time spent in stretching is not wasted at all if it keeps people healthy and better prepares them for their activity.

CONCLUSION

Flexibility is the range of motion at a joint. The body has various types of joints. Common tests for flexibility include the sit-and-reach test, wall test, shoulder elevation test, and the overhead squat assessment. Many factors can

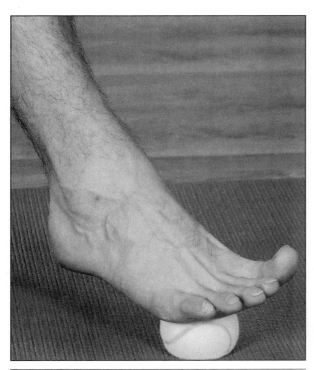

Figure 23.18 Using a ball for self-administered myofascial release.

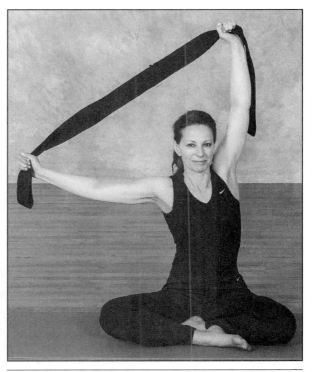

Figure 23.19 Using a band to enhance stretching.

affect flexibility, including the type of joint moving, body shape, activity level, age, and weight training.

Personal trainers can use several types of stretches on their clients. These stretches can be static, dynamic, ballistic, or they can involve the use of various proprioceptors such as PNF stretching. Stretching can be performed before, during, or after training, but it is most commonly performed after training because a client is warmed up and any potential loss of power will not negatively affect performance at that time. Personal trainers can incorporate a variety of tools to improve their clients' flexibility. These tools consist of yoga straps, foam rollers, balls, and exercise bands and tubes.

Flexibility is one of the fundamental components of fitness. Abnormal ranges of motion can predispose a client to injury. Personal trainers should have a solid understanding of what flexibility is, what affects it, and how to modify a client's current flexibility level.

Study Questions

1. Which type of joint displays a greater range of motion?
   a. synovial joint
   b. cartilaginous joint
   c. fibrous joint
   d. fused joint

2. When performed before activity, which type of stretching is most associated with a loss of strength and power?
   a. dynamic stretching
   b. ballistic stretching
   c. static stretching
   d. PNF stretching

3. What is the principle behind PNF stretching?
   a. A muscle will contract hardest immediately after it has been stretched.
   b. A muscle is most flexible immediately after it contracts.
   c. Contracting one muscle will force its antagonist to relax.
   d. Stimulating the muscle spindles results in a stronger muscular contraction.

4. As we age, our bodies lay down more collagen fibers in the muscle tissue. What is this process called?
   a. sarcolemma
   b. collagen remodeling
   c. fibrosis
   d. sarcopenia

5. When first introducing myofascial release to the client, what type of tool should be used?
   a. relatively soft, broad, and not dense—a low-density foam roller
   b. relatively firm, broad, and quite dense—a high-density foam roller
   c. relatively soft, small, and pinpoint—a tennis ball
   d. relatively hard, small, and pinpoint—a lacrosse ball

Power and Speed Development

In addition to the five components of fitness previously studied, a few additional subcomponents of fitness—speed and power—are important for personal trainers to understand, especially if they have clients who are preparing for a sport-related event or desiring to improve performance in a sport-related activity.

TERMS RELATED TO POWER AND SPEED

A helpful first step is to define the various subcomponents that a client might wish to improve. The definitions might seem a bit weighty and unwieldy at first, but they serve as an important starting point. The principle of specificity tells us that to produce a specific adaptation, people must train in a precise way. A wide receiver, a 100-meter sprinter, an Olympic weightlifter, and a powerlifter cannot all follow the same training program and expect to excel in their chosen sports. As people advance in their sports, the more specific their programs must become.

Strength

Strength, the ability of the muscle to contract maximally one time, does not consider a person's body size, weight, or composition. Therefore, it can be referred to as absolute strength or maximum strength.

Relative Strength

The absolute strength of a person in proportion to his or her body size, weight, or composition is called relative strength. To calculate it, divide the weight lifted by the person's body weight. This formula usually favors lighter people. Other formulas, such as the Wilk and Schwartz formulas, have been developed to counteract this bias. The Wilk formula looks like this:

$$Coeff = \frac{500}{a + b * x + c * x^2 + d * x^3 + e * x^4 + f * x^5}$$

where

x is the body weight of the person (in kilograms) and the coefficients for men are

a = −216.0475144

b = 16.2606339

c = −0.002388645

d = −0.00113732

e = 7.01863×10^{-6}

f = $−1.291 \times 10^{-8}$

The coefficients for women are

a = 594.31747775582

b = −27.23842536447

c = 0.82112226871

d = −0.00930733913

e = 0.00004731582

f = −0.00000009054

Larger people usually express greater absolute strength, and smaller people usually express greater relative strength. Absolute strength is more important in sports such as football and rugby, and relative strength is more important in sports such as gymnastics, sprinting, and basketball.

Maximal Speed

The highest velocity that a person can achieve while sprinting is called maximal speed. Most people can sprint over 15 miles per hour (24.1 km/h), faster people will be in the range of 20 to 25 miles per hour (32.2–40.2 km/h), and elite sprinters might be close to 30 miles per hour (48.3 km/h) (208). Note that these speeds are not average speeds attained during a race, in a 100-meter dash, for example, but are momentary top speeds that are generally not maintained for a significant time.

Agility

A person's ability to decelerate, change direction (or at least have the option to do so), and then accelerate again is agility. This ability is related to maximal speed, but the correlation is not perfect. The most agile person is not necessarily the fastest and vice versa. High levels of agility are demonstrated by wide receivers, racquetball players, and tennis players. Agility is measured by the shuttle run or T-test (155).

Speed Strength and Strength Speed

These two terms are sometimes interchanged, but they have separate meanings. Speed strength is the ability to perform work quickly against an unloaded or light resistance, whereas strength speed is the ability to move quickly against a heavy resistance.

Starting Strength and Acceleration Strength

The ability of the muscles to develop force in the beginning of a movement, before a concentric action occurs, is referred to as starting strength. This ability is contrasted to acceleration strength, which is the ability to achieve maximal external force quickly. Concentric movement is produced after the movement has already started (125).

Explosive Strength, or Power

The ability of muscles to produce maximal force in a minimal time is explosive strength,

or power. The classic physics definition of power is

$$\text{Power (P)} = \text{Work (W)} \div \text{Time (T)}$$

Work

Work is the amount of effort performed, and it increases not only with greater effort but also when that effort is given through a greater distance (range of motion). The classic physics definition of work is

$$W = \text{Force (F)} \times \text{Distance (D)}$$

Force

A force is the muscular effort given by a person to push or pull on an object, typically an external load or resistance. The classic physics definition of force is

$$F = \text{Mass (M)} \times \text{Acceleration (A)}$$

Mass is commonly considered to be the weight or load lifted, although in a pure physics sense, there is more to that definition.

Although you, as a personal trainer, should know the classic physics formulas, you should recognize that because the force produced in muscular work is almost never constant, the precise nature of those formulas limits their usefulness in a practical context. You should focus more on the following key concepts:

- The highest levels of force are not generated by lifting a maximal weight because the weight is moved slowly (at low acceleration).

- The highest levels of force are not generated by lifting a light weight as fast as possible because the weight lifted is low.

- The highest levels of force are generated by lifting a medium weight (about 40 to 60 percent of 1RM in most instances) as fast as possible.

- The more work that is performed, the more difficult the action or exercise is. Longer limbed and taller people usually have a greater ROM in most exercises and thus are at a disadvantage when attempting to demonstrate maximal strength.

- To generate high levels of power, the action must be executed rapidly, decreasing the time needed to complete the movement (any number divided by a smaller number yields a larger quotient).

FOUR CATEGORIES OF MOVEMENTS

A useful approach for personal trainers is to separate all movements into one of four categories, based on the speed of movement and the external resistance involved. This approach can aid you in allocating the appropriate time to training specific abilities and developing the best program for your clients.

Low Speed, Light Resistance

In category 1, a person uses light or no resistance coupled with a low speed. Fitness level and strength have little bearing on this ability. This ability is not improved in the gym. Movements of this type are referred to as skill, and that skill must be practiced repeatedly with proper technique to achieve mastery. Examples include drawing, painting, typing, billiards, shuffleboard, dribbling a soccer ball or basketball, and putting in golf (187).

High Speed, Light Resistance

In category 2, a person generates a high level of speed (the body or involved limb is moving rapidly) and is working against relatively light resistance. This movement is primarily a representation of a person's speed strength, although starting strength and acceleration strength also contribute. Examples of this type of movement include pitching a baseball, swinging a baseball bat, throwing a ball, punching, kicking, driving a golf ball off the tee, swinging a racket, and maintaining speed in sprinting (maintaining maximal speed after it has been achieved). This type of activity is common in sport but is not usually trained in the gym. Guidelines for improving this ability are provided in this chapter (187).

Low Speed, Heavy Resistance

In category 3, a person works against high external resistance and is moving the resistance relatively slowly, not necessarily intentionally. The high weight simply forces the person to lift it slowly. This type of activity is commonly performed in the gym. Examples of this type of movement include lifting heavy weights, playing tug of war, pushing against an opposing lineman, arm wrestling someone of similar ability, dragging a weighted sled, pushing the prowler, lifting a heavy object, or resisting the movement of a heavy object (an eccentric muscle action). Training to improve this ability should follow the guidelines for increasing maximal strength (187).

High Speed, Heavy Resistance

Category 4 movements are also referred to as power movements. They require a person to work against high external resistance and move that resistance rapidly. This type of training can be performed in the gym, although untrained beginners and general fitness exercisers often do not focus on improving this ability. A person's explosive strength combined with acceleration strength and strength speed are important to this ability. Examples of this type of movement include Olympic weightlifting exercises such as the snatch, clean, jerk, and push press. Additional examples are running into and tackling someone, wrestling and throwing an opponent to the ground, putting the shot, the start phase of a sprint, squat jumps, and a variety of plyometric exercises. Training to improve this ability should follow the guidelines to improve Olympic lifting and power provided in this chapter (187).

DIFFERENCES BETWEEN STRENGTH AND POWER

Many people use the terms *strength* and *power* interchangeably, but in the fitness world, the meanings are different. Strength is demonstrated by lifting a heavy weight without any consideration of the time required to lift the weight. A person who can bench press

400 pounds (181.4 kg) demonstrates a high level of strength, even if eight seconds are needed to complete the concentric portion of the lift. If another person benches 400 pounds, his or her level of strength would be the same because the total weight lifted is equal. But if the lift takes the second person only two seconds to complete, the second person would have demonstrated significantly greater power than the first person.

The difference between power and strength is important because in many real-life events outside the gym and in many events on the field, court, mat, or ring, power is a better predictor of ability than pure maximal strength. This difference is explained by a concept called the rate of force development (RFD), which describes how rapidly a person's force is developed. For a more detailed look at this concept, refer to figure 24.1.

Note that the figure has four curved lines. They indicate people who are untrained and people who train for strength, power, and endurance. Force is measured on the vertical axis of the graph, and time is measured on the horizontal axis.

This concept should help explain what we often see in everyday life. Baseball pitchers

and American football quarterbacks do not usually have exceptional 1RM bench presses, yet they can throw a ball better than someone who can lift heavier loads in that exercise. Sprinters and high jumpers are not necessarily able to lift high loads in the squat, yet they will outsprint and outjump a person who can squat more than they can. The strength generated in those two examples (the bench press and the squat) does not have a dramatic effect on athletic performance. That is not to say that strength is irrelevant; instead, the point is that strength is not the only factor to consider when trying to improve those abilities.

TRAINING TO IMPROVE POWER

Power is a neuromuscular-specific activity. In addition to the simple power that muscle fibers can generate, two other factors contribute to the expression of power (figure 24.2). The first factor is the elastic properties in muscle tissue and its fascia, which allow the tissue to stretch and return to its original shape (8). These properties are referred to as the series elastic components (SEC) of the muscle. The second factor is proprioceptors, namely the muscle spindles, which detect any stretch on the muscle and cause a resulting contraction.

Powerful activities involve three movements performed in a set sequence. The first movement is the eccentric, or lengthening, phase. This phase serves to stretch out the SEC and stimulate the muscle spindles. Remember that the spindles do not have to be stretched to the maximum to cause the contraction; in fact, they are more sensitive to the speed of the stretch than to the range of motion of the stretch. A fast eccentric phase, even if it involves a small range of motion, will still elicit a strong stretch reflex (25). Almost all powerful movements involve this initial stretch phase. When throwing a football, the first movement produced is to pull back the arm. Swinging a golf club, pitching a baseball, throwing a punch, kicking a ball, swinging a bat, and jumping all involve

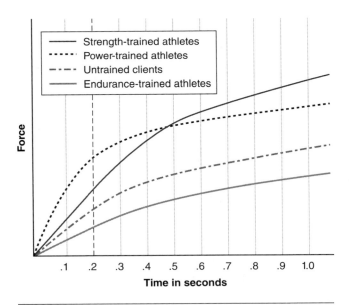

Figure 24.1 Rate of force development among trained and untrained populations.
Based on Häkkinen and Komi 1985.

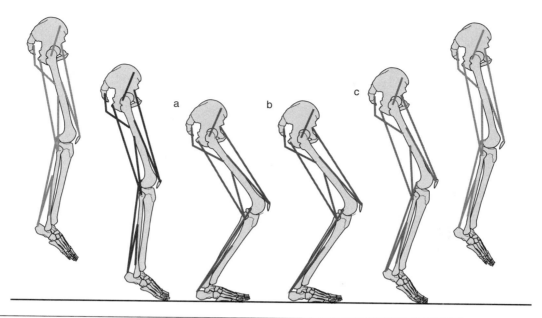

Figure 24.2 Three phases in a plyometric movement.

Reproduced with permission of *Annual Review of Biomedical Engineering,* Volume 11: 81-107, © Annual Reviews, www.annualreviews.org.

this quick eccentric phase. Eliminating this phase will significantly compromise the power produced in the movement.

The second phase is called the amortization, or transition, phase. This phase describes the switch from the previous eccentric movement to the ensuing concentric phase. To produce a high level of power, the amortization phase must be short. Otherwise, the SEC and stretch reflex will begin to dissipate and the subsequent power produced will be compromised. In other words, adding a lengthy pause (for example, three seconds or longer) between the eccentric and concentric phases of all the activities listed in the previous paragraph would cause a significant decrease in performance.

The third phase is the concentric, or shortening, phase. This is the phase when the action seems to happen, but coaches and personal trainers should focus on all three phases of movement, not just the concentric phase.

When considering training for power, you need to know which type of power you are looking to improve. A shot putter and a baseball pitcher both display tremendous power, but logic dictates that their two training programs will be quite different. Again, the movement classification system applies. Two

of the categories of movement involve high expressions of power: category 2 (high speed, light resistance) and category 4 (high speed, heavy resistance).

NPTI's system of exercise program design can be used to design a resistance program for increasing power. The system will be used twice—first to increase power in category 2 movements and second to increase power in category 4 movements. Additionally, plyometric training will increase power.

Define and Clarify the Goal: Increasing Power With High-Speed, Light Resistance Exercises

The purpose of this program is to improve the client's ability to generate high speed (the body or involved limb is moving rapidly) while working against relatively light resistance.

List the Expected Outcomes

After following a program designed for power, the client should be able to move light resistance objects significantly faster, thus generating more force.

List the Expected Physiological Adaptations

Specific changes take place in the body when a client follows a category 2 power training program:

- Increased neuromuscular coordination
- Increased rate of force development
- Decreased reaction time

Analyze the Program Setup

Creating a program to build power will generally have the client training two to four times a week and hitting each area or movement two to four times a week.

Select the Specific Routine

The most common routines to improve power are total-body routines; push–pull or upper–lower setups can be used as well (see table 24.1 for examples).

Select the Number of Resistance Training Exercises per Workout

Training for power against a light resistance will usually include four to eight resistance training exercises per workout.

Select the Number of Resistance Training Exercises per Body Part or Movement

Typically, one or two exercises are performed for each body part.

Select the Specific Exercises

To build power against light resistance, exercises should be selected that the client can complete safely at high speed (table 24.2).

Traditional machines are less likely to be incorporated, but medicine balls, barbells, body weight, and band exercises can be used. When training for power, smaller muscle groups such as biceps or triceps are usually not isolated, so few exercises will be listed for those areas. Most exercise selections are based on movements rather than muscles when the goal is increased power.

Put the Exercises in Their Proper Order

Exercise order is important when training for power. Clients should start with the bigger, higher-skill exercises first, but you may choose to have the client alternate exercises to avoid fatigue and maximize performance.

Select the Number of Reps per Work Set

The number of reps can vary when training for power against a light resistance; performing 5 to 20 reps per set is common.

Select the Load per Set

The load will be light because the client is working on improving power against light resistance; five out of every six sessions should use 20 percent of 1RM, and the remaining session (out of six) should use 40 percent of 1RM.

Select the Number of Work Sets per Exercise

When training for category 2 power, performing two to four work sets per exercise is suggested.

Table 24.1 Specific Light Resistance Power Routines and Their Corresponding Frequency

Total training sessions per week	Frequency of each area per week	Specific routine
4	2	Upper–lower repeated or push–pull repeated
4	4	Total body
3	3	Total body
2	2	Total body

Table 24.2   Ideal Exercises for Body Areas to Build Power Against Light Resistance

Chest	Back
Med ball chest pass	Med ball overhead throw
Med ball drop and catch	Standing band row
Bench press	Bent-over row
Push-up	Inverted row
Standing cable chest press	DB row
Shoulders and arms	**Total body**
Push press	Clean
Band face pull	Med ball thruster
Band lateral raise	Sprints

Clients are not expected to train only on these exercises or to perform all the exercises in every session.

Select the Number of Warm-Up Sets per Exercise

Warm-up sets are useful to get the mind and body ready to act quickly, but because the load is low, they are not as important as when training for strength or power against heavy resistance. For the first exercise in the session, one to three warm-up sets are usually used, and zero to two warm-up sets are used for each subsequent exercise.

Choose the Desired Weight Progression

Progression during the workout usually consists of straight sets. The client works on improving speed and form with that weight and fighting fatigue.

Confirm That the Selected Number of Reps per Set Matches the Goal Time Under Tension

Power exercises have a limited time under tension because the reps should be performed explosively; each set should be 10 seconds or less in duration.

Select the Appropriate Rest Time Between Sets

The typical rest time assigned is 30 seconds to 1 minute between sets.

Implement Any Tricks of the Trade to Elicit Faster Adaptations

When training for power a few tricks of the trade might be useful:

- Peripheral heart action
- Pairing a resistance exercise with a plyometric exercise for the same movement
- Using bands to build explosiveness (being careful that they do not completely change the motor pattern of the exercise)

Program an Appropriate Progressive Overload

Progressive overload is not as significant when training for power against a light resistance. It is more important for the client to increase his or her speed of movement and form and learn to fight fatigue. As the client gets stronger, the resistance can be increased slightly, but 20 percent of the 1RM even for strong people is still quite light. Mel Siff in *Supertraining* suggests that people can increase unloaded category 2 movement speeds by up to 150 percent with training (180).

Define and Clarify the Goal: Increasing Power with High-Speed, Heavy Resistance Exercises

The purpose of this program is to improve the client's ability to work against high external resistance and move that resistance rapidly.

List the Expected Outcomes

After following a program designed for power, the client should be able to move heavy resistance objects significantly faster, thus generating more force. The client may also increase maximal strength.

List the Expected Physiological Adaptations

Specific changes take place in the body when a client follows a category 4 power training program:

- Increased neuromuscular coordination
- Increased rate of force development
- Decreased reaction time
- Increased bone density
- Increased flexibility

Analyze the Program Setup

Creating a program to build power will generally have the client training two to four times a week and performing each exercise two to four times a week. Elite athletes often train several times a day on most days of the week.

Select the Specific Routine

The most common routines to improve power are total-body routines; push–pull or upper–lower setups can be used as well (see table 24.3 for examples). Routines are often centered on specific movements (such as the snatch or the clean) rather than parts of the body.

Select the Number of Resistance Training Exercises per Workout

Programs designed to improve power against a heavy resistance usually incorporate two to six resistance training exercises per workout.

Select the Number of Resistance Training Exercises per Body Part or Movement

One to four exercises per movement are usually selected.

Select the Specific Exercises

To build power against heavy resistance, exercises should be selected that allow the client to use a heavy weight, move that weight rapidly, and demonstrate a high degree of skill involvement (see table 24.4). Most commonly, free-weight barbell exercises are selected to build power against heavy resistance.

Put the Exercises in Their Proper Order

Exercise order is important when training for power. Clients should begin the session with the exercises that require the most skill, use the most speed, and involve the heaviest weight and then progress to the more standard exercises.

Select the Number of Reps per Work Set

The number of reps is usually low when training for power against heavy resistance. Performing one to five reps per set is common.

Select the Load per Set

The load needs to be heavy to build up power against heavy resistance. But if the load is too heavy, the speed of movement will be too slow. Loads of 75 to 90 percent of 1RM are usually recommended when training for power.

Table 24.3   Specific Heavy Resistance Power Routines and Their Corresponding Frequency

Total training sessions per week	Frequency of each area per week	Specific routine
4	2	Upper–lower repeated or push–pull repeated
4	4	Total body
3	3	Total body
2	2	Total body

Table 24.4 Ideal Exercises for Body Areas to Build Power Against Heavy Resistance

Chest	Back		Legs
Bench press Bench press throw Plyometric push-up	Pull-up Plyometric pull-up Bent-over row		Squats Jump squat Front squat Overhead squat

Shoulders and arms		Total body	
Push press Overhead press Power curl		Clean Jerks Snatch Jump Sprint Box jump	

People are not expected to train only on these exercises or to perform all the exercises in every session.

Select the Number of Work Sets per Exercise

When training for category 4 power, three to five work sets per exercise are recommended.

Select the Number of Warm-Up Sets per Exercise

Warm-up sets are important when training for category 4 power because the speed is high, the skill level is high, and the weight is heavy. For the first exercise in the session, three to six warm-up sets are commonly used. Two to four warm-up sets are usually used for each following exercise.

Choose the Desired Weight Progression

Weight progression during the workout usually consists of ascending weight as the client builds to heavy resistance. Wave loading can be used with more advanced clients.

Confirm That the Selected Number of Reps per Set Matches the Goal Time Under Tension

Power exercises have a limited time under tension because the reps are to be performed explosively; each set should be 10 seconds or less in duration. The time under tension per rep is generally less than 2 seconds, and a short break then occurs.

Select the Appropriate Rest Time Between Sets

Rest time is two to five minutes between sets to allow the muscle, energy substrates, and neuromuscular system to recharge so that performance is high on each set.

Implement Any Tricks of the Trade to Elicit Faster Adaptations

The standard program is followed when training to improve category 4 power; personal trainers can also make use of the following methods:

- Pairing a resistance training exercise with a lighter explosive exercise for the same movement
- Using plyometrics to build power
- Using various psych methods to raise arousal level

Program an Appropriate Progressive Overload

Progressive overload is important when training for power against heavy resistance. The end goal is to move something heavy, often something as heavy as possible. Initially, clients train with light weights, but as their strength increases, they can follow a linear progression. Intermediate and advanced clients can use other periodization and progression schemes to continue to lift heavier loads.

In addition, we can look at the athletes who generate the most explosive strength—Olympic weightlifters. Their training generally has them lifting with relatively high frequency, performing each exercise at least twice a week and often three to four times a week, performing several shorter workouts each day to be as fresh as possible, and choosing exercises that allow a high level of speed. These people rarely do machine-based training, and most of their exercises present little eccentric stress, which facilitates recovery.

A.S. Prilepin was a Soviet coach who examined the journals of hundreds of successful weightlifters to see what they had in common. He developed a chart (table 24.5) that became known as Prilepin's table, a guideline about how to set up a training program to increase Olympic weightlifting prowess.

Although traditional strength training recommendations have the greatest effect on category 3 movements (low speed, heavy resistance), note that strength and power have a relationship. If strength is very low, then power will be limited. If a client cannot lift much weight, he or she will not be able to lift much weight fast. For clients in the early to intermediate stages of training, simply getting stronger will cause a significant improvement in their ability to express power.

Plyometric Training

Plyometrics are another popular method of increasing power. Plyometric exercises can be selected for category 2 or category 4 movements, depending on the resistance used. Note that plyometric training has minimal effect on maximal strength or muscle size. Originally, plyometric exercises were not intended to be used as conditioning drills, but that type of application has recently become more popular as a form of high-intensity training to promote loss of body fat.

Types of Exercises

Plyometric exercises are divided into three categories based on the area of the body most involved: upper-body plyometrics, trunk plyometrics, and lower-body plyometrics. Upper-body plyometrics usually involve some sort of throws, often with a medicine ball, or a version of a push-up, usually involving some type of clapping between reps. Trunk plyometrics usually involve drills with a medicine ball or kettlebell in which the person rapidly flexes the trunk forward; rotates left or right, or flexes laterally or diagonally; or performs a combination of both movements against a resistance. Lower-body plyometrics usually involve some sort of jumping or bounding drills. A person's jumping ability is generally considered the best expression of lower-body power (211).

Intensity

Plyometrics, when performed correctly, are a high-intensity activity. Because the goal is to increase power, reasonable rest time between sets should be given to maximize performance on each set and rep. Plyometric exercises are usually high impact, so the program should include adequate rest between sessions (two days or more) to allow the client to recover. They are generally performed early in the workout because the focus is explosive movement, which is not effective or possible when a client is fatigued. Plyometrics will not create the same level of muscular fatigue as traditional exercises, and care must be taken not to overtrain the client with plyometric exercises. Clients may not feel the intensity of a plyometric workout until the following day, when their joints may be stiff. Consult table 24.6 for guidelines when prescribing plyometrics.

A rep is any contact or impact; thus, jumping five times on each foot would count as five reps for the left leg and five reps for the right leg,

Table 24.5   Prilepin's Table

% of 1RM	Reps per set	Optimal total reps	Range of total reps
<70%	3–6	24	18–30
70–80%	3–6	18	12–24
81–90%	2–4	15	10–20
>90%	1–2	7	4–10

Table 24.6 Recommended Volume of Plyometric Drills per Session Based on Training Age

Beginner volume	80–100 reps per session
Intermediate volume	100–120 reps per session
Advanced volume	120–140 reps per session

Reprinted, by permission, from NSCA, 2008, Plyometric training, by D.H. Potach and D.A. Chu. In *Essentials of strength training and conditioning*, 3rd ed., edited by T. Baechle and R.W. Earle (Champaign, IL: Human Kinetics), 421.

for a total of 10 reps. The suggested volume is easily reached in a few minutes with certain drills. As you can see, the volume does not build significantly. Instead, the emphasis is on progressing the exercises so that they are more challenging instead of simply performing huge quantities of easier exercises.

General Guidelines

Plyometric training has many of the same technique, safety, and program design guidelines as resistance training (11):

- Technique. Do clients know how to perform the exercise adequately at a high rate of speed? Do they know how to land or correct a potential fall? If not, these techniques need to be taught and learned.

- Body weight. Because clients are often lifting their own weight, body weight is a big factor in plyometrics. Heavier clients (more than 220 pounds [100 kg]) should use care with plyometric training because the impact on their bodies is greater.

- Footwear. Clients need to wear footwear suitable to the drill; a shoe with good ankle and lateral support is critical.

- Landing surface. Ideally, the landing surface will have some slight give; examples include an outdoor track, an aerobics studio, or grass. Asphalt, pavement, and concrete will create more shock.

- Level of fitness. Plyometrics are generally not considered ideal for new clients and are usually incorporated into a program after a reasonable level of fitness has been established.

- Initial strength. Plyometrics involve a minimum necessary level of strength. The NSCA suggests that people should be able to bench press and squat 1.5 times their body weight before performing plyometrics. The NSCA's recommendations for females are the same as those for males and are thus unattainable for almost all females (less than .01 percent of the female population can bench press 1.5 times their body weight). A more reasonable recommendation is that females should be able to bench press .75 times their body weight and squat their body weight.

- Order. Power exercises should be practiced early in the session because the movements require a high degree of skill and clients should be relatively fresh when performing them (43).

- Training time. Athletes may have an entire workout session dedicated to improving their power. Personal-training clients rarely devote that much time to improving power; instead, power exercises might make up 10 to 20 minutes of the overall session.

- Frequency. Plyometrics are usually performed one or two times a week per area. The area trained should be allowed adequate recovery time (48 hours or more) before training it again (222).

- Speed. A more accurate determination of beginning plyometric ability is the ability to lift weights with a certain speed. The NSCA suggests that people should be able to bench press or squat 60 percent of their body weight and be able to complete five reps with that weight in five seconds. This guideline is reasonable for both males and females and is much easier to attain than the strength recommendations (5).

- **Balance.** If clients are going to perform jumps and will land on just one leg, it is important to establish that they have the balance necessary to complete those exercises with minimal risk:
  - Beginner single-leg plyometric exercises—stand on one leg for 30 seconds
  - Intermediate single-leg plyometric exercises—stand on one leg in a quarter squat (figure 24.3) for 30 seconds
  - Advanced single-leg plyometric exercises—stand on one leg in a half squat (figure 24.4) for 30 seconds

- **Training area.** With any reactive, high-speed exercise, something could go wrong, even with a highly trained client. As a personal trainer, you are responsible for ensuring that the training area is reasonably safe and secure for the client. You should also be aware of other members in a fitness facility, both to make sure that the actions of your client do not injure them (for example, an overthrown medicine ball that hits another user) and to make sure that other users do not injure your client (for example, allowing another user to perform high box jumps right next to a client who is squatting with a barbell) (42).

- **Depth jumps.** A depth jump is a jump from a height in which a client stands on a box or similar sturdy structure, jumps off it, lands, and rapidly performs another explosive movement, usually a second jump. The theory behind a depth jump is that the increased force on the way down from the additional height of the fall further triggers the stretch reflex, allowing the person to experience a greater muscle contraction on the concentric phase (10). Depth

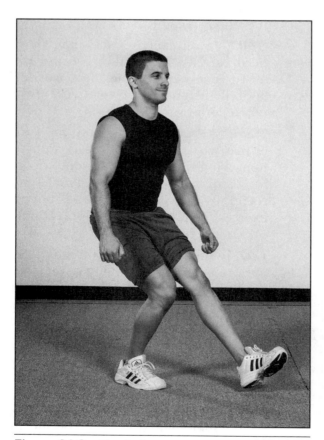

Figure 24.3 Single-leg quarter squat and hold balance test.

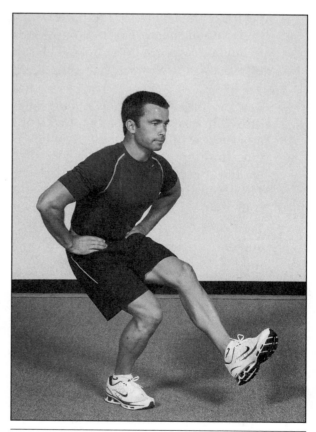

Figure 24.4 Single-leg half squat and hold balance test.

jumps have their purpose, but if the box is too high, it is hard for the person to overcome the force of his or her body falling. The standard recommendation is to avoid depth jumps over 42 inches (106 cm) in height. Heavier people generally use a lower height. A maximum height of 18 inches (45 cm) is recommended for those who weigh over 220 pounds (100 kg).

TRAINING TO IMPROVE SPEED

The ability to run fast is a recurring theme in discussions of human fitness, and in most sports sprinting ability is crucial to success. Sprinting involves a large number of muscles, including the largest muscles in the body. It is a functional movement (in any definition of functional), broadly applicable in almost all sports, targets the fast-twitch muscle fibers and motor units, is extremely intense and time efficient, builds lean tissue, creates EPOC, and likely releases some anabolic hormones in the body (116).

Sprinting speed is clearly heavily influenced by genetics. Some people can run extremely fast with little or no training, whereas others remain comparatively slow after significant training. As with most aspects of fitness, training will improve this capacity, and people will not reach elite status without training it. Sprinting speed comes from a synergistic combination of technique, stride length, and stride frequency.

Technique

This book cannot qualify a personal trainer as an elite-level track coach, but because sprinting is fundamental to many fitness-related activities, a brief analysis of proper technique is provided. Technique is the first thing to look at when attempting to improve a person's sprinting ability. A sprint has two main phases—the start, or acceleration, phase and the maintenance of maximal speed. The ideal technique varies depending on the phase.

Start, or Acceleration, Phase

At the start, people lean forward with their center of gravity in front of them. They are pushing powerfully off the ground, the chest is in front of the feet, and the gaze is likely down at the ground (135, 147, 148). This start, or acceleration, phase is shown in figure 24.5.

Maintenance, or Maximal Velocity, Phase

As people build speed, they enter the maintenance, or maximal velocity, phase. Here, clients are running at full speed, or very near it, and are trying to increase their speed slightly or maintain it. The technique has now changed. Clients will be more upright, and the head and hips will generally be in line. The chest will be behind the lead foot, except at the time of ground contact. Clients will likely be looking straight ahead (27). See figure 24.6 for an example of the form used during this phase of the sprint.

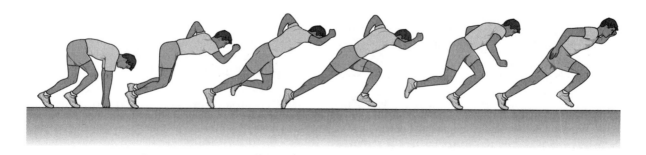

Figure 24.5 Acceleration phase of a sprint.

Reprinted, by permission, from G. Schmolinsky, 2000, *Track and field: The East German textbook of athletics* (Toronto: Sport Books Publisher).

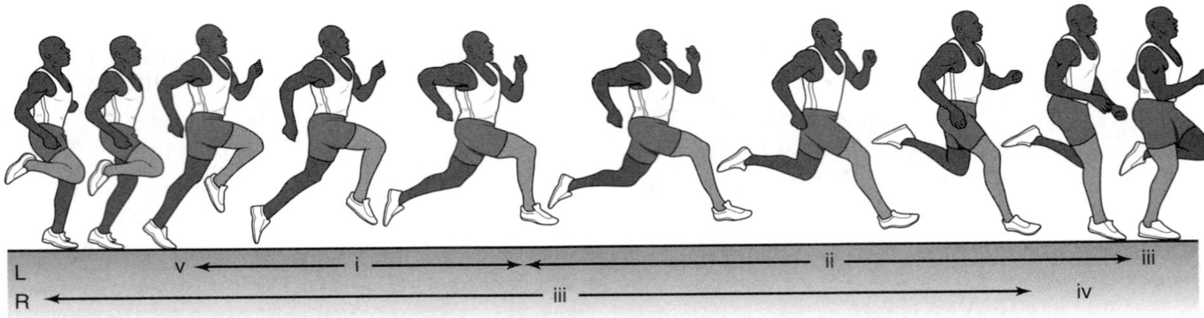

Figure 24.6 Maintenance phase of a sprint.

Reprinted, by permission, from G. Schmolinsky, 2000, *Track and field: The East German textbook of athletics* (Toronto: Sport Books Publisher).

Common Errors

Pumping the arms during both phases of a sprint is important. The significance of the arms can be demonstrated by asking clients to run fast with their arms held straight down by their sides. This form will feel awkward, and their running speed will be significantly reduced. Clients should be cued to swing their arms, particularly to drive back on the backward part of the arm swing. After they reach the maximal velocity phase, the hands will rarely rise above the eyes on the upswing and they will rarely go behind the body on the backswing. The hand should not cross the midline of the body, which would create excessive rotational movement at the core. Clients should be focused but relaxed when sprinting. Novices commonly try to contract and squeeze every muscle in the body to go faster, but this usually prevents them from reaching maximal speed (140).

Sometimes, the first step is backward—the lead foot shifts back a few inches from a start in a standing position—which means that the initial position was not correct. Clients may simply try to run fast instead of sprint; they may use a heel-to-toe foot strike that results in a much longer ground contact time (thus increasing the amortization phase) (37). Clients should be cued to get up on the balls of their feet with their heels either never or very minimally contacting the ground.

If a client becomes serious about sprinting, it can be valuable to film a sprint from various angles, such as the client running toward the camera, away from the camera, and past the camera from the side. Video can provide important feedback about what the client's sprinting form looks like.

Stride Length

Another key variable that affects sprinting speed is stride length. Stride length is defined as the distance between each step. A small stride length limits maximal speed, but a very large stride length tends to increase ground contact time and also limits maximal speed. Stride length is affected primarily by three factors: limb length, flexibility, and power production. Limb length is unchangeable. Proper flexibility allows the leg to travel relatively far in front of the runner as well as trail behind him or her, but extreme flexibility may not provide the necessary tightness and stretch reflex required to achieve a high-speed sprint. Stride length is heavily affected by power production, which is trainable. The more power that people can generate against the ground, the farther they will propel the body forward (46). Several types of training will help increase power:

- Traditional strength training. Lift weights and perform exercises such as the squat, deadlift, bench press, pull-up, row, and so on.
- High-speed strength training. Lift weights and perform explosive power exercises such as the clean, jerk, snatch, push press, and so on.
- Plyometrics. Focus primarily on lower-body plyometrics and include drills such as depth jumps, pike jumps, frog jumps, and bounds (41).
- Resisted sprinting. Run against or with a resistance such as dragging a sled, towing a person, running against a parachute, or running uphill.

Stride Frequency

The final variable that affects sprinting speed is stride frequency. Stride frequency is defined as how fast the feet are able to move; faster feet yield a higher frequency. As with stride length, the sprinter must find a happy medium. A person could move the feet as fast as possible, but if horizontal travel is not significant, the runner will not go anywhere. At the other extreme, a person could take a series of huge, slow steps, but that would also result in a poor sprint time. The runner must balance stride length and stride frequency and try to find an optimal level.

Stride frequency is generally considered the toughest of the three variables to improve. The action is highly neuromuscular, and, as such, the training must be specific. Some authorities suggest performing general footwork drills such as running through tires or jumping rope, but other experts believe that those activities are not specific enough to teach the brain to make the feet move faster during a full-speed sprint (122).

The primary method of training to improve stride frequency is to use assisted sprinting. Resisted sprinting, as mentioned earlier, makes the sprinting harder. Assisted sprinting, in turn, must mimic the actual sprint but make the sprinting easier. Clients will be able to run faster than they are usually capable of, which, at least in theory, should push the brain to learn a faster foot speed.

Two methods are commonly used for assisted sprinting. The simplest is to have clients sprint downhill, but the decline must be such that it allows them to run with their usual form, just faster. If the decline is too steep, clients will lean backward and apply the brakes to prevent themselves from falling forward when they sprint. The general recommendation is to keep the decline at 5 percent or less. The second mode of assisted sprinting is to tow the client. This method requires two sprinters, connected to each other by a bungee cord. The first sprinter takes off and experiences some drag from the trailing sprinter, thus performing resisted sprinting. A short while later, the second sprinter takes off and feels some pull as he or she is towed toward the lead sprinter, thus performing assisted sprinting. In the ideal scenario, the bungee pulls on the second sprinter enough to make him or her run faster than normal, but not enough to alter form.

Pros and Cons of Sprinting

Personal trainers must be extremely cautious when using sprinting as a mode of exercise. Most clients will be 30 years old or older. Many may have never, or at least not since high school, engaged in a full-speed sprint. Most beginning clients lead a relatively sedentary lifestyle that does not leave the body prepared for a full-speed sprint. Taking untrained, slightly older clients and asking them to sprint as fast as possible is a recipe for injury. Indeed, even trained clients are at risk, especially if most of their training has been primarily resistance-based training. Lifting weights and performing traditional cardio training sessions is great, but those programs do not prepare the body to engage in an all-out sprint (50).

Any client who has not sprinted for a long time (six months or longer; usually, the interval will have been several years or more), even a relatively strong one, may be at increased risk for injury (49). Now the client will be exerting the stronger muscles, which can generate a lot of force in a way that the body is unprepared for.

One of the simplest ways to help clients modulate their sprinting speed is to ask them to sprint at a certain percentage of their maximum speed. Exactly how accurately clients are able to match the percentage is not the point; you just want to direct clients to leave some speed in the tank. Sprinting at a slightly reduced speed is significantly safer. In general, most personal trainers give their clients a goal speed expressed in terms of a percentage, which is then increased by 5 or 10 percentage points, starting at about 50 percent. A 50 percent sprint is usually a fast jog. Then you can instruct clients to proceed to 60 percent, then 70 percent, and so on.

If clients have not performed sprint training recently, you should have them spend four to eight weeks in this acclimation phase before they sprint at 100 percent of full speed. Clients should be kept at 95 percent intensity or less, often at 90 percent or less in the beginning of that phase. In addition, if clients are going to engage in any type of full-speed sprinting, you should have them perform two to five warm-up sprints, usually in the range of 50 to 80 percent intensity, to help prepare them for the activity.

Types of Sprints

The many types of sprints are usually broken up by distance covered. Modifying the length of the sprint will change the effect of the sprint significantly. Sprints of the following distance are the most common:

- 5-meter sprints—helps clients work on the start of the sprint, helps build power, can be performed inside, has a lower injury rate, can be combined with short rest to create a conditioning effect, can alternate the lead foot for a more symmetrical workout, and takes about 1 second to complete
- 40-meter sprints—teaches clients to burst to full speed, common test in sports, good for conditioning, often sport specific, and usually takes 4.5 to 7 seconds to complete
- 60-meter sprints—similar to the 40-meter sprint, more time spent at full speed, can usually be run at full speed all the way, and usually takes 6 to 9 seconds to complete
- 100-meter sprints—somewhat challenging to maintain full speed all the way, moderately draining physically and mentally, tough to couple this with short rest periods, creates significant EPOC, and usually takes 12 to 20 seconds to complete
- 200-meter sprints—takes extra effort to be able to sprint the full distance, somewhat hard on the body, can be slowed to create more of a conditioning effect for more advanced sprinters, creates significant EPOC, and usually takes 25 to 40 seconds to complete

- 400-meter sprints—very effective at building lactate threshold, very draining, keeps the volume of this work relatively low, creates significant EPOC, and usually takes 55 to 90 seconds to complete

Programming Sprints

Sprints are high-speed and high-power exercises and are generally incorporated early into a workout session. The exception occurs when they are being used solely as a means of conditioning, in which case they can be performed at the end of the workout. You can easily overtrain a person who is not adapted to sprinting. A good guideline to follow is to have clients sprint for a total distance of 80 to 1,200 meters during the entire workout. Sprinting is ideally performed on a field or grass, but watch for uneven terrain where a client might twist an ankle. Sprinting on pavement and asphalt is not as ideal because the surface will produce a strong impact on the body. If you are training a group of people, keep in mind that many people, particularly athletes, can be competitive. Sprinting alone is different from sprinting against another person. Until people are fully acclimated to sprinting, setting up a situation in which they race others is not advisable. The competitive spirit may get the best of them, and they will try to go faster than would be good for the body (9).

Training for power and speed can provide a valuable benefit to clients, particularly those who participate in field sports. In addition, many clients who are not involved in competitive sport still enjoy being trained with these types of exercises; it makes them *feel* like athletes. But this type of training needs to be used with caution. You should not rush to employ these methods with all clients. Establish a base level of fitness and gradually introduce relatively easy power exercises to see how they handle them. After clients have established that base and are responding well to the training, you can employ more advanced methods.

CONCLUSION

People can develop a variety of power and speed abilities. Personal trainers should know which abilities are important for their clients to improve. Familiarity with the equations of force, work, and power will help personal trainers grasp the nuances of the terms. Clients will develop the most power by lifting a medium weight as fast as possible.

All movements can be separated into four categories based on speed of movement and resistance used. Low-speed, low-resistance movements are purely skill based. High-speed, low-resistance movements involve using power against minimal load. Low-speed, heavy resistance is most commonly trained in the gym with resistance training. High-speed, high-resistance movements are reflected in the Olympic lifts. Rate of force development has a significant effect on how useful maximal strength is in certain movements.

Plyometrics are exercises designed to increase power. Power movements generally consist of eccentric, amortization, and concentric phases. Personal trainers should consider a client's technique, body weight, footwear, environment, level of fitness, strength, speed, and balance before incorporating plyometrics into a workout program.

Some clients may wish to improve their maximal sprinting speed. Speed is highly affected by technique, stride length, and stride frequency. Technique should be the initial focus. Attention should be paid to proper arm movement, body lean, and foot strike. Stride length is most affected by power, and it can be improved by resisted sprinting. Stride frequency is most affected by neuromuscular coordination, and it can be improved by assisted sprinting. Sprinting is a tremendous exercise available to trainers, but it should be used with care because the chance for injury is elevated, particularly with clients who have not sprinted for an extended time.

Study Questions

1. What is the physic equation for work?
   a. mass × acceleration
   b. (force × distance) ÷ time
   c. (time × acceleration) ÷ mass
   d. force × distance

2. Approximately how long does an athlete have to interact with an object in most sporting events?
   a. .02 seconds
   b. .2 seconds
   c. 2 seconds
   d. 20 seconds

3. In which category of movement would a maximal attempt on the power clean be classified?
   a. category 1
   b. category 2
   c. category 3
   d. category 4

4. Which proprioceptors are particularly important in helping produce maximal power?
   a. muscle spindles
   b. golgi tendon organs
   c. golgi apparatus
   d. mitochondria

5. What is the transition phase in a plyometric movement called?
   a. eccentric phase
   b. amortization phase
   c. concentric phase
   d. power phase

Advanced Concepts in Program Design

Chapter 17 presented the NPTI system of creating exercise programs for your clients. This chapter delves into some of the deeper aspects of program design such as creating a weekly exercise routine, understanding current training philosophies, and comparing and contrasting the many ways to vary training intensity.

EXERCISE ROUTINE SELECTION

In selecting a weekly routine for a client, the two main variables that personal trainers must balance are the frequency of training and the intensity of the exercise. Frequency refers to how often the stimulus is presented, and intensity refers to the difficulty of the activity.

There are two types of intensity. Relative intensity refers to how hard the activity is for the client. If clients are training until failure or really pushing themselves, they are training at a maximum relative intensity. Absolute intensity refers to how hard the activity is compared with others. In general, beginners and weaker people tend to perform at low absolute intensity. For example, lifting an empty bar (45 pounds, or 20.4 kg) for 5 reps in the bench press involves low absolute intensity, but that activity might be hard for an untrained client so it would have high relative intensity. Bench pressing 315 pounds (142.9 kg) for 5 reps involves high absolute intensity—few people can complete that activity—but if the

person could bench 315 pounds for 12 reps but performed only 5 reps with that weight, the activity is at low or moderate absolute intensity. Having a proper balance of frequency and intensity is important to achieving success in the fitness world, although intensity is likely the single most important factor in an exercise program. Many faulty programs can be overcome with hard work, but a perfectly designed program combined with minimal effort will not produce positive results (9).

Some fitness professionals tend to favor high-frequency, total-body training in their programs, whereas others favor low-frequency split routines. Both systems have pros and cons. Outlined here are some things to consider when setting up an exercise routine.

Pros of Total Body Training

- Total-body training (TBT) allows more frequent training, which may be better for increased neuromuscular coordination. Practice makes perfect, and people generally get a better practice effect from frequent shorter sessions than from one long session (29).

- A client is relatively fresh for each exercise because each body area is trained only once; therefore, there is not much of an accumulated specific fatigue effect from performing many exercises.

- It is easier to incorporate total-body exercises such as the Olympic lifts, gymnastic movements, and strongman-based exercises into this type of routine.

- Essentially all fitness professionals agree that TBT is ideal for beginners.
- TBT may be better than split training in preparing a client to handle total-body fatigue.
- TBT hits a higher percentage of the total motor units in the body per day than split training does.
- Because a client is training the whole body, TBT may be better at burning calories and promoting fat loss.
- A client who misses a workout or two during the week still receives some training stimulus to the whole body instead of neglecting parts of the body for that week.
- Greater frequency can help prevent undertraining.
- Implementing supersets (antagonistic sets) is easy, which can reduce the length of the training session.
- Easy total-body days are harder than easy split days; for example, an arms-only split routine session trains only the arm muscles, but a TBT session trains the whole body, even though the intensity is lower (42).
- Clients do not get the deep soreness from a TBT routine that they get from a split routine because they are performing fewer sets for any single muscle group.
- Clients can have a good overall training routine while working out only three days a week.
- Many people find it is easier to do a hard TBT program without a partner than a hard split routine without a partner.

Pros of Split Training

- Split training allows maximum intensity during most sessions regardless of the level of advancement (61).
- Repeated sets on a fatigued muscle build muscular endurance (particularly multiple-set endurance) more effectively.
- Split training allows clients to work out more than three days a week.

- Extra training days allow clients to devote more time to weak points in physique or performance.
- Split training gives muscles more time to recover, which can help prevent overtraining.
- Essentially all fitness professionals agree that split training is better for bodybuilders and fitness-oriented clients.
- Split training hits more total motor units in the body per week than a TBT plan does; as a muscle becomes fatigued, more motor units are recruited, which is better for increasing muscular size.
- The hardest split day is usually harder than the hardest total-body day; for example, a legs-only split routine session uses more sets and exercises for the legs than the limited number of sets and exercises for the legs in a TBT session (39).
- It is easy to follow the intensity techniques (e.g., drop sets and compound sets) during a split training workout because of the greater number of sets and exercises performed.
- Split training may do a better job of teaching a client to lift intensely.
- Clients tend to become sore and feel the muscle that they trained for several days afterward; some people like this feeling, but others do not.
- Split training is better if your clients have to work out multiple days in a row (for instance, if Tuesday, Wednesday, and Thursday are the only days that a client can train).

Cons of Total-Body Training

- High frequency combined with high intensity may overtrain certain areas of the body (for example, shoulders and elbows become susceptible to tendonitis from pressing three days a week).
- Most split programs allow a person to work out four or more times a week; doing more than three days per week is

difficult on a TBT plan because training must occur on sequential days.

- TBT may not allow enough recovery time, particularly if your clients train at high relative intensity or high absolute intensity (15).

- TBT may not allow enough training to improve or correct weak points. If weak points are addressed along with regular training, overtraining may occur.

- Clients may be tempted to decrease intensity because they are doing the same workout again in a few days.

- TBT may not build up local muscular endurance or resistance to fatigue as expressed by lactate threshold as much as split training does.

- Implementing intensity techniques such as drop sets and compound sets is difficult because of the short recovery time between training sessions.

- With TBT, clients do not get much of a pump in a specific muscle group (which some people enjoy and some experts think is beneficial to promoting muscular growth).

Cons of Split Training

- The reduced frequency for a given body part may not provide enough training stimulus to increase neuromuscular coordination, which may, in turn, limit strength.

- A client will be somewhat fatigued after the first exercise for a certain body part, so continuing to train that area forces a slight reduction in the weight lifted.

- A split routine must be planned properly to prevent overtraining of susceptible body parts or areas, such as the lower back and front delts.

- It is hard to fit total-body exercises or combination exercises, such as thrusters and Olympic lifts, into a split training routine.

- A split routine may not promote total-body fatigue, so the client may not be prepared for activities that require that type of stress.

- A client may not be stimulating the muscle intensely enough to require a long recovery time between training sessions.

- A split routine takes more time out of a client's schedule than TBT does.

- A client may need a regular workout partner to have good split training workouts. Of course, this might be a benefit because a personal trainer is always available to spot and motivate the client.

OPTIMAL TRAINING FREQUENCY

Both systems can clearly work, but which one is optimal? That is the dilemma, and there is no specific answer. What is optimal for a client now may not be optimal for him or her in one year and may not have been optimal a year ago. Figure 25.1 illustrates the optimal training frequencies compared with a client's training age, not chronological age.

The upper area suggests the range for the total number of sessions per week. Beginners should start with three sessions a week, although two is doable, and over time the number of workouts that they perform per week should rise, often hitting five workouts a week. Advanced clients sometimes perform multiple workouts per day to raise their total.

The lower area suggests the number of sessions per week that each area of the body, muscle part, or type of movement is trained. Beginners usually start on a total-body routine two to three times a week and then often progress to reduced frequency and increased intensity as time goes by. But as clients become more advanced and have trained for many years, increasing the frequency again may become necessary because advanced clients can outwork their recovery capacity if they push themselves too hard. For these types of clients, you may need to reduce the intensity slightly and make up for it with significantly increased frequency. This plan also facilitates

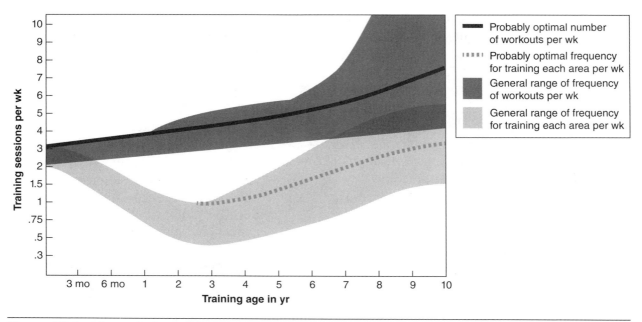

Figure 25.1 Theoretical optimal range of frequency per week versus training age.

neuromuscular coordination, which is important to high-performing clients (7).

As a personal trainer, you do not need to reinvent the wheel. Many good training routines that you can use with your clients have already been used and tested over time. Table 25.1 provides examples of routines based on how frequently clients are lifting per week (first number) and how frequently they are training each area of the body (second number). For example, 4/2 means that the client is training four days a week and hitting each area of the body two times per week.

PERIODIZATION

Periodization is planned variation in a workout routine. It involves intentionally manipulating the key variables in a workout routine (weight, sets, reps, rest, exercise selection, volume, intensity, and so on) with the purpose of maximizing performance and avoiding plateaus. Periodization helps intermediate and advanced athletes avoid overtraining and peak for certain events or activities. When a workout program is periodized, that entire program is then broken down into various cycles.

A macrocycle is a relatively long (about six months) block of time devoted to one primary fitness goal. It is generally associated with long-term goals, something the client would love to achieve but isn't that close to doing yet. Running a marathon, bench pressing 315 pounds (142.9 kg) (if a client was currently at 250 pounds [113.4 kg]), or losing 50 pounds (22.7 kg) would all be examples of a macrocycle.

Within each macrocycle are two or more mesocycles. Mesocycles are typically two to four months long and they are associated with short-term goals. The focus of the mesocycle must be related to the main goal outlined in the macrocycle. If a client wants to run a marathon, spending two months working on their vertical jump is unlikely to help with that goal. If a client wants to bench press 315 pounds (142.9 kg), she doesn't need to spend three months devoting most of her energy to an intense lower-body stretching regimen. Instead, our running client might work on increasing her $\dot{V}O_2$max, increasing her sustainable running speed, or decreasing her body weight. Our strength client might focus on increasing muscle size, perfecting his technique on the bench press, or building up a synergistic muscle that might be a weak spot (e.g., his shoulders).

Inside each mesocycle are two or more microcycles. *Micro* refers to something small—

Table 25.1 **Frequency of Training and Corresponding Workout Programs**

Routine*	Day 1	Day 2	Day 3	Day 4	Day 5
1/1			Total body		
2/2		Total body		Total body	
2/1		Push		Pull	
2/1		Upper body		Lower	
3/3	Total body		Total body		Total body
3/2	Push		Pull		Total body
3/1.5	Push		Pull		Push
3/1.5	Upper		Lower		Upper
3/1	Chest Back		Legs LB and abs		Shoulders Arms
3/1	Push		Pull		Legs
4/2	Push	Pull		Push	Pull
4/2	Upper	Lower		Upper	Lower
4/1	Chest Abs	Back Biceps		Legs LB	Shoulders Triceps
4/1	Legs Abs	Chest Biceps		Back LB	Shoulders Triceps
4/1	Chest Back	Legs LB		Shoulders Abs	Biceps Triceps
4/1	Chest Biceps	Legs LB		Back Abs	Shoulders Triceps

Note: LB = lower back.

*The first number is how often a client is training each week, and the second number is how often each muscle group is trained each week.

this is our shortest time period. Microcycles generally last from one to four weeks and they are focused around daily or weekly goals. While most athletes and clients are happy to spend their time daydreaming about the completion of the macrocycle, the microcycle is where all of the action happens. This is where the personal trainer will actually create the specific program to accomplish the client's fitness goals. If the client wants to improve his or her $\dot{V}O_2$max or decrease body weight, the trainer must come up with a plan to do that. Remember, it is ideal to direct your client's energy toward process goals (i.e., goals that one has control over). Successful completion of multiple microcycles will lead to completion of the mesocycle and ultimately completion of

the macrocycle. It is an exciting time when the microcycle goal for that day is the completion of the macrocycle—when you wake up that morning and say "This is it; today is the day I run the marathon," or "Today is the day I bench press 315 pounds (142.9 kg)." If your training has been going well, the completion of that microcycle should not be any harder than the completion of all of the other microcycles that lead you to that point.

TRAINING PHILOSOPHIES

Many training philosophies that have a base in exercise science can be used when designing a client's training program. You should have an understanding of these philosophies because a gym or fitness center may follow a particular philosophy and expect you to do the same, your peers may be drawn to these philosophies, you may find that one of them clicks with you, or you may desire to blend aspects of different philosophies together. By understanding each of these philosophies, you can choose the best plan for you and your clients.

High-Intensity Training

High-intensity training, or HIT training, was developed by Arthur Jones (the founder of Nautilus equipment) and followed by bodybuilders Mike Mentzer (in the 1970s and 1980s) and Dorian Yates (in the 1990s). In the last 10 or 15 years, HIT training has spread out to the masses and is popular among the general population and personal trainers.

Many HIT philosophies have developed as people have tweaked the idea to meet their own needs. In general, however, HIT training can be summarized this way: Perform one high-intensity work set until failure per exercise and then change exercises.

This philosophy includes two primary aspects. First, clients complete only one work set per exercise. You can use as many warm-up sets as you like for your clients, normally from zero to three warm-up sets on each exercise, with relatively light weight. But when it comes time to work hard, you just have your clients complete one set per exercise, and then you move on to another exercise (39). The number of reps performed is typically 6 to 12 per set with a load of at least 70 percent of 1RM. The rest period varies; one to three minutes are needed between warm-up sets, but minimal rest is needed between exercises because only one work set is performed. Generally, the whole workout is relatively short, often less than an hour.

Second, you should have your clients perform as many reps as possible until failure and beyond. In other words, when your clients are performing their work sets, they should continue lifting the weight until their form breaks down considerably or until they can no longer complete the reps on their own. Then you, as the personal trainer, assist them with one or two

forced reps, in which you help them lift several extra reps to stimulate the muscle further (47).

To understand and evaluate HIT training, we need to examine each of those two points. To begin, the idea of going to failure on each exercise will be analyzed, and then the idea of performing just one work set per exercise will be discussed.

Train to Failure

The purpose of training until failure is to stimulate the muscle fully. If your clients do not go until failure, how do you know how many reps they could have completed? Many people simply do not train hard enough to get the best results, and going to failure forces them to increase their intensity. Physiologically, training until failure will recruit and fatigue a large number of motor units and muscles fibers, and only the motor units recruited and fatigued will adapt to the exercise. This point is a strong positive on the side of training until failure, and it correlates with increased intensity.

Training to failure, however, does have its problems. First, the practicality is that a person needs a personal trainer for this method to work, especially if the client is performing forced reps. Second, when people fail, they are tempted to put the body in a more mechanically advantageous position to finish the exercise. For example, people may start swinging on those last few reps of a bicep curl, or lean forward during a tricep push-down, or cut the depth on a squat. That is just human nature. A saying in weightlifting goes "If you aren't cheating, you aren't trying hard enough," meaning that as people lift heavier, the body tries to find a way to make it easier, which is not always safe and is not part of the proper approach to training to failure. In addition, failing during an exercise like a heavy squat or a bench press can be dangerous, for both the client and the personal trainer (50). Traditionally, what happens is that when smaller muscles are being trained and those muscles fail, the body recruits larger muscles to spot the fatigued muscle. For example, the body recruits the erector spinae muscles to start swinging the torso to help the biceps finish the reps of a bicep curl exercise. This approach is often considering cheating on an exercise, but if some basic guidelines of body mechanics are followed, this method is usually not dangerous. If a big muscle fails, however, the body does not have anything else to recruit to perform the work, so it will attempt to change the lifting position (shorten or alter the moment arm of the resistance force and lengthen or change the moment arm of the muscle force) to complete the rep. These alterations are often cause for concern and may place the client at greater risk for injury.

Other issues with failing are that having to go until failure on every exercise can be mentally defeating or tiring. If a client is supposed to perform a leg press for 10 reps but gets 12 all on his or her own, there is no reward. Instead, the person must try for 13 or 14 reps just to see where failure occurs. Over time, the body wants to take the lazy way out and say, "Well, I could have completed 10 reps, but because I have to go until failure anyway, I will fail at 8 reps." If you make your clients fail on each exercise, that attitude may eventually come out.

Reaching failure on each exercise does not build confidence. Although it does build up a person's constitution, which is desirable, one of the great things about lifting weights is that it builds confidence. Generally, you foster that confidence in clients by helping them reach their goals. They feel good about themselves. Clients are empowered when they complete a hard set of 10 reps and walk out of the gym knowing that they could have done 1 or 2 more if they had to. That does not make the set too easy. Then, when clients approach the weight the next time, they are confident and ready to go because they think that they can reach a new goal. If they failed on the set the last time, they know what their limits are and face the

difficult task of trying to break past those limits. People who do not know what their limits are can convince themselves that they are stronger than they might have initially thought. Therefore, they can improve their performance (by having an optimal state of mind).

Training until failure can also be detrimental to learning proper form on the exercise. Most experts agree that beginners should not go until failure, but even intermediate or advanced clients have breakdowns in form when they are at or near failure. But this occurs when they are trying their hardest. The memory is often strongest when a significant event is occurring, and if that fact carries over to weightlifting, people are going to be remembering their form the most when they are trying their hardest and, in this case, failing (19).

What is the answer? Unfortunately, there is no perfect answer for all people; table 25.2 provides a list of pros and cons of training until muscular failure. A reasonable guideline is that clients should not regularly train until failure, but they should be willing to fail as they train. The difference is that instead of seeking failure for your clients, you let the goal reps and goal weight guide you and allow clients to fail within that structure. For example, if your advanced client squatted 400 pounds (181.4 kg) for 10 reps last time and you want him or her to make progress this time, you will have your client try either 400 pounds for 11 reps or 405 pounds (183.7 kg) for 10 reps. Both of those sets will be hard, but you pick one and have your client go after it. He or she may fail on that 11th rep, but you do not want to let that possibility stop the client or you. But after the client reaches the goal, you stop the set. That is the reward. Your goal is to avoid failure with your clients, but you do that by

Table 25.2 Pros and Cons of Training Until Muscular Failure

Pros	Cons
Forces a client to train hard	Usually requires a spotter
Recruits a large number of motor units	May have a greater chance of injury
Recruits primarily Type IIb motor units	May cause form to break down
Promotes intensity, which is likely the single most important variable in achieving results	May lead to overtraining
Unlikely to undertrain	Mentally fatiguing to take all sets to failure in a workout
	May not build confidence
	Not ideal for beginners or older adults

encouraging them to attack the weight. This method may be taking the easy way out in the beginning, but if you consistently follow progressive overload with your clients, their workouts will continue to get tougher. In addition, performing something and then stopping is more natural and rewarding, and people are more likely to perform a rewarding activity.

To summarize, having your clients train until they reach failure on each exercise is not generally necessary or desirable. Reaching failure occasionally during intense weightlifting is acceptable and is a by-product of pushing your clients hard. People who have never reached failure are probably not working out hard enough. Beginners should not train until failure on any exercise.

Perform One Set per Exercise

The second idea behind HIT training is to perform only 1 main set per exercise. A logical response to that is to ask why. Why do just 1 set and not 3? Of course, HITers might ask why weightlifters stop at 3 sets. Why not always complete 5, 10, or 20 sets per exercise?

The one-set protocol was established because the people who developed HIT training believed that many people were overtraining. Keep in mind that HIT training developed as a response to the high-volume programs of the 1970s such as those described in Arnold Schwarzenegger's *Encyclopedia of Bodybuilding*. Bodybuilders often performed multiple exercises (four to six per muscle group) and many sets (five or six work sets per exercise) while training each muscle twice per week. The system obviously worked for Arnold, but most experts agree that without good genetics and some assistance with recovery through steroids, most people will not be able to tolerate that kind of workout. Thus, the pendulum swung the other way. The one-set protocol asserted that people could get results as good or better by completing just one set per exercise and that they did not need to perform multiple sets per exercise.

Common Questions

The first question on most people's minds is, "Does HIT work?" Can people really do just one set for each exercise? The answer is yes;

it does work. Put simply, people can see good results by performing just one intense set per exercise. The most well-known recent HITer is Dorian Yates, a six-time Mr. Olympia. During his reign he had a physique that had not been seen before. No one could argue that he did not get good results by completing one set per exercise. He did not always perform one set, but as he progressed through the years, he eventually dropped down to one set per exercise. His book *Dorian Yates: A Warrior's Story* provides more information about his workouts.

The second question is, "Does HIT work better than doing three sets?" The answer is generally no; it does not. Most studies show that average people improve their strength and size more rapidly with three sets than with one set (36). The consensus is that the first work set is the most important set; not all sets are equally important. For example, if three sets provide 100 percent of the results, each set does not contribute 33 percent of the total. Rather, the client might receive 85 percent of the results after the first set, 95 percent of the results after the second set, and 100 percent of the results after the third set. This idea that each subsequent work set provides diminishing returns is highlighted in figure 25.2.

Pros and Cons

What are the benefits of performing only one set per exercise? First, it is generally considered a good strategy for a size-building program, and it helps avoid overtraining, which was the reason that this training program was developed. Normally, one-set training is combined with a once-a-week split routine, but it does not have to be. It does not work as well on a total-body routine, particularly for men.

Another benefit of one-set training is that it is a great time saver. Completing one set per exercise instead of the traditional three sets often cuts the workout time in half. Now your clients have extra time to head back to the office or do whatever they want to do. If they chose to reinvest that time by staying in the gym, you have the option of training them with more exercises. Given that the first set is the most important set, it is likely that performing one set of three different exercises is

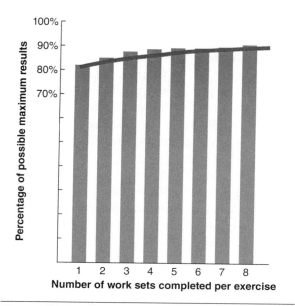

Figure 25.2 Theoretical valuation of results based on work sets performed per exercise.

better than completing three sets of the same exercise.

A HIT program is most effective for large-muscle groups or hard, intense exercises. One hard set of squats or deadlifts may be all that a person needs to do. A HIT program also helps your clients learn how to train intensely, if they do not know already. People who are performing just one set can easily convince themselves that they do not have to save their energy and can go all out.

The biggest flaw in the HIT program is that it does not adequately target neuromuscular coordination (NMC). Remember that the two factors that contribute most to strength are neuromuscular coordination and muscle size. HIT training is good for increasing muscle size, but it does not do much for neuromuscular coordination (NMC), particularly if your clients need to work on that aspect. Neuromuscular coordination is improved through practice and repetition, and this plan allows limited time for that. Imagine that you are a basketball coach. You hold basketball practice and set a goal of having everyone learn how to shoot foul shots. You line everybody up and say, "OK. We are going to shoot one round of 15 foul shots, and then that is it for the week. I expect us to be good in a month." Clearly, that approach would be foolish. If you want to improve on

something like foul shots, you have to practice all the time. The idea of shooting 60 total foul shots in a month is absurd; you would want to shoot more like several hundred every day. This idea is true with almost any sport. But if you have your clients follow the HIT routine and your goal is to have them become proficient at the bench press, doing a few warm-up sets and one set of 10 reps once a week is only 50 sets a year of practicing the bench press—a training stimulus insufficient to improve NMC. If your client's NMC is already good, performing only one set is generally adequate to maintain NMC. For example, if a client already knows how to perform the bench press exercise, then completing one set each week may be enough to maintain that form.

HIT training is not effective in increasing muscular endurance, particularly multiple-set muscular endurance, which is the ability to complete a set, rest, and complete a second set (50). A high-intensity training program does not provide your clients with that level of practice because they always stop after one set. Their bodies will not become used to having to repeat a difficult set. In most sports and daily activities, people have to repeat something that is challenging several times.

HIT training does not offer an effective stimulus for losing body fat. If your clients are lifting weights with the goal of burning as many calories per minute as possible, you generally want them to complete a high volume of work. The HIT program yields a low volume of work, although it can create EPOC when used effectively (39, 47).

The goal of HIT training is to prevent over-training, but in some cases it can promote undertraining. As mentioned previously, most studies show that results are better when a person completes three sets instead of just one. The workout takes more time, but all else being equal your clients will get slightly better results that way. Many clients are willing to put in extra time and effort for that small improvement in performance.

HIT training works well for large-muscle groups or large exercises, but it does not work nearly as well for small-muscle groups or small exercises. The nature of small muscles is that they are designed to be used repeatedly and recover quickly. Using just one set on muscles like the rear delts, abs, calves, forearms, and, to some extent, biceps and triceps, is not a good idea. Your clients likely cannot fatigue the muscle enough in one set for the workout to be maximally effective. Imagine doing just one set of abs for maybe three exercises and then being done for the week. The muscles that are primarily slow-twitch muscles need a high volume to make significant improvements. In addition, if your clients have weak points that they need to work on, one set per exercise may not be enough. If your clients need to work on their rear delts or their left biceps, performing multiple sets for those types of muscles is ideal. Further, in a rehab setting, clients usually perform more than one set.

Another issue with HIT training is that it does not adequately build up work capacity, sometimes referred to as general physical preparedness (GPP). The very nature of a HIT program is that it is a low-volume program. Traditional plans involve more work and therefore better improve work capacity.

The final issue with HIT training is that although it is effective for advanced or late intermediate clients, it is not well suited for beginners or early intermediates. Those clients need to complete multiple sets on the exercises to build work capacity, increase NMC, and tax the muscle fully. One set per exercise just is not right for them. See table 25.3 for a list of the pros and cons of performing only one set per exercise.

So what is the answer then? Should HIT be declared not acceptable, a tried and failed experiment? Definitely not. HIT training is still appropriate in many circumstances. As an overall theory of weightlifting, it may leave something to be desired, but in terms of practical application, it has many positives and should be included in most training programs, particularly for advanced clients who are looking to improve their size. Training HIT-style makes for a great shock set, shock day, or shock week. A client can regularly follow this routine for six to eight weeks to explore how the body responds to low-volume, high-intensity training. But a high-intensity training workout followed for months on end often leads to a tired, overtrained client who is making only small gains (or, even more likely, an unemployed personal trainer).

Westside

Another important philosophy to examine is the way that the Westside Barbell Club sets up its training programs. Westside was started by Louie Simmons, an elite powerlifter who had in-depth knowledge about resistance training and the willingness to try new ideas.

The idea behind the Westside workouts is to train four days per week. This particular program focuses on maximal strength. It is most popular among powerlifters and other strength-focused clients, but anyone except beginners can use this type of program.

Table 25.3 Pros and Cons of Performing One Set per Exercise

Pros	Cons
Less likely to overtrain	May not be enough stimulus to create adaptation; may result in undertraining
Saves time by shortening the workout	Does little to improve neuromuscular coordination and technique
Allows the client to perform more exercises in the same amount of time	May not work as well for small-muscle groups
Produces most of the benefits in a single work set on each exercise	May not work as well for isolation exercises
Works better with clients who are more experienced	May not work as well with clients who have less experience
Works better when combined with larger muscles or compound exercises	May yield better results than performing single sets
Works well if the total training time is limited	May do little to build muscular endurance (particularly multiple-set endurance)
	May not build work capacity or GPP as well as multiple-set routines

Training Days

Each training day of the Westside routine has a particular theme. Instead of focusing on muscle groups, this program focuses on the exercises that will be performed. In terms of a routine, this program is an upper–lower split, and each day is performed twice a week. The days do not have to be performed in a specific order, but two days for the same exercise cannot be performed consecutively. Each day normally consists of about four main exercises and is completed in about an hour (training a large group may increase that time).

Day 1—Dynamic Effort Squat Day (DE Lower-Body Day or Speed Squat Day) On this day, you start the routine by having clients squat, normally on a box. Your clients perform 10 to 12 sets of 2 reps and have a short rest after each set. The weight is relatively light, normally 60 to 70 percent of their 1RM on squats, and they should attempt to lift the weight as fast as possible. The rest after each set is a minute or less. Then you have them perform two or three assistance exercises for the squat. The assistance portion of the training includes exercises that emphasize the muscles used in the squat (glutes, quads, hamstrings, erectors). Normally, clients perform three sets of 8 to 12 reps on those exercises, but that can vary depending on need. Finally, you finish the day with weighted abdominal training, not the common high-rep, body-weight training.

Day 2—Maximum Effort Bench Press Day (ME Upper-Body Day) On this day, clients start by performing an exercise similar to the bench press without performing the bench press itself. A few examples might be a partial bench press, a close-grip bench, an incline bench press, or a floor press. Clients perform several warm-up sets on this exercise (about five to eight sets) and then perform approximately three heavy sets, each set progressing in weight until they max out on the exercise. Each of the heavy sets is usually one rep, so they are essentially performing a 1RM in this exercise; the goal is to get used to lifting a heavy weight. Then you have them perform a back exercise as assistance for the bench press. You

follow that with a shoulder exercise, usually for the middle or rear delts. Finally, you end with a triceps exercise. For most assistance exercises, they perform three sets of 8 to 12 reps, although you can add more or less as needed. More sets are often completed for the triceps; six sets is most common. Triceps are heavily emphasized in this program.

Day 3—Maximum Effort Squat or Deadlift Day (ME Lower-Body Day) On this day, you choose an exercise that is like a squat or deadlift for your clients. You have them perform a reasonable number of warm-up sets (about five to eight), and then they attempt to max out on that exercise. This day is similar to the ME upper-body day. Examples of exercises you might choose are the box squat, good morning, 13-inch-high (33 cm) deadlift, or a squat with bands. The assistance work is the same for this day as it is for day 1, although your clients do not have to perform the same exercises if you do not want them to.

Day 4—Dynamic Effort Bench Press Day (DE Upper-Body Day or Speed Bench Day) On this day your clients start with the bench press. They complete eight sets of three reps with 60 to 70 percent of 1RM for the bench press, often changing their grip and focusing on a closer grip than normal. They have short rest after each set, and they should attempt to lift the weight as fast as possible. The assistance work is the same for this day as it is for day 2. Again, you may or may not choose to change exercises for them.

Each week your clients follow this routine. You rotate the exercises that you use on ME days for them every one to three weeks. After two or three months you have them come back to those exercises and try to hit a new max to show that they have made progress. The speed days are pretty much the same each day. Sometimes the weight is changed in a wavelike pattern, but it is always relatively light. You change their assistance exercises as necessary, normally every few weeks, and the general idea is to try to bring up their weak points. Occasionally, instead of having them perform a 1RM on the max day, you can choose a lighter weight and have them perform one to three sets of as many reps as they can perform, often in the 20-rep range.

Common Questions

The Westside routine may prompt many questions. The first question is often, "Why is the program set up this way?" Strength can be improved in three main ways. The first is by lifting heavy weights with relatively few reps. This approach is termed *maximal effort*, which is where the term *maximal effort* (or ME) *day* originates. The second way to gain strength is to lift a moderate weight for as many reps as possible, usually going to or near failure. This method is termed *repetitive effort*, which is what most programs (for example, HIT training) use to gain strength. The third way to improve strength is to take a light weight and lift it as fast as possible, thereby generating a maximal amount of force. This method is termed *dynamic effort* or *speed day*. The maximal effort and the dynamic effort have the most beneficial effect on the neuromuscular system, thereby increasing NMC.

Why twice a week? Once a week is not enough practice, especially if you think of working out as a sport instead of a healthy activity. Also, the body generally needs 72 hours to adapt to the training session; after that time, detraining can occur.

Why use assistance exercises? The exercises are designed to improve the muscles that are involved in the main exercises. For example, a stronger triceps will lead to a stronger bench press.

Why eight sets of three for bench? Three reps were chosen because a person should be able to perform 3 light reps in the same time it takes to perform a 1RM on the bench. The Westside routine uses 20 to 30 reps for most exercises because it follows Prilepin's chart (see chapter 24), which makes a similar recommendation ($8 \times 3 = 24$ reps).

Why 10 to 12 sets of two reps for the squat? Two reps were chosen for the same reason that 3 reps were used for the bench press. A client should be able to squat 2 reps with light weight in the same time that it takes

to squat 1 rep with heavy weight. Ten to 12 sets are used because clients should be performing 20 to 30 working reps, and it follows the principle of specificity, which states that when a person is trying to become stronger, performing many singles or doubles (i.e., training with very heavy weights) is more effective than doing one set of 10 reps, all else being equal.

Why short rest on the speed day? The idea is that short rest induces some fatigue, thus requiring greater motor unit recruitment as the workout progresses. A lifter might also release more hormones from training in a rapid fashion. A practical advantage is that the workout won't take forever with this method (10 sets with a five-minute rest after each would take an hour to complete).

Why no speed deadlift day? The deadlift requires the least skill of the three powerlifting exercises, so it does not need to be practiced as much as the other two exercises. In addition, regularly practicing the squat helps to maintain deadlift form. The program allows you to add the deadlift if desired. A general recommendation is to use 5 to 10 total reps, usually performed as singles, at about 50 to 60 percent of the 1RM. This is normally done after the DE squat exercise.

Why no biceps exercises? Westside believes that biceps are not used much in the three powerlifting exercises and that people frequently overtrain that muscle. The thought is that the back exercises offer sufficient stimulus to the biceps.

Are two exercises per week really enough for the shoulders? The Westside philosophy is that the shoulders, particularly the front delts, receive heavy stimulus during any pressing movement, so they do not need additional training. The goal is to bring up the middle and rear delts for support and stability.

Isn't lifting one rep dangerous? Generally, lifting one heavy rep is not much more dangerous than lifting eight reps with a slightly lighter weight, assuming that the lifter knows how to perform the exercise, has a qualified spotter, and takes the proper safety precautions (such as performing the exercise in a squat rack). It also assumes that the person has some idea of how to judge how much weight he or she can lift and how to make proper increases in weight. But any time clients push themselves to the extreme, injury can occur. In addition, powerlifters have to lift just one rep in competition, so the principle of specificity calls for them to practice that by lifting just one rep in training.

Pros and Cons

The Westside theory of weightlifting was developed because the traditional philosophy at the time was becoming less effective. Elite clients got to a point where they just could not add another 5 pounds (2.3 kg) to an exercise. They plateaued, and neither the traditional model nor the HIT training model offered any solutions. This program is significantly different from what most people are using (which is why some people do not like it), but therein lies its strength. If a program can be different and effective at the same time, the body will respond to that.

The Westside program puts significant focus on neuromuscular coordination, which is important for all clients. This program also attempts to fight overtraining of the nervous system. The stronger that people get, the more they can tax their nerves; that is the training paradigm. The better shape that people are in, the more work they need to do to improve their fitness and the more recovery time they need after a hard workout. Lifting very heavy week after week will eventually cause burnout; the body becomes stale from lifting maximally all the time. Alternatively, if people do not regularly lift heavy, they will not get stronger. Westside's way around that problem is to rotate exercises on a regular basis, normally every one, two, or three weeks. Using that method postpones the burnout of the central nervous system and allows people to lift heavier longer.

The program is not time consuming. Like the HIT training program, it promises high-level results without extensive time commitment. Most high-level Olympic weightlifters train three hours a day, five or six days a week. Few personal-training clients would have the time or money to train at that level. Westside proposes that, in just four one-hour workouts a week, a person can achieve a high level of success. That type of time commitment is much more feasible for people who live in the real world, and clients could learn to perform some of those days (particularly the DE days) on their own after some guidance by the personal trainer.

Although the Westside system can be effective, the system has some potential flaws. The first is readily acknowledged; the program is heavily biased towards the squat, bench press, and deadlift exercises. Although those movements are extremely beneficial to almost all people, not everyone is focused on improving their performance in those exercises. In addition, although the Westside system may initially cause increases in muscle size, it is mainly a strength and power training program, not a hypertrophy training program. Similarly, the Westside system is not a muscular endurance training program; it is not designed to burn a maximal number of calories per minute, despite the intensity of the workouts.

Two additional weaknesses of the Westside system are its complexity and its unequal treatment of muscle groups. For example, bar speed is an important factor that is extremely hard to measure, and exercises do not emphasize the biceps, calves, and lats. The result is that clients may develop weak spots, but trying to include exercises for those muscle groups in addition to the exercises already prescribed in the workout can create too much overall stress and compromise the effectiveness of the main program. In other words, it is hard to add exercises to this program without needing to exclude other exercises at the same time. Also, this program might create a slightly higher chance of injury. Lifting weights fast is jarring on the joints, even with good form, and going heavy on an unfamiliar exercise can be dangerous. Because this program focuses on people who use powerlifting equipment, some of the programming and technique advice is not pertinent to regular personal-training clients, even those interested in developing maximal strength, because those clients will never use that equipment.

Although this program is effective for breaking plateaus created by the other methods of training, people can also plateau on this program. After two to six months of following programs like the Westside system, many people report that they are ready to move on to something else.

The Westside program has much to offer clients who are interested in strength training. The idea that working out can be thought of as practice instead of just exercise can help change perceptions about fitness. The idea that neuromuscular coordination, skill, and technique are all central to success is valuable. When something stops working, people have to step outside the box, but do it in a scientific way, to continue to get results. That concept is really what fitness is all about.

CrossFit

CrossFit was founded in 1995 by Greg Glassman, a gymnast who starting training fire fighters and police officers with the perspective that agents of the law had to be prepared for anything. He believed that specializing in one aspect of fitness was a negative because it usually meant that people were weak in another aspect of fitness.

CrossFit as a system is made up of the workout of the day (WOD), or "constantly varied, high-intensity, functional movements" that are posted online or created each day. The workouts are built on a foundation of nutrition, metabolic conditioning, gymnastics movements, and sport, which includes the key exercises of the squat, deadlift, military (shoulder) press, clean and jerk, snatch, gymnastics moves, body-weight exercises, running, jumping, and rowing. In other words, CrossFit focuses on the large-muscle groups, compound movements, and rarely, if ever, on isolation exercises. The workouts train all the energy systems, giving special attention to the fast and slow glycolytic energy systems because, CrossFit asserts, they are typically neglected in fitness programs.

CrossFit is known for relatively short workouts; the workouts can often be completed in 5 to 30 minutes, and rarely are they as long as 60 minutes. CrossFit promotes intense workouts and makes no apologies for it. Traditionally, CrossFit workouts are held as group sessions. A class of 5 to 20 people might show up, and all would perform the WOD. Often, the entire workout is timed, a feature not incorporated by most other philosophies. Instead of having the fitter people in the group perform more work or lift more weight, they simply complete the workout faster. For example, if a WOD was to complete 100 push-ups, a fit person might complete that in 90 seconds with no rest, whereas an out-of-shape person might need to do 10 sets of 10 push-ups with 90 seconds of rest after each set. That person would need 15 or 20 minutes to complete the workout.

One of the goals of a CrossFit program is to reduce body fat, a goal that appeals to the vast majority of exercisers. CrossFit accomplishes this by creating high EPOC, not strictly through the caloric burn of the actual workout (because it is relatively short). Most of the workouts stress and train the glycolytic energy system, which has been shown to create EPOC, and all the workouts involve high intensity, which raises EPOC further.

CrossFit's general philosophy is this:

Eat lean meats and veggies, nuts and seeds, some fruit, little starch, and no sugar. Keep intake to levels that will support exercise but not body fat. Practice and train the major lifts: deads, clean, squat, presses, clean and jerk, and snatch. Similarly, master the basics of gymnastics: pull-ups, dips, rope climb, push-ups, sit-ups, presses to handstands, pirouettes, flips, splits, and holds. Bike, run, swim, row, etc. hard and fast. Five or six days a week mix these elements in as many combos and patterns as creativity will allow. Routine is the enemy. Keep workouts short and intense. Regularly learn and play new sports.

CrossFit has a variety of key tests, which are generally named workouts. The workouts, often named after females or soldiers killed in action, represent measuring sticks that cross-Fitters (what those who follow the programs are typically called) complete periodically to see how they compare with others. The most common test is the timed workout called Fran, which consists of performing 21 thrusters (men use a 95-pound [43.1 kg] barbell, and women use a 65-pound [29.5 kg] barbell), performing 21 pull-ups, then 15 thrusters followed by 15 pull-ups, and then 9 thrusters followed by 9 pull-ups.

Pros and Cons

If you find the CrossFit philosophy appealing, you can become CrossFit certified. This process usually involves going to a weekend workshop, becoming familiar with CrossFit exercises and workout regimes, and taking a test to measure competency. The workshops cost approximately $1,000, which at over $60 per hour is expensive compared with other courses of similar nature.

A positive attribute of CrossFit training is that it encourages hard work; in fact, intensity is the single most important factor in a CrossFit workout. Also, because workouts are short, many clients are able to fit them into their busy schedules. CrossFit workouts are often performed in groups, although this is not a necessity. The group training makes each session more affordable than a standard one-on-one personal training session, so more people are able to access it. Group workouts help build a sense of teamwork and community, which can lead to increased exercise program adherence.

CrossFit promotes competition, which leads to increased performance. CrossFit routines attempt to target 10 key aspects of fitness (cardiovascular and respiratory endurance, stamina, strength, flexibility, power, speed, agility, balance, coordination, and accuracy), so it tends to promote a relatively well-rounded person. CrossFit pushes the primary exercises and key body-weight movements that are functional and tend to yield good results. Females often take particularly well to CrossFit, likely because of the emphasis on flexibility, relative strength, and endurance. CrossFit seems to be effective at reducing body fat, and many clients find it to be fun, at least compared with traditional cardiovascular or resistance training.

Many professionals believe that the programming behind CrossFit routines is haphazard. The training includes no periodization, and little thought seems to go into the day-to-day sequencing of the WODs. Too much volume or too much loading on the joints may occur, and progression may not be maximized. Stronger people generally perform well in CrossFit workouts if they have some endurance.

CrossFit is intense; they make no claims to the contrary. But it may be too intense for some people, and that attitude may turn off some people. People often need to work out for a while and learn to love exercise before they perform intense workouts; going too intense too fast can turn some people away from exercising altogether. One negative of this intense training is that CrossFit can lead to rhabdomyolysis (rhabdo) in some individuals, particularly when excessively high-volume workouts are used with relative novices to that style of training. Rhabdo can be a debilitating condition that requires immediate medical attention and it can leave one in pain and discomfort for months (from just one workout). It can even be fatal in some circumstances. Beginners should be eased into CrossFit-style workouts and their WOD should be altered as necessary by a knowledgeable and qualified coach to appropriately match their current fitness level. See chapter 1 for more information on rhabdo.

CrossFit workouts can involve high volume on exercises such as push-ups, pull-ups, and body-weight squats. This program can be tough on the joints, particularly for larger people. CrossFit workouts are difficult to scale and are not specialized. Many personal trainers do not like the idea of their clients performing a large number of reps on the Olympic lifting exercises. When fatigue sets in, form will deteriorate, and the lifter may start to learn new movement patterns in a fatigued state. CrossFit does little to work on aesthetic weak points. Isolation exercises that can help clients increase the size of their biceps or improve their calves are not emphasized and are often actively discouraged. Adding exercises to the WODs is not a realistic option because the additional volume might lead to more overtraining.

In summary, CrossFit can be an exciting training philosophy to follow, but personal trainers should approach the program with their eyes open and realize that everything has pros and cons to it.

EVALUATION OF TRAINING PROGRAM OR PHILOSOPHY

A variety of training programs or philosophies are available to choose from, and each claims to have solved all the problems associated with other methods. Because of space considerations, they cannot all be listed here. In addition, new ones are constantly being developed. New exercise programs can add variety and present new challenges to the body. But performing something new for the sake of novelty rather than effectiveness can waste time that could be devoted to exercises known to be beneficial. When considering a new program, philosophy, or even exercise, ask these questions:

How hard is the activity? The program should be as hard or harder than what clients are currently doing if you want them to increase their fitness level.

How long will the activity take to master? Mastering or becoming truly proficient at the activity should take years.

What else will people be able to do if they master this activity? What carryover will this activity have? Mastering this activity should improve many other aspects of fitness and life in general.

Does this activity help people achieve their goals? Any new program or activity should take people closer to their goals.

Is the activity awesome? Only you (or your client) can answer this subjective question. Jim Wendler, author of *The Simplest and Most Effective Training System for Raw Strength*, suggested this simple litmus test, and it works well. If the activity is awesome, by your definition, it is likely beneficial and would enhance your clients' fitness. If it is not awesome or if it does not help people become awesome, why spend time on it?

INTENSITY TECHNIQUES

When a person spends years working out, trying something different or doing something unusual to spice up the routine can be appealing. A new activity can reignite enthusiasm for training, and occasionally shocking the muscle with a new stimulus can boost results. Intensity techniques can be used to provide this variety and novel stimulus. Generally, these techniques are not recommended for beginners. Also, they are not designed to be performed all the time, and using them too frequently can lead to burnout and overtraining.

Making a blanket recommendation about how often to use these methods is difficult, but some aspects should be incorporated every three to eight workouts for a muscle group or body area, not added or used every workout. Some are intense and should be used sparingly, and others can be used more regularly.

Superset

A superset involves performing one set of one exercise and then, usually immediately, performing a second set of another exercise for an opposite or unrelated muscle before the rest period begins. The intensity of this varies with the size of the muscle and the difficulty of the set. Using this technique with larger muscles is more exhausting.

- Positives: excellent time saver, can almost double amount of work completed, good for size and endurance, elevates the heart so it is useful as cardio and for burning calories, good when working out alone, provides a good pump, good way to fit in small muscles such as calves and abs without increasing time in the gym (3)
- Negatives: is hard, not good for strength because of insufficient recovery between sets, cannot lift as much weight as normal, may be difficult in a crowded gym

Examples

EZ-bar bicep curl and skull crusher superset

Leg extension and leg curl superset

Bench press and pull-up superset

Bicep curl and crunch superset (unrelated muscles)

Compound Set

A compound set involves performing one set of one exercise and then immediately performing a second set of another exercise for the same muscle. People can complete two or more exercises in a row; three is common. They rest and then repeat, usually for one to three total sets, often called a giant set. The intensity varies with the size of the muscle and the difficulty of the set; sets that use the larger muscles are more exhausting. Because the lifter is working the same muscle, compound sets are more challenging than supersets (56).

Positives: fully stimulates the muscle so it is good for size, builds endurance and constitution, elevates the heart rate, provides a good pump, builds work capacity and lactate threshold, saves time

Negatives: hard and draining, may lead to overtraining if used too often, not good for strength because recovery between sets is incomplete, cannot lift as much weight as normal on subsequent sets, may be difficult in a crowded gym

Examples

Bench press, dumbbell bench press, dumbbell fly compound set

Squat, leg press, leg extension compound set

EZ-bar bicep curl, hammer curl, cable curl compound set

Drop Set

A drop set involves performing one set of an exercise and then immediately decreasing the weight and performing a second set of that same exercise. The weight is normally dropped one to four times, so two to five total sets are completed, which is considered one drop set. The full drop set is usually repeated one to three times per exercise. A drop set is often used as a last set after completing the traditional sets. The weight is dropped 5 to 50 percent; a 10 to 20 percent drop is the most common choice. The number of reps performed is whatever the person is capable of (until failure) or is chosen based on the specific goals. To make this intensity technique effective, the first set in the sequence must be challenging. These are sometimes called strip sets.

Positives: fully stimulates the muscle so it is good for muscle size; builds endurance, work capacity, and lactate threshold

Negatives: hard, may lead to overtraining if done too often, not good for strength because recovery between sets is incomplete, cannot lift as much weight as normal on subsequent sets

Examples

Bench press 275 pounds (124.7 kg) × 10, 225 pounds (102.1 kg) × 6, 185 pounds (83.9 kg) × 6, 155 pounds (70.3 kg) × 10

Leg press 630 pounds (285.8 kg) × 12, 540 pounds (244.9 kg) × 8, 450 pounds (204.1 kg) × 6, 360 pounds (163.3 kg) × 8, 270 pounds (122.5 kg) × 10

Dumbbell bicep curl 50 pounds (22.7 kg) × 12, 40 pounds (18.1 kg) × 8, 30 pounds (13.6 kg) × 8, 20 pounds (9.1 kg) × 12

High Reps

This approach involves performing a higher number of reps on an exercise than normal, usually 20 or more reps, up to 500 reps. The most common choice is 20 to 50 reps. One to three sets are usually performed, using a much lighter weight than usual (45).

Positives: builds endurance, builds speed in the early reps, builds lactate threshold, high volume

Negatives: can decrease maximal strength, may promote the laying down of collagen instead of muscle tissue

Examples

Bench press the bar as many reps as possible

Complete 100 push-ups

Bicep curl 70 pounds (31.8 kg) as many times as possible

Squat 135 pounds (61.2 kg) as many reps as possible

Low Reps

This approach involves performing an unusually low number of reps, coupled with higher weight, on a regularly performed exercise. For example, a person who normally uses 10 reps can try doing 3 reps. One or two extra sets can be added at the end of the workout, or this approach can be used for the whole workout. Doing one to six reps for one to five sets is common, although the number of sets can be higher, if desired. The client can take long breaks, such as two to five minutes (which is similar to a strength program). People should perform this method only on familiar exercises; they should not use it on a new exercise, particularly a high-skill exercise. If a client has never used this method, add 10 percent to the weight that he or she can lift for 8 to 12 reps and have the person try 1 to 3 reps. If that is easy, add another 5 to 10 percent and have the client do the same thing. People should not try to lift more than 20 percent of the most weight they have ever lifted (for a set of reps) without building up to it gradually (63).

Positives: allows a much heavier weight to be used, good to build mental confidence and break through plateaus, good for strength

Negatives: doesn't build much endurance, may not be suited for a client's particular goal although can be used occasionally even if that is the case, results in longer workout, often requires a spotter, can cause injury if too much weight is used

Examples

Bench press 95 pounds (43.1 kg) for 3 reps after doing 80 pounds (36.3 kg) for 10 reps

Bicep curl 105 pounds (47.6 kg) for 1 rep after doing 75 pounds (34.0 kg) for 12 reps

Chest press 250 pounds (113.4 kg) (the whole stack) just to see if it's possible

Short Rest

For this technique, people perform their normal workout but with a significantly decreased rest time, generally half of what they are used to. You will probably have to decrease the client's weight as a result, but do not start out with lighter weight. This method is a good shock to the client's cardio and recovery system. You will probably need to watch the clock to monitor the rest time accurately.

Positives: improves endurance, improves recovery, improves cardio, builds lactate threshold and stamina, saves time

Negatives: cannot use heavier weight so it is not good for strength, not good for size if the weight is too light, will be fatiguing, the rest time is no longer goal specific

Examples

Use 30 seconds of rest instead of the normal 60 seconds of rest

Use 90 seconds of rest instead of the normal 3 minutes of rest

Long Rest

For this technique, people perform their normal workout but use a significantly longer rest time, generally double their current rest time, or they use the rest protocol for strength, which is two to five minutes. The weight should probably be increased.

Positives: good for strength, allows the person to lift heavier weight, good for breaking plateaus and building mental confidence, may be good for size

Negatives: not good for muscular endurance or $\dot{V}O_2max$, does not help improve recovery ability between sets, takes a long time, rest time is no longer goal specific

Examples

Allow two minutes of rest between sets instead of just one minute

Allow a four-minute break between tough leg press sets instead of just two minutes

Negatives

This approach involves lifting a heavier weight than normal and focusing only on the eccentric (negative) portion of the repetition. People spot themselves (in exercises such as a dumbbell curl) or, more commonly, a partner provides assistance on the concentric part of the range of motion. Generally people lift the negative portion using a 6 to 10 count for one to four reps. This can be done at the end of a usual set or as a set all by itself.

> Positives: can lift more weight than normal, good for strength, can break through mental plateaus, gets the body used to lifting a lot of weight
>
> Negatives: usually requires a strong spotter, can cause extreme soreness, hard to do safely on some exercises such as squats, not sport-specific in that most events focus on the concentric part of the movement

Examples

Do a one-rep max weight on bench press and lower it only to the chest for one to four reps with a spotter

Lower the curl bar extra slowly during the bicep curl exercise

Partials

To do a partial, people focus on just a portion of the range of motion for any exercise. For example, they could bring the bar only halfway down on a bench press. Clients can perform an entire set of partials, or they can use them at the end of a set when they are too tired to complete the full ROM but still have some strength left.

> Positives: can lift more weight in an easy part of the range of motion, can focus on weak points in the range of motion, can be sport specific, good for strength and size, further stimulates muscle
>
> Negatives: builds strength only in the range of motion trained in, tendency of people

to focus only on the easy part of the range of motion (see discussion of power factor training)

Examples

Rack press three sets of eight reps

After a set of the dumbbell chest fly exercise, perform only the last 6 inches (15.2 cm) of the range of motion for six reps

Perform the bottom quarter of the range of motion on the back squat to work on form

Holds

A hold during a rep occurs when the person performs an isometric contraction during the exercise, at the end of the set, or as a set all by itself. Holds usually last 15 to 60 seconds, but they can be longer or shorter depending on the goal and the intensity. Normally, the hold is done at the hardest part of the exercise. People should take short, small breaths during the hold; they do not hold their breath.

> Positives: strong muscle contraction, may be sport specific, further stimulates muscle
>
> Negatives: can be hard on the joints, raises blood pressure, builds strength only in the range of motion trained in, form can change during the hold and cause injury

Examples

Hold dumbbells with arms held straight out to the side for 30 seconds for the delts

Hold the bicep curl in the midpoint for 1 minute

Perform a wall sit for 1 minute

Complete a plank on the elbows for 2 minutes

Cluster Set

A cluster set involves performing one rep of an exercise, resting for 10 to 30 seconds, performing another rep of the exercise with the same weight, resting again, and repeating as desired. Generally, people rerack the weight when resting, although that is not mandatory. The weight lifted is typically relatively heavy (85 to 95 percent).

Positives: good for strength because it allows a higher number of reps to be completed at a given percentage of 1RM, which builds NMC

Negatives: can be draining, less time under tension, cannot use the reps completed in this fashion with a conversion chart

Examples

Bench press 90 percent of 1RM for as many reps as possible with a 30-second rest after each set (might get 10 or more reps)

Perform one rep of the weighted pull-up exercise, rest on the ground for 15 seconds, perform another rep, rest, and repeat as many reps as desired

21s

This intensity technique is called 21s because the total number of reps in the set is 21. People consecutively complete three sets of 7 reps, most often using the following order: the full range of motion, the top half range of motion, and then the bottom half range of motion. The order is not incredibly important, but to lift the most weight people should complete the hardest part first, which is usually the full ROM, and the easiest part last. No rest occurs between the sets of the 21 total reps. This method is commonly used on bicep curls, but it can be performed on many exercises. The number of reps does not have to be 7; for example, clients could do 24s (three sets of 8 reps) or 15s (three sets of 5 reps).

Positives: high intensity, stimulates more muscle, ultimately trains the full range of motion, builds lactate tolerance, is good to use occasionally, better for muscles that are slow to fatigue and have a decent range of motion

Negatives: is hard, cannot use as much weight as normal, does not feel as natural on some exercises, form can change on partials

Example

A client who can bicep curl 90 pounds (40.8 kg) for 10 reps uses 75 pounds (34.0 kg) to perform 21s (7 full, 7 top half, 7 bottom half)

Complexes

A traditional complex involves performing a series of exercises with the same load without any rest between exercises. A complex is usually performed with a barbell. A common instruction is that after the hands are on the bar, they do not leave the bar until the complex is finished. A complex usually consists of four to seven exercises in a row of any number of reps, but 3 to 10 reps is a common choice. Usually, one to five sets of the complex is performed. The term is sometimes used to describe any series of exercises performed in a row that are not for the same muscle group (22).

Positives: causes a high level of fatigue, can be somewhat sport specific in that the work time on the complex can match the work time of the sport, can create EPOC, can be a good warm-up

Negatives: because weight on the bar is constant, it is limited to weight that can be lifted in the weakest exercise; breakdown in form possible as fatigue builds; not ideal for developing strength

Examples

Load a barbell with 85 pounds (38.6 kg) and perform the following exercises in order with no rest:

- Clean: 85 pounds (38.6 kg) × 8
- Front squat: 85 pounds (38.6 kg) × 8
- Shoulder press: 85 pounds (38.6 kg) × 8
- Back squat: 85 pounds (38.6 kg) × 8
- Good morning: 85 pounds (38.6 kg) × 8
- Bent-over row: 85 pounds (38.6 kg) × 8

Rest two minutes after the complex is finished and repeat two more times.

Active Rest

Instead of passively resting between sets, people make it an active rest by performing some sort of activity. They usually perform a total-body movement for 15 to 60 seconds or 10 to 30 reps. This approach elevates the heart rate and challenges the recovery system (44).

Positives: burns more calories per workout, does not waste time, builds $\dot{V}O_2$max, builds endurance, improves recovery ability, builds work capacity, builds lactate threshold

Negatives: cannot lift as much weight as normal, thus limiting strength and size development; not as good at building $\dot{V}O_2$max as pure cardio; can be hard depending on activity chosen; may not be as fun as traditional resistance training

Examples

Insert 30 seconds of jumping rope during the rest period for the first four exercises of the workout

Alternate between 10 burpees and 20 jumping jacks after completing each resistance training set

Forced Reps

The goal of forced reps is to train until failure and beyond; generally, two to four forced reps are performed at the end of the regular set when this technique is used.

Positives: stimulates and fatigues a large number of motor units, recruits Type IIb motor units, builds lactate threshold and pain tolerance, teaches people to train intensely

Negatives: requires a good spotter, form may break down, may have a greater chance for injury, often causes soreness, failing regularly can be mentally defeating

Examples

After the client bench presses 185 pounds (83.9 kg) for eight reps, which is all that he or she can do, the personal trainer helps the client complete two more reps by spotting him or her

After the client performs six pull-ups without assistance, which is all that he or she can do, the personal trainer spots the client and helps him or her complete three more reps by pushing up on the client's back or lifting at the waist

Preexhaustion

To use the preexhaustion method, a person performs an isolation exercise before performing a compound exercise for the same muscle group (such as a dumbbell chest fly before a bench press or a leg extension before a squat). This term can also be applied if a strict exercise is performed before a looser but similar exercise (such as a preacher curl before a power curl).

Positives: good for size, forces the preexhausted muscle to work harder, good for teaching the client to feel the muscle working, can be useful if total weights available are limited, can be useful if the spotter doesn't feel comfortable spotting the lifter using maximal weights

Negatives: not good for strength, undertrains the synergistic muscles, less weight lifted after exhaustion, can alter form on an exercise

Examples

Perform three sets of 12 of the cable fly exercise and then perform the bench press exercise

Perform three sets of 10 of the machine pullover exercise and then perform the lat pull-down exercise

Perform two sets of 20 of the hyperextension exercise and then perform the deadlift exercise

Circuit Training

This technique can have a variety of names, but the classic definition of circuit training is the performance of a series of exercises (usually 4 to 12) in a row, one set of each, with minimal rest. Completing a full circuit is one round. Multiple rounds are often performed (three rounds is common).

Positives: little down time, useful when time available to exercise is limited, elevates heart rate, provides a better than normal cardiovascular benefit from lifting weights, might build lactate threshold

Negatives: often involves lifting relatively light weights, less intense on the heart than hard cardio, less intense on the muscles than hard lifting, tends to accomplish two things mediocrely rather than one thing well, often set up on machines (50)

Example

Perform the following five exercises in a row, one set of each, and then repeat:

- Chest press: 80 pounds (36.3 kg) × 10
- Lat pull-down: 70 pounds (31.8 kg) × 10
- Machine shoulder press: 55 pounds (24.9 kg) × 10
- EZ-bar cable bicep curl: 40 pounds (18.1 kg) × 10
- V-grip tricep push-down: 50 pounds (22.7 kg) × 10

Reverse Sets and Reps

With this technique, the personal trainer reverses the standard set and rep scheme. For example, if a client usually performs three sets of eight reps on an exercise, now he or she performs eight sets of three reps.

Positives: allows more weight to be lifted, builds strength, builds confidence with the lighter weights, better for bone growth, often considered fun

Negatives: promotes longer rest times, can take longer, may not be goal specific, not as effective at increasing muscular endurance or lactate threshold

Examples

Lat pull-down: Instead of lifting 70 pounds (31.8 kg) for three sets of eight, lift 80 pounds (36.3 kg) for eight sets of three

Dumbbell bicep curl: Instead of lifting 12 pounds (5.4 kg) for three sets of eight, lift 20 pounds (9.1 kg) for eight sets of three

Super Slow

With this method, people perform each rep with a super slow cadence, usually by following a 10:10 tempo (i.e., 10 seconds for the concentric phase, 10 seconds for the eccentric

phase). An isometric pause can be added as well if desired.

Positives: makes light weight feel heavy, uses no momentum, builds mind–muscle connection, can build lactate threshold, works better with isolation exercises and machines

Negatives: must use a light weight, can promote high blood pressure while lifting, harder to do on bigger and compound exercises, cannot be performed with explosive power exercises, may shift emphasis to other muscles like the lower back, often not considered fun if performed regularly, not sport specific

Example

Perform a bicep curl with a tempo of 10:10 for three sets of eight reps

Explosive Training

An important aspect of explosive training is performing each rep rapidly by accelerating the weight during the concentric portion. This action is sometimes referred to as compensatory acceleration.

Positives: sport specific, builds power, targets Type IIb motor units, may prime the muscle spindles for a rapid firing, works well on bigger muscles and compound exercises (17)

Negatives: may cause form to break down, not for beginners, allows too much momentum to be used, does not work well with small muscles and isolation exercises, not effective in building muscle size because the time under tension is short, can lead to the joints forcefully locking out under load, forces the lifter to decelerate significantly at the end of the range of motion

Examples

Perform a dynamic effort bench or squat day (see the section "Westside")

Perform the power clean and snatch exercises

Perform the jumping squat and clap push-up exercises

Continuous Tension

The continuous tension technique requires the personal trainer to ensure that the client's skeletal system or the apparatus does not bear the weight of the exercise, thereby forcing the client's muscles to maintain tension the entire time to support the weight.

> Positives: good for size, builds lactate threshold, helps build mind–muscle connection, reinforces slow and controlled movements with excellent technique
>
> Negatives: eliminates some of the range of motion, usually uses lighter weight than normal, muscle does not learn to recharge with short rest

Examples

> Leg press: Do not allow the client to lock the knees to rest at the end of the movement; instead, force the client to press up until near full extension and then immediately begin another rep
>
> Bench press: Have the client press the bar 7/8ths of the way up, not to full extension of the elbows, and then begin another rep

Pause Reps

The pause reps method involves implementing a pause between the eccentric and the concentric phase of the exercise, thus making the exercise harder.

> Positives: eliminates momentum, makes the lift easier to judge, may build starting strength, may add tension on the working muscle
>
> Negatives: can weaken the stretch reflex, may teach the muscle to develop force slowly, usually requires lighter weight to be used

Examples

> Perform a set of five reps of the bench press exercise but pause the bar on the chest for one second before pressing it

Perform the dead hang pull-up exercise by fully relaxing and allowing the arms to fully extend; rest for one second before performing the next rep

Rest Pause

To perform a rest pause, the client completes a certain number of reps, rests for a brief time (usually 10 to 30 seconds), and then continues the set to complete a few more reps. The short rest allows the client to recharge somewhat (50).

> Positives: allows the muscle to perform more work, teaches recovery in short breaks, helps increase muscle size, recruits additional motor units
>
> Negatives: for an equal number of reps, easier than just going straight through without stopping; becomes two separate sets if the rest is too long; if the first part of the set is not hard enough, rest not warranted before the second part

Example

> If the goal is to complete a set of 12 reps on the bench with 70 pounds (31.8 kg) and the client reaches the point of fatigue at 8 reps, the bar is racked. The client rests for about 20 seconds and then completes the remaining 4 reps

Unstable Training

For this type of training, the personal trainer removes an element of stability from the exercise or adds an element of instability such as requiring the client to stand on one leg, use one arm, lie on a stability ball, use gymnastics rings, or use suspension.

> Positives: is a form of progression because the exercise is harder, may have high skill transfer to the lower-skill versions, may require the core and stabilizing muscles to work harder (6)
>
> Negatives: requires use of lighter weights, may cause the client to become weaker if used too frequently, possible issues of safety and joint stability, not effective in increasing muscular size, usually not

effective in increasing strength as demonstrated by a barbell lift, reduced muscle activation resulting from instability (14)

Examples

Perform the dumbbell bench press exercise on a stability ball instead of a bench (figure 25.3)

Perform dips with gymnastics rings instead of a dip bar

Stand on a Bosu ball to perform the dumbbell hammer curl exercise

Tabata

Tabata training uses a specific work and rest interval. The work period is 20 seconds, and the rest period is 10 seconds. Generally, people perform four to eight sets or circuits of this protocol, which means that one tabata protocol will last two to four minutes.

Positives: builds lactate threshold, builds conditioning and stamina and toughness, works better on some exercises than others, induces strong fatigue level in short time, creates EPOC (9)

Negatives: uses light weights, may promote unhealthy form, not ideal for building maximal strength

Example

Perform a front squat with 95 pounds (43.1 kg) for 20 seconds (about eight reps), rest for 10 seconds, and repeat eight times (4 minutes total)

Combination Exercises

Personal trainers often like to combine two or more exercises into one exercise. This approach can be productive, but equal or superior results can often be achieved by supersetting the same exercises (60).

Positives: fatigues many muscles at once, raises the heart rate, saves time

Negatives: weight for one exercise likely not appropriate for other exercises, resulting in undertraining on one exercise

Examples

A dumbbell squat combined with a bicep curl

A dumbbell step-up combined with a shoulder press

A leg press and a calf raise on the leg press machine

A dumbbell row and a dumbbell tricep kickback (figure 25.4)

A squat and a shoulder press

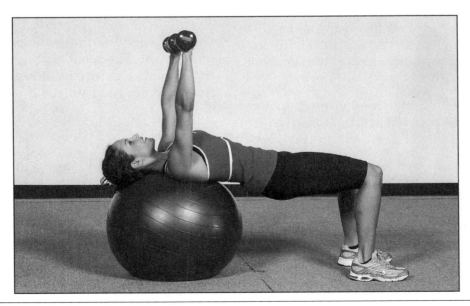

Figure 25.3 Example of an unstable exercise.

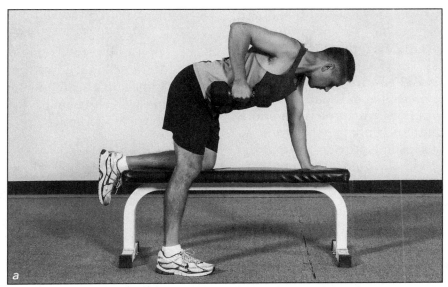

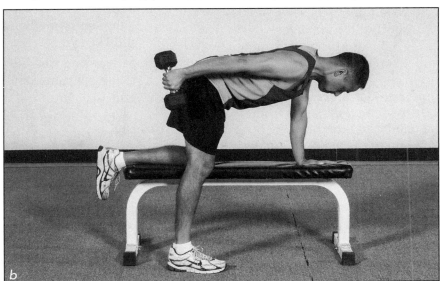

Figure 25.4 Example of a combination exercise: *(a)* ending position of dumbbell row and *(b)* ending position of tricep kickback.

CONCLUSION

An important part of designing a resistance training program is choosing the exercise routine. Simply stated, routines are either total-body programs or split programs. Total-body routines typically include less volume per movement or body part in a workout but allow greater frequency of training of those areas. Split routines typically include a higher volume and intensity per movement or body part in a workout but do not allow as much frequency of training of that specific area. Split

routines are common among advanced clients who want to train on consecutive days.

Personal trainers often develop fitness philosophies as they progress in their careers. Some philosophies have become quite popular. High-intensity training involves performing one all-out work set until failure for each exercise; the goal is to promote size and strength without overtraining. Westside Barbell Club focuses on training movements, not muscles, and trains each key area twice per week. One time each week is focused on going heavy and hard, and the other training session is a dynamic effort day to develop speed and power. CrossFit does not focus on one area of fitness; it aims to develop proficiency in all aspects of fitness. The goal of the CrossFit program is to prepare clients for whatever fitness activity may be presented to them.

Personal trainers can incorporate various intensity techniques to enhance the workout, achieve results faster, and provide physical and mental variation in the gym. Intensity techniques tend to focus on improving a certain component of fitness. Cluster sets, negatives, partials, low reps, reverse sets and reps, long rest, holds, pause reps, explosive training, and rest pause reps tend to focus on building strength. Supersets, compound sets, drop sets, 21s, forced reps, preexhaustion, super slow, and continuous tension tend to focus on building size. High reps, short rest, complexes, active rest, circuit training, tabatas, unstable training, and combination exercises tend to promote muscular endurance.

Personal training program design is a combination of art and science. Personal trainers should learn the science behind how the body adapts to exercise and then combine that with their own philosophy to create an individualized but highly optimal workout program for their clients.

Study Questions

1. What is the philosophy of high-intensity training?
   a. to take all sets until failure
   b. to train all muscles on a once-a-week split
   c. to perform one all-out work set per exercise until failure
   d. to specialize in maximizing muscular endurance

2. According to the Westside philosophy, what is *not* one of the three main ways to build strength?
   a. to lift as heavy a weight as possible
   b. to lift a light weight slowly and in a controlled way for a limited number of reps

   c. to lift a moderate weight for as many reps as possible
   d. to lift a moderate weight as fast as possible

3. Which of the following clients would most likely benefit from following a CrossFit workout?
   a. competitive powerlifter
   b. football offensive lineman
   c. a 40-year-old intermediate-level female looking to tone up
   d. a 75-year-old beginning male with hypertension and diabetes

4. Which of the following is an example of a compound set?
   a. performing one set of bicep curls followed immediately by one set of skull crushers
   b. performing one set of bench press followed immediately by one set of pull-ups
   c. performing one set of squats followed immediately by one set of leg press
   d. performing one set of squats followed immediately by one set of calf raises

5. You are going to set up a double drop set for your male client on the bench press. Which of the following weights represent a logical progression if the client's first challenging set is 200 pounds (90.7 kg) × 10 reps?
   a. 170 pounds (77.1 kg), 140 pounds (63.5 kg)
   b. 170 pounds (77.1 kg), 200 pounds (90.7 kg)
   c. 100 pounds (45.4 kg), 45 pounds (20.4 kg)
   d. 195 pounds (88.5 kg), 190 pounds (86.2 kg)

Training Special Populations

Most of this book is geared to providing personal trainers with information about how to train clients within their scope of practice—the generally healthy adult population. But a small portion of a personal trainer's clients may require special care when exercising. These people include older adults, children, and women who are pregnant or have recently delivered a child. General information on training women is also included, not because women are outside a personal trainer's scope of practice but because resistance training has historically focused on males. Therefore, specific information regarding resistance training for women is needed. In general, personal trainers should communicate effectively, use common sense, involve other health professionals when necessary, and error on the side of caution when training clients who have special needs and considerations.

OLDER ADULTS

Older adults are typically defined as people aged 65 years old and over. The number of older adults in America continues to grow as medical advances and safety conditions improve. Older adults commonly turn to personal trainers for advice on exercise programs to keep them feeling young, mobile, and healthy.

The body generally starts to show signs of aging around the age of 30 years old, but the progression is slow and ideally the body is coming down from a high level of fitness. Ten or 20 years of regular training is often needed for the body to peak in terms of physical performance, and people need to be old enough to express that training time, which is why many athletes seem to peak in their 30s, even after the body starts to age. Performance is usually still quite strong in the 40s, but as people enter their 50s the effects of aging become more noticeable. Still, we don't need to look too far to find adults of a broad age range excelling at various sports and activities, often at a level the typical 20-year-old could not come close to matching (329).

Many physical effects occur as the body ages. Maximum muscle strength decreases, as does maximum power (power is usually more significantly affected than strength). Overall muscle mass decreases, muscle endurance decreases, $\dot{V}O_2max$ decreases, bone density decreases, flexibility decreases, circulation decreases, reaction time and balance decrease, and rate of force development decreases. Two things increase, but unfortunately they are body fat and recovery time.

The good news is that exercise can reverse or at least slow down the effects of aging. Exercise increases strength and power, muscle mass, muscle endurance, $\dot{V}O_2max$, bone density, flexibility, circulation, reaction, balance, and rate of force development. Exercise also decreases body fat and recovery time. It is a cliche, but there is some truth to the idea that exercise is the best fountain of youth available, and it comes with little or no side effects. Of course, exercise cannot fully stave off the effects of aging, but it can have a significant effect on health and fitness (23, 87).

It is wise for a personal trainer to seek a medical clearance when training older adults. An older adult will automatically have on CAD risk factor due to age and is very likely to have two or more risk factors, placing the client in the moderate risk category and requiring a clearance for vigorous exercise. The client is also more likely to have signs or symptoms and thus be classified as high risk. The personal trainer should still perform an initial consultation to understand the client's health history, but the client should receive a medical clearance and the personal trainer should follow any indications and contraindications provided by the doctor.

Program Guidelines

Those who train older adults may ask several reasonable questions: "At what age does the body stop responding to exercise? When does training become essentially useless? When should people call it quits?" The good news in response to those questions is that as long as the body is alive, it is an adaptable organism that can respond to training (4). A client who is 80 years old and has osteoporosis can still build bone. Of course, the adaptation rate of an older adult is slower than that of a younger adult, but the body can adapt at any age. Personal trainers should keep in mind that at an older age, the hormonal response of clients is likely to be subdued, so the hypertrophic response to exercise will be less. In short, older clients will have a harder time putting on significant muscle mass, and a typical bodybuilding program is likely not optimal for older adults.

Most older adults do well training twice a week for 60 minutes each time. The training days should be spread apart to allow adequate recovery. As the older adults' fitness improves, the training frequency can be increased, and they do not need to reduce training frequency simply because they are older if the body is already adapted to the current workload. The purpose of the reduced frequency is to provide the body with greater recovery time.

Many older adults find they like a longer warm-up because they need more time to get their blood flowing and their joints and muscle loose. They often prefer to double the standard warm-up time and go for 10 minutes or so, and they might want to include stretching as part of that warm-up procedure. The guideline for stretching holds true. If people

have trouble performing the normal range of motion without stretching before the exercise, they should stretch before performing the exercise. Because many older adults are less flexible (because of both aging and a general decrease in flexibility), they will need to stretch before lifting weights. If clients have the time, the personal trainer can show them how to warm up and then suggest that clients arrive 15 minutes early for their sessions. Clients can perform the warm-up and some basic stretches on their own time. If clients are unable to do this, the personal trainer needs to incorporate an adequate warm-up into the training session (18).

By the time people reach 65 years of age, they are likely to have one or more significant injuries that the personal trainer should be aware of. Generally, these injuries will be preexisting conditions. The main goal of the personal trainer is to work around the injuries. Small adjustments to the form of an exercise can either exacerbate or alleviate the discomfort of an injury. Many times the range of motion has to be slightly limited; for example, older adults may not need to touch the chest on a bench press if doing so bothers the shoulder joint. Often a change in grips will feel better. For example, if an older adult switches to a neutral grip dumbbell press from the standard pronated grip, that movement often feels more comfortable. The personal trainer will use his or her knowledge of anatomy and exercise, combined with communication from the client, to devise the most appropriate exercise program. Even the most beneficial exercise should not be forced on a client if the client cannot perform it in a pain-free way.

As people age, they often lose flexibility, particularly in the hips, trunk, and shoulder girdle (29). Most older adults benefit from spending a certain amount of time in each session to improving or at least maintaining flexibility. Partner stretches and PNF stretches can be particularly valuable in this instance. They feel good for the client, the client often looks forward to that activity, these types of stretches tend to be effective, and they are ideal to be performed with a personal trainer. Physical human contact tends to decrease as people age. The client can benefit by being touched and stretched by another person.

The personal trainer will likely want to incorporate some balance-related exercises into the program. As people age, balance decreases, which increases the likelihood of a fall and increases the chance of injury or possibly death (20 percent of older adults who break their hips die within one year). Improving balance is an admirable goal, but the personal trainer must take care that the client does not fall while working on balance. If a client is very unstable, machines can generally provide stability so that the personal trainer can work on improving the client's basic musculature. As clients advance, they can move to more functional exercises, but if the chance of falling is reasonable, the personal trainer should provide clients with an easy out—meaning a bar or hand or something stable to provide immediate assistance. The risk–reward ratio of each exercise should be evaluated before clients perform it (17).

The personal trainer should attempt to avoid making the client excessively sore. Keep in mind that soreness is related to intensity (percentage of 1RM), volume (too much work), intensity techniques (drop sets, preexhaustion, and so on), and changing exercises. The personal trainer should start slow and light, gradually increase the overload, and err on the side of caution.

Older adults often have some issue with their blood pressure. Because of these issues and because they are usually focused more on health than performance, as a personal trainer, you should avoid invoking the Valsalva maneuver with clients. Instruct clients to breathe on each rep. If they report feeling dizzy or seeing stars or the face gets extremely red, decrease the intensity. In addition, blood pressure can be position dependent. Avoid positions in which the head is below the body (declines) or in which some part of the body is above the head (leg press).

Summary of Guidelines to Consider When Training Older Adults

- Have clients obtain medical clearance for exercise.

- Include a longer warm-up (10 or more minutes).
- Have clients stretch before resistance training.
- Follow the guidelines presented with the beginner workout including performing a total-body routine, one to two exercises per muscle, one to three sets per exercise, 10 to 15 reps per set, and a 2:4 count.
- Start with a stable movement and progress to a more unstable, challenging movement as clients' ability improves.
- Keep clients as comfortable as possible.
- Emphasize safety and minimize risk of falling as the number one priority.
- Avoid invoking the Valsalva maneuver and exercises that unduly increase blood pressure (e.g., with the feet above the head).
- Focus on improving clients' balance.
- Focus on exercises that improve clients' ability to perform their activities of daily living.
- Finish the session with partner stretching.
- Allow rest during the session as needed if clients become short of breath.
- Start light and follow progressive overload.

CHILDREN

Children are another group that personal trainers commonly work with. In this context, children, who are outside the scope of practice for personal trainers, are people under the age of 16 years old. Children need to receive medical clearance to be placed in the scope of practice of personal trainers.

A logical question to ask is whether children respond to physical training. The answer, of course, is that children can respond and adapt in a positive fashion to physical training. But they may not respond in the same manner because of their lower hormonal levels, particularly in the testosterone levels of boys.

Adult men usually have 10 or more times as much testosterone in the body as young boys do, which indicates that children are unlikely to see the large hypertrophic response that adult men are capable of. Put simply, children will generally not add significant amounts of muscle to their frames, even if they work out extremely hard. They can add some muscle, but they will not look like mini-bodybuilders even if they wanted to (assuming that they are not given steroids). Instead, children respond in a more neuromuscular manner, and the type of training selected for them should reflect that (10).

The most common concern, usually from parents or other well-meaning adults, is that children will stunt their growth if they lift weights too early. Put simply, this is a myth. No scientific evidence indicates that weight-lifting or other forms of sensible exercise will stunt a child's growth. Although the idea of having children regularly engage in resistance training is relatively new, children have performed simple physical labor (such as carrying buckets of water from the well to the kitchen or moving bales of hay on the farm) for centuries. We can imagine the reaction that we might get if we approached a farmer and suggested that his or her children not perform any physical labor until the age of 16 or so. Simply placing a load on the skeleton does not stunt growth. Extreme, long-term exercise or manual labor (many hours a day for many years) combined with (and likely a contributing factor to) long-term deprivation of essential nutrients (starvation for a long time) could stunt a person's growth, but this type of situation would not occur in a personal training setting (34, 35).

A more valid concern is how to deal with growing pains. Bones grow from an epiphyseal growth plate located at the end of the long bones. Bones grow from their ends, not from their middle. Bone growth does not occur uniformly and consistently; for example, children do not grow .1 millimeter every day. Instead, bones can grow a measurable amount literally overnight. If a child experiences a growth spurt (which can vary from one person to another but might be characterized as growth

of several inches in a short time), he or she may experience growing pains, which is pain in the joints and muscles. Personal trainers should know that the bones grow first. This growth, in turn, will stretch out the muscles, tendons, ligaments, and fascia that surround that area. Those tissues will adapt to the new length of bone over time. This rapid growth can also explain why kids seem to go through an awkward or gangly stage in which they often appear uncoordinated; they are still learning where their bodies are in space. If somehow your femurs grew 1 inch (2.5 cm) longer overnight, your coordination would decrease until you adapted to the new you (43).

Intense exercise and a high volume of activity seem to exacerbate growing pains (6). If a child is experiencing growing pains, the personal trainer should listen to what the child is saying (adults sometimes downplay the information they receive from a child). During this time, the personal trainer should focus on flexibility, muscle balance, and a moderate level of exercise, as tolerated by the client.

Children can vary greatly in physical and mental maturity. When designing a program for a child, the personal trainer should take into account the child's attention span. A 5-year-old would probably not be able to follow a structured one-hour workout routine and stay on task, but a 15-year-old would likely be able to complete something like that. The more physically mature and physically developed a child is, the more intensity and structure he or she will be able to handle in training. In addition, the personal trainer should consider the training age of the client, that is, how long the client has been performing similar activity.

Program Guidelines

When it comes to creating exercise programs for children, personal trainers should consider some specific guidelines. First, the child should receive medical clearance to exercise. The personal trainer can tell parents to ask for a sports physical instead of just a regular physical, which may not go into enough depth to determine whether the child is ready for physical activity.

Most children do well performing regular exercise two to three times a week to begin. Children can perform both compound and isolation exercises for one to three work sets of 6 to 15 reps. Machines work well for most beginners, but kids can be an exception for the simple reason that they often do not fit well into machines, which are made for average-sized adults. Children can work with barbells and dumbbells after they have learned proper form. Personal trainers need to be able to modify the weight; a 45-pound (20.4 kg) barbell is likely too heavy for most children to work out with. Training bars, body bars, lighter preloaded bars, EZ-bars, which are often 15 to 20 pounds (6.8 to 9.1 kg), or even broomsticks or PVC pipes can be used as tools with kids. Barbells and dumbbells can be effective because they automatically match the person's size. But barbell and dumbbell exercises often require more skill and may require a spot (99).

Calisthenics (body-weight exercises) are probably the ideal exercises for kids. Children often display relatively poor absolute strength, but their relative strength can be acceptable. Body-weight exercises take advantage of relative strength. As children grow in weight, body-weight exercises become more challenging. Therefore, progressive overload will be followed, which is important with kids just as it is with adults. Body-weight exercises can be regressed (performing a push-up on the knees instead of the toes) and progressed (performing a push-up on gymnastics rings instead of the ground). Most body-weight exercises are extremely functional because they teach clients how to use their own bodies in various activities and they take place in three dimensions so they develop balance and coordination. They can be performed easily in groups and usually do not require a spotter or equipment (10, 26).

Safety

Practicing proper safety techniques should be a priority for personal trainers who work with children. Children tend to lack the body awareness of adults, so their form can deteriorate quickly. As a personal trainer, you should be continually monitoring their form and cor-

recting any deviations from proper technique. You should also take time in the beginning to ensure that children know proper form with the lighter weights. If a child is unable to learn or demonstrate the correct form, go to another similar exercise and revisit that exercise on a later date.

In general, you should have children make small jumps in weight between sets and use the smallest amount of weight possible for progressive overload. You may want to look into securing .75-pound (.3 kg) or 1.25-pound (.6 kg) weight plates to add to a bar because the lightest plate in most gyms is 2.5 pounds (1.1 kg), which results in a 5-pound (2.3 kg) increase because you have to use one plate on each side of the bar.

Injury rarely occurs in a gym from performing the exercises, but the gym environment itself can be dangerous. Children should be instructed on proper form and etiquette for the gym. The number one hazard, horseplay, cannot be tolerated. This danger is more likely to occur in a group setting.

Personal trainers need to watch and ensure that the proper range of motion is followed on exercises. Children are more flexible than adults are because some of their bones are not yet fused and they have much less tissue surrounding the joints. This flexibility can be a benefit, but it can also mean that they can get out of position when exercising. For example, in performing a dumbbell fly, a child might take the dumbbells all the way down to the floor if not cued properly. Children should perform the same maximal range of motion as adults do. They should be monitored, particularly when performing exercises for the shoulders and lower back because of their frequently excessive flexibility in those joints.

Exercise can go a long way to building a child's confidence and health. Unfortunately, the number of children who play outside several hours a day is small, so exercise must replace that play. Children play because it is fun. Adults play because it is fun. The presence of fun is the number one reason that people continue to do an activity. Having fun is more powerful than receiving money or seeing results. You must make the personal training session fun for the child, at some level, so that he or she will want to continue the activity for a lifetime. To help do that, you need to think outside the box to make the training session less structured and more creative. Instead of telling a child, "We are going to do 15 minutes of conditioning exercises," you say, "Let's throw the football for 15 minutes, and I will have you run some patterns." Both activities accomplish the same thing, but the first one seems like exercise and the second one seems like fun. Strive for the second one, and the physical results will come.

Summary of Guidelines to Consider When Training Children

- Have the client obtain medical clearance for exercise.
- Focus on proper form and technique.
- Provide constant supervision.
- Be in a position to spot the child if necessary.
- Ensure that children avoid excess range of motion during resistance training exercises.
- Properly align exercise machines to a child's body dimensions.
- Incorporate lighter implements when necessary; standard barbells and plates may be too heavy for children to lift or warm-up with.
- Include calisthenic exercises.
- Focus on all aspects of fitness; do not just specialize in one area.
- Make the training fun and build a life-long love of fitness.

WOMEN

Women are not typically classified as a special population, but it is still important to address specific issues or concerns that might arise when training female clients.

At the most basic level, muscle tissue and muscle cells are not sex specific. A woman's muscle fiber and a man's muscle fiber are essentially the same; it is not necessary to write one book on the fundamentals of fitness and personal training for men and a second book on the fundamentals of fitness and personal training for women. That is the good news; all the anatomy and exercise information you have been learning while studying this information applies to both men and women. Even so, men and women are not identical in all respects. Well-qualified personal trainers should be aware of some of the differences (233).

Women usually have less lean mass and more fat mass than men do at a given weight. Women usually have lower absolute strength than men do. The greatest difference is displayed in upper-body strength. A woman's relative strength is closer to that of a man, particularly if compared in relation with total lean mass. But men, on average, are still stronger and more powerful than women, on average, likely because of varying hormone levels, neuromuscular coordination, and joint stability, among other factors (233).

Women have slightly smaller and thinner bones than men, and they are more likely to develop osteoporosis. The average American woman is approximately 5 feet, 4 inches (162.6 cm) tall and weighs 163 pounds (73.9 kg). Note that this average weight does not indicate the ideal healthy weight for that height; an ideal weight is likely closer to 115 to 125 pounds (52.2 to 56.7 kg) at that height. A woman's heart and lungs tend to be slightly smaller than a man's, and her $\dot{V}O_2$max is usually 5 to 6 points lower than a man's. Although world record $\dot{V}O_2$max scores are hard to validate, the highest $\dot{V}O_2$ scores reported for women usually range between 75 and 78 milliliters per kilogram per minute.

Women are likely to be more flexible than men are. On average, women score 2 to 3 inches (5.1 to 7.6 cm) higher in the sit-and-reach test, likely because they have less lean mass, different hormones, more flexible joints, and lower body mass in general. Women are also more likely to experience hypermobility.

Women express a slower basal metabolic rate than men do, likely because of smaller amounts of muscle tissue, smaller organs, and greater amounts of body fat. Women also live longer than men do—six to eight years longer, on average. Whether the two variables (metabolism and lifespan) are linked or not is unknown.

Program Guidelines

As previously mentioned, women sometimes lack upper-body strength, particularly when compared with men. Women in general and female athletes in particular can often benefit by training with weights to increase upper-body strength. That type of training will make many of the activities of daily living easier, and a strong woman will have a significant advantage over her competitors. A well-rounded resistance training program that focuses on foundational barbell and body-weight exercises is suggested.

Women are significantly more likely to incur serious knee injuries than men (157). The reason for this is not clear. A leading hypothesis is that the angle that the femur makes contact with the tibia in a woman is sharper (not as straight) than it is in a man (figure 26.1). If the bones connect at a steeper angle, the structure at the knee is less sound and more likely to become injured. This circumstance combined with some other variables such as poorer neuromuscular coordination (which may result simply from less practice time), unstable ankles or hips, less muscle mass surrounding the joint,

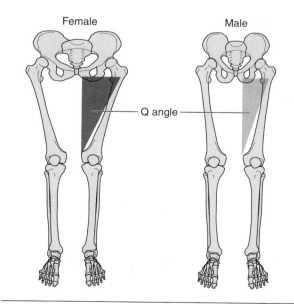

Figure 26.1 Differing Q angles between men and women.

and more flexible ligaments and joints seems to explain why women suffer a higher percentage of knee injuries than men do. Strengthening the quads, hamstrings, abductors, adductors, calves, and other muscles that surround and protect the knee is suggested. Working on improving neuromuscular coordination through practice and improving ankle proprioception is also likely to help (212).

Women should be discouraged from displaying excess range of motion when resistance training. The same form and technique guidelines that apply to training men apply to training women. Common areas where this excess range of motion is seen include the machine chest fly (the handles are moved too far back behind the body), lateral raise (the arms are raised too high above the shoulders), rear delt raise (the arms are raised too far back behind the body), and deadlift (the lower back is allowed to round). Excess range of motion is often more a problem with dumbbells and machines than with a barbell because the barbell often contacts the body as a natural stopping point (199, 248).

Women can take advantage of their greater flexibility by working on some of the more classic power exercises (clean, snatch, thruster) and other exercises that require a high level of flexibility (turkish get-up and pistol squat). Personal trainers often find that women take well to the power exercises for several reasons. First, women are often flexible enough to get into the proper positions; many men, particularly those 30 years old and older, often struggle to achieve the proper position. Second, because women have less total strength than men, they end up using the proper muscles in a power exercise to complete the exercise (76). Men, who are stronger, can often muscle through a lightweight version of the exercise but ultimately never learn the proper form. Finally, many personal trainers find women to be better listeners and more receptive to instruction than men.

Common Concerns

A common concern that women express to their personal trainers is the fear of getting big or gaining too much muscle. Women worry that if they lift weights too hard for too long they will develop big, bulky muscles similar to those of male bodybuilders. Personal trainers need to handle this topic properly to develop and maintain good relationships with their female clients. First, the personal trainer should seek to understand the client and find out what "too big" means to her. Often, it means looking like a male bodybuilder. Professional male bodybuilders in general and the vast majority of those who appear in the magazines and on stage competing for the Mr. Olympia title are on steroids and other drugs. Men who train hard cannot come close to looking like those bodybuilders, and women who are drug free have no chance of becoming that muscular. Large muscles are not built overnight. If a woman finds that she is becoming too muscular for her preference, she can simply stop lifting as hard. Her muscles will then start to shrink (but will not turn into fat). Women have much lower levels of testosterone than men do, so they have to train harder to compensate for this lack of hormonal influence if they want to gain muscle tissue (61, 159, 293).

A personal trainer may want to learn about the female client's perception of her ideal appearance. Women often turn to fitness or figure athletes, soccer players, dancers, gymnasts, or celebrities as role models. Most of these athletes train extremely hard. Learning more about the client's role model may be useful; although the role model is not big and bulky, she may be able to perform seven pull-ups! The client may not be able to perform a single pull-up, but knowing that her role model can do that many may help her work hard to match the performance of her role model.

Women can develop a high level of strength and athleticism without becoming big and bulky. Jennifer Thompson, the greatest pound-for-pound drug-free female bench presser and a math teacher from Denver, has benched over 300 pounds (136.1 kg) at a body weight of 132 pounds (59.9 kg) and a height of 5 feet, 5 inches (165 cm). Another example is Li Ping from China. She weighs 120 pounds (54.4 kg) and snatched 230 pounds (104.3 kg) and clean and jerked 280 pounds (127.0 kg). The

human body, both male and female, is capable of impressive feats of strength without needing to have a tremendous amount of muscle.

Goal of Being Toned

A common goal of women is to become toned. This goal is challenging because it is vague. Each woman has her own definition, and unfortunately, becoming toned is not a component of fitness. Becoming toned might mean losing body fat and revealing the muscle under that layer of fat; in this instance, the client wants to get smaller. Becoming toned might mean increasing the amount of muscle so that it becomes visible; in this case, the client might be thin but have no visible muscle, a condition sometimes referred to as "skinny fat." Becoming toned to this person might mean adding size to the arms or legs. The personal trainer needs to find out which goal applies to each client.

Although women can select exercises that are ideal for achieving a toned look, they often use a weight that is too light to achieve their goal simply because they are not strong enough (yet) to use enough weight to reshape the body. Women first need to develop a base of strength before moving on to exercises that might be classified as shaping exercises. With bones, a minimal essential strain is the minimum weight necessary to build bone. A similar concept applies here: A minimum weight is necessary to build and shape a muscle. Although providing ranges for all women is difficult, a woman who can full squat 105 pounds (47.6 kg), bench press 75 pounds (34.0 kg), and deadlift 135 pounds (61.2 kg)—all for one rep—is likely strong enough to use weights in other exercises that will have a positive effect on her body.

The NPTI's system of exercise program design can be used to create an effective workout program to tone a woman's body.

Define and Clarify the Goal: Increase Muscle Tone

The purpose of this program is to improve the client's aesthetic appearance and health by improving the look and shape of the primary skeletal muscles and by improving body composition.

List the Expected Outcomes

After following a program designed for toning, the client should experience better body composition (if combined with a good nutrition plan), increased firmness of the muscle when the muscle is contracted, improved posture by training through a full range of motion, increases in strength and muscular endurance, improved visibility of the external muscles as measured by pictures, improved waist-to-hip ratio, and greater self-confidence as aesthetic appearance improves.

List the Expected Physiological Adaptations

Specific changes take place in the body when a client follows a toning program:

- Actin, myosin, and related filaments thicken and increase in relative strength.
- Neuromuscular coordination improves.
- Motor units may begin to switch over to Type IIa motor units.
- Bone, tendons, and ligaments generally increase in strength, along with the muscle.
- Myoglobin density and capillary density increase.
- Blood volume and anaerobic capacity increase.

Analyze the Program Setup

A program that has the goal of toning can vary because the term means different things to dif-ferent people. Normally, people will resistance train two to four times per week and stimulate each area or movement one to three times per week.

Select the Specific Routine

Common routines to achieve toning are total-body routines, push–pull routines, and upper–lower routines (table 26.1).

Select the Number of Resistance Training Exercises per Workout

Training to improve tone usually incorporates 6 to 12 resistance training exercises per workout (see table 26.2).

Select the Number of Resistance Training Exercises per Body Part or Movement

One to three exercises per muscle group or movement are usually selected.

Select the Specific Exercises

Guidelines for exercise selection for this goal are based on a certain targeted area of the body and performed through a full range of motion. These exercises are decidedly less useful if a woman is unable to lift the recommended weight previously described—a strength level that usually requires at least two to six months of dedicated resistance training.

Clients are not expected to train only on these exercises or to perform all the exercises in every session.

Put the Exercises in Their Proper Order

Exercise order is somewhat important in achieving a toned look. The traditional guidelines of starting the workout with high-skill,

Table 26.1 Specific Toning Routines and Their Corresponding Frequency

Total training sessions per week	Frequency of each area per week	Specific routine
4	2	Upper–lower repeated or push–pull repeated
3	3	Total body
3	1	Chest and back, legs, shoulders and arms
2	2	Total body

Table 26.2　Ideal Exercises per Body Area to Create a Toned Look

Chest	Back	Shoulders	Total body
Incline press	Chin-up	DB shoulder press	Snatch
DB press	DB row	Arnold press	Power clean
Cable crossover	Pullover	DB lateral raise	Thruster
DB fly	Straight arm	DB front raise	Yoga
Push-up	Lat pull-down	DB rear delt raise	Gymnastic movements
	Cable row		

Biceps	Triceps	Legs	Abs
Incline DB curl	Overhead tricep extension	Single-leg squat	Hanging leg raise
Concentration curl	Pullover skull crusher	Single-leg leg press	Inverted sit-up
Double DB preacher curl	DB tricep kickback	RDL or stiff-legged deadlift	Ab wheel
Cross-body curl	Rope tricep push-down	Hip thrust	L-hold
Supinated DB curl	Bench dip	Hyperextension	Pike

compound, free-weight exercises and then moving to lower-skill, isolation machine exercises still apply. Advanced clients might perform preexhaustion sets, compound sets, or supersets to increase the challenge of the workout.

Select the Number of Reps per Work Set

For training to improve tone, the number of reps can vary considerably, but it usually falls between 6 and 20 per set.

Select the Load per Set

The load does not have to be super heavy when toning, but it needs to be heavy enough to elicit adaptations. Clients with this goal tend to error on the side of lifting too lightly. Generally, 40 to 70 percent of the 1RM is used.

Select the Number of Work Sets per Exercise

Commonly, two to five work sets per exercise are used when training for toning.

Select the Number of Warm-Up Sets per Exercise

Warm-up sets are less significant when training for this goal because the load is light, the skill required is often low, and the number of reps is high. Warming up for the first exercise of the day usually involves performing one or two warm-up sets; on subsequent sets, zero or one warm-up set is usually performed.

Choose the Desired Weight Progression

Strategies to increase the weight lifted progression can vary when the goal is toning, but the most common arrangement is to perform straight sets; thus, the weight remains the same during the exercise.

Confirm That the Selected Number of Reps per Set Matches the Goal Time Under Tension

Toning workouts need some time under tension, although the load is usually not great and the exercise is rarely continued until failure. Typically, 15 to 45 seconds under tension is used.

Select the Appropriate Rest Time Between Sets

Rest time is usually limited to one minute or less between sets for training to become toned.

Implement Any Tricks of the Trade to Elicit Faster Adaptations

With each training goal, tricks or specific tools can be used to help reach that goal. Several techniques can be used for training to improve tone:

- Preexhaustion
- Supersets
- Compound sets
- Active rest

- Peripheral heart action
- Continuous tension
- Super slow
- Circuit training

Program an Appropriate Progressive Overload

Progressive overload is most commonly incorporated into a toning workout through progression in rep range. After a client hits the top number of reps, the weight is increased, the number of reps is lowered, and the process begins anew. Decreased rest, increased time under tension, use of intensity techniques, and progressing to more challenging exercises are all used to produce positive physiological adaptations in clients.

Sample One-Month Toning Training Workout Program

The application of the program design variables to design a resistance training program to create a toned look can be seen in table 26.3.

Total-body workouts two days per week

Cardio two to four days per week

Client—150-pound (68.0 kg) female, intermediate level

Starting 1RMs—95-pound (43.1 kg) bench, 150-pound (68.0 kg) squat, 185-pound (83.9 kg) deadlift

Exercises to tone the chest. Incline bench press, DB press, DB fly, cable crossover, pec deck, push-up.

Table 26.3 Sample One-Month Toning Program for an Intermediate Female Client

Total-body day 1						
Exercise	**Day 1**	**Day 3**	**Day 5**	**Day 7**	**Day 9**	**Day 11**
Incline bench press	45 lb (20.4 kg) x 10 55 lb (24.9 kg) x 8 60 lb (27.2 kg) x 5	45 lb (20.4 kg) x 12 55 lb (24.9 kg) x 10 60 lb (27.2 kg) x 6	45 lb (20.4 kg) x 15 55 lb (24.9 kg) x 12 60 lb (27.2 kg) x 7	50 lb (22.7 kg) x 10 60 lb (27.2 kg) x 6 65 lb (29.5 kg) x 4	50 lb (22.7 kg) x 10 60 lb (27.2 kg) x 7 65 lb (29.5 kg) x 5	50 lb (22.7 kg) x 10 60 lb (27.2 kg) x 8 65 lb (29.5 kg) x 6
Cable crossover	15 lb (6.8 kg) x 12	15 lb (6.8 kg) x 15	15 lb (6.8 kg) x 20	20 lb (9.1 kg) x 12	20 lb (9.1 kg) x 15	20 lb (9.1 kg) x 20
Chin-ups with light band	4 x 6	4 x 8	4 x 10	3–4 neg	3–4 neg	3–4 neg
Straight-arm lat pull-down	40 lb (18.1 kg) x 8 3 sets	40 lb (18.1 kg) x 10 3 sets	40 lb (18.1 kg) x 12 3 sets	45 lb (20.4 kg) x 8 3 sets	45 lb (20.4 kg) x 10 3 sets	45 lb (20.4 kg) x 12 3 sets
Arnold press	15 lb (6.8 kg) x 12 3 sets	15 lb (6.8 kg) x 15 3 sets	15 lb (6.8 kg) x 18 3 sets	20 lb (9.1 kg) x 10 3 sets	20 lb (9.1 kg) x 12 3 sets	20 lb (9.1 kg) x 15 3 sets
Rope face pull	30 lb (13.6 kg) x 12 3 sets	30 lb (13.6 kg) x 15 3 sets	30 lb (13.6 kg) x 20 3 sets	35 lb (15.9 kg) x 12 3 sets	35 lb (15.9 kg) x 15 3 sets	35 lb (15.9 kg) x 20 3 sets
DB incline curl	12 lb (5.4 kg) x 12 3 sets	12 lb (5.4 kg) x 15 3 sets	12 lb (5.4 kg) x 20 3 sets	15 lb (6.8 kg) x 10 3 sets	15 lb (6.8 kg) x 12 3 sets	15 lb (6.8 kg) x 15 3 sets
Overhead rope tricep extension	30 lb (13.6 kg) x 12 3 sets	30 lb (13.6 kg) x 15 3 sets	30 lb (13.6 kg) x 20 3 sets	35 lb (15.9 kg) x 12 3 sets	35 lb (15.9 kg) x 15 3 sets	35 lb (15.9 kg) x 20 3 sets
Pistols with strong or average band	3 x 8	3 x 10	3 x 12	3 x 8	3 x 10	3 x 12
One-leg leg press	45 lb (20.4 kg) x 12 70 lb (31.8 kg) x 10 95 lb (43.1 kg) x 8	55 lb (24.9 kg) x 12 80 lb (36.3 kg) x 10 105 lb (47.6 kg) x 8	65 lb (29.5 kg) x 12 90 lb (40.8 kg) x 10 115 lb (52.2 kg) x 8	70 lb (31.8 kg) x 12 95 lb (43.1 kg) x 10 120 lb (54.4 kg) x 8	75 lb (34.0 kg) x 12 100 lb (45.4 kg) x 10 125 lb (56.7 kg) x 8	80 lb (36.3 kg) x 12 105 lb (47.6 kg) x 10 130 lb (59.0 kg) x 8
Stability ball leg curl	3 x 10	3 x 12	3 x 15	2 x 15	2 x 20	2 x 25
Fire hydrant with leg kick	3 x 20	3 x 25	3 x 30	2 x 35	2 x 40	2 x 45
Ball crunch with tube	3 x 20	3 x 25	3 x 30	4 x 20	4 x 25	4 x 30
Bench L-hold	ALAP 3 sets	ALAP 3 sets	ALAP 3 sets	ALAP 3 sets	ALAP 3 sets	ALAP 3 sets

(continued)

Table 26.3 *(continued)*

Exercise	Day 2	Day 4	Day 6	Day 8	Day 10	Day 12
Total-body day 2						
Weighted step-ups with hip extension	35 lb (15.9 kg) x 12 3 sets	35 lb (15.9 kg) x 15 3 sets	35 lb (15.9 kg) x 20 3 sets	45 lb (20.4 kg) x 12 3 sets	45 lb (20.4 kg) x 15 3 sets	45 lb (20.4 kg) x 20 3 sets
Lateral lunge	3 sets of 10	3 sets of 12	3 sets of 14	4 sets of 10	4 sets of 12	4 sets of 14
Good morning	45 lb (20.4 kg) x 8 3 sets	45 lb (20.4 kg) x 10 3 sets	45 lb (20.4 kg) x 12 3 sets	55 lb (24.9 kg) x 8 3 sets	55 lb (24.9 kg) x 10 3 sets	55 lb (24.9 kg) x 12 3 sets
Penguin walk	Up–back 2 times	Up–back 2 times	Up–back 3 times	Up–back 3 times	Up–back 4 times	Up–back 4 times
Standing one-arm cable row	30 lb (13.6 kg) x 12 3 sets	30 lb (13.6 kg) x 15 3 sets	30 lb (13.6 kg) x 20 3 sets	35 lb (15.9 kg) x 12 3 sets	35 lb (15.9 kg) x 15 3 sets	35 lb (15.9 kg) x 20 3 sets
DB pullover	20 lb (9.1 kg) x 20 2 sets	20 lb (9.1 kg) x 20 3 sets	20 lb (9.1 kg) x 20 4 sets	25 lb (11.3 kg) x 20 2 sets	25 lb (11.3 kg) x 20 3 sets	25 lb (11.3 kg) x 20 4 sets
Shins on ball push-up	30	35	40	45	50	55
Standing DB press, alt hand up	15 lb (6.8 kg) x 10 3 sets	15 lb (6.8 kg) x 12 3 sets	15 lb (6.8 kg) x 15 3 sets	20 lb (9.1 kg) x 8 3 sets	20 lb (9.1 kg) x 10 3 sets	20 lb (9.1 kg) x 12 3 sets
Shoulder series	8 lb (3.6 kg) x 12 3 sets	8 lb (3.6 kg) x 15 3 sets	8 lb (3.6 kg) x 20 3 sets	10 lb (4.5 kg) x 12 3 sets	10 lb (4.5 kg) x 15 3 sets	10 lb (4.5 kg) x 20 3 sets
Double DB preacher curl	15 lb (6.8 kg) x 12 3 sets	15 lb (6.8 kg) x 15 3 sets	15 lb (6.8 kg) x 20 3 sets	20 lb (9.1 kg) x 10 3 sets	20 lb (9.1 kg) x 12 3 sets	20 lb (9.1 kg) x 15 3 sets
Pullover skull crushers	15 lb (6.8 kg) x 12 20 lb (9.1 kg) x 10 25 lb (11.3 kg) x 8	15 lb (6.8 kg) x 15 20 lb (9.1 kg) x 12 25 lb (11.3 kg) x 10	15 lb (6.8 kg) x 18 20 lb (9.1 kg) x 15 25 lb (11.3 kg) x 12	20 lb (9.1 kg) x 12 25 lb (11.3 kg) x 10 30 lb (13.6 kg) x 8	20 lb (9.1 kg) x 15 25 lb (11.3 kg) x 12 30 lb (13.6 kg) x 10	20 lb (9.1 kg) x 18 25 lb (11.3 kg) x 15 30 lb (13.6 kg) x 12
Clams	30	35	40	45	50	55
Dead bugs with ball	20	25	30	35	40	45

ALAP = as long as possible.

Women often prefer to target the incline bench press over regular chest press exercises because the female breast tissue sits on top of the pectoralis muscle. Therefore, even if that muscle is built up, it remains unseen under the breast tissue. Dumbbells allow a slightly greater range of motion and stretch and use less than optimal weight compared with a barbell. Cable crossovers and the pec deck focus significantly on the chest, and many females have a hard time feeling their chest working during an exercise. Most lean, athletic, fit females are capable of performing a large number of military style push-ups.

Exercises to tone the back. Straight-arm lat pull-down, chin-ups, DB rows, pullovers. Women are usually more interested in getting that V-shape in their lats (which makes the waist appear smaller) as opposed to getting thicker from front to back. Wide-grip rows and pull-downs tend to do the latter, but shoulder extension exercises tend to focus more on the lats themselves and help with the V-shape. The straight-arm pull-down and pullover exercises also target the abs, rear delts, and long head of the triceps—all common trouble spots for women. Lean and fit women are able to do several chin-ups; five reps is a good goal to strive for.

Exercises to tone the delts. DB military press, Arnold press, all shoulder raise exercises. The deltoid exercises are not as limited because the goal is often to build some size in the delts. Larger delts also makes the waist look thinner (similar to wearing shoulder pads in a jacket or blazer). Raises by their nature involve lighter loads, so no added effort is needed to reduce the weight lifted on raises.

Exercises to tone the triceps. Overhead tricep extension, pullover and skull crusher combo exercise, kickback, rope push-down.

Most women want firmness in their posterior upper arm, which is where the long head of the triceps is located. As a personal trainer, you do not want to indicate that performing these exercises will burn the fat off that area (known as spot reduction), because that won't happen. But an area can be spot improved by building muscle under the area to firm it up. Again, improving body composition is an important goal. Overhead exercises and the pullover skull crusher combination do a good job of hitting the long head. Remember that the tricep kickback and rope push-down involve lighter weights.

Exercises to tone the biceps. Incline bicep curl, concentration curl, double dumbbell preacher curl, cross-body curl.

For biceps training, most women want to focus on the biceps brachii in general and specifically on the long head of the biceps brachii, which contributes to the peak (bump) of the biceps. Women are often not as interested in training the brachioradialis or brachialis because those muscles tend to provide a thicker, blockier look to the arm or forearm. The biceps exercises in table 26.2 emphasize the long head of the biceps.

Exercises to tone the legs. One-leg leg press, lunge, step-up, one-legged squat, stiff-legged deadlift, RDL, good morning, hip extension, glute–ham raise, hip thrust, stability ball leg curl, stability ball bridge, jumps, sprints.

Many women want toned and strong legs, but they do not want their legs to get too big. Women have more muscle in their lower body, so hypertrophy is more likely to occur in the legs than in the upper body. Squats and leg presses are good exercises, but they can create muscular growth in the hip and thigh area. One-legged leg presses, lunges, step-ups, and one-leg squats stimulate the glutes and quads but use lighter loads. The stiff-legged deadlift, romanian deadlift, good morning, and hyperextension exercises train the erectors, glutes, and hamstrings well and still promote flexibility. Glute–ham raises greatly emphasize the hamstrings. Hip thrusts, stability ball leg curls, and stability ball bridges are effective at targeting the glutes and hamstrings without targeting the quads, which is the way to go if a client wishes to increase her hip measurement (add muscle to her glutes) without increasing the size of her quads or thighs. Finally, various jumps and sprints train the muscles without inducing large amounts of hypertrophy. They build power and speed, stimulate the Type II muscle fibers, and improve athleticism.

Exercises to tone the abs. Knee and leg raises (hanging), stability ball crunch, ab wheel, L-hold, inverted sit-up, pikes.

Most women want to tone and tighten their waists and at the same time maintain or decrease its circumference. Most of these exercises target the rectus abdominis. In the figure and fitness world, women are often discouraged from doing exercises specifically for their obliques for fear of building up those muscles and creating a more blocky, thick-waisted look. If a woman wishes to train her obliques more directly, torso rotations are a more effective choice than trunk abductions (side bends). The abs respond well when stretched, and the lower abs are usually the hardest part of the muscle to emphasize. The exercises listed in table 26.2 target the rectus abdominis, stretch the abs at the end range, and produce good results.

Exercises to tone the whole body. Snatch, power clean, thruster, Pilates, yoga, dance, gymnastics.

Women often perform well on total-body or power-related exercises. Snatches, power cleans, and thrusters all require good flexibility along with strength and coordination, but enough weight needs to be used to elicit results. Pilates, yoga, and dance all build flexibility and strength and promote lower levels of body fat. Gymnastics is great for developing relative strength, power, speed, coordination, and flexibility. Although elite-level gymnastic movements are most often performed by small, younger females, many women can perform those types of movements. Gymnastic training, under proper supervision, can be beneficial at most ages.

Other Considerations

On average, women tend to have a healthier diet than men do, if healthier is defined as eating fewer processed foods and more fruits and vegetables. But women may need to be encouraged to add protein to their diets to get up to 20 percent or more protein. Healthy fat does not need to be avoided, and protein and healthy fat often travel together. Light or low-calorie foods may claim to be healthier alternatives but often are not. Natural, whole, unprocessed organic foods are usually ideal. Whole eggs, whole milk, organic meats, fish, organic butter, natural starch, fruit, and vegetables are excellent foods to consume on a regular basis (323).

Women often do well in group settings that focus on group or team goals. Men often like the idea of individualized accomplishment and recognition. Men often, but not always, respond to negative feedback. By telling a person that he or she cannot do something, personal trainers might motivate the person to do just that. Women often, but not always, respond to positive feedback. By indicating that they believe in the client and know that he or she can do it, personal trainers can empower the client. Women are capable of training just as hard as men can. Male personal trainers sometimes think that they need to coddle female clients, but that approach is unnecessary and inappropriate. Indeed, because women often have smaller muscles than men do and often have a training history that is more cardiovascularly based, women often recover faster between sets than men do. Women have a lower conversion rate than men do, which means that small jumps in weight (which will represent large percentages) will significantly alter how many reps they can perform. On the flip side, a slight decrease in weight will often allow female clients to perform many more reps. For example, if a man can bench press 225 pounds (102.1 kg) for two reps as a max and the personal trainer gives that man 215 pounds (97.5 kg) to lift, he will likely complete three or four reps with that weight. If a woman can bench press 75 pounds (34.0 kg) for two reps as a max and the personal trainer

gives that woman 65 pounds (29.5 kg) to lift, she will likely complete five to eight reps—a much greater difference.

PRE- AND POSTNATAL WOMEN

For a woman, discovering that she is pregnant can be an extremely exciting and slightly anxious time. Her body will go through significant changes in the coming months. Her focus is likely to be on the health of the fetus as well as her own health, and many women who become pregnant look to a personal trainer for advice on how to exercise properly both to improve their own health and to decrease any possible risk to their unborn child.

Regular exercise can be helpful during pregnancy. Mothers who are fit tend to have slightly easier and shorter childbirths, resulting in quicker recovery times. They tend to gain less weight during pregnancy and are likely to have more energy during pregnancy. Increased blood flow can deliver additional nutrients, and the fetus can experience the same hormones that the mother does while exercising. Exercise is generally considered an effective method to help control stress, and being in a calm environment (as opposed to being carried by a mother who is feeling stressed out all the time) is likely beneficial for the fetus (6).

Possible Exercise Stressors

If a woman is going to exercise during pregnancy, she should first consult with her medical doctor. Her pregnancy has placed her outside the scope of practice for personal trainers, so her doctor must place her back inside that scope of practice. Most doctors encourage pregnant women to engage in a moderate exercise program. The concerns usually focus on four key issues (7):

• Insufficient oxygen to the fetus—If the mother exercises to the point of very high intensity, she might not provide enough oxygen for her fetus if she herself is oxygen deprived.

• Fetal hyperthermia—As people exercise, body temperature rises. The body temperature of the mother is unlikely to overheat excessively, but because the fetus is at the core of the woman's body, it cannot dissipate heat in the same way that an adult can. The negative effects of fetal hyperthermia can vary and often depend on how hot the fetus gets and the duration that the fetus spends in that environment. Hyperthermia generally starts when the fetal body temperature rises by about 2 degrees Celsius. It can produce fetal abnormalities, birth defects, or death.

• Increased contractions—Certain exercises and movements may increase the number and strength of the uterine contractions in females, which can be uncomfortable and might lead to premature labor.

• Trauma to the abdomen—Certain movements or activities can have a higher risk of injury than others. Of course, engaging in a full-contact football or a boxing match would present significant risk of trauma to the abdomen, which might endanger the fetus. Although common sense would preclude these activities, women and their personal trainers will have to use their own judgment when considering activities like riding a bicycle, inline skating, running, and other similar activities. Erring on the side of caution is likely the best approach.

Exercise Contraindications

If a doctor clears a woman for exercise, certain situations may later arise that would make exercise contraindicated for that session until she is reexamined by her doctor:

• Vaginal bleeding
• Leakage of amniotic fluid
• Preterm labor
• Dyspnea (a hard time breathing before activity begins)
• Heart palpitations or chest pain
• Headache, nausea, vomiting
• Dizziness of fainting
• Muscle weakness
• Sudden change in temperature
• Swelling or pain in the calves
• Decreased fetal movement

Program Modifications

The significant majority of pregnant women will be able to engage in activity during pregnancy, but even if exercise is not contraindicated, modifications may have to be made to the exercise program.

First, a woman's heart rate while pregnant is not as reliable a measure of exercise intensity. Instead of measuring heart rate, personal trainers should use the RPE scales to assess intensity. As such, moderate intensity is the most common guideline for how hard a female should exercise while pregnant. Second, the client should not lie supine (on her back) for any length of time after the beginning at the second trimester because that position compresses the inferior vena cava of the mother and disrupts blood flow. Standing, seated, or side-lying exercises are therefore the ones most commonly used. Also, personal trainers should be aware that a pregnant female will release more of the hormone relaxin, which helps prepare the pelvis for birth and, as the name implies, loosens up the tendons and ligaments. That increased flexibility, however, means less stability and a greater chance for injury. Combined with the fact that a woman's body is changing and her center of gravity is different, the enhanced flexibility increases the chance of falls. Further, pregnant women should avoid the regular use of the Valsalva maneuver when exercising because it can place too much pressure on the pelvic floor. Last, personal trainers need to make sure that pregnant women are able to regulate their body temperature. They should exercise indoors in a temperature-controlled environment, particularly if the external environment is at either end of the spectrum (too cold or too hot). Pregnant women should wear appropriate clothing and take regular water breaks. Personal trainers should look for signs of overheating from pregnant clients (red or flushed face, excessive sweating, weakness, dizziness, skin hot to the touch, and so on) and reduce or stop activity if they present themselves (25).

If a client was exercising previously, she likely will be able to continue a similar exercise program after she becomes pregnant. She need not decrease intensity of exercise to just above resting levels simply because she is pregnant. But she should not decide to start training intensely during her pregnancy. Clients who are currently engaged in a fitness program should focus on maintaining their current fitness level for as long as possible instead of pushing to improve it.

If a pregnant woman is going to begin an exercise program after becoming pregnant, she should ease herself into the program because the pregnancy itself is going to be a big change for her body. Many women find themselves extremely tired during certain phases of pregnancy, particularly in the first trimester, so exercise should be balanced with their other activities. The sample beginner workout program provided in chapter 18, modified as necessary, would be a good starting point for the pregnant woman. The American Congress of Obstetricians and Gynecologists (ACOG) suggests that pregnant women can safely engage in 30 minutes or more of moderate exercise on most, if not all, days of the week (13).

Program Guidelines

During pregnancy and afterward, two groups of muscles undergo significant changes. The first group is the muscles that help control the pelvic floor, which generally run from the pubic bone in the front to the coccyx bone in the back. These muscles help hold in the structures of the lower abdomen when standing, but as pregnancy progresses those structures undergo a great deal of stress. Weak pelvic floor muscles can lead to issues related to urinating or having bowel movements and might contribute to backaches. The most common exercises to work the pelvic floor muscles are the Kegel exercises.

The second group of muscles that is likely to change is the rectus abdominis. As the fetus grows, it pushes out on the abdominal wall, and a situation called diastasis recti can occur (figure 26.2). This condition occurs when the two sides of the rectus abdominis separate from each other. Often, but not always, this condition improves after the baby is delivered. When diastasis recti occurs, the abs are no longer able to perform one of their key functions, to compress the abdominal contents, and those abdominal contents can protrude through the tear in the abs. Having strong abdominal muscles before becoming pregnant can help prevent and control this. Attempting to maintain a neutral pelvis while standing or seated is also beneficial because pregnancy tends to shift the woman to an anterior pelvic tilt, which puts added stress on the rectus abdominis. A pregnant woman should avoid performing any movements that seem to exacerbate the separation of the abs. Working to activate the transverse abdominis first can help hold everything in (the bracing maneuver). The client should be encouraged to use her legs to squat down to pick things up and to avoid the Valsalva maneuver (13).

Ideal choices for exercising while pregnant include the following (note that supine exercises are contraindicated beginning in the second trimester):

- Everyday exercises
  - Kegel exercises
  - Pelvic tilt
  - Bridge
  - Bird dog
- Cardio exercises
  - Walking
  - Swimming
  - Stationary biking or other cardiovascular machines
- Resistance training exercises
  - Push-ups or seated chest press machine
  - One-arm DB row or cable row with handle to accommodate the abdomen
  - Lateral raise with dumbbells, cables, or bands
  - Rear delt raise with cables or bands
  - Bicep curl
  - Tricep push-down
  - Squat (body weight, goblet, dumbbell, ball)

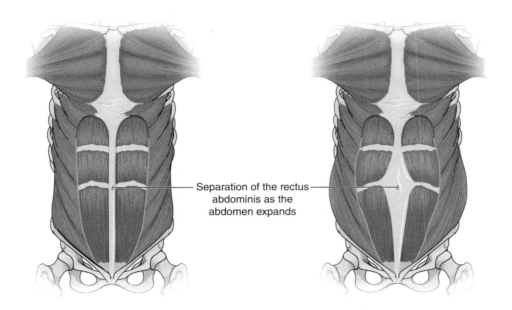

Separation of the rectus abdominis as the abdomen expands

Figure 26.2 Illustration of diastasis recti.

- Lunge (watch balance)
- Torso rotation (within a smaller range of motion as pregnancy progresses)

Other Considerations

Females need a period of recovery after giving birth. Exactly how much time a woman needs depends on her fitness level, her motivation, and the complexity of the birthing process. Generally, this period lasts for four to six weeks for a normal vaginal birth and six to eight weeks for birth by cesarean section. Regular personal training sessions will likely not take place during this time, but women can return to light activity as soon as they feel ready (13). The exercises listed as everyday exercises can be performed as soon as the client feels ready for them after giving birth. Light walking can also have a restorative effect.

If a client experiences heavy bleeding or pain, or has an infection after giving birth, she should see a doctor and should not exercise. If a client had a cesarean section, she should wait six weeks before starting an exercise routine. If a client has significant breast discomfort or significant pelvic pressure during exercise, the exercise session should be discontinued until the pain goes away. Most clients find that if they express their breast milk and use the restroom before exercising, they will be more comfortable during the workout.

Clients should start out light and easy, as would any client who has taken significant time off from regular intense exercise, and gradually build back up to previous workout levels. The combination of regular exercise combined with breast feeding (which raises the metabolism by 500 kilocalories per day) can have a highly positive effect on body composition and help the client return to a prepregnancy fitness level in a reasonable time (three to six months is common).

CONCLUSION

This chapter provided training information geared toward specific types of clients commonly referred to as special populations. The special populations covered in this chapter are older adults, children, and women.

Older adults are defined as those over 65 years old. A properly programmed exercise routine can be extremely valuable to older adults in improving their health, fitness, and quality of life. The human body can respond to exercise at any age, so it is never too late to begin a workout routine. Programs geared toward older adults should focus on all aspects of fitness, particularly balance and flexibility.

Older adults often need a longer recovery time between workouts, and they may need a longer time to warm up before the exercise session begins. Personal trainers need to be able to work around any injuries or medical conditions that clients have developed. Using proper risk stratification procedures to screen clients with is crucial. Exercise can help reverse and delay many of the effects of the aging process.

Children under the age of 16 can benefit significantly from an exercise program. Pre-adolescent children have not reached puberty yet, so their results will be primarily neuromuscular in nature. Programs for all children should focus on being fun, providing general adaptations, being a positive experience for the child, and building confidence and a lifelong love of fitness. Children can lift weights at any age, but this activity should be done under qualified supervision. Body-weight exercises are excellent choices for children. There is no research to suggest that resistance training stunts a child's growth.

Women may require exercise programs slightly different from those of their male counterparts, primarily because of different goals and different hormone levels. Women have lower testosterone and are unlikely to build as much muscle as men do, even with heavy resistance training. Women have lower absolute strength than men do, particularly in the upper body. Women may be more predisposed to knee injuries, so personal trainers should work to ensure that the surrounding areas are strong and in balance with each other. The goal of toning is not specific and measurable, so personal trainers should establish what toning means to the individual client.

Pre- and postnatal clients may also participate in exercise programs. Such participation may ease the delivery and recovery process. Prenatal clients should be on the lookout for low oxygen levels for the baby, fetal hyperthermia, increased contractions during exercise, and trauma to the abdomen. Any unusual signs or symptoms such as a vaginal discharge should be immediately checked out by a doctor.

Most women need about a month or more after giving birth before they return to vigorous activity, although every person will respond differently to that experience.

Personal trainers will likely work with some or all of the special populations during their careers. All these groups can benefit from a properly programmed exercise program, but each population has its own needs that must be considered. With just a few modifications, these clients can enjoy all the benefits of a regular fitness program.

Study Questions

1. Which of the following statements is most true when training older adults?

    a. Older adults should warm up longer and may want to stretch statically before they begin the workout program.

    b. Older adults should strictly follow the target heart rate predicted by the standard heart rate formula.

    c. Older adults should always train with descending sets.

    d. Older adults should perform a minimum of 20 reps on all resistance training exercises.

2. Which joint on a female is more prone to significant injury than on a male?

    a. ankle

    b. lower back

    c. knee

    d. acromioclavicular joint

3. Children are closer in _____ strength when compared with adults. Therefore, good choices of exercises for them include _____.

    a. absolute strength; machines

    b. absolute strength; calisthenics

    c. relative strength; machines

    d. relative strength; calisthenics

4. Which one of the following is *not* a concern when training pregnant females?

    a. a stronger uterus causing injury to the baby during delivery

    b. increased fetal temperature

    c. decreased oxygen blood flow to the fetus

    d. increased contractions

5. Which of the following clients would likely produce the most testosterone on a daily basis?

    a. a 30-year-old male

    b. a 30-year-old female

    c. a 75-year-old male

    d. an 8-year-old male

Injury and Rehabilitation

This chapter provides information about common sport-related injuries and suggests methods for prevention and rehabilitation. Exercise and resistance training are relatively safe activities, but anyone who trains over a lifetime will likely experience some sort of injury. In addition, clients may sustain injuries outside the gym that end up affecting their fitness routines inside the gym.

Note that the advice and recommendations in this chapter are general guidelines. Any moderate or severe injury should be examined by a medical doctor. This chapter is designed not to replace a doctor's guidelines but to supplement them. Injuries can vary greatly from person to person. Personal trainers should listen carefully to the words of their clients, and under no circumstances should personal trainers allow clients to do anything that causes immediate pain. Erring on the side of caution and leaving the area alone is the prudent approach.

TYPES OF INJURIES

All injuries can be broken into two categories. Macrotraumas are acute, specific injuries. When people experience a macrotrauma, they know it the instant it happens. If while you are playing basketball, you land from a jump, hear a snap in your ankle, and feel a shooting pain, you know immediately that you have injured your ankle. Macrotraumas can occur in many forms:

• A fracture is a break in the bone. In an open, or compound, fracture, the bone breaks through the skin. In a closed fracture, the bone does not break through the skin. Open

fractures are generally more serious because of the risk of infection.

• A dislocation is an injury to a joint in which a bone moves and stays out of place. Dislocations at the fingers and shoulder are relatively common, but dislocations can occur at all major joints. A subluxation is a partial dislocation in which the bone pops out of the joint and then pops back in on its own. It is not as serious as a dislocation. Repeated dislocations of the same joint can leave the joint loose and unstable. This condition usually requires surgery to treat. From a rehabilitation standpoint, a dislocated joint must be allowed to recover fully before the person can resume intense activity. Returning to intense activity too soon can reinjure the area, delay the recovery process, and ultimately cause permanent damage to the joint.

• A contusion is a bruise on the skin, muscle, or bone, normally from a direct injury or blow. Contusions that affect exercise are usually to the deeper tissues. In this instance, pain should be the guide. If movement or contraction of the injured area hurts, the person should avoid working that area. But if the person has no pain when working the bruised area, he or she can train as usual (9).

• A strain is an injury to a tendon or muscle, and a sprain is an injury to the ligament. There are three degrees of strains or sprains. A first-degree strain or sprain involves an overstretching of the tissue and possibly some tearing, up to a 10 percent tear. These injuries can be painful, but the muscle and joint are still relatively stable. First-degree strains or sprains are the least severe injuries of this type. A second-degree strain or sprain has definite tearing, normally an 11 to 50 percent tear. This kind of injury is painful. Because their integrity is compromised, the joint and muscle are now weak. A third-degree strain or sprain has a full or almost full tear of the tissue, generally 51 to 100 percent. Surgery is often required to fix this injury because the joint and muscle are weak and unstable. A third-degree strain or sprain is the most severe, but it is not necessarily the most painful (1).

The second type of an injury is a microtrauma. This chronic injury often results from overuse. The person is usually not aware of exactly when the injury occurred. When you wake up in the morning and something hurts but you can't remember what you did to make it feel that way, the injury is a microtrauma. Microtraumas can be annoying to people involved in fitness because they can keep reappearing if they do not heal fully, and they often force people to take time off from the activities that they enjoy doing. The two most common forms of microtrauma are the following:

• Stress fractures are hairline fractures of the bone that result from overuse or overstress. Marathon runners and soldiers often get stress fractures in their feet from the repeated pounding of running, and gymnasts get them in their

wrists from the repeated stress of landing on their hands (106).

• Tendinopathy is an injury to the tendon. There are two types of tendon injuries. Tendinitis, the swelling and inflammation of the tendon, is often considered the more significant injury. Tendinosis is chronic degeneration without inflammation. Some professionals use the term *tendinitis* to describe most injuries to the tendon. After the tendon becomes irritated, it swells and is sensitive if the muscle is used at all. This injury can be bothersome, because even seemingly insignificant movement can cause a sharp pain as the muscle contracts (26).

The two most common forms of tendinitis are tennis elbow and golfer's elbow (figure 27.1). Tennis elbow occurs on the lateral side of the proximal forearm, and golfer's elbow occurs on the medial side of the proximal forearm. These two injuries are overuse injuries that occur when the muscle is not adapted to performing a specific repetitive movement (30).

TISSUE HEALING PROCESS

When the body is injured, it goes through three phases to reach full recovery. The length

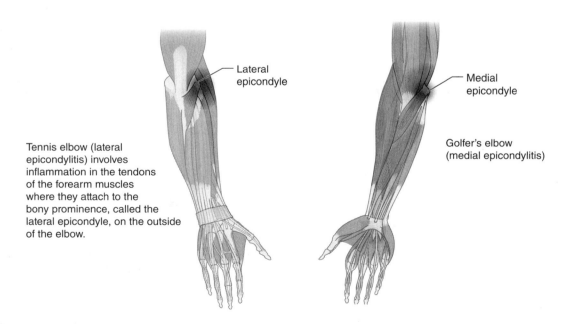

Tennis elbow (lateral epicondylitis) involves inflammation in the tendons of the forearm muscles where they attach to the bony prominence, called the lateral epicondyle, on the outside of the elbow.

Lateral epicondyle

Medial epicondyle

Golfer's elbow (medial epicondylitis)

Figure 27.1 Illustration of tennis and golfer's elbow.

of each phase varies, depending on the injury itself. Of course, serious injuries require a longer time to heal. The body needs to progress through these phases in the order listed; it cannot skip from the first phase to the last phase. As a personal trainer, you need to estimate what phase your client is currently in because that will have a big influence on how you train the injured area.

Phase 1: Inflammation

The first phase after injury is the inflammation phase. This phase occurs immediately after the injury happens. As the name indicates, inflammation, or edema (swelling), occurs. Inflammation serves several functions. The swelling can act like a splint, reducing the range of motion in the joint. This condition is beneficial in the short term when additional movement can produce further damage to the injured area. In addition, swelling increases blood flow, which brings in nutrients and other cells that assist in the healing process. Some cells come in and look for foreign organisms or debris and attempt to eradicate them through a process called phagocytosis (cell eating). During the inflammation stage, the injured area is often painful. Attempts to use the injured area will range from uncomfortable to agonizing, and sometimes the area will simply be unusable (43).

The inflammation stage lasts anywhere from an hour to two weeks; two to three days is the most common duration of this stage for moderate injuries. Few people enjoy being in the inflammation stage—it hurts and you can't do anything—but it is vital to the healing process.

Each stage of injury should have a training goal. The training goal for the inflammation stage is, "Do not make the affected area worse." That instruction is simple to follow if you can just get your client to comply. You do not want your clients to do anything that involves the affected area. Your client can train another body part or area and that activity if it is pain free. For example, if your client sprained an ankle, he or she may be able to sit down and perform dumbbell curls.

Clients often ask for your advice when it comes to injury. Do not step outside your scope of practice and start suggesting radical treatments in an effort to be helpful. You might end up making the injured area worse. But you are not powerless when a client asks for suggestions to make the injured area feel better. You will not train the area, and you will not stretch the area because stretching might make the injury worse, but you can recommend applying the RICE guideline to the area, which advises using rest, ice, compression, and elevation.

The rest part is easy. Injured clients need to take some time off from working the affected area. For most injuries, one week of no activity is sufficient, but occasionally a few weeks off are required.

Ice is useful during the inflammation phase to help control the inflammation and improve blood flow. Several methods can be used to ice an injured area, but a common one is to place a good amount of ice in a bag and then wrap the bag in something relatively thin such as a paper towel or a few napkins. The injured person then places the covered ice bag directly on the affected area. Putting something between the ice and the skin can help prevent injury to the skin that may result from direct application. But a wrap that is too thick will not allow the coldness of the ice to penetrate to the body. Typically, the ice is left on for about 20 minutes. The area is then left alone for about 40 minutes and allowed to return to normal temperature. The ice can then be reapplied. Icing immediately after the injury and then for 20 minutes each hour is the best way to maximize this treatment. This method can be continued as long as desired and will be useful for as long as the swelling remains.

A more recent suggestion for the use of ice is called the four by numb rule. In this instance the injury is iced until it becomes numb (which usually occurs sooner than 20 minutes). Then the ice is removed. This process is repeated four times during the day. Excessive icing may slow the healing rate of some injuries.

Compression is also useful during the inflammation stage. A simple wrap or brace is used to keep the injured area under some pressure. If clients injure themselves, such as by spraining an ankle, you can suggest that they purchase and wear a basic ankle wrap. The wrap will add compression, limit movement, and provide some added structural support to the area. In addition, the wrap can serve as a reminder, for both the injured person and those nearby, to treat the area with care (83).

Finally, elevation is the act of raising the injured area, normally above the heart. This position can help control the swelling and keep blood flowing out of the wound. Ice, elevation, and compression can all be used at the same time. Most injuries don't require constant elevation, but when sitting or sleeping, elevating the injured areas as much as possible is a good idea. The injured person should try to avoid spending prolonged time in the opposite position, where the injured area is well below the heart. For example, a person with an injured knee should not stand constantly.

Phase 2: Repair

As the inflammation stage winds down and ends, the repair phase begins. As the name indicates, in this stage the body is beginning to repair the injured area. The goal of the body during the repair phase is to return to basic functioning. During this phase, the tissue that has been injured is regenerated, and scar tissue forms as well. Both personal trainers and clients need to understand that the regenerated tissue is being laid down in a haphazard function. The injured area is returning to basic functioning, but it is still weak, unsteady, and susceptible to reinjury (71).

During the repair phase, the pain in the injury generally subsides, especially when the area is at rest. Certain movements or pressure may still hurt, but the area should not hurt all the time. The swelling and redness also dissipate. The repair phase lasts anywhere from one or two weeks to as long as a couple of months for severe injuries.

Training during the repair phase is often crucial, and extreme care must be taken during this time. Clients tend to become anxious during the repair phase because the pain is gone and they can return to basic activities

such as walking and getting around. After they can perform the basics, clients usually want to get back to working out as soon as possible. In addition, clients who have achieved a high level of fitness know that any extended time off will cause their fitness level to drop significantly. Because those gains didn't come easily, they often try to rush back to a preinjury fitness level.

At this point, you must really caution your clients against doing that. The key thing to remember during the repair phase is that the tissue is still weak. Although the tissue has likely become strong enough for everyday activities, it is not ready for any kind of high-intensity activities. If clients perform those types of activities, they run a strong risk of reinjuring the tissue, which means even more down time in the long run.

The training plan should have three main goals during the repair phase. The first goal is to maintain, or possibly even improve, areas unrelated to the injured area. The second goal is to prevent atrophy of the injured area. To accomplish that goal, the personal trainer wants to stimulate the area somewhat with resistance but keep it light. The third goal is to return the injured area to a full, natural range of motion. If an injured area is allowed to remain immobile for a prolonged time, or if enough effort is not placed on regaining normal range of motion, then the new limited range of motion can become permanent. If a client is unable to attain a full normal range of motion two months or so after the injury, he or she should seek the further advice of a doctor or physical therapist. If the range of motion does not return, the injury will likely limit the client in the future.

If you want to introduce a new exercise, first have the client perform that same range of motion with just body weight. If you want a client to perform the bench press, simply have him or her mimic the motion of a bench press, horizontal shoulder adduction and elbow extension, with the arms and no resistance at all. If using no resistance causes the client pain, using some resistance will cause more pain, which indicates that the client is not yet ready for that movement.

Generally, the best approach is to start with light isolation exercises for the injured area to give it a little bit of stimulus. Temporarily reducing the range of motion for the injured area is fine. If a client who is dealing with an injured shoulder feels pain when performing a full front raise, he or she should stay in a pain-free range of motion. The client can lift the arm up halfway and use that range of motion for a week. Then the person can gradually increase the range of motion each week until at some point, even if it is two months later, he or she is performing the full range of motion.

The repair phase is also a good time to use isometric contractions. When a muscle or joint is injured, certain positions may cause pain while others are pain free. Have the client take a position in which the injured area feels the best and then perform a light isometric contraction. For example, most injured knees feel best when they are fully extended and hurt when they are bent. The injured person begins by performing straight-leg isometric contractions with no weight or a very light weight and holding for 15 to 30 seconds. As the client progresses week to week, increase the weight gradually, increase the time under tension gradually (two minutes is normally the max), or add greater range of motion. Continuing with the previous example, if after two weeks the client's knee is feeling a little better, you might incorporate both a straight-leg isometric contraction and one with the knee slightly bent.

The biggest thing to remember in the repair phase is that the body is healing but is doing a quick-fix job. It is just trying to get itself back to normal, not back to optimal. You must instill patience in this phase and use lighter weights and lower levels of force with your clients. A good rule of thumb is to use less than 50 percent of the 1RM for any area that is affected by the injury. Even if lifting feels good to the client, which it probably will after a time, stay light. Remember that the tissue is being repaired haphazardly, and if you allow the client to rush it, he or she is likely to reinjure it and be back to square one. Sticking with low force also means using slow speed. Activities such as sprinting, quick movements, hitting,

throwing, and agility drills are probably out during this phase. When training in the repair phase, you need to remember that you are rebuilding the client's foundation. Hold off on progressing rapidly now so that you can progress the client more rapidly in the future. With this approach, you may help the client surpass all previous training levels once the client is fully healed.

Phase 3: Remodeling

The remodeling phase is the last phase of injury that the body goes through. As the repair phase ends, the remodeling phase begins. The remodeling phase is normally the longest phase, often lasting two to four months. But this phase is generally pleasant for the client because the body is beginning to feel like its old self. The client will be making noticeable physical progress and will be feeling optimistic about returning to the previous fitness level.

Physiologically, the body is now attempting to fix the injury properly. The collagen fibers that were initially laid down randomly begin to align themselves correctly, which causes an increase in strength in the injured area. Over time, the tissue attempts to heal fully. Some injuries will heal so well that the client will feel as if nothing ever happened. Others, unfortunately, will limit the ability of the person even after they have healed. The outcome depends on the severity of the injury, the quality of the treatment, and the person's ability to heal.

Training during the remodeling phase is crucial to the health of the client. Training will help place the proper stimulus on the body to cause it to adapt positively and thus help correct the injury. The main goal of training during the remodeling phase is to return to previous (preinjury) levels of performance. Still, caution must be taken not to rush progress.

Luckily, progress will occur faster now than it did the first time, but that does not mean the process should be rushed. Also, remember that after perhaps two months of being in the inflammation and repair phases, a person's fitness level may have dropped, especially if it was high to begin with. So if a client who is used to benching 300 pounds (136.1 kg) hurts his shoulder playing football and then takes two months off to let it heal, don't expect him to come back and bench the same weight right away. Taking two months off from training will reduce performance in any case; a person coming back from an injury is likely to have an even greater falloff.

In the remodeling phase, your clients should be able to perform pretty much any exercise you choose for them. They should have a pain-free range of motion with their body weight in any direction, so now it is time to build back their fitness level. If your client has been using primarily machines and isolation exercises in the repair phase, you can reintroduce free weights and compound movements in the remodeling phase. Still, begin light, but progress moderately quickly back to the weight that the client was lifting. An increase of 2 to 5 percent in weight each week is normally acceptable, assuming that the person was starting with less than 50 percent of the 1RM. Always remember to cause no pain. If something flares up or hurts, it simply means that the client isn't yet ready and you need to back off for a while (6).

Test the balance of the injured area and work to improve the proprioceptors in that area. If a client hurt an ankle, begin by having him or her stand on the injured ankle and perform easy movements to get it used to handling all the weight. If a client hurt a shoulder, have him or her perform isolateral (one-sided) movements, such as a dumbbell press, to make sure that each side of the body is lifting the weight evenly and that the client is not relying more on the strong side to move the weight.

Finally, add high-speed, sport-specific movements. The client can begin performing the Olympic lifts if he or she was using them previously. Throws, kicks, jumps, and other high-speed movements can be added during this phase. A general rule to follow is to employ high-speed or plyometric type activities only when the injured side is as least 90 percent as strong as the uninjured side. The closer that strength level gets to 100 percent, the better off the client will be.

You need to remember the order in which the body proceeds through the phases of injury. A simple way to remember this is to understand that you would repair something first before you would remodel it. People occasionally get those two ideas confused.

Table 27.1 presents a summary of the phases of injury, the training goal for each phase, and indications and contraindications for each phase.

OPEN- AND CLOSED-CHAIN MOVEMENTS

Movements can be classified as either open- or closed-chain movements. The definition depends on whether the involved limb moves during the movement or not. In an open-chain exercise, the distal end of the involved

Table 27.1 Phases of Injury and Corresponding Training Information

Phase of injury	Training goal	Typical duration	Indications	Contraindications
Inflammation	Do not make the injury worse	Up to 2 weeks	RICE	No activity for the injured area
Repair	Prevent atrophy	Up to 2 months	Very light weight Isometric exercises Pain-free range of motion Flexibility exercises Proprioception exercises if appropriate	Heavy weight High speed Explosive movements High-impact movements Pain with movement
Remodeling	Return to normal and beyond	Up to 4 months	Full range-of-motion exercises Progressive overload Gradual return to sport-specific speed of movement	Large jumps in weight, intensity, or volume Pain with movement

limb moves during the exercise. That sounds complex, but in simple terms it means that the hand or foot moves during the exercise. Imagine if you were to grab a client's wrist (for upper-body exercises) or ankle (for lower-body exercises). If the client performs the exercise and the wrist or ankle moves through space, that is an open-chain exercise. Common examples include the bench press, dumbbell press, dumbbell row, lateral raise, bicep curl, and tricep push-down for the upper body; examples for the lower body are the leg extension and leg curl.

If the client's wrist or ankle would not move during the exercise, and if it stays rooted in place, then the exercise is considered to be a closed-chain exercise. Technically the definition of a closed-chain exercise is when the distal end of the involved limb does not move. Common examples include the push-up, pull-up, and dip for the upper body; examples for the lower body are the squat and hip thrusts.

Not all exercises are easily defined as closed or open chain. Something like a deadlift can be challenging, but assuming the erectors are the main muscle working (the agonist), the distal end of the involved area becomes the superior region of the trunk (and by default, the hand and arm). When one performs a deadlift, that area is moving through space. Imagine hugging a client's chest and then asking him or her to do a deadlift; you would go along for the ride. Thus, a deadlift is an open-chain exercise, much like a hyperextension exercise. A leg press can be variable depending on the type of apparatus used; some leg presses involve a stationary platform and the client's body will move back and forth, much like a squat. In this instance, that type of leg press—sometimes referred to as a horizontal leg press—is a closed-chain exercise. Other leg presses (usually referred to as plate-loaded leg presses) involve the sled itself moving as the client pushes against it. Thus, the ankles and feet do move through space, in which case that type of leg press is an open-chain exercise.

Stereotypically (but not a rule set in stone), open-chain exercises are often more isolated in nature and involve fewer muscles. Closed-chain exercises tend to be compound in nature and involve more muscles. These terms are often applied to clients dealing with injuries. Clients in the repair phase of injury will incorporate mainly isolated, open-chain exercises to gradually rehabilitate the injured area. Once the client moves into the remodeling phase and feels comfortable with larger movements and more weight, the client can progress to closed-chain exercises if appropriate.

ROLE OF OTHER HEALTH CARE PROFESSIONALS

In the unfortunate instance that a client is seriously injured, that person should seek professional help. Personal trainers should know the general scope of practice for other professionals so that everyone can work well together as a team (58).

• Doctor (MD). When a client gets hurt, a doctor, either the person's regular doctor or a specialist, is normally the first person the client should see. The doctor's main job is to diagnose the injury and then, if possible, tell the client what to do to fix it. If the client is an athlete, he or she may want to find a doctor who specializes in athletes and sports medicine and has a better understanding of how the activity and the injury might relate.

• Physical therapist (PT). If a client needs to go through rehab from a serious injury, the client may work with a physical therapist. As this chapter has detailed, the body is more fragile after an injury, and the more serious the injury is, the more specialized the care must be to help the client recover from it. A PT's job is to help the client recover from that injury. A PT will normally work with the client during the inflammation and repair phases of the injury.

• Registered dietitian (RD). Under normal circumstances, simply being injured will not necessitate a meeting with a registered dietitian, but if an underlying abnormality is present, such as a disease, or if a client has had a heart attack, stroke, or something similar, dietary modifications may be necessary. An RD is a special nutritionist who is particularly trained to deal with people suffering from disease or recovering from serious health problems.

• Athletic trainer (AT). An athletic trainer is trained to help people, normally athletes, work through and deal with injuries. When someone gets hurt in a football game, those who run out on the field to help are normally team doctors and athletic trainers. The AT tapes up or braces a joint if necessary. ATs also work with athletes after an injury has occurred to help them recover. A personal trainer and an athletic trainer are not the same, and the two are not interchangeable.

• Chiropractors (DC). Chiropractors are doctors who have specialized in the spine. They often help people with posture problems and chronic pains such as backaches. They adjust or manipulate the body into proper alignment and normal functioning. Some people have excellent success with chiropractors, but others do not. Working with a knowledgeable chiropractor can be valuable in recovering from and preventing injury.

• Strength coach (CSCS). A strength coach is much like a personal trainer, but a strength coach works primarily with athletes whereas a personal trainer works mainly with nonathletes. A strength coach generally works with a team or school and has the job of making the athletes as fit as possible and setting up their workouts to improve their performance on the field or in the game.

• Personal trainer (CPT). The scope of practice for a personal trainer is to enhance the components of fitness for the general, healthy population. After someone has been seriously injured, he or she often falls outside that scope of practice, even if just temporarily. The person needs to be evaluated by a doctor or physical therapist and then, if appropriate, placed back in the scope of practice to continue under the guidance of the personal trainer. A personal trainer is not trained to deal with immediate, acute injuries. In addition, the personal trainer should not diagnose injuries. If you believe that you know what is wrong with a client, you can offer your opinion as a starting point, but you should always follow that up with the statement that the client should have a doctor look at any serious injury. Personal trainers should not attempt to brace or tape any injury, nor should they attempt to adjust someone's spine or any other joint. As a personal trainer, you have not received formal training in those modalities.

Whenever possible, a personal trainer should work with the doctor and the therapist to help the client receive the best possible care. The various health care professionals will explain the indications and contraindications to the client, so you need to understand the meaning of those terms. An indication is something that the client should perform, such as exercises or movements to facilitate the healing process. A contraindication is something that the client should not do. These exercises or movements are not appropriate for the client at this time. As the client heals, he or she may be able to use those exercises again, or those exercises may be forever contraindicated.

Unlike the four contraindicated exercises described in chapter 17, no specific indications apply to all people. Rather, when new clients are starting out on a fitness program, you should emphasize and improve each aspect of fitness instead of focusing on just one. If a client is starting with an existing injury, rely on a doctor or physical therapist for specific instructions. Encourage your injured client to be proactive and ask his or her doctor specifically for the contraindications and indications for the injury. In addition, if you have a specific movement or exercise in mind that you want your client to perform, then definitely encourage him or her to ask the doctor about it.

STAYING INJURY FREE

An important goal for you as a personal trainer is to keep your clients free from injury. Following some general guidelines can help prevent that first injury from happening in the gym. You want to help your clients get stronger and fitter, which in turn will help avoid future injury; you never want their training to set them up for injury somewhere down the line.

Shoulder

The shoulder is the most flexible joint in the body, but it sacrifices some stability for its great mobility. Without taking certain precautions, it can be injured or aggravated during training. Here are some guidelines to provide your clients to help prevent a shoulder injury:

- **Warm up.** Make sure that your client is warmed up before you have him or her try a heavy upper-body exercise, particularly any pressing motion.

- **Avoid excessive range of motion.** Because the shoulders are highly flexible, people are often inclined to use excessive range of motion with them. Performing exercises correctly significantly reduces the chance of injury. A guideline for most shoulder exercises is to stop the range of motion when the hand comes in line with the body.

- **Use a moderate grip width.** Super-wide grips for the lat pull-down, pull-up, and bench press exercises can place extra stress on the shoulders. If you do try a new grip with a client, start light and give the client a few weeks to work up to his or her usual weight. Narrow grips may well be harder, so going a little bit lighter with a narrower grip is natural on most exercises.

- **Learn how to bench press.** The bench press is arguably the most popular exercise, and most clients can lift a moderate amount of weight on it. For a complete review of the bench press, see chapter 20. The key to protecting the shoulders is to keep the arms tucked in at a 45- to 60-degree angle to the side.

- **Develop muscle balance.** Train all the muscles that affect the shoulder. The lats and pecs, front and rear delts, biceps and triceps, rhomboids and serratus anterior, and rotator cuff all need to be in balance and able to work harmoniously with each other (7).

- **Stretch the shoulders.** Shoulder injuries are often caused by tight muscles in the front of the body or the internal rotators, such as the pecs, front delts, biceps, and to a lesser extent the pec minor, lats, teres major, and subscapularis. On a regular basis, have clients stretch these muscles using both static and dynamic stretching after they train them.

- **Work on thoracic spine mobility.** The thoracic spine is the section of the vertebral column associated with the ribs, sometimes called the T-spine for short. Maintaining good mobility in this area is important. T-spine extensions and other mobility drills that affect this area are useful in attempting to correct the problem.

- **Strengthen the upper back.** This guideline goes along with stretching the muscles in the front of the body; strengthening the muscles in the back will help with posture and general muscular balance. Stretching is particularly important for the midback and external rotators, including the middle and lower traps, rhomboids, teres minor and infraspinatus, and the rear delt. Wide-grip rows with the elbows flared out are excellent exercises to target those muscles.

- **Strengthen the rotator cuff.** Do not forget that the rotator cuff is a muscle, so spending a few minutes on it at the end of the workout might help the client. Most of the work in this area should focus on internal and external rotations (14).

- **Design a proper exercise routine.** Many people overtrain the front delt and coracoid process of the body because they don't allow those muscles to recover from one day to the next. When you are designing workouts for your clients, don't forget to allow the shoulders and biceps to recover not only when they are the agonist but also when they are a synergist in the exercise.

- **Do not do any of the four contraindicated exercises.** Chapter 17 described them and provided a photo of each nonrecommended exercise; three of them are known to bother the shoulder.

If a client's shoulder is bothering him or her, you can use a few simple guidelines to help the person get through the injury. Remember that a doctor should look at any serious injury.

- Don't cause any pain.
- Make the grip narrower on any pressing exercises.

- Have the client press with a neutral grip, although you should first test this idea with light weight; this modification will make the discomfort either better or worse, likely better.
- Temporarily limit the range of motion by having the client perform rack presses or board presses instead of the bench press or military press; make an effort to increase the range of motion back to normal as the injury feels better and goes away.
- Have the client lift lighter loads while the injury heals; a client's strength will not disappear in two weeks!
- Train the rotator cuff muscles and any other weak points such as rear delts, rhomboids, and external rotators (17).

Lower Back

The lower back is an area of the body that often bothers people, and unfortunately, when that area is injured, it seems prone to reinjury (63). Here are some general guidelines to follow with your clients that can help keep their backs strong and healthy:

- Maintain a flat or slightly arched spine. The spine has natural curves in it, and clients will want to maintain that position or increase the arch in the lower back slightly when lifting. Clients should not excessively arch or round the back, particularly under loads, because serious injury can result. If you see a client's back get out of alignment during the exercise, instruct him or her to stop lifting, even in the middle of a set. Some personal trainers like to work through a spinal positioning hierarchy with their clients. These positions are listed from number 1, considered ideal, to number 4, considered less than ideal and slightly less safe.
  - Braced neutral (1)—The core is braced and held in a neutral position without movement.
  - Global fixed extension (2)—The core is held tight and the lower back is locked in a slightly arched position. Some authorities believe that this position

is even safer than the braced neutral position.
  - Global fixed flexion (3)—The core is held tight, and the lower back is locked in a slightly flexed position.
  - Movement or translation under load (4)—The core is not held tight, and the lower back moves significantly under the load. Movement into significant flexion is generally considered the most dangerous position to be in under load.

- Lift with the legs. Many people injure their backs by trying to lift something that is too heavy for them. Have clients bend their knees as in a squat and go about halfway down, keep the back flat, look straight ahead, and lift something up. One reason that deadlifts are valuable is that they teach clients how to lift something off the ground properly. Even with light weight, using good lifting form is important.

- Use good form in the gym. When clients are lifting heavy weights, they tend to swing the body too much, particularly on rows or curls, or arch the back on presses. They should avoid such motions. First, by swinging the body or arching the back, they are increasing their risk of injury. Second, they are cheating and not performing the correct form on the exercise anyway, so the weight they are lifting does not count in the sense of comparing it with what others are lifting.

- Maintain normal flexibility. Some muscles are prone to get tight, particularly as we age. Those muscles are the hamstrings, erectors, glutes, and hip flexors. Maintaining flexibility in those areas allows clients to continue to have proper form as they go through the movements required for everyday life. The sit and reach is the most popular lower-body flexibility exercise and test because it assesses most of those muscles (73).

- Strengthen the surrounding areas. A lower-back injury may occur because the lower back itself is weak or because some of the stabilizing muscles such as the abs, obliques, transverse abdominis, glutes, and hip flexors are weak. Strengthening those muscles will help carry the load.

- Help clients lose weight. A big contributing factor to back pain is excess body weight, which can alter posture and set people up for back problems down the road.

- Wear a belt. If you are training a strong client who is using heavy weight, particularly with squats, deadlifts, and good mornings, you can allow the person to try a weightlifting belt. Belts can be helpful in keeping the back flat while using heavy weights. Don't let clients wear a belt all the time.

- Perform the cat and cow movements. The cat and cow (sometimes called cat and dog) are yoga moves that involve bending the spine and tilting the hips. For the cat, the person rounds the spine as much as possible, like a cat stretching itself out, and creates a posterior pelvic tilt with the hips by tucking the glutes up underneath. For the cow, the person arches the back by imagining that water running down the back would gather in a pool in the lower-back area. The person also creates an anterior pelvic tilt by pushing the hips out and back. These positions are shown in figure 27.2. These moves help maintain or increase the flexibility of the spine. They can also be used as tools to teach your clients how to position the spine and hips when they exercise. Generally, when clients lift, they should be in a slight cow position, and they should definitely avoid being in a cat position under load.

- Let the area rest. Train the client for a few weeks using basic exercises that do not specifically target the lower back. How does the person feel? If the client feels fine with this type of workout, that is a good sign and you can progress with him or her. If this workout hurts, then either the injury is worse than initially realized or the client is doing something that you are unaware of that is bothering the back. Encourage the client to consult with a doctor and make sure that the client is using good form on all exercises. If the client can lift with no pain, then you should be able to target and strengthen the lower back. Start with the lower-back machine, go light, and have the client perform that for a week or two. If that feels good, have the client keep doing that, gradually increasing the weight, or progress to hyperextensions. If the client can perform both the lower-back machine and the hyperextension with no pain, then he or she is probably ready to try deadlifts, if they are not contraindicated. Some authorities disagree with the idea of performing deadlifts if a person has a sensitive lower back, but a client has to perform deadlifts all the time in real life, such as when they pick up groceries, laundry baskets, kids, dogs, book bags, suitcases, or anything off the floor. Attempting a deadlift doesn't mean lifting 500 pounds (226.8 kg). Choose a light weight and have the client perform a set or two with good form. The empty bar is often a good place to start. If the client feels OK with this weight and feels fine the next day, chances are that deadlifts are not going to be a problem and you can use them to build up lower-back strength. If you want to be extra cautious, have the client do a rack pull with the bar elevated, which makes a deadlift even easier (but still stay light with the weight) (16, 78).

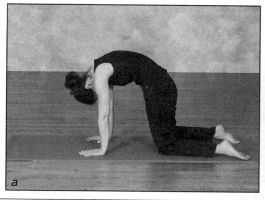
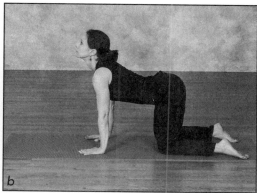

Figure 27.2 Illustration of the *(a)* cat and *(b)* cow yoga poses.

One thing to be aware of with the lower back is that a client may feel fine while performing an exercise but have a sore back the next day. When you add new exercises into a routine, add only one new exercise each time. That way, if a person's back ever flares up, you know which exercise caused it. If you add 10 new exercises and the client's back hurts the next day, you don't know which of those 10 exercises caused the problem.

Knee

The knee is another problematic joint, and many people aggravate or injure their knees at some point in their lives. The muscles around the knee can generate high levels of force. The knee is precariously positioned between two long bones, and it is considered the most complex joint in the body. Generally, two main kinds of injury occur to the knee—compression forces and shearing forces. A compression force occurs when the femur and the tibia are forced together, compressing the cartilage and soft tissue in the area. This type of injury causes pain when weight goes through the leg (as in the start position in a squat or a leg press). A shearing force occurs when the lower part of the leg and the upper part of the leg want to go in two different directions. This action can often damage the ligaments in the knee that attach the femur to the tibia. A shearing injury would usually hurt when performing leg extensions. To help prevent knee damage, particularly during training, you can take several steps (2):

• Develop balance in the muscles around the knee. Several sets of muscles around the knee act on it either directly or indirectly. The opposing muscles should be in balance to one another. They do not need to have exactly the same strength, but they should be in proportion to each other. Those sets of muscles are the following:

   • Quadriceps and hamstrings
   • Abductors and adductors
   • Calves and tibialis anterior

• Develop balance in the quadriceps muscle. The quad pulls on the patellar tendon, which causes the patella (kneecap) to slide up and down. If the patella is not pulled in a straight line, problems can develop over time. If one part of the quad is much stronger than another, the patella can be pulled in that direction. The two main muscles here are the ones on each side of the patella, the vastus medialis and vastus lateralis. They should be relatively even in strength and size. If one dominates the other, injury can develop over time. To strengthen the vastus medialis, focus on the lockout portion of the range of motion. In addition, leg exercises that use an extrawide stance might shift additional emphasis to the vastus medialis. To hit the vastus lateralis, focus on the bottom of the range of motion. Have the client take a narrower stance, shoulder-width or narrower, and point the toes straight ahead to place more emphasis on the vastus lateralis.

• Maintain flexibility in the muscles around the knee. Clients should stretch the surrounding muscles, particularly the quads, hamstrings, hip flexors, calves, and adductors.

• Strengthen and stretch the hip flexors. Some research shows that weak or tight hip flexors can contribute to knee problems. This muscle is often neglected in the gym because of the emphasis on hip extension exercises and the move away from sit-ups. Good exercises to target the hip flexor include mountain climbers, particularly with a band around the ankle to make the upward phase harder, weighted knee and leg raises, decline sit-ups, and sled drags with the strap tied around the ankles.

• Use proper foot wear. During both exercise and everyday life, people need to wear appropriate shoes. They should choose something that is comfortable and designed for the activity in question. Worn-out shoes should be replaced.

• Use a proper surface. When performing impact exercise such as running and jumping, people should use a surface that has some give to it. Natural grass is best, but most tracks and aerobics floors have some built-in cushioning. People should try to avoid regularly running and jumping on concrete and asphalt if possible. In addition, clients should be instructed on proper landing technique (have soft knees and hips, contact first with the balls of the feet, absorb the impact with the legs, keep the chest over the knees and the hips back) if they will be performing a lot of jumping.

• Avoid reliance on machines. Surprisingly, machines are more likely to lead to injury of the knee than free weights are. Machines allow some of the key stabilizers to relax, and the joint doesn't move in a completely natural way. When free weights are used, all the necessary muscles have to contract. The Smith machine commonly bothers lifter's knees. The leg extension, particularly when going heavy, can also add to the problem. Remember that these machines, especially the Smith machine, if used at all, should be a transition exercise to build up strength and flexibility to prepare for free weights. They should not be an end in themselves; the machines are too low skill to provide much positive transfer to the real world. When training the lower body with machines and even with free weights, a good approach is to perform more functional exercises simultaneously, such as mobility drills, sprints, and, if appropriate, agility drills. This practice will ensure that the strength developed in the gym can be applied outside the gym.

• Gait and bone structure can affect the health of the knees. An unusual or uneven walk may place pressure on the knees. Flat feet or an excessive arch can affect structures of the body above it, in this case the knees and even all the way up to the neck. Being bow legged or knock kneed also increases the chance of knee injury. If the client experiences any foot pain when he or she walks or runs, or if the client is noticeably bow legged or has an unusual walk, you should suggest that the client have that issue checked out by a qualified doctor. The client might be able to use inserts or other corrective wear to help fix the issue. A simple way to tell whether a client has an uneven walk is to look at the bottom of a pair of shoes that he or she has worn out. If one side is much more worn down than the other, the client's feet are not hitting the ground evenly.

Women are significantly more likely than men to suffer knee injuries. A multitude of factors likely contribute to this disparity, but a leading theory is that the Q angle, which describes the angle of the hips and the knee, is larger on a female than it is on a male. A woman's hips are wider than a man's (of the same size), so the femur must come down at a sharper angle inward to reach the lower leg. A man's femur is more up and down, whereas a woman's femur is more slanted, and this angle creates instability. A personal trainer can't do anything to change this Q angle, but by training the legs, particularly the involved areas around the knees, you can strengthen the surrounding tissue and make it more able to withstand pressure. This sort of work is no guarantee against injury, but it does reduce the likelihood of it.

Wrist

The wrist is another major joint that is prone to exercise-related injuries. Weight training in particular can put a lot of stress on the wrists. Many people, especially older adults, have weak wrists and forearms. If you follow a few simple guidelines, you can help your clients strengthen their wrists and often relieve pain and prevent injury (19, 35):

• Strengthen the wrist. The wrist is a joint crossed by muscles, like any other joint, and it benefits from strength training just as any other part of the body does. To strengthen the wrist with the primary goal of simply improving wrist health, consider including these five simple exercises:

- Wrist curl—have clients use a light weight (3–10 lb or 1.4–4.5 kg) and flex the wrist—palms up, moving the wrist toward themselves—for three sets of 10 to 20 reps.

- Reverse wrist curl—have clients use a light weight (3–10 lb or 1.4–4.5 kg) and extend the wrist—palms down, moving the back of the hand upward—for three sets of 10 to 20 reps.

- Upward wrist curl—have clients use a light weight (3–10 lb or 1.4–4.5 kg), hold it at the bottom of the dumbbell with a neutral grip, and move the wrist down and up. The motion is similar to using a fishing rod or shaking someone's hand. They perform three sets of 10 to 20 reps.

- Downward wrist curl—have clients hold a light dumbbell with a neutral grip at the top of the dumbbell, lift the weight so that the bottom of the dumbbell moves toward the elbow, let it go back down, and repeat. They do three sets of 10 to 20 reps.
- Squeeze a tennis ball—have clients hold a regular tennis ball (it doesn't have to be new) and squeeze it so that the ball compresses. They should do 100 reps. A client who can't complete them consecutively can rest when necessary.

• Stretch the forearm muscles. Many clients have tight wrists with a limited range of motion. Performing the preceding exercises will help stretch the wrists, but actively stretching them can help improve the range of motion. You should instruct the client to stretch the forearm flexors by bending the fingers and the wrist backward (putting those joints in extension) and to stretch the forearm extensors by bending the wrist forward (putting the wrist in flexion).

• Avoid repetitive overuse movements. Like any joint, the wrist is susceptible to injury from overuse. A common problem is carpal tunnel syndrome. Carpal tunnel syndrome normally arises from continually using the wrist in the same motions repeatedly, such as typing on a computer. If a person uses a computer often or performs other sorts of repetitive movements, you might suggest having a specialist in ergonomics examine the person's work space.

• Use good form when lifting weights. Many clients do not align their wrists properly when lifting weights, particularly on pressing exercises and curling exercises. You need to ensure that your clients align their bodies properly, from head to toe. In general, the wrist should always be a continuation of the forearm; the forearm and wrist should be in a straight line. Many people allow their wrists to extend backward as they lift. This configuration will cause a decrease in power and over time can aggravate the wrists. Sometimes this occurs

because the wrist and forearm are too weak to handle the weight that the prime mover is capable of using. While exercising, the wrist should not be significantly flexed or extended. Sometimes during back or biceps exercises, clients flex their wrists, particularly at the end of the range of motion in an effort to move the bar another inch or two. That movement is unnecessary. Unless they are specifically training their forearms, they should keep their wrists in a straight line with their forearms.

• Try wrist wraps. A wrist wrap is a piece of lifting apparel that goes around the wrist. It is usually up to 1 meter long and about 8 centimeters wide. The lifter can make the wrap as tight or as loose as desired. Wrist wraps can be beneficial on heavy squats, especially when using the lower bar position, cleans, front squats, curls, lateral raises, and any presses. Wrist wraps are not just for elite lifters. If a client is older, has already suffered an injury to the wrist, or has arthritis in the wrist, the wrist wrap can help take some pressure off the wrist joint itself.

A key part of being fit is being healthy, and part of that equation is staying relatively injury free. If a client becomes injured, the knowledge gained from this chapter will help you better understand how the body is healing and what you can do to facilitate the recovery process. The best plan of attack is not to get hurt, and following the guidelines outlined in the chapter can go a long way to preventing any fitness-related injury. Even if the worst happens and a client suffers an injury, either inside or outside the gym, know that humans are tough and adaptable creatures. By helping your client maintain a positive attitude and motivating them to work hard, he or she will be fit and happy again.

CONCLUSION

The body can experience two broad types of injuries. Macrotraumas are acute injuries that immediately affect performance; microtraumas are chronic injuries that develop over time. After the body is injured, it goes through three phases of healing. The inflammation phase lasts up to two weeks, and the personal trainer should not allow the client to perform any activity in this phase. The training goal is not to make the injury worse. Clients are often advised to RICE the injured area. The repair phase lasts up to two months. During this time the body is repairing the injury with collagen fibers laid down haphazardly. The training goal in this phase is to prevent atrophy. Clients should work on regaining range of motion and mobility in the injured area. Any resistance training should incorporate light weight and slow-speed exercises. The remodeling phase lasts up to four months. Now the body is attempting to return to its previous status. The training goal is to return to normal and beyond. Clients can begin to lift heavier weights and, when appropriate, return to sport-specific activities. Personal trainers will likely work with other health professionals if a client has a serious injury. Knowing the scope of practice of those involved in the process is useful.

Some areas of the body are particularly prone to injury. The shoulder is the most flexible joint in the body. Personal trainers should watch for excess range of motion during exercise, poor form on upper-body exercises such as a bench press, and a client's overall posture. The lower body is often troublesome for clients. Personal trainers should teach and enforce braced neutral and braced extension spinal positions, as well as proper form on exercises like squats and deadlifts. Clients should maintain adequate flexibility and should use their legs when lifting things off the ground. The knee is the most complex joint in the body and is often injured. Personal trainers should ensure good form during lower-body exercises, and they should work with their clients on ankle and hip strength and mobility as well the muscles that surround the knee joint. The wrist can also cause problems, so the muscles of the forearms should be both strengthened and stretched to maintain wrist health.

Injuries are bound to happen over the course of a client's life. The more active a person is, especially in activities of an intense nature, the more orthopedic those injuries may be. Working in conjunction with other health professionals, personal trainers who have a solid knowledge of anatomy and an understanding of how the body heals itself can greatly aid and speed up the recovery process.

Study Questions

1. What is the primary concern when clients perform the behind-the-neck military press and lat pull-down?

   a. greater stress on the elbow joint

   b. significant stress on the wrists

   c. compounding stress on the sternum

   d. impingement of the rotator cuff

2. During which stage of tissue repair are the collagen fibers laid down haphazardly?

   a. inflammation

   b. repair

   c. reconstruction

   d. remodeling

3. What training goal for the affected area is associated with the inflammation stage?

   a. Don't make it worse.

   b. Prevent atrophy.

   c. Return to normal level of functioning.

   d. Maximize hypertrophy.

4. In which stage of injury are isometrics most commonly performed?

   a. inflammation

   b. repair

   c. reconstruction

   d. remodeling

5. Which of the following is an example of an open-chained movement and a closed-chained movement (note that order is important)?

   a. dumbbell press; bench press

   b. push-up, pull-up

   c. leg press, leg extension

   d. leg curl, squat

A

Study Questions Answer Sheet

Chapter	Question 1	Question 2	Question 3	Question 4	Question 5
1	c	c	b	c	a
2	c	a	d	a	b
3	b	b	a	d	c
4	d	b	a	b	b
5	c	a	c	b	d
6	c	d	a	b	c
7	b	a	a	c	c
8	a	b	d	a	c
9	d	b	a	d	b
10	a	b	a	c	d
11	b	a	d	b	a
12	c	d	a	a	d
13	d	c	c	a	b
14	a	b	a	c	c
15	c	a	a	a	d
16	b	c	c	a	c
17	b	c	a	a	d
18	b	d	c	a	b
19	d	a	b	c	a
20	d	b	a	b	d
21	d	c	b	c	a
22	b	d	a	c	d
23	a	c	b	c	a
24	d	b	d	a	b
25	c	b	c	c	a
26	a	c	d	a	a
27	d	b	a	b	d

For true or false questions, a = true and b = false.

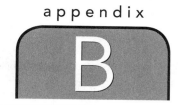

a p p e n d i x

B

Exercise List

Table B.1 Back Exercises

Exercise	Agonists	Synergists	Movement	Plane of movement
Wide-grip lat pull-down	Latissimus dorsi	Rhomboids, brachialis, posterior deltoid, lower traps	Shoulder adduction Elbow flexion	Frontal
Reverse-grip lat pull-down	Latissimus dorsi	Biceps, rhomboids, posterior deltoid, lower traps	Shoulder extension Elbow flexion	Sagittal
V-grip cable row	Latissimus dorsi	Rhomboids, brachialis, posterior deltoids, middle traps	Shoulder extension Elbow flexion	Sagittal
Hammer strength row	Latissimus dorsi	Rhomboids, brachialis, posterior deltoid, middle traps	Shoulder extension Elbow flexion	Sagittal
Wide-grip cable row	Latissimus dorsi	Rhomboids, posterior deltoid, brachialis, middle traps	Horizontal shoulder abduction Elbow flexion	Transverse
Hammer strength lat pull-down	Latissimus dorsi	Biceps, rhomboids, posterior deltoid, lower traps	Shoulder extension Elbow flexion	Sagittal
90-degree pronated bent-over row	Latissimus dorsi	Rhomboids, brachialis, rear delts, middle traps	Horizontal shoulder abduction Elbow flexion	Transverse
45-degree supinated bent-over row	Latissimus dorsi	Biceps, rhomboids, posterior deltoids, middle and upper traps	Shoulder extension Elbow flexion	Sagittal
Dumbbell row	Latissimus dorsi	Rhomboids, brachialis, rear delts, middle traps	Shoulder extension Elbow flexion	Sagittal
Pull-up (BW or assisted)	Latissimus dorsi	Rhomboids, posterior deltoid, brachialis, lower traps	Shoulder adduction Elbow flexion	Frontal
Chin-up (BW or assisted)	Latissimus dorsi	Biceps, rhomboids, posterior deltoid, lower traps	Shoulder extension Elbow flexion	Sagittal
Straight-arm lat pull-down	Latissimus dorsi	Triceps long head, posterior deltoid, rectus abdominis	Shoulder extension	Sagittal

(continued)

465

Table B.1 *(continued)*

Exercise	Agonists	Synergists	Movement	Plane of movement
Pullover machine	Latissimus dorsi	Triceps long head, posterior deltoid, rectus abdominis	Shoulder extension	Sagittal
Wide-grip supported T-bar row	Latissimus dorsi	Rhomboids, brachialis, rear delts, middle traps	Horizontal shoulder abduction / Elbow flexion	Transverse
Narrow-grip supported T-bar row	Latissimus dorsi	Rhomboids, brachialis, posterior deltoids, middle traps	Shoulder extension / Elbow flexion	Sagittal
Old school T-bar row V-grip	Latissimus dorsi	Rhomboids, brachialis, posterior deltoid, middle traps, erectors	Shoulder extension / Elbow flexion	Sagittal
Two-arm dumbbell row	Latissimus dorsi	Rhomboids, brachialis, rear delts, middle traps, erectors	Shoulder extension / Elbow flexion	Sagittal
Standing cable row	Latissimus dorsi	Rhomboids, brachialis, rear delts, middle traps, erectors	Shoulder extension / Elbow flexion	Sagittal
Body-weight row (also called inverse push-up)	Latissimus dorsi	Rhomboids, brachialis, rear delts, middle traps	Horizontal shoulder abduction / Elbow flexion	Transverse
Ball shoulder extension	Latissimus dorsi	Triceps long head, posterior deltoid, rectus abdominis	Shoulder extension	Sagittal

Note: Teres major always works with the lats; the elbow flexor listed is the one most involved; all three are always working.

Table B.2 Chest Exercises

Exercise	Agonists	Synergists	Movements	Plane of movement
Chest press machine	Pectoralis major	Anterior deltoid, triceps, lats	Horizontal shoulder adduction Elbow extension	Transverse
Hammer strength bench press	Pectoralis major	Anterior deltoid, triceps, lats	Horizontal shoulder adduction Elbow extension	Transverse
Incline press machine	Clavicular pectoralis major	Anterior deltoid, triceps	Horizontal shoulder adduction Elbow extension	Transverse*
Hammer strength incline press	Clavicular pectoralis major	Anterior deltoid, triceps	Horizontal shoulder adduction Elbow extension	Transverse*
Bench press	Pectoralis major	Anterior deltoid, triceps, lats	Horizontal shoulder adduction Elbow extension	Transverse
Incline bench press	Clavicular pectoralis major	Anterior deltoid, triceps	Horizontal shoulder adduction Elbow extension	Transverse*
Dumbbell press	Pectoralis major	Anterior deltoid, triceps, lats	Horizontal shoulder adduction Elbow extension	Transverse
Incline dumbbell press	Clavicular pectoralis major	Anterior deltoid, triceps	Horizontal shoulder adduction Elbow extension	Transverse*
Push-up	Pectoralis major	Anterior deltoid, triceps, lats	Horizontal shoulder adduction Elbow extension	Transverse
Smith machine push-up Modified push-up	Pectoralis major	Anterior deltoid, triceps	Horizontal shoulder adduction Elbow extension	Transverse
Smith machine bench press	Pectoralis major	Anterior deltoid, triceps, lats	Horizontal shoulder adduction Elbow extension	Transverse
Pec deck	Pectoralis major	Anterior deltoid	Horizontal shoulder adduction	Transverse
Chest fly machine	Pectoralis major	Anterior deltoid, biceps	Horizontal shoulder adduction	Transverse
Decline bench press	Sternal pectoralis major	Triceps, anterior deltoid	Horizontal shoulder adduction Elbow extension	Transverse*
Decline dumbbell bench press	Pectoralis major	Triceps, anterior deltoid	Horizontal shoulder adduction Elbow extension	Transverse*
Cable fly	Pectoralis major	Anterior deltoid, biceps	Horizontal shoulder adduction	Transverse
Cable incline fly	Clavicular pectoralis major	Anterior deltoid, biceps	Horizontal shoulder adduction	Transverse*
Cable crossover	Sternal pectoralis major	Front deltoid, biceps	Shoulder adduction	Frontal

(continued)

Table B.2 (continued)

Exercise	Agonists	Synergists	Movements	Plane of movement
Dumbbell fly	Pectoralis major	Anterior deltoid, biceps	Horizontal shoulder adduction	Transverse
Incline dumbbell fly	Clavicular pectoralis major	Anterior deltoid, biceps	Horizontal shoulder adduction	Transverse*
Ball dumbbell press	Pectoralis major	Anterior deltoid, triceps	Horizontal shoulder adduction Elbow extension	Transverse
Dips	Pectoralis major	Anterior deltoid, triceps	Shoulder flexion Elbow extension	Sagittal
Power dumbbell fly	Pectoralis major	Anterior deltoid, biceps, triceps	Horizontal shoulder adduction Elbow extension	Transverse
Ball push-up, feet on ball	Pectoralis major	Anterior deltoid, triceps	Horizontal shoulder adduction Elbow extension	Transverse

*Note: All inclines and declines take place in between planes, so their movements and planes are the closest ones to that exercise.

Table B.3   Biceps Exercises

Exercise	Agonists	Synergists	Movements	Plane of movement
Cybex machine curl	Biceps brachii, brachialis	Brachioradialis	Elbow flexion	Sagittal
Icarian machine curl	Biceps brachii, brachialis	Brachioradialis	Elbow flexion	Sagittal
Strive machine curl	Biceps brachii, brachialis	Brachioradialis	Elbow flexion	Sagittal
EZ cable curl	Biceps brachii, brachialis	Brachioradialis	Elbow flexion	Sagittal
FM cable curl	Biceps brachii, brachialis	Brachioradialis	Elbow flexion	Sagittal
EZ-bar curl	Biceps brachii, brachialis	Brachioradialis	Elbow flexion	Sagittal
Dumbbell curl	Biceps brachii, brachialis	Brachioradialis	Elbow flexion	Sagittal
Dumbbell hammer curl	Brachialis	Brachioradialis, biceps brachii	Elbow flexion	Sagittal
EZ preacher curl	Biceps brachii, brachialis	Brachioradialis	Elbow flexion	Sagittal
Dumbbell preacher curl	Biceps brachii, brachialis	Brachioradialis	Elbow flexion	Sagittal
Dumbbell concentration curl	Biceps brachii, brachialis	Brachioradialis	Elbow flexion	Sagittal
Hercules curl High-pulley curl	Biceps brachii, brachialis	Brachioradialis	Elbow flexion	Frontal
Spider curl	Biceps brachii, brachialis	Brachioradialis	Elbow flexion	Sagittal
EZ reverse curl	Brachioradialis	Brachialis, biceps brachii	Elbow flexion	Sagittal
EZ reverse cable curl	Brachioradialis	Brachialis, biceps brachii	Elbow flexion	Sagittal
Parallel bar curl	Brachialis	Brachioradialis, biceps brachii	Elbow flexion	Sagittal
Incline dumbbell curl	Biceps brachii, brachialis	Brachioradialis	Elbow flexion	Sagittal
Standing dumbbell incline curl	Biceps brachii, brachialis	Brachioradialis	Elbow flexion	Sagittal
21s	Biceps brachii, brachialis	Brachioradialis	Elbow flexion	Sagittal
Barbell hold	Biceps brachii, brachialis	Brachioradialis, anterior deltoid, erectors	Elbow flexion (isometric)	Sagittal

Note: Muscle listed first is considered the most important, main agonist for the exercise.

Table B.4 Triceps Exercises

Exercise	Agonists	Synergists	Movements	Plane of movement
Machine overhead tricep extension	Triceps long head	Triceps lateral and medial heads	Elbow extension	Sagittal
V-grip tricep push-down	Triceps lateral head	Triceps long and medial heads	Elbow extension	Sagittal
Straight-bar tricep push-down	Triceps lateral and long head	Triceps medial head	Elbow extension	Sagittal
Rope tricep push-down	Triceps medial and lateral heads	Triceps long head	Elbow extension	Sagittal
Skull crusher	Triceps long head	Triceps lateral and medial heads	Elbow extension	Sagittal
Pullover skull crusher	Triceps long head	Triceps lateral and medial heads	Shoulder extension Elbow extension	Sagittal
Reverse-grip skull crusher	Triceps long head	Triceps lateral and medial heads	Elbow extension	Sagittal
Dumbbell tricep extension	Triceps long head	Triceps lateral and medial heads	Elbow extension	Sagittal
Dumbbell tricep kickback	Triceps long and medial heads	Triceps lateral heads	Elbow extension	Sagittal
Dumbbell overhead tricep extension	Triceps long and lateral head	Triceps medial head	Elbow extension	Sagittal
Reverse-grip tricep pull-down	Triceps long head	Triceps lateral and medial head	Elbow extension	Sagittal
Close-grip bench press	Pectoralis major, long and lateral triceps	Anterior deltoid, triceps medial head	Shoulder flexion Elbow extension	Sagittal
Bench dips	Triceps long head	Triceps lateral and medial, anterior deltoid	Shoulder flexion Elbow extension	Sagittal
Overhead rope tricep extension	Triceps long and medial heads	Triceps lateral head	Elbow extension	Sagittal
Decline skull crusher	Triceps long head	Triceps lateral and medial heads	Elbow extension	Sagittal
Dips	Pectoralis major	Triceps, anterior deltoid	Shoulder flexion Elbow extension	Sagittal
Cable skull crusher	Triceps long head	Triceps lateral and medial	Elbow extension	Sagittal
Reverse-grip bench press	Pectoralis, triceps long head	Triceps lateral and medial, anterior deltoid	Shoulder flexion Elbow extension	Sagittal
Rack or board press	Pectoralis major	Triceps, anterior deltoid	Horizontal shoulder adduction Elbow extension	Transverse
Ball dumbbell tricep pullover	Triceps long and lateral head	Triceps medial head	Shoulder extension Elbow extension	Sagittal
Ball push-up, hands on ball	Pectoralis major, triceps long and lateral head	Triceps medial head, anterior deltoid	Horizontal shoulder adduction Elbow extension	Transverse
JM press	Triceps long head	Triceps lateral and medial head	Elbow extension	Sagittal

Table B.5   Shoulder Exercises

Exercise	Agonists	Synergists	Movements	Plane of movement
Hammer strength military press	Anterior deltoid	Medial deltoid, triceps	Shoulder abduction Elbow extension	Frontal
Military press machine	Anterior deltoid	Medial deltoid, triceps	Shoulder abduction Elbow extension	Frontal
Dumbbell military press	Anterior deltoid	Medial deltoid, triceps	Shoulder abduction Elbow extension	Frontal
Dumbbell front raise	Anterior deltoid	Clavicular pec major	Shoulder flexion	Sagittal
Barbell front raise	Anterior deltoid	Clavicular pec major	Shoulder flexion	Sagittal
Cable front raise	Anterior deltoid	Clavicular pec major	Shoulder flexion	Sagittal
Barbell military press	Anterior deltoid	Medial deltoid, triceps	Shoulder abduction Elbow extension	Frontal
Push press	Anterior deltoid	Medial deltoid, triceps, legs	Shoulder abduction Elbow extension	Frontal
Handstand push-up	Anterior deltoid	Medial deltoid, triceps, core	Shoulder abduction Elbow extension	Frontal
Cable lateral raise	Medial deltoid	Supraspinatus	Shoulder abduction	Frontal
Lateral raise machine	Medial deltoid	Supraspinatus	Shoulder abduction	Frontal
Dumbbell lateral raise	Medial deltoid	Supraspinatus	Shoulder abduction	Frontal
Dumbbell leaning lateral raise	Medial deltoid	Supraspinatus	Shoulder abduction	Frontal
Dumbbell power lateral raise	Medial deltoid	Supraspinatus	Shoulder abduction	Frontal
Lateral hold	Medial deltoid	Supraspinatus	Shoulder abduction (isometric)	Frontal
Dumbbell rear delt raise	Posterior deltoid	Middle trapezius	Horizontal shoulder abduction	Transverse
Rear delt machine	Posterior deltoid	Middle trapezius, latissimus dorsi	Horizontal shoulder abduction	Transverse
Cable rear delt raise	Posterior deltoid	Middle trapezius	Horizontal shoulder abduction	Transverse
One-arm rear delt cable row	Posterior deltoid	Middle trapezius, lats, biceps	Horizontal shoulder abduction Elbow flexion	Transverse
Dumbbell power rear delt raise	Posterior deltoid	Middle trapezius, lats, biceps, erectors	Horizontal shoulder abduction	Transverse
Rope face pull	Posterior deltoid	Middle delt, biceps, middle traps	Horizontal shoulder abduction Elbow flexion	Transverse

Table B.6 Leg Exercises

Exercise	Agonists	Synergists	Movements	Plane of movement
Leg press	Gluteus maximus, quadriceps	Hamstrings	Hip extension Knee extension	Sagittal
Horizontal leg press	Gluteus maximus, quadriceps	Hamstrings	Hip extension Knee extension	Sagittal
Bridge	Gluteus maximus	Hamstrings	Hip extension	Sagittal
Hack squat	Gluteus maximus, quadriceps	Hamstrings	Hip extension Knee extension	Sagittal
Bench squat with body weight	Gluteus maximus, quadriceps	Hamstrings	Hip extension Knee extension	Sagittal
Smith machine squat	Gluteus maximus, quadriceps	Hamstrings	Hip extension Knee extension	Sagittal
Wall squat	Gluteus maximus, quadriceps	Hamstrings	Hip extension Knee extension (isometric)	Sagittal
Barbell squat	Gluteus maximus, quadriceps	Hamstrings, erector spinae	Hip extension Knee extension Trunk extension	Sagittal
Lunges	Gluteus maximus, quadriceps	Hamstrings	Hip extension Knee extension	Sagittal
Sissy squat	Gluteus maximus, quadriceps	Hamstrings	Hip extension Knee extension	Sagittal
Step-ups	Gluteus maximus, quadriceps	Hamstrings	Hip extension Knee extension	Sagittal
Butt blaster	Gluteus maximus	Quadriceps, hamstrings	Hip extension Knee extension	Sagittal
Front squat	Gluteus maximus, quadriceps	Hamstrings, erector spinae	Hip extension Knee extension Trunk extension	Sagittal
Pistol	Gluteus maximus, quadriceps	Hamstrings	Hip extension Knee extension Trunk extension	Sagittal
Leg extension	Quadriceps	–	Knee extension	Sagittal

Note: Adductor magnus often performs hip extension.

Table B.7   Hamstring Exercises

Exercise	Agonists	Synergists	Movements	Plane of movement
Prone leg curl	Hamstrings	Gastroc	Knee flexion	Sagittal
Seated leg curl	Hamstrings	Gastroc	Knee flexion	Sagittal
Single-leg curl	Hamstrings	Gastroc	Knee flexion	Sagittal
Ball leg curl	Hamstrings, gluteus maximus	Gastroc	Hip extension Knee flexion	Sagittal
Glute–ham raise	Hamstrings	Glute maximus, gastroc, erectors	Knee flexion Hip extension (isometric)	Sagittal

Table B.8   Calf Exercises

Exercise	Agonists	Synergists	Movements	Plane of movement
Seated calf machine	Soleus	Gastrocnemius	Ankle plantar flexion	Sagittal
Standing calf machine	Gastrocnemius	Soleus	Ankle plantar flexion	Sagittal
Rotary calf machine	Gastrocnemius	Soleus	Ankle plantar flexion	Sagittal
45-degree calf machine	Gastrocnemius	Soleus	Ankle plantar flexion	Sagittal
Standing barbell calf raise	Gastrocnemius	Soleus	Ankle plantar flexion	Sagittal
Leg press calf raise	Gastrocnemius	Soleus	Ankle plantar flexion	Sagittal
Smith machine calf raise	Gastrocnemius	Soleus	Ankle plantar flexion	Sagittal

Table B.9   Lower-Back Exercises

Exercise	Agonists	Synergists	Movements	Plane of movement
Lower back machine	Erector spinae	Quadratus lumborum	Trunk extension	Sagittal
Conventional deadlift	Erector spinae	Hamstrings, trapezius, grip, gluteus maximus, quadriceps	Trunk extension Hip and knee extension	Sagittal
Sumo deadlift	Erector spinae	Gluteus maximus, adductors, trapezius, grip, hamstrings, quadriceps	Trunk extension Hip and knee extension	Sagittal
Hyperextensions	Erector spinae, hamstrings	Gluteus maximus	Trunk extension	Sagittal
Stiff-legged deadlift	Hamstrings, erector spinae	Trapezius, grip, gluteus maximus	Trunk extension Hip extension	Sagittal
Romanian deadlift	Hamstrings, erector spinae	Trapezius, grip, gluteus maximus	Trunk extension Hip and knee extension	Sagittal
Rack pull	Erector spinae	Hamstrings, trapezius, grip, gluteus maximus, quadriceps	Trunk extension Hip and knee extension	Sagittal
Deadlift off a step (deficit deads)	Erector spinae	Hamstrings, trapezius, grip, gluteus maximus, quadriceps	Trunk extension Hip and knee extension	Sagittal
Good morning	Erector spinae, hamstrings	Gluteus maximus	Trunk extension Hip extension	Sagittal

Note: Quadratus lumborum is always working with the erector spinae.

Table B.10   Trapezius Exercises

Exercise	Agonists	Synergists	Movements	Plane of movement
Dumbbell shrug	Upper trapezius	Grip	Scapula elevation	Frontal
Barbell shrug	Upper trapezius	Grip	Scapula elevation	Frontal
Smith machine shrug	Upper trapezius	Grip	Scapula elevation	Frontal
Hammer strength shrug	Upper trapezius	Grip	Scapula elevation	Frontal
Trap bar shrug	Upper trapezius	Grip	Scapula elevation	Frontal
Protraction*	Serratus anterior	Pec minor	Scapula protraction	Transverse
Retraction	Middle trapezius	Rhomboids	Scapula retraction	Transverse
Depression	Lower trapezius	–	Scapula depression	Frontal

*Note: Protractions do not work the traps.

General Resume Format

NAME—NICE AND BIG, TOP MIDDLE (CAN BE IN THE HEADER SECTION)

Contact information—phone, address, e-mail (beware of inappropriate e-mail names)

Objective or mission statement—in one sentence, why do you want the job or why are you a PT? *My goal is to share my passion, enthusiasm, and education in fitness with others to show them how rewarding leading a healthy, active lifestyle can be.*

Education

College and postgraduate schooling (even if you didn't finish): year, major(s), minor(s), focus of study
- NPTI
- Other courses, specialties
- High school

Work Experience

Practicums and internships can be included here.
Job title, date held
List main duties in bullet style; focus on
- Dependability
- Interpersonal interactions
- Sales (even minor stuff)
- Responsibility (handling money)
- Creativity
- Progression (promotions, new duties, and so on)
- Work ethic
- Obviously, fitness related is a plus but not necessary.

Repeat for each job.

Certifications

- NPTI certified personal trainer, CPT
- NPTI certified in basic nutrition
- CPR or AED, first-aid certified
- Anything additional you have

Volunteer Work

Such as volunteer work in sports and fitness-related organizations

Extracurricular Activities

Such as sports and fitness-related stuff

Awards Won

Such as employee of the month, fitness related, and so on
If you have a personal story about fitness (lost a bunch of weight, recovered from an accident, or other), you can include a short version here if you wish.

References

Resumes can be two pages. Name, education, experience, and certifications (if room allows) are on the first page; everything else is on the second page. Also, include the resume addendum for NPTI as a third page (provided upon graduation).

1 pg outline of NPTI requirement

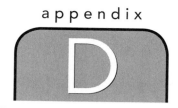

Interviewing
for Fitness-Related Jobs

After you have assembled your resume and sent it out, you will (you hope) be called in for an interview. The purpose of a well-written resume is to give a potential employer some background information and impress them enough to give you an interview. The purpose of the interview is to sell yourself to the employer and reassure them that you are the right choice for the job.

The many steps to conducting an impressive interview are outlined here. The first step is to be prepared, and this means being prepared on many levels.

• **Know where the interview is**. Be sure that you know where the interview is and what time it is to take place. You will likely be interviewing at a place you have never been to before. Always overestimate how long you will need to find the location. Recognize that you might get lost. If you are late to an interview, you can probably kiss the job goodbye. Try to plan to arrive in the parking lot at least 15 minutes before the interview starts; 30 minutes is even better. If you do arrive early, use the time to relax in your car and mentally rehearse some of the questions that you have prepared and what you want to say.

• **Have a professional appearance**. When going for an interview, make an effort to make yourself look good. This means being showered and shaved. Or, if you have facial hair, have it well groomed. Most fitness jobs will not require you to wear a suit, but you should make an effort to dress up. Wear nice, clean clothes, not what you just worked out in or your favorite sweats. Some interviews may have a practical component, so you want to be prepared by bringing presentable workout clothes and shoes to wear if necessary. When in doubt, call the interviewer. Ask whether the interview includes a practical portion and what you should wear for the interview. This kind of question is not inappropriate. Always error on the side of being too dressed up. If you are coming from your current job, let the person know that you are dressed the way you are for that reason.

• **Have your paperwork ready**. Do not walk into an interview empty handed. You should bring a folder and some pertinent papers with you for every interview. You should always bring an extra copy of your resume for the interviewer to look over. You should bring with you a list of references that you can leave with the interviewer. Bringing extra stuff and then ending up not handing it out doesn't hurt. Other items are optional but will often help your cause. If you have a favorable job review from your past employer, bring that with you. If you have positive client evaluations or testimonial letters from clients, bring copies of those for your potential employer. Leaving letters of recommendation with the interviewer is appropriate, and, of course, you should have a list questions that you want to ask the interviewer. Finally, bring some blank paper so that you can take notes during the interview. Doing so looks professional.

• **Practice the interview beforehand**. You cannot know exactly what questions the interviewer might ask you, but you do know what you want to say during an interview. Ask a close friend or family member to pretend to be the interviewer in a half hour session with you. He or she should ask you whatever questions he or she wants to ask, and you should do your best to answer them as if you were in a real interview. This session may feel cheesy or corny while you are doing it, but when you do the real interview, the payoff will be significant. Think of interviewing like a sport or activity. How many athletes wait until an important competition to try something that they have never done before? None, more than likely. Instead, they practice repeatedly until they are good at it. Then, when the competition comes, they are ready.

• **Be on time.** This point is simple but important. If you are late, you are telling the interviewer that the job isn't important to you and that you will be late to work a lot. Nobody wants to hire a person like that, even someone who has a good reason for being late. Try to walk in the door between 0 and 5 minutes early. No one will fault you for being 5 minutes early, and no one will fault you for being on time. Obviously, you don't want to be late, but less obviously, you don't want to be super early either. You don't want to appear desperate for the job or that you have nothing better to do. So if you arrive early to the site, and you should (remember to arrive 15 to 30 minutes early), stay in your car until you are 0 to 5 minutes early for the interview and then enter the building.

After you have arrived, on time and dressed professionally, you are ready for the interview itself. Chances are that you will not know exactly what the interviewer is going to ask you during your interview, but that is OK. If you are given an interview, the employer has probably decided from your resume that you are capable of doing the job. Now they are trying to find out what kind of person you are, whether you will do the job well, whether you will be a good fit for the company, and whether you will complement the company. In a nutshell, they are looking for the best person to do the job.

When you go into an interview, your goal is to sell yourself to the prospective employer. Keep in mind that the interviewer doesn't know you at all. He or she doesn't know whether you are a good person or not, whether you are honest or not, whether you are hard working or not, whether you know what you are talking about or not. The list goes on and on. Making an important judgment about a person based on a conversation that lasts a half hour or less is difficult, so the interviewer must read into the answers that you give. Therefore, you want to give the "right" answers during the interview.

Before you go for the interview, you should try to analyze yourself. Try to think about what strengths you have, either relating to the fitness profession specifically or just to your strengths in general. These strengths can be broad. Do you know a lot about bodybuilding? Did you raise your baby sister when you were 12? Are you a single parent? Are you hard working? As you analyze yourself, try to find at least five qualities that you are proud of and that you think would benefit a prospective employer. Make it your mission to have the interviewer be aware of those five qualities at the end of the interview.

The key to a successful interview is understanding what the interviewer is really asking. Interview questions can take many forms. Some questions are direct; some are not. Here is an example: "Do you handle responsibility well?" This direct question does not require a direct answer. What you must ask yourself after every question is what the interviewer really wants to know. Here it is clear. The interviewer wants to know if you handle responsibility well. Now you must provide examples to him or her that show how well you handle responsibility. Answering yes or no will get you nowhere here. You need to give specific examples, such as that the boss in your past job gave you a task and then left you alone because he or she knew that you would complete it on time.

Another example might be a question like this: "What do you think of resistance training for weight loss?" Again, when you hear the question, ask yourself what the interviewer is trying to discover about you. Here, it seems as if the interviewer is trying to assess your knowledge of resistance training versus cardiovascular training. The question has no right or wrong answer, depending on the evidence that you provide, but saying "I think it's good," doesn't tell the interviewer much. Instead, you need to say something like "Resistance training is effective for weight loss because it burns calories during the workout and builds muscle, which cardio doesn't do. Every pound of muscle burns about 12 to 20 calories per day, so resistance training is the only way to change a person's basal metabolic rate. Thus it is effective for long-term weight loss."

A more abstract example is this question: "What is your favorite animal?" Again, you hear the question and ask yourself what the interviewer is trying to learn about you. Here it seems that the interviewer is trying to learn something about your personality, so now you want to answer accordingly. If you say, "I would be a cat because they are cute," the interviewer learns nothing important about you, so you waste the opportunity to promote yourself. If you say, "I would be a cat because they get to sit around all day and everything is provided for them," you would be telling the interviewer that you envy laziness and that you would like to do nothing all day if you could. If you say, "I would be a cat because they are clever. It seems that my cat can eventually figure out any problem or challenge that I give her. Now she can go around and open doors in my house. I really respect something or someone who faces a challenge that at first might seem impossible but sticks with it and eventually figures it out. I would like to think that I have that quality myself. I know my cat does, so I would like to be a cat if I could." Now you are telling the interviewer that you respect hard work and that you are someone who doesn't quit if you fail the first time you do something. Now you have told the interviewer something valuable about yourself.

The final thing to think about when answering an interview question is this: You have to say what you mean to say. This means that you have to explain to the interviewer what point it is that you are trying to get across. Don't expect the interviewer to infer anything positive about you. For example, if you are asked whether you are hardworking, don't say, "Yeah, I am

a roofer. I am hardworking." You may be thinking in your mind that roofing is surely hard work, but don't expect the interviewer to infer that. You need to tell him or her that you get up at 5:00 a.m. in the morning every day, that you carry heavy things up and down ladders, that you work in the hot sun or the cold weather all day long, and that you still smile and look forward to work and generally make any job fun. Now the interviewer has some idea that you are a hard worker when before he or she didn't. If you are asked whether you are responsible, don't just say, "Well, I have a daughter and I am a single parent," and assume that the person will infer that you are responsible. Tell the interviewer about what you have done for your daughter and how much you have learned about yourself while raising her. Then throw in the fact that on top of all, you worked a full-time job and didn't miss any days. Now you have impressed the person even more by saying that you are both responsible and hardworking!

Remember, follow these steps for every question that you are asked:

- Listen to the question intently and alertly.
- Ask yourself what the interviewer is really trying to learn.
- Provide an answer that addresses what the interviewer is really trying to learn about you.
- When possible, provide specific examples and use the question as an opportunity to tell the employer about one or more of the five qualities that you want to convey.
- Remember that you have to say what you mean to say.

After asking all of his or her questions, the interviewer will give you an opportunity to ask questions of your own. You should have spent some time beforehand to come up with several questions that you want to ask the employer. Write these questions down. Many of them will be answered during the course of the interview, but some of them will not. Even if most of your questions have been answered, take the time to ask a few questions of the interviewer. When the interviewer asks you whether you have any questions, you do yourself no favor by sitting there and saying no.

Below is a list of questions that you might want to ask a prospective employer. The list is not comprehensive, so feel free to develop your own questions.

- What are the hours expected of this job?
- How flexible is the schedule? Who determines the schedule?
- Does the staff work well as a team here?
- What kind of manager are you? Are you hands on, or do you take a laissez-faire approach?
- What type of employee excels in this company?
- What is the biggest challenge that most of your employees face?
- Does this position have a high turnover ratio?
- How will I be evaluated, and who will perform that evaluation?
- If an employee works hard for one year and has a positive evaluation, what kind of compensation might he or she expect to receive at the end of the year?
- Does this position offer any insurance or benefits?
- How does sick leave or vacation time work?
- How does the cancellation policy for a personal training session work?
- What kind of employee are you looking for?
- What is the biggest challenge that you as the manager face (what keeps you up at night)?

The last two questions are important. You will want to ask them almost every time because they will set up your closing statement. The first question asks the person what kind of employee he or she wants working for the organization. The interviewer will then list several qualities that he or she thinks are important. Ideally, you have those qualities

and have already highlighted them during the interview, but if you haven't, you still have time to save yourself. This question is useful because it induces the interviewer to lay down his or her cards, so that you can discover what is important. Then all you have to do is feed that information back to the interviewer so that he or she knows that you have the desired qualities.

The second question asks what the main challenge is for the manager. Is it having dependable employees—knowing that someone who opens the gym at 5:00 a.m. will actually show up? Is it having employees who are good at sales? It is having employees who will please their customers with effective programs and good customer service? Whatever the problem is, you want to remember it because you will be bringing it back up in just a few moments.

After you have asked the interviewer all your questions, you are ready to sum up your case, to present your closing arguments. You want to reiterate all those qualities that you believe you have. This is the time to create a lasting impression in the person's mind to make him or her want to hire you. The beauty is that the interviewer has already given you all the information you need to succeed. After the interviewer has told you what kind of employee the organization is looking for and what the biggest problem is, you can respond by saying that you have the qualities that the organization is looking for (assuming that you do; this is not a time to lie just to get the job) and that you can help solve the problem. Even if you have already mentioned in the interview that you are hardworking, honest, dependable, and good at sales, say it all again. Repetition within reason is a good thing in an interview; more than one mention is often needed for a statement to stick in a person's head. Then tell the interviewer how you will do your best to solve the organization's biggest problem or at least that you will not be an employee who exacerbates that problem.

After you have said everything that you want to say, thank the interviewer for taking the time to interview you, shake the person's hand (firmly, no dead fish), and exit as appropriate. If the job is important to you, which it should be, then send a note through the mail (not e-mail) thanking the person for the interview. This old-school tactic still impresses people. If the employer makes you an offer monetarily during the interview, do not accept or reject it right away. Tell the interviewer that you will consider it. If the offer is much too low for you to accept, you can try to negotiate the offer right there. If you are excited about the offer and know that you will accept it, you should still say that you need a day or two to think about it. Then call back and accept the offer if you wish. Accepting the offer on the spot may cause the employer to think that the offer was excessive. You do not want the employer to have the feeling that they are overpaying you.

Interviewing is a complex process. Of course, the spotlight is on you as a candidate, but the interviewer faces a challenge as well in trying to gather a lot of information about you in a relatively short time. Therefore, you need to give pertinent information in response to open-ended questions. If you are saying yes or no for most of your responses, you are shooting yourself in the foot. A good interview is often a half hour to an hour long, so giving longer responses is not a problem. Longer is often better, assuming that you are keeping the person's interest and are not messing up his or her schedule.

Finally, if you still want more information about the job, the best thing to do is to talk to an employee who works there, preferably someone who works in your prospective position. If you want to be a personal trainer at a gym, just ask a personal trainer at that gym about the job. Does the person like the job? What is the worst part of the job? What is the best part of the job? How does the person like his or her boss? What is the stress level on the job? Ask the personal trainer whatever you want to know, but be careful about asking about salary because that issue is often too personal. After you have all the information, you just have to make the best decision you can.

Good luck with your interviews. Like anything else, interviewing is a skill. Some people are naturally good at interviews, and some are not. As with anything else, anyone can become better with practice. The more interviews you do, both mock interviews and real ones, the better prepared you will be for the future.

/

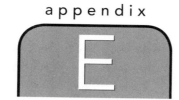
Sample Introductory Workout

Routine

- Warm-up: cardio or calisthenics for five minutes.
- Shoulder series: front, lateral, and rear DB raises for 10 to 15 reps, light weight.
- Bench press: one or two warm-up sets, 10 to 15 reps. Then two or three work sets, moderate intensity.
- Fly machine: one warm-up set, two to three work sets, 10 to 15 reps.
- Wide-grip lat pull-down: one warm-up set, two to three work sets, 10 to 15 reps.
- Cable row or DB row: one warm-up set, two to three work sets, 10 to 15 reps.
- V-grip push-downs or skull crushers: one warm-up set, two to three work sets, 10 to 15 reps.
- EZ-bar curl: one warm-up set, two to three work sets, 10 to 15 reps. Try super-sets with triceps if appropriate.
- Abs: Show clients something new that they will feel—ball crunches, clams, leg thrusts, incline crunches, leg raises, planks, whatever is appropriate.
- Stretch: Do a partner stretch with clients. Try chest or shoulder stretch or hamstring stretch.

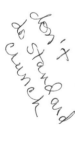

At the end, remind clients that you are heading down to the office to discuss which program is best for them. This workout should take 30 to 40 minutes. Remember that you have about 10 to 15 minutes of stuff to do in the beginning and then you have about 10 minutes of stuff to do at the end, so don't plan a 60-minute workout.

Things to Do

- Be picky about form. Point out things that clients are doing wrong. Watch for shoulders, wrists, grip placement, being jerky, breathing, and rounded shoulders.
- Be knowledgeable; use some fancy muscle names and terms so that they believe that you know what you are doing.
- Be friendly and respectful.
- Make them work hard but don't kill them. Causing them to feel the burn will release endorphins, which will put them in a better mood and make them more receptive to the sale.
- Make them feel as if they need you to succeed and that they can't do it on their own.
- Act as if they have already signed up.

Things *Not* to Do

- Describe how to set up the machine.
- Take detailed notes on the workout. Clients will ask for the workout that you just gave them and you don't want them to understand it that well. Use obscure abbreviations or write things down after they leave.
- Tell them that they have been doing everything right all along.
- Explain how they should set up their workout program.
- Explain how many sets and reps they should do.
- Give them detailed nutrition advice. Just throw out a few samples of information

so that they believe that you know what you are doing.

- If they can go through the same workout that you just took them through at the end of the workout, you were too thorough. Remember that you are using this hour to give them an idea of how they like working with you, not so that they can learn some stuff and do it on their own.

F

Sample Pricing

Like other professionals, personal trainers need to have a price sheet for all of their services. Unless you are working for a company that has predetermined prices, you need to have a price sheet that covers all the services that people may want to buy. Many elements go into the design of a price sheet. Do you want to sell a certain number of sessions, or do you want to sell a program for a certain length of time? Does a customer get a discount for buying longer sessions? These are just two of the many options to consider when setting up your price sheet.

Personal trainers commonly set a base price for one session. This price is normally a little higher than what they usually charge, but it serves as a base to establish all the other prices. A common base price for a personal trainer is $60 to $70 per hour. Clients normally have two or three program lengths to choose from. For example, a client might wish to purchase a program for three months or six months in duration. Prices are often set depending on how many sessions per week a client purchases, from 1 session per week to 5 sessions per week. Some trainers may offer a short introductory period involving a set number of sessions such as 8 sessions or 16 sessions.

When setting up your price sheet, the most important thing is to be comfortable with your prices. Of course, if they are too high, few people will sign up, but if they are too low, you will not feel as if you are being adequately compensated for your services. Keep in mind that if you work for a gym, 50 percent of your price per hour will commonly be taken by the gym or the company that you work for. If you are charging $40 per hour, you personally will only make $20 per hour.

Here is a sample price sheet. Feel free to use this as a guideline or start your own.

Base Price

1 session: $65 per hour

4 sessions: $255 total

8 sessions: $505 total

12 sessions: $760 total

16 sessions: $1,000 total

All block sessions must be used within three months from the date of purchase.

IN-HOME TRAINING

Base Price

One session per week: $80 per hour

Two sessions per week: $75 per hour

Three sessions per week: $70 per hour

Location within a 15-mile radius is included; each additional 5 miles is an additional $5 per hour.

You might want to have less expensive options that you can use as a last resort or for your nutrition programs.

PROGRAM DESIGN*

Beginner workout: a workout to follow for one to three months—$40

Intermediate workout: a workout to follow for three to six months—$60

Advanced workout: a workout to follow indefinitely—$80

*All programs include unlimited e-mail access to answer any of your questions.

Three-month program			
Sessions per week	**Price per hour**	**Sessions per month, price per month**	**Total sessions, total price**
1x week	$60	4 sessions $240 per month	12 sessions $720 total
2x week	$57	8 sessions $456 per month	24 sessions $1,368 total
3x week	$54	12 sessions $648 per month	36 sessions $1,944 total
4x week	$51	16 sessions $816 per month	48 sessions $2,448 total
5x week	$48	20 sessions $960 per month	60 sessions $2,880 total

Six-month program			
Sessions per week	**Price per hour**	**Sessions per month, price per month**	**Total sessions, total price**
1x week	$57	4 sessions $228 per month	24 sessions $1,368 total
2x week	$54	8 sessions $432 per month	48 sessions $2,592 total
3x week	$51	12 sessions $612 per month	72 sessions $3,672 total
4x week	$48	16 sessions $768 per month	96 sessions $4,608 total
5x week	$45	20 sessions $900 per month	120 sessions $5,400 total

EQUIPMENT ORIENTATION

The perfect program to learn about all the equipment in the gym:

One session: $70

Three sessions: $200, includes a free beginner workout

Calculating Lean Body Mass and Fat Weight

Start with two pieces of information:

Body weight _____ Body fat % _____

Take 100 – body fat % = _____ body lean %

Take body weight × body fat % = _____ lb (kg) of fat on body

Take body weight × body lean % = _____ lb (kg) of lean on body

Example 1

200 lb (90.7 kg) male 15% body fat

100 – 15% = 85% body lean

200 lb (90.7 kg) × 15% (15% is 0.15 in decimal form) = 30 lb (13.6 kg) of fat

200 lb (90.7 kg) × 85% (85% is 0.85 in decimal form) = 170 lb (77.1 kg) of lean

Example 2

145 lb (65.8 kg) female 25% body fat

100 – 25% = 75% body lean

145 × 25% (0.25) = 36.25 lb (16.4 kg) of fat

145 × 75% (0.75) = 108.75 lb (49.3 kg) of lean

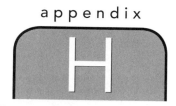

appendix

H

Skinfold Formulas

DURNIN–WOMERSLEY FORMULA

Age (years)	Males	Females
<17	D = 1.1533 − (0.0643 × L)	D = 1.1369 − (0.0598 × L)
17–19	D = 1.1620 − (0.0630 × L)	D = 1.1549 − (0.0678 × L)
20–29	D = 1.1631 − (0.0632 × L)	D = 1.1599 − (0.0717 × L)
30–39	D = 1.1422 − (0.0544 × L)	D = 1.1423 − (0.0632 × L)
40–49	D = 1.1620 − (0.0700 × L)	D = 1.1333 − (0.0612 × L)
≥50	D = 1.1715 − (0.0779 × L)	D = 1.1339 − (0.0645 × L)

D is then converted to body fat with the Siri equation, which is

Percent body fat = (495 ÷ body density) − 450

The Siri equation is commonly used in formulas that attempt to find percent body fat. It is based on the idea that all tissues in the body are either fat mass or fat-free mass. Fat mass and fat-free mass tissue do not have the same density. Fat-free mass tissue is denser and has a value of 1.1 grams per cubic centimeter. Fat mass is less dense and has a value of .9 grams per cubic centimeter. Density equals mass divided by volume, which can also be expressed as volume equals mass divided by density, and mass equals all the fat mass plus all the fat-free mass in the body.

JACKSON–POLLOCK SEVEN-SITE FORMULA

Body density = 1.112 − (0.00043499 × S) +
(0.00000055 × S^2) − (0.00028826 × age)

Body fat is then calculated using the Siri equation.

JACKSON–POLLOCK THREE-SITE FORMULA

Male Formula

Body density = 1.10938 −
(0.0008267 × sum of chest, abdomen, and thigh skinfolds in mm) +
(0.0000016 × square of the sum of chest, abdomen, and thigh) −
(0.0002574 × age in years)

(Jackson AS, Pollock ML, 1978, based on a sample aged 18–61)

Body density is then converted in percent body fat using the Siri equation.

Female Formula

Body density = 1.0994921 −
(0.0009929 × sum of triceps, thigh, and suprailiac skinfolds in mm) +
(0.0000023 × square of the sum of triceps, thigh, and suprailiac skinfolds) −
(0.0001392 × age in years)

(Jackson, et al., 1980, based on a sample aged 18–55)

Body density is then converted in percent body fat using the Siri equation.

PARILLO NINE-SITE FORMULA

Percent body fat = (27 × S) ÷ body weight (in pounds)

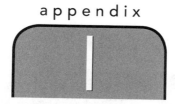

NPTI Resting Fitness Assessments

The following table is a sample resting fitness assessment record.

Name: _____

Assessment	Test 1 date	Test 2 date	Test 3 date
Sex			
Age			
Height			
Weight			
Body mass index			
Resting pulse			
Heart rate reserve			
Blood pressure			
Chest BF			
Axilla BF			
Bicep BF			
Triceps BF			
Abdominal BF			
Suprailiac BF			
Thigh BF			
Calf BF			
Subscapular BF			
Lower-back BF			
Durnin–Womersley Body-fat calculation			
Jackson–Pollock seven-site body-fat calculation			
Jackson–Pollock three-site body-fat calculation			
Parrillo nine-site Body-fat calculation			
Bioelectrical BF			
Neck	R/F	R/F	R/F
Shoulders	R/F	R/F	R/F
Chest	R/F	R/F	R/F
Waist (thinnest part)	R/F	R/F	R/F
Waist (belly button)	R/F	R/F	R/F
Hips	R/F	R/F	R/F
Thigh (thickest part)	R/F	R/F	R/F
Thigh (halfway)	R/F	R/F	R/F
Calf	R/F	R/F	R/F
Upper arm	R/F	R/F	R/F
Forearm	R/F	R/F	R/F
Wrist			
Waist–hip ratio			

R = relaxed measurement; F = flexed measurement (optional).

Key Concept References

Key reference entries for each chapter are listed here. For a complete list of all the references cited in this book, visit www.HumanKinetics.com/products/all-products/NPTIs-Fundamentals-of-Fitness-and-Personal-Training.

Chapter 1

1. Alter MJ. *Science of Flexibility*. 2nd ed. Champaign, IL: Human Kinetics; 1996.
2. American College of Sports Medicine. Position stand: The recommended quantity and quality of exercise for developing and maintaining cardiorespiratory and muscular fitness in healthy adults. *Med Sci Sports Exerc*. 1990;22:265-274.
3. Amundson EP. Scope of practice: Overly cautious or professional vigilance? *S D Med*. 2010 Mar;63(3):107. PubMed PMID: 20301875.
4. Baechle TR, Groves BR. *Weight Training: Steps to Success*. Champaign, IL: Human Kinetics; 1992.
5. Baechle TR, Earle RW, eds. *NSCA's Essentials of Strength Training and Conditioning*. 3rd ed. Champaign, IL: Human Kinetics; 2008.
6. Blair SN, Kohl HW, Barlow CE, Paffenbarger RS Jr, Gibbons LW, Macera CA. Changes in physical fitness and all-cause mortality. A prospective study of healthy and unhealthy men. *J Amer Med Assoc*. 1995;273(14):1093-1098.
7. Chu DA. Plyometrics: The link between strength and speed. *Nat Strength Cond Assoc J*. 1983;5(2):20-21.
8. Clark MA. *Integrated Training for the New Millennium*. Thousand Oaks, CA: National Academy of Sports Medicine; 2001.
9. Enoka RM. Muscle strength and its development. New perspectives. *Sports Med*. 1988;6:146-168.
10. Fischer DV, Bryant J. Effect of certified personal trainer services on stage of exercise behavior and exercise mediators in female college students. *J Am Coll Health*. 2008 Jan-Feb;56(4):369-76. PubMed PMID: 18316279.
11. Hansen J. *Natural Bodybuilding*. Champaign, IL: Human Kinetics; 2005.
12. Marsh HW. The multidimensional structure of physical fitness: Invariance over gender and age. *Res Q Exerc Sport*. 1993 Sep;64(3):256-73. PubMed PMID: 8235047.
13. McCauley SM, Hager MH. Why are therapeutic diet orders an issue now and what does it have to do with legal scope of practice? *J Am Diet Assoc*. 2009 Sep;109(9):1515-9. PubMed PMID: 19699824.
14. Nieman DC. The exercise test as a component of the total fitness evaluation. *Prim Care*. 1994 Sep;21(3):569-87. PubMed PMID: 9132759.
15. O'Shea P. Effects of selected weight training programs on the development of strength and muscle hypertrophy. *Res Q*. 1966;37:95-102.
16. Rippetoe M, Kilgore L. *Starting Strength: A Simple and Practical Guide for Coaching Beginners*. Wichita Falls, TX: Aasgaard; 2005.
17. Smeltzer CH, Fewster L. Getting your own personal trainer. *Mich Health Hosp*. 2002 Mar-Apr;38(2):30. PubMed PMID: 11968989.
18. Starr, B. *The Strongest Shall Survive: Strength Training for Football*. 1st ed. Washington: Fitness Products; 1978.
19. Trudelle-Jackson E, Jackson AW, Morrow JR Jr. Relations of meeting national public health recommendations for muscular strengthening activities with strength, body composition, and obesity: The Women's Injury Study. *Am J Public Health*. 2011 Oct;101(10):1930-5. doi: 10.2105/AJPH.2011.300175. Epub 2011 Aug 18. PubMed PMID: 21852647; PubMed Central PMCID: PMC3174351.
20. Verkhoshansky YV, Siff MC. *Supertraining*. 6th ed. Denver CO: Supertraining International; 2003.
21. Wilmore JH, Costill DL. *Training for Sport and Activity*. 3rd ed. Dubuque, IA: Brown; 1988.
22. Zatsiorsky VM. *Science and Practice of Strength Training*. Champaign, IL: Human Kinetics; 1995.

Chapter 2

1. Baechle TR, Earle RW, eds. *NSCA's Essentials of Strength Training and Conditioning*. 3rd ed. Champaign, IL: Human Kinetics; 2008.
2. Campos GE, Luecke TJ, Wendeln HK, Toma K, Hagerman FC, Murray TF, Ragg KE, Ratamess NA, Kraemer WJ, Staron RS. Muscular adaptations in response to three different resistance-training regimens: Specificity of repetition maximum training zones. *Eur J Appl Physiol*. 2002;88:50-60.
3. Dick FW. *Sports Training Principles*. 5th ed. London: A&C Black; 2007.
4. Durstine JL, Davis PG. Specificity of exercise training and testing. In: Roitman JL, ed. *American College of Sports Medicine Resource Manual for Guidelines for Exercise Testing and Prescription*. 3rd ed. Baltimore: Lippincott Williams & Wilkins; 1998:472-479.
5. Gillam GM. Effects of frequency of weight training on muscle strength enhancement. *J Sports Med Phys Fitness*. 1981;21:432-436.
6. Harre D, ed. *Principles of Sports Training*. Berlin: Sportverlag; 1982.
7. Hartmann J, Tunnemann H. *Fitness and Strength Training*. Berlin: Sportverlag; 1989.
8. O'Shea P. *Scientific Principles and Methods of Strength Fitness*. Reading, MA: Addison-Wesley; 1976.

9. Plisk SS. *Theories, concepts and methodology of speed development as they relate to sports performance.* Presented at the NSCA Certification Commission's Essential Principles of Strength Training and Conditioning Symposium. Phoenix, AZ; 1995 June.

10. Rippetoe M, Kilgore L. *Starting Strength: A Simple and Practical Guide for Coaching Beginners.* Wichita Falls, TX: Aasgaard; 2005.

11. Stone MH, Collins D, Plisk S, Haff G, Stone ME. Training principles: Evaluation of modes and methods of resistance training. *Strength Cond J.* 2000;22(3):65-76.

12. Stone MH, Stone M, Sands WA. *Principles and Practice of Resistance Training.* Champaign, IL: Human Kinetics; 2007.

13. Verkhoshansky YV, Siff MC. *Supertraining.* 6th ed. Denver, CO: Supertraining International; 2003.

14. Weir JP, Cramer JT. Principles of musculoskeletal exercise programming. In: Kaminsky LA, senior ed., Glass S, section ed. *ACSM Resource Manual for Exercise Testing and Prescription.* 5th ed. American College of Sports Medicine. Philadelphia: Lippincott Williams & Wilkins; 2005:350-365.

15. Zatsiorsky VM. *Science and Practice of Strength Training.* Champaign, IL: Human Kinetics; 1995.

Chapter 3

1. American College of Sports Medicine. *ACSM's Health/Fitness Facility Standards and Guidelines.* 2nd ed. Champaign, IL: Human Kinetics; 1997.

2. American College of Sports Medicine. *ACSM's Resource Manual for Guidelines for Exercise Testing and Prescription.* 3rd ed. Baltimore: Lippincott Williams & Wilkins; 1998.

3. American College of Sports Medicine. *ACSM's Guidelines for Exercise Testing and Prescription.* 6th ed. Philadelphia: Lippincott Williams & Wilkins; 2000.

4. Anderson RE. Body composition assessment. In: Cotton RT, ed. *Lifestyle and Weight Management Consultant Manual.* San Diego, CA: American Council on Exercise; 1996:70-92.

5. Baechle TR, Earle RW, eds. *NSCA's Essentials of Strength Training and Conditioning.* 3rd ed. Champaign, IL: Human Kinetics; 2008.

6. Baechle TR, Earle RW, Wathen D. Resistance training. In: Baechle TR, Earle RW, eds. *NSCA's Essentials of Strength Training and Conditioning.* 2nd ed. Champaign, IL: Human Kinetics; 2000:395-425.

7. Baumgartner TA, Jackson AS. *Measurement for Evaluation in Physical Education and Exercise Science.* Boston: McGraw-Hill; 1999.

8. Brzycki M. Strength testing: Predicting a one rep max from reps-to-fatigue. *J Phys Educ Rec Dance.* 1993;64(1):88-90.

9. Caspersen CJ, Heath GW. The risk factor concept of coronary heart disease. In: *ACSM's Resource Manual for Guidelines for Exercise Testing and Prescription.* 2nd ed. Philadelphia: Lea & Febiger; 1993:151-167.

10. Committee on Diet and Health, Food and Nutrition Board, Commission on Life Sciences, National Research Council. *Diet and health: Implications for reducing chronic disease risk.* Washington, DC: National Academy Press; 1989.

11. Cotton RT. Testing and evaluation. In: Cotton RT, ed. *Personal Trainer Manual.* San Diego, CA: American Council on Exercise; 1996:168-205.

12. De Vries HA, Housh TJ. *Physiology of Exercise for Physical Education, Athletics and Exercise Science.* 5th ed. Madison, WI: Brown and Benchmark; 1994.

13. Drought HJ. Personal training: The initial consultation. *Conditioning Instructor.* 1990;1(2):2-3.

14. Durnin JVGA, Womersley J. Body fat assessed from total body density and its estimation from skinfold thickness measurements on 481 men and women aged 16-72 years. *Br J Nutr.* 1974;32:77-97.

15. Esquerre R. *Legal liability issues for personal trainers.* Presentation at the NSCA's Personal Trainer's Clinic. Fort Lauderdale, FL; 2001, May.

16. Franklin BA, Whaley MH, Howley ET, eds. *ACSM's Guidelines for Exercise Testing and Prescription.* 6th ed. Philadelphia: Lippincott Williams & Wilkins; 2000.

17. Golding LA, Myers CR, Sinning WE, eds. *Y's Ways to Physical Fitness: The Complete Guide to Fitness Testing and Instruction.* Champaign, IL: Human Kinetics; 1989.

18. Harman E, Pandorf C. Principles of test selection and administration. In: Baechle TR, ed. *NSCA's Essentials of Strength Training and Conditioning.* Champaign, IL: Human Kinetics; 1994:275-286.

19. Herbert DL. Legal and professional responsibilities of personal training. In: Roberts SO, ed. *The Business of Personal Training.* Champaign, IL: Human Kinetics; 1996:53-63.

20. Howley ET, Franks BD. *Health Fitness Instructor's Handbook.* 3rd ed. Champaign, IL: Human Kinetics; 1997.

21. Johnson B, Nelson J. *Practical Measurements for Evaluation in Physical Education.* 2nd ed. Minneapolis, MN: Burgess; 1974.

22. Kannel WB, Cordon T. *The Framingham Study: An epidemiological investigation of cardiovascular disease.* Section 30. Public Health Service, NIH, DHEW Pub. No. 74-599. Washington, DC: U.S. Government Printing Office; 1974.

23. Kraemer WJ, Fry AC. Strength testing: Development and evaluation of methodology. In: Maud PJ, Foster C, eds. *Physiological Assessment of Human Fitness.* Champaign IL: Human Kinetics; 1995:115-138.

24. Mcinnis KJ, Balady CJ. Higher cardiovascular risk clients in health clubs. *ACSMs Health Fit J.* 1999;3(1):19-24.

25. Morrow JR Jr, Jackson AW, Disch JG, Mood DP. *Measurement and Evaluation in Human Performance.* 4th ed. Champaign, IL: Human Kinetics; 2011.

26. Olds T, Norton K. *Pre-Exercise Health Screening Guide*. Champaign, IL: Human Kinetics; 1999.

27. Prochaska JO, Norcross JC, DiClemente CC. *Changing for Good: A Revolutionary Six-Stage Program for Overcoming Bad Habits and Moving Your Life Positively Forward*. New York: Avon Books; 1994.

28. Rozenek R, Storer TW. Client assessment tools for the personal trainer. *Strength Cond*. 1997;June:52-63.

29. Thomas S, Reading J, Shephard RJ. Revision of the Physical Activity Readiness Questionnaire (PARQ). *Can J Sports Sci*. 1992;17:338-345.

30. U.S. Department of Health and Human Services. *Physical Activity and Health: A Report of the Surgeon General*. Atlanta, GA: U.S. Department of Health and Human Services, Centers for Disease Control and Prevention; 1996.

31. Whaley MA, Kaminsky LA. Epidemiology of physical activity, physical fitness, and selected chronic diseases. In: American College of Sports Medicine, ed. *ACSM's Resource Manual for Guidelines for Exercise Testing and Prescription*. 3rd ed. Baltimore: Lippincott Williams & Wilkins; 1998.

Chapter 4

1. Baechle TR, Earle RW, eds. *NSCA's Essentials of Strength Training and Conditioning*. 3rd ed. Champaign, IL: Human Kinetics; 2008.

2. Gallagher, M. *The Purposeful Primitive: Using the Primordial Laws of Fitness to Trigger Inevitable, Lasting and Dramatic Physical Change*. Dragon Door Publications; 2008.

3. Gould D. Goal setting for peak performance. In: Williams JM, ed. *Applied Sport Psychology: Personal Growth to Peak Performance*. Mountain View, CA: Mayfield; 1998:182-196.

4. Hall HK, Kerr AW. Goal setting in sport and physical activity: Tracing empirical developments and establishing conceptual direction. In: Roberts GC, ed. *Advances in Motivation in Sport and Exercise*. Champaign, IL: Human Kinetics; 2001:183-234.

5. Kyllo LB, Landers DM. Goal setting in sport and exercise: A research synthesis to resolve the controversy. *J Sport Exercise Psy*. 1995;17:117-137.

6. O'Block FR, Evans FH. Goal setting as a motivational technique. In: Silva JM, Weinberg RS, eds. *Psychological Foundations of Sport*. Champaign, IL: Human Kinetics; 1984:188-196.

7. Roberts GC, Treasure DC. Achievement goals, motivation climate and achievement strategies and behaviors in sport. *Int J Sport Psychol*. 1995;26:64-80.

8. Siedentop D, Ramey G. Extrinsic rewards and intrinsic motivation. *Motor Skills: Theory Into Practice*. 1977;2:49-62.

9. Vallerand RJ, Losier GF. An integration analysis of intrinsic and extrinsic motivation in sport. *Journal of Appl Sport Psychol*. 1999;11:142-169.

10. Weinberg RS, Fowler C, Jackson A, Bagnall J, Bruya L. Effect of goal difficulty on motor performance: A replication across tasks and subjects. *J Sport Exerc Psychol*. 1991;13:160-173.

Chapter 5

1. Armstrong CA, Sallis JF, Howell MF, Hofstetter CR. Stages of change, self-efficacy, and the adoption of vigorous exercise: A prospective analysis. *J Sport Exercise Psy*. 1993;15:390-402.

2. Cardinal BJ. The stages of exercise scale and stages of exercise behavior in female adults. *J Sport Med Phys Fit*. 1995;35:87-92.

3. De Vries HA, Housh TJ. *Physiology of Exercise for Physical Education Athletics and Exercise Science*. Madison, WI: Brown; 1994.

4. Deci EL, Ryan RM. *Intrinsic Motivation and Self-Determination in Human Behavior*. New York: Plenum Press; 1985.

5. Duda JL. Relationships between task and ego orientation and the perceived purpose of sport among high school athletes. *J Sport Exercise Psy*. 1989;11:318-335.

6. Feltz DL, Landers DM. The effects of mental practice on motor skill learning and performance: A meta-analysis. *J Sport Psychol*. 1983;5:25-57.

7. Gould D. Goal setting for peak performance. In: Williams JM, ed. *Applied Sport Psychology: Personal Growth to Peak Performance*. Mountain View, CA: Mayfield; 1998:182-196.

8. Hatfield BD, Walford GA. Understanding anxiety: Implications for sport performance. *Nat Strength Cond Assoc J*. 1987;9(2):60-61.

9. Landers DM, Arent SA. Physical activity and mental health. In: Singer RN, Hausenblas HA, Janelle CM, eds. *Handbook of Sport Psychology*. 2nd ed. New York: Wiley; 2001:740-765.

10. Marcus BH, Eaton CA, Rossi JS, Harlow LL. Self-efficacy, decision making, and stages of change: An integrative model of physical exercise. *J Appl Soc Psychol*. 1994;24:489-508.

11. Roberts CC. Understanding the dynamics of motivation in physical activity: The influence of achievement goals on motivational processes. In Roberts GC, ed. *Advances in Motivation in Sport and Exercise*. Champaign, IL: Human Kinetics; 2001:1-50.

12. Siedentop D, Ramey G. Extrinsic rewards and intrinsic motivation. *Motor Skills: Theory Into Practice*. 1977;2:49-62.

13. U.S. Department of Health and Human Services. *Physical Activity and Health: A Report of the Surgeon General*. McLean, VA: International Medical; 1996.

Chapter 6

1. Baechle TR, Earle RW, eds. *NSCA's Essentials of Strength Training and Conditioning*. 3rd ed. Champaign, IL: Human Kinetics; 2008.

2. Bergman RA, Afifi AK. *Atlas of Microscopic Anatomy*. Philadelphia: Saunders; 1974.

3. Durstine JL, Davis PG. Specificity of exercise training and testing. In: Roitman JL, ed. *American College of Sports Medicine Resource Manual for Guidelines for Exercise Testing and Prescription*. 3rd ed. Baltimore: Lippincott Williams & Wilkins;1998:472-479.

4. Gray H. *Gray's Anatomy: The Unabridged Running Press Edition of the American Classic.* Unabridged ed. Philadelphia: Running Press; 1974.

5. Guyton AC, Hall JE. *Textbook of Medical Physiology.* 10th ed. Philadelphia: Saunders; 2000.

6. Johnson MA, Polgar J, Weightman D, Appleton D. Data on the distribution of fiber types in thirty-six human muscles. *J Neural Sci.* 1973;18:111-129.

7. Luttgens K, Hamilton N. *Kinesiology: Scientific Basis of Human Motion.* 9th ed. Dubuque, IA: Brown & Benchmark; 1997.

8. McArdle WD, Katch FI, Katch VI. *Exercise Physiology.* 6th ed. Philadelphia: Lippincott Williams & Wilkins; 2007.

9. McComas AJ. *Skeletal Muscle: Form and Function.* Champaign, IL: Human Kinetics; 1996.

10. McKinley M, O'Loughlin V. *Human Anatomy.* 1st ed. New York: McGraw-Hill Science/Engineering/Math; 2005.

11. Norkin CC, Levangie PK. *Joint Structure and Function: A Comprehensive Analysis.* 2nd ed. Philadelphia: Davis; 1992.

12. Rohen JW, et al. *Color Atlas of Anatomy: A Photographic Study of the Human Body.* 7th ed. Baltimore: Lippincott Williams & Wilkins; 2010.

13. Rosse C, Gaddum-Rosse P. *Hollinshead's Textbook of Anatomy.* 5th ed. Baltimore: Lippincott Williams & Wilkins; 1997.

14. Sieg WK, Adams SP. *Illustrated Essentials of Musculoskeletal Anatomy.* 3rd ed. Gainesville, FL: Megabooks; 1996.

15. Verkhoshansky YV, Siff MC. *Supertraining.* 6th ed. Denver, CO: Supertraining International; 2003.

16. Watkins J. *Structure and Function of the Musculoskeletal System.* Champaign, IL: Human Kinetics; 1999.

Chapter 7

1. Baechle TR, Earle RW, eds. *NSCA's Essentials of Strength Training and Conditioning.* 3rd ed. Champaign, IL: Human Kinetics; 2008.

2. Buller AJ, Eccles JC, Eccles RM. Interaction between motor neurons and muscles in respect of the characteristic speeds of their responses. *J Physiol* (Lond). 1960;150:139-417.

3. Deschenes MR, Covault J, Kraemer WJ, Maresh CM. The neuromuscular junction: Muscle fibre type differences, plasticity and adaptability to increased and decreased activity. *Sports Med.* 1994;17:358-372.

4. Enoka RM. Neural adaptations with chronic physical activity. *J Biomech.* 1997;30:447-455.

5. Enoka RM. *Neuromechanics of Human Movement.* Champaign, IL: Human Kinetics; 2001.

6. Ghez C. The control of movement. In: Kandel E, Schwartz J, Jessel T, eds. *Principles of Neuroscience.* New York: Elsevier Science; 1991.

7. Häkkinen K, Pakarinen A, Kyrolainen H, Cheng S, Kim DH, Komi PV. Neuromuscular adaptations and serum hormones in females during pro-longed power training. *Int J Sports Med.* 1990;11:91-98.

8. Häkkinen K, Pakarinen A, Alen M, Kauhanen H, Komi PV. Relationships between training volume, physical performance capacity, and serum hormone concentrations during prolonged training in elite weight lifters. *Int J Sports Med.* 1987;8:61-65.

9. Häkkinen K, Komi PV, Alen M, Kauhanen H. EMG, muscle fibre and force production characteristics during a one year training period in elite weightlifters. *Eur J Appl Physiol.* 1987;56:419-427.

10. Hellebrandt FA, Parrish AM, Houtz JJ. Cross education: The influence of unilateral exercise on the contralateral limb. *Arch Phy Med.* 1947;28:76-85.

11. Milner-Brown A. *Neuromuscular Physiology.* Thousand Oaks, CA: National Academy of Sports Medicine; 2001.

12. Sale DG. Neural adaptation to strength training. In: Komi PV, ed. *Strength and Power in Sport: The Encyclopedia of Sports Medicine.* Oxford, England: Blackwell Scientific; 1992:249-265.

13. Schmidt RA, Wrisberg CA. *Motor Learning and Performance.* 2nd ed. Champaign, IL: Human Kinetics, 2000.

14. Verkhoshansky YV, Siff MC. *Supertraining.* 6th ed. Denver, CO: Supertraining International; 2003.

15. Zatsiorsky VM. *Science and Practice of Strength Training.* Champaign, IL: Human Kinetics; 1995.

Chapter 8

1. Baechle TR, Earle RW, eds. *NSCA's Essentials of Strength Training and Conditioning.* 3rd ed. Champaign, IL: Human Kinetics; 2008.

2. Barnard RJ, Edgerton VR, Furakawa T, Peter JB. Histochemical, biochemical and contractile properties of red, white and intermediate fibers. *Am J Physiol.* 1971;220:410-411.

3. Brooks GA, Fahey TD, Baldwin KM. *Exercise Physiology: Human Bioenergetics and Its Application.* 4th ed. New York: McGraw-Hill; 2005.

4. Craig BW, Lucas J, Pohlman R, Stelling H. The effects of running, weightlifting and a combination of both on growth hormone release. *J Appl Sport Sci Res.* 1991;5(4):198-203.

5. Creer AR, Ricard MD, Conlee RK, Hoyt GL, Parcell AC. Neural, metabolic, and performance adaptations to four weeks of high intensity sprint-interval training in trained cyclists. *Int J Sports Med.* 2004;25:92-98.

6. Edington OE, Edgerton VR. *The Biology of Physical Activity.* Boston: Houghton Mifflin; 1976.

7. Fleck SJ, Kraemer WJ. *Designing Resistance Training Programs.* 3rd ed. Champaign, IL: Human Kinetics; 2003.

8. Garrett RH, Grisham CM. *Biochemistry.* 2nd ed. Fort Worth, TX: Saunders College; 1999.

9. Gastin PB. Energy system interaction and relative contribution during maximal exercise. *Sports Med.* 2001;31(10):725-741.

10. Hadmann R. The available glycogen in man and the connection between rate of oxygen intake and carbohydrate usage. *Acta Physiol Scand.* 1957;40:305-330.

11. Hirvonen J, Ruhunen S, Rusko H, Harkonen M. Breakdown of high-energy phosphate compounds and lactate accumulation during short submaximal exercise. *Eur J Appl Physiol.* 1987;56:253-259.

12. Hultman E, Sjoholm H. Biochemical causes of fatigue. In: Jones NL, McCartney N, McComas AJ, eds. *Human Muscle Power.* Champaign, IL: Human Kinetics; 1986:215-235.

13. Kindermann W, Simon G, Keul J. The significance of the aerobic-anaerobic transition for the determination of work load intensities during endurance training. *Eur J Appl Physiol.* 1979;42:25-34.

14. Robergs RA, Ghiasvand F, Parker D. Biochemistry of exercise-induced metabolic acidosis. *Am J Physiol Regul Integr Camp Physiol.* 2004;287:R502-R516.

15. Sahlin K, Tonkonogy M, Soderlund K. Energy supply and muscle fatigue in humans. *Acta Physiol Scand.* 1998;162:261-266.

16. Sjodin B, Jacobs I. Onset of blood lactate accumulation and marathon running performance. *Int J Sports Med.* 1981;2:23-26.

17. Tesch PA, Colliander B, Kaiser P. Muscle metabolism during intense, heavy resistance exercise. *Eur J Appl Physiol.* 1986;55:362-366.

18. Verkhoshansky YV, Siff MC. *Supertraining.* 6th ed. Denver, CO: Supertraining International; 2003.

19. Weir JP, Beck TW, Cramer JT, Housh TJ. Is fatigue all in your head? A critical review of the central governor model. *Br J Sports Med.* 2006;40:573-586.

20. Zatsiorsky VM. *Science and Practice of Strength Training.* Champaign, IL: Human Kinetics; 1995.

Chapter 9

1. Baechle TR, Earle RW, eds. *NSCA's Essentials of Strength Training and Conditioning.* 3rd ed. Champaign, IL: Human Kinetics; 2008.

2. Boule NG, Weisnagel SJ, Lakka TA, Tremblay A, Bergman RN, Rankinen T, Leon AS, Skinner JS, Wilmore JH, Rao DC, Bouchard C. Effects of exercise training on glucose homeostasis: The HERITAGE Family Study. *Diabetes Care.* 2005;28:108-114.

3. Clarkson P, Tremblay I. Exercise-induced muscle damage, repair, and adaptation in humans. *J Appl Physiol.* 1988;65(1):1-6.

4. Fahey TD, Rolph R, Moungmee P, Nagel J, Mortar S. Serum testosterone, body composition, and strength of young adults. *Med Sci Sports Exerc.* 1976;8:31-34.

5. Fiorini JR. Hormonal control of muscle growth. *Muscle Nerve.* 1987;10:577-598.

6. Fleck SJ, Kraemer WJ. *Designing Resistance Training Programs.* 3rd ed. Champaign, IL: Human Kinetics; 2003.

7. Fry AC, Kraemer WJ, Ramsey LT. Pituitary-adrenal-gonadal responses to high-intensity resistance exercise overtraining. *J Appl Physiol.* 1998;85(6):2352-2359.

8. Fry AC, Kraemer WJ, van Borselen F, Lynch JM, Marsit JL, Triplett NT, Koziris LP. Catecholamine responses to short term, high intensity resistance exercise overtraining. *J Appl Physiol.* 1994;77(2):941-946.

9. Galbo H. *Hormonal and Metabolic Adaptation to Exercise.* Stuttgart, Germany: Georg Thieme Verlay; 1983.

10. Gotshalk LA, Lobel CC, Nindl BC, Putukian M, Sebastianelli WJ, Newton RU, Häkkinen K, Kraemer WJ. Hormonal responses of multiset versus single-set heavy resistance exercise protocols. *Can J Appl Physiol.* 1997;22(3):244-255.

11. Guezennec Y, Leger L, Lhoste F, Aymonod M, Pesquies PC. Hormone and metabolite response to weight-lifting training sessions. *Int J Sports Med.* 1986;7:100-105.

12. Häkkinen K, Pakarinen A, Kyrolainen H, Cheng S, Kim DH, Komi PV. Neuromuscular adaptations and serum hormones in females during prolonged power training. *Int J Sports Med.* 1990;11:91-98.

13. Kraemer WJ, Fleck SJ, Evans WJ. Strength and power: Physiological mechanisms of adaptation. *Exer Sport Sci Rev.* 1996;24:363-397.

14. Kraemer WJ, Fry AC, Warren BJ, Stone MH, Fleck SJ, Kearney JT, Conroy BP, Maresh CM, Weseman CA, Triplett NT, Gordon SE. Acute hormonal responses in elite junior weightlifters. *Int J Sports Med.* 1992;13(2):103-109.

15. Kraemer WJ, Patton JF, Gordon SE, Harman EA, Deschenes MR, Reynolds K, Newton RU, Triplett NT, Dziados JE. Compatibility of high-intensity strength and endurance training on hormonal and skeletal muscle adaptations. *J Appl Physiol.* 1995;78(3):976-989.

16. Kraemer WJ, Staron RS, Karapondo D, Fry AC, Gordon SE, Volek JS, Nindl B, Gotshalk L, Newton RU, Häkkinen K. The effects of short-term resistance training on endocrine function in men and women. *Eur J Appl Physiol.* 1998;78(1):69-76.

17. Kraemer WJ, Fleck SJ, Dziados JE, Harman EA, Marchitelli LJ, Gordon SE, Mello R, Frykman PN, Koziris LP, Triplett NT. Changes in hormonal concentrations following different heavy resistance exercise protocols in women. *J Appl Physiol.* 1993;75(2):594-604.

18. Okayama T. Factors which regulate growth hormone secretion. *Med J.* 1972;17(1):13-19.

19. Rogol AD. Growth hormone: Physiology, therapeutic use, and potential for abuse. In: Pandolf KB, ed. *Exercise and Sport Sciences Reviews.* Baltimore: Lippincott Williams & Wilkins; 1989:353-377.

20. Tapperman J. *Metabolic and Endocrine Physiology.* Chicago: Year Book Medical; 1980.

21. Verkhoshansky YV, Siff MC. *Supertraining.* 6th ed. Denver, CO: Supertraining International; 2003.

22. Wikkinen K, Pakarinen A, Alen M, Kauhanen H, Komi PV. Neuromuscular and hormonal adaptations in athletes to strength training in two years. *J Appl Physiol.* 1988;65(6):2406-2412.

23. Zatsiorsky VM. *Science and Practice of Strength Training.* Champaign, IL: Human Kinetics; 1995.

Chapter 10

1. Astrand P, Rodahl K, Dahl HA, Stromme SB. *Textbook of Work Physiology.* 4th ed. Champaign, IL: Human Kinetics; 2003.

2. Baechle TR, Earle RW, eds. *NSCA's Essentials of Strength Training and Conditioning.* 3rd ed. Champaign, IL: Human Kinetics; 2008.

3. Challis JH. Muscle-tendon architecture and athletic performance. In: Zatsiorsky VM, ed. *Biomechanics in Sport: Performance Enhancement and Injury Prevention.* London: Blackwell Science; 2000:33-55.

4. Fleck SJ, Kraemer WJ. *Designing Resistance Training Programs.* 3rd ed. Champaign, IL: Human Kinetics; 2003.

5. Garhammer J. Weight lifting and training. In: Vaughn C, ed. *Biomechanics of Sport.* Boca Raton, FL: CRC Press; 1989:169-211.

6. Gowitzke BA, Milner M. *Scientific Bases of Human Movement.* 3rd ed. Baltimore: Lippincott Williams & Wilkins; 1988.

7. Hamill J, Knutzen JM. *Biomechanical Basis of Human Movement.* Baltimore: Lippincott Williams & Wilkins; 1995.

8. Harman EA, Rosenstein RM, Frykman PN, Nigro GA. Effects of a belt on intra-abdominal pressure during weight lifting. *Med Sci Sports Exerc.* 1989;21(2):186-190.

9. Hay JG, Reid JG. *The Anatomical and Mechanical Bases of Human Motion.* Englewood Cliffs, NJ: Prentice Hall; 1982.

10. Knuttgen H, Kraemer W. Terminology and measurement in exercise performance. *J Appl Sport Sci Res.* 1997;(1):1-10.

11. Luttgens K, Hamilton N. *Kinesiology: Scientific Basis of Human Motion.* 9th ed. Dubuque, IA: Brown & Benchmark; 1997.

12. McComas AJ. *Skeletal Muscle: Form and Function.* Champaign, IL: Human Kinetics; 1996.

13. Norkin CC, Levangie PK. *Joint Structure and Function: A Comprehensive Analysis.* 2nd ed. Philadelphia: Davis; 1992.

14. Siff M. Biomechanical foundations of strength and power training. In: Zatsiorsky VM, ed. *Biomechanics in Sport: Performance Enhancement and Injury Prevention.* London: Blackwell Science; 2000:103-139.

15. Stauber WT. Eccentric action of muscles: Physiology, injury, and adaptation. In: Pandolf KB, ed. *Exercise and Sports Sciences Reviews,* vol. 17. Baltimore: Lippincott Williams & Wilkins; 1989:157-185.

16. Verkhoshansky YV, Siff MC. *Supertraining.* 6th ed. Denver, CO: Supertraining International; 2003.

17. Zatsiorsky VM. *Science and Practice of Strength Training.* Champaign, IL: Human Kinetics; 1995.

Chapter 11

1. Bhatia DN, de Beer JF, van Rooyen KS, Lam F, du Toit DF. The "bench-presser's shoulder": An overuse insertional tendinopathy of the pectoralis minor muscle. *Br J Sports Med.* 2007 Aug;41(8):e11. Epub 2006 Nov 30. PubMed PMID: 17138640.

2. Cogley RM, Archambault TA, Fibeger JF, Koverman MM, Youdas JW, Hollman JH. Comparison of muscle activation using various hand positions during the push-up exercise. *J Strength Cond Res.* 2005 Aug;19(3):628-33. PubMed PMID: 16095413.

3. Dark A, Ginn KA, Halaki M. Shoulder muscle recruitment patterns during commonly used rotator cuff exercises: An electromyographic study. *Phys Ther.* 2007 Aug;87(8):1039-46. Epub 2007 Jun 19. PubMed PMID: 17578940.

4. de Oliveira AS, de Morais Carvalho M, de Brum DP. Activation of the shoulder and arm muscles during axial load exercises on a stable base of support and on a medicine ball. *J Electromyogr Kinesiol* 2008; 18:472-479.

5. Delavier, F. *Strength Training Anatomy.* 3rd ed. Champaign, IL: Human Kinetics, 2010.

6. Gentil P, Oliveira E, de Araújo Rocha Júnior V, do Carmo J, Bottaro M. Effects of exercise order on upper-body muscle activation and exercise performance. *J Strength Cond Res.* 2007 Nov;21(4):1082-6. PubMed PMID: 18076251.

7. Gjøvaag TF, Dahl HA. Effect of training with different intensities and volumes on muscle fibre enzyme activity and cross sectional area in the m. Triceps brachii. *Eur J Appl Physiol.* 2008 Jul;103(4):399-409. PubMed PMID: 18351376.

8. Gray H. *Gray's Anatomy: The Unabridged Running Press Edition of the American Classic.* Unabridged ed. Philadelphia: Running Press; 1974.

9. Kolber MJ, Beekhuizen KS, Cheng MS, Hellman MA. Shoulder joint and muscle characteristics in the recreational weight training population. *J Strength Cond Res.* 2009 Jan;23(1):148-57. PubMed PMID: 19077737.

10. McKinley M, O'Loughlin V. *Human Anatomy.* 1st ed. New York: McGraw-Hill Science/Engineering/Math; 2005.

11. Newton RU, Kraemer WJ, Häkkinen K, Humphries BJ, Murphy AJ. Kinematics, kinetics and muscle activation during explosive upper body movements. *J Appl Biomech.* 1996;12:31-43.

12. Patton KT, Thibodeau GA. *Anatomy & Physiology.* 6th ed. St. Louis, MO: Mosby; 2006.

13. Rohen JW, et al. *Color Atlas of Anatomy: A Photographic Study of the Human Body.* 7th ed. Baltimore: Lippincott Williams & Wilkins; 2010.

14. Saeterbakken AH, van den Tillaar R, Fimland MS. A comparison of muscle activity and 1-RM strength of three chest-press exercises with different stability requirements. *J Sports Sci.* 2011 Mar;29(5):533-8. PubMed PMID: 21225489.

15. Sieg, WK, Adams SP. *Illustrated Essentials of Musculoskeletal Anatomy.* 3rd ed. Gainesville, FL: Megabooks; 1996.

16. Youdas JW, Amundson CL, Cicero KS, Hahn JJ, Harezlak DT, Hollman JH. Surface electromyographic activation patterns and elbow joint motion during a pull-up, chin-up, or perfect-pull-up rotational exercise. *J Strength Cond Res.* 2010 Dec;24(12):3404-14. PubMed PMID: 21068680.

Chapter 12

1. Augustsson J, Thomeé R, Hörnstedt P, Lindblom J, Karlsson J, Grimby G. Effect of pre-exhaustion exercise on lower-extremity muscle activation during a leg press exercise. *J Strength Cond Res.* 2003 May;17(2):411-6. PubMed PMID: 12741886.

2. Ayotte NW, Stetts DM, Keenan G, Greenway EH. Electromyographical analysis of selected lower extremity muscles during 5 unilateral weight-bearing exercises. *J Orthop Sports Phys Ther.* 2007 Feb;37(2):48-55. PubMed PMID: 17366959.

3. Boudreau SN, Dwyer MK, Mattacola CG, Lattermann C, Uhl TL, McKeon JM. Hip-muscle activation during the lunge, single-leg squat, and step-up-and-over exercises. *J Sport Rehabil.* 2009 Feb;18(1):91-103. PubMed PMID: 19321909.

4. Caterisano A, Moss RF, Pellinger TK, Woodruff K, Lewis VC, Booth W, Khadra T. The effect of back squat depth on the EMG activity of 4 superficial hip and thigh muscles. *J Strength Cond Res.* 2002 Aug;16(3):428-32. PubMed PMID: 12173958.

5. Clark BC, Manini TM, Mayer JM, Ploutz-Snyder LL, Graves JE. Electromyographic activity of the lumbar and hip extensors during dynamic trunk extension exercise. *Arch Phys Med Rehabil.* 2002 Nov;83(11):1547-52. PubMed PMID: 12422323.

6. Crossley KM, Zhang WJ, Schache AG, Bryant A, Cowan SM. Performance on the single-leg squat task indicates hip abductor muscle function. *Am J Sports Med.* 2011 Apr;39(4):866-73. Epub 2011 Feb 18. PubMed PMID: 21335344.

7. Delavier, F. *Strength Training Anatomy.* 3rd ed. Champaign, IL: Human Kinetics; 2010.

8. Ebben WP, Feldmann CR, Dayne A, Mitsche D, Alexander P, Knetzger KJ. Muscle activation during lower body resistance training. *Int J Sports Med.* 2009 Jan;30(1):1-8. Epub 2008 Oct 30. PubMed PMID: 18975260.

9. Escamilla RF, Francisco AC, Kayes AV, Speer KP, Moorman CT 3rd. An electromyographic analysis of sumo and conventional style deadlifts. *Med Sci Sports Exerc.* 2002 Apr;34(4):682-8. PubMed PMID: 11932579.

10. Felício LR, Dias LA, Silva AP, Oliveira AS, Bevilaqua-Grossi D. Muscular activity of patella and hip stabilizers of healthy subjects during squat exercises. *Rev Bras Fisioter.* 2011 May-Jun;15(3):206-11. English, Portuguese. PubMed PMID: 21829984.

11. Gray H. *Gray's Anatomy: The Unabridged Running Press Edition of the American Classic.* Unabridged ed. Philadelphia: Running Press; 1974.

12. Hassani A, Patikas D, Bassa E, Hatzikotoulas K, Kellis E, Kotzamanidis C. Agonist and antagonist muscle activation during maximal and submaximal isokinetic fatigue tests of the knee extensors. *J Electromyogr Kinesiol.* 2006 Dec;16(6):661-8. Epub 2006 Jan 24. PubMed PMID: 16434213.

13. Helgerud J, Wang E, Mosti MP, Wiggen ØN, Hoff J. Plantar flexion training primes peripheral arterial disease patients for improvements in cardiac function. *Eur J Appl Physiol.* 2009 May;106(2):207-15. Epub 2009 Feb 24. PubMed PMID: 19238425.

14. Hudelmaier M, Wirth W, Himmer M, Ring-Dimitriou S, Sänger A, Eckstein F. Effect of exercise intervention on thigh muscle volume and anatomical cross-sectional areas—quantitative assessment using MRI. *Magn Reson Med.* 2010 Dec;64(6):1713-20. doi: 10.1002/mrm.22550. Epub 2010 Jul 27. PubMed PMID: 20665894.

15. Kellis E, Galanis N, Natsis K, Kapetanos G. Validity of architectural properties of the hamstring muscles: Correlation of ultrasound findings with cadaveric dissection. *J Biomech.* 2009 Nov 13;42(15):2549-54. Epub 2009 Jul 31. PubMed PMID: 19646698.

16. Marieb EN, Hoehn KN. *Human Anatomy & Physiology With Mastering A&P.* 8th ed. San Francisco: Benjamin Cummings; 2010.

17. McKinley M, O'Loughlin V. *Human Anatomy.* 1st ed. New York: McGraw-Hill Science/Engineering/Math; 2005.

18. Pandy MG, Andriacchi TP. Muscle and joint function in human locomotion. *Annu Rev Biomed Eng.* 2010 Aug 15;12:401-33. Review. PubMed PMID: 20617942.

19. Paoli A, Marcolin G, Petrone N. The effect of stance width on the electromyographical activity of eight superficial thigh muscles during back squat with different bar loads. *J Strength Cond Res.* 2009 Jan;23(1):246-50. PubMed PMID: 19130646.

20. Patton KT, Thibodeau GA. *Anatomy & Physiology.* 6th ed. St. Louis, MO: Mosby; 2006.

21. Rohen JW, et al. *Color Atlas of Anatomy: A Photographic Study of the Human Body.* 7th ed. Baltimore: Lippincott Williams & Wilkins; 2010.

22. Rosse C, Gaddum-Rosse P. *Hollinshead's Textbook of Anatomy.* 5th ed. Baltimore: Lippincott Williams & Wilkins; 1997.

23. Sieg WK, Adams SP. *Illustrated Essentials of Musculoskeletal Anatomy.* 3rd ed. Gainesville, FL: Megabooks; 1996.

Chapter 13

1. Axler CT, McGill SM. Low back loads over a variety of abdominal exercises: Searching for the safest abdominal challenge. *Med Sci Sports Exerc.* 1997 Jun;29(6):804-11. PubMed PMID: 9219209.

2. Behm DG, Leonard AM, Young WB, Bonsey WA, MacKinnon SN. Trunk muscle electromyographic activity with unstable and unilateral exercises. *J Strength Cond Res.* 2005 Feb;19(1):193-201. PubMed PMID: 15705034.

3. Beim G, Giraldo JL, Pincivero DM, Borror MJ, Fu FH. Abdominal strengthening exercises: A comparative EMG study. *J Sports Rehab.* 1997;6:11-20.

4. Bittenham D, Brittenham G. *Stronger Abs and Back.* Champaign, IL: Human Kinetics; 1997.

5. Brown SH, Ward SR, Cook MS, Lieber RL. Architectural analysis of human abdominal wall muscles: Implications for mechanical function. *Spine.* 2011 Mar 1;36(5):355-62.

6. Chek P. *Scientific Abdominal Training. Correspondence Course.* La Jolla, CA: Paul Chek Seminars; 1992.

7. Delavier, F. *Strength Training Anatomy.* 3rd ed. Champaign, IL: Human Kinetics; 2010.

8. Drake JD, Fischer SL, Brown SH, Callaghan JP. Do exercise balls provide a training advantage for trunk extensor exercises? A biomechanical evaluation. *J Manipulative Physiol Ther.* 2006 Jun;29(5):354-62. PubMed PMID: 16762662.

9. Duncan M. Muscle activity of the upper and lower rectus abdominis during exercises performed on and off a Swiss ball. *J Body Mov Ther.* 2009 Oct;13(4):364-7. Epub 2009 Feb 26. PubMed PMID: 19761961.

10. Ekstrom RA, Donatelli RA, Carp KC. Electromyographic analysis of core trunk, hip, and thigh muscles during 9 rehabilitation exercises. *J Orthop Sports Phys Ther.* 2007 Dec;37(12):754-62. Epub 2007 Aug 29. PubMed PMID: 18560185.

11. Gray H. *Gray's Anatomy: The Unabridged Running Press Edition of the American Classic.* Unabridged ed. Philadelphia: Running Press; 1974.

12. Hamlyn N, Behm DG, Young WB. Trunk muscle activation during dynamic weight-training exercises and isometric instability activities. *J Strength Cond Res.* 2007 Nov;21(4):1108-12. PubMed PMID: 18076231.

13. Imai A, Kaneoka K, Okubo Y, Shiina I, Tatsumura M, Izumi S, Shiraki H. Trunk muscle activity during lumbar stabilization exercises on both a stable and unstable surface. *J Orthop Sports Phys Ther.* 2010 Jun;40(6):369-75. PubMed PMID: 20511695.

14. Kohler JM, Flanagan SP, Whiting WC. Muscle activation patterns while lifting stable and unstable loads on stable and unstable surfaces. *J Strength Cond Res.* 2010 Feb;24(2):313-21. PubMed PMID: 20072068.

15. Konrad P, Schmitz K, Denner A. Neuromuscular evaluation of trunk-training exercises. *J Athl Train.* 2001 Jun;36(2):109-118. PubMed PMID: 12937449; PubMed Central PMCID: PMC155519.

16. Lehman GJ, McGill SM. Quantification of the differences in electromyographic activity magnitude between the upper and lower portions of the rectus abdominis muscle during selected trunk exercises. *Phys Ther.* 2001 May;81(5):1096-101. PubMed PMID: 11319934.

17. Marieb EN, Hoehn KN. *Human Anatomy & Physiology With Mastering A&P.* 8th ed. San Francisco: Benjamin Cummings; 2010.

18. Marshall PW, Desai I. Electromyographic analysis of upper body, lower body, and abdominal muscles during advanced Swiss ball exercises. *J Strength Cond Res.* 2010 Jun;24(6):1537-45. PubMed PMID: 20508456.

19. McKinley M, O'Loughlin V. *Human Anatomy.* 1st ed. New York: McGraw-Hill Science/Engineering/Math; 2005.

20. Patton KT, Thibodeau GA. *Anatomy & Physiology.* 6th ed. St. Louis, MO: Mosby. 2006.

21. Richardson CA, Jull G, Toppenberg R, Comerford M. Techniques for active lumbar stabilization for spinal protection. *Austr J Physiother.* 1992;38:105-112.

22. Rohen, JW, et al. *Color Atlas of Anatomy: A Photographic Study of the Human Body.* 7th ed. Baltimore: Lippincott Williams & Wilkins; 2010.

23. Rosse C, Gaddum-Rosse P. *Hollinshead's Textbook of Anatomy.* 5th ed. Baltimore: Lippincott Williams & Wilkins; 1997.

24. Saeterbakken AH, Fimland MS. Muscle activity of the core during bilateral, unilateral, seated and standing resistance exercise. *Eur J Appl Physiol.* 2012;112(5):1671. PubMed PMID: 21877146.

25. Sieg WK, Adams SP. *Illustrated Essentials of Musculoskeletal Anatomy.* 3rd ed. Gainesville, FL: Megabooks; 1996.

26. Styf J. Pressure in the erector spinae muscle during exercise. *Spine.* 1987 Sep;12(7):675-9. PubMed PMID: 3686219.

27. Vera-Garcia FJ, Grenier SG, McGill SM. Abdominal muscle response during curl-ups on both stable and labile surfaces. *Phys Ther.* 2000 Jun;80(6):564-9. PubMed PMID: 10842409.

28. Workman JC, Docherty D, Parfrey KC, Behm DG. Influence of pelvis position on the activation of abdominal and hip flexor muscles. *J Strength Cond Res.* 2008 Sep;22(5):1563-9. PubMed PMID: 18714231.

Chapter 14

1. Ascherio A, Willett WC. Health effects of trans fatty acids. *Am J Clin Nutr.* 1997;66(4 Suppl):1006S-1010S.

2. Baechle TR, Earle RW, eds. *NSCA's Essentials of Strength Training and Conditioning*. 3rd ed. Champaign, IL: Human Kinetics; 2008.

3. Below PR, Mora-Rodriguez R, Gonzalez-Alonso J, Coyle EF. Fluid and carbohydrate ingestion independently improve performance during 1 h of intense exercise. *Med Sci Sports Exerc*. 1995;27:200-210.

4. Berdanier CD. *Advanced Nutrition: Macronutrients*. Boca Raton, FL: CRC Press; 1995.

5. Binkoski AE, et al. Balance of unsaturated fatty acids is important to a cholesterol-lowering diet: Comparison of mid-oleic sunflower oil and olive oil on cardiovascular disease factors. *J Am Diet Assoc*. 2005;105(7):1080.

6. Brown RC, Cox CM. Effects of high fat versus high carbohydrate diets on plasma lipids and lipoproteins in endurance athletes. *Med Sci Sports Exerc*. 1998;30:1677-1683.

7. Burke LM, Collier GR, Davis PG, Fricker PA, Sanigorski AJ, Hargreaves M. Muscle glycogen storage after prolonged exercise: Effect of the frequency of carbohydrate feedings. *Am J Clin Nutr*. 1996;64:115-119.

8. Clark N. *Nancy Clark's Sports Nutrition Guidebook*. 4th ed. Champaign, IL: Human Kinetics; 2008.

9. Dreon DM, Fernstrom HA, Williams PT, Krauss RM. A very-low-fat diet is not associated with improved lipoprotein profiles in men with a predominance of large, low-density lipoproteins. *Am J Clin Nutr*. 1999;69:411-418.

10. Ernst ND, Obarzanek E, Clark MB, Briefel RR, Brown CD, Donato K. Cardiovascular health risks related to overweight. *J Am Diet Assoc*. 1997;97(7 Suppl):S47-S51.

11. Food and Nutrition Board, Institute of Medicine. *Dietary Reference Intakes for Energy, Carbohydrate, Fiber, Fat, Fatty Acids, Cholesterol, Protein, and Amino Acids*. Washington, DC: National Academies Press; 2002.

12. Gastelu D, Hatfield F. *Dynamic Nutrition for Maximum Performance: A Complete Nutritional Guide for Peak Sports Performance*. Garden City Park, NY: Avery; 1997.

13. Jacobs KA, Sherman WM. The efficacy of carbohydrate supplementation and chronic high-carbohydrate diets for improving endurance performance. *Int J Sport Nutr*. 1999;9(1)92-115.

14. Jeukendrup A, Gleeson M. *Sport Nutrition: An Introduction to Energy Production and Performance*. 2nd ed. Champaign, IL: Human Kinetics; 2010.

15. Leddy J, Horvath P, Rowland J, Pendergast D. Effect of a high or a low fat diet on cardiovascular risk factors in male and female runners. *Med Sci Sports Exerc*. 1997;29:17-25.

16. Lemon PWR. Effects of exercise on dietary protein requirements. *Int J Sport Nutr*. 1998; 8:426-447.

17. MacDougall CR, Ward DC, Sale DC, Sutton JR. Muscle glycogen repletion after high intensity intermittent exercise. *J Appl Physiol*. 1977;42:129-132.

18. National Research Council. *Recommended Dietary Allowances*. 10th ed. Washington, DC: National Academy Press; 1989.

19. Nix S. *Williams' Basic Nutrition & Diet Therapy*. 13th ed. St. Louis, MO: Mosby/ Elsevier; 2009.

20. Price WA. *Nutrition and Physical Degeneration*. 6th ed. New Canaan, CT: Keats; 2003.

21. Sherman WM. Metabolism of sugars and physical performance. *Am J Clin Nutr*. 1995;62(Suppl):228S-241S.

22. Sherman WM, Doyle JA, Lamb DR, Strauss RH. Dietary carbohydrate, muscle glycogen, and exercise performance during 7 d of training. *Am J Clin Nutr*. 1993;57:27-31.

23. Starr B. *The Strongest Shall Survive: Strength Training for Football*. 1st ed. Washington, DC: Fitness Products; 1978.

24. Tarnopolsky MA, Atkinson SA, MacDougall JD, Chesley A, Phillips S, Schwarcz HP. Evaluation of protein requirements for trained strength athletes. *J Appl Physiol*. 1992;73(5):1986-1989.

25. Tato F. Trans-fatty acids in the diet: A coronary risk factor? *Eur J Med Res*. 1995;1(2):118-122.

26. U.S. Department of Health and Human Services. *Healthy People 2010: Understanding and Improving Health*. Washington, DC: U.S. Government Printing Office; 2000.

27. Verkhoshansky YV, Siff MC. *Supertraining*. 6th ed. Denver, CO: Supertraining International; 2003.

28. Wardlaw GM, Insel PM. *Perspectives in Nutrition*. St. Louis: Mosby Year Book; 1996:76.

Chapter 15

1. American College of Sports Medicine. Position stand. Exercise and fluid replacement. *Med Sci Sports Exerc*. 1996;28:i-vii.

2. American Dietetic Association. Position of the American Dietetic Association: Fortification and nutritional supplements, *J Am Diet Assoc*. 2005;105(8):1300-11.

3. Baechle TR, Earle RW, eds. *NSCA's Essentials of Strength Training and Conditioning*. 3rd ed. Champaign, IL: Human Kinetics; 2008.

4. Berning JR, Steen SN. *Nutrition for Sport and Exercise*. Gaithersburg, MD: Aspen; 1998.

5. Clark N. *Nancy Clark's Sports Nutrition Guidebook*. 4th ed. Champaign, IL: Human Kinetics; 2008.

6. Gastelu D, Hatfield F. *Dynamic Nutrition for Maximum Performance: A Complete Nutritional Guide for Peak Sports Performance*. Garden City Park, NY: Avery; 1997.

7. Greenleaf JE, Harrison MH. Water and electrolytes. In: Layman OK, ed. *Nutrition and Aerobic Exercise*. Washington, DC: American Chemical Society; 1986:107-124.

8. Groff JL, Gropper SS, Hunt SM. *Advanced Nutrition and Human Metabolism*. St. Paul, MN: West; 1995.

9. Jeukendrup A, Gleeson M. *Sport Nutrition: An Introduction to Energy Production and Performance*. 2nd ed. Champaign, IL: Human Kinetics; 2010.

10. Maughan RJ, Leiper JB, Shirreffs SM. Restoration of fluid balance after exercise-induced dehydration: Effects of food and fluid intake. *Eur J Appl Physiol*. 1996;73:317-325.

11. Maughan RJ, Owen JH, Shirreffs SM, Leiper JB. Post-exercise rehydration in man: Effects of electrolyte addition to ingested fluids. *Eur J Appl Physiol*. 1994;69:209-215.

12. McArdle WD, Katch FI, Katch VL. *Sports and Exercise Nutrition*. Baltimore: Lippincott Williams & Wilkins; 1999.

13. Nix S. *Williams' Basic Nutrition & Diet Therapy*. 13th ed. St. Louis, MO: Mosby/ Elsevier; 2009.

14. Penniston KL, Tanumihardjo SA. Vitamin A in dietary supplements and fortified foods: Too much of a good thing? *J Am Diet Assoc*. 2003;103:1185-7.

15. Price, WA. *Nutrition and Physical Degeneration*. 6th ed. New Canaan, CT: Keats; 2003.

16. Sizer FS, Whitney EN. *Nutrition Concepts and Controversies*. 9th ed. Belmont, CA: Wadsworth Thomson Learning; 2002.

17. Starr B. *The Strongest Shall Survive: Strength Training for Football*. 1st ed. Washington, DC: Fitness Products; 1978.

Chapter 16

1. American College of Sports Medicine, American Dietetic Association, Dietitians of Canada. Joint position statement: Nutrition and athletic performance. *Med Sci Sports Exerc*. 2000;32(12):2130.

2. American College of Sports Medicine. Position stand: The recommended quantity and quality of exercise for developing and maintaining cardiorespiratory and muscular fitness, and flexibility in healthy adults. *Med Sci Sports Exerc*. 1998;30:975-91.

3. American Dietetic Association. Position of the American Dietetic Association: Nutrition intervention in the treatment of anorexia nervosa, bulimia nervosa, and other eating disorders. *J Am Diet Assoc*. 2006;106:2073-82.

4. Baechle TR, Earle RW, eds. *NSCA's Essentials of Strength Training and Conditioning*. 3rd ed. Champaign, IL: Human Kinetics; 2008.

5. Buemann B, Tremblay A. Effects of exercise training on abdominal obesity and related metabolic complications. *Sports Med*. 1996;21(3):191-212.

6. Clark N. *Nancy Clark's Sports Nutrition Guidebook*. 4th ed. Champaign, IL: Human Kinetics; 2008.

7. Coyle EF, Hagberg JM, Hurley BF, Martin WH, Ehsani AA, Holloszy JO. Carbohydrate feeding during prolonged strenuous exercise can delay fatigue. *J Appl Physiol*. 1983;55(1 Pt 1):230-235.

8. Flegal KM, Carroll MD, Kuczmarski RJ, Johnson CL. Overweight and obesity in the United States: Prevalence and trends, 1960-1994. *Int J Obes Relat Metab Disord*. 1998;22(1):39-47.

9. Gallagher M. *The Purposeful Primitive: Using the Primordial Laws of Fitness to Trigger Inevitable, Lasting and Dramatic Physical Change*. Dragon Door Publications; 2008.

10. Gastelu D, Hatfield F. *Dynamic Nutrition for Maximum Performance: A Complete Nutritional Guide for Peak Sports Performance*. Garden City Park, NY: Avery; 1997.

11. Hansen J. *Natural Bodybuilding*. Champaign, IL: Human Kinetics; 2005.

12. Hofmekler O. *The Warrior Diet: Switch on Your Biological Powerhouse for High Energy, Explosive Strength, and a Leaner, Harder Body*. 2nd ed. Berkeley, CA: Blue Snake Books; 2007.

13. Jeukendrup A, Gleeson M. *Sport Nutrition: An Introduction to Energy Production and Performance*. 2nd ed. Champaign, IL: Human Kinetics; 2010.

14. Karlsson J, Saltin B. Diet, muscle glycogen, and endurance performance. *J Appl Physiol*. 1971;31:203-206.

15. Lemon PW, Mullin JP. Effect of initial muscle glycogen levels on protein catabolism during exercise. *J Appl Physiol*. 1980;48(4):624-629.

16. Nix S. *Williams' Basic Nutrition & Diet Therapy*. 13th ed. St. Louis, MO: Mosby/ Elsevier; 2009.

17. Pollan M. *The Omnivore's Dilemma: A Natural History of Four Meals*. New York: Penguin Press; 2006.

18. Price WA. *Nutrition and Physical Degeneration*. 6th ed. New Canaan, CT: Keats; 2003.

19. Schlosser E. *Fast Food Nation*. New York: Harper Perennial; 2005.

20. Sears B, Lawren B. *The Zone: A Dietary Road Map*. 1st ed. New York: Regan Books; 1995.

21. Sizer FS, Whitney EN. *Nutrition Concepts and Controversies*. 9th ed. Belmont, CA: Wadsworth Thomson Learning; 2002.

22. Spruce N. Plateaus and energy expenditure. Increased difficulty in attending fat or weight loss goals in healthy subjects. *J Natl Intramural Recreat Sports Assoc*. 1997;22(1):24-28.

23. Starr B. *The Strongest Shall Survive: Strength Training for Football*. 1st ed. Washington, DC: Fitness Products; 1978.

24. Tarnopolsky MA, Atkinson SA, MacDougall JD, Chesley A, Phillip S, Schwarcz HP. Evaluation of protein requirements for trained strength athletes. *J Appl Physiol*. 1992;73(5):1986-1995.

25. The Apex Fitness Group. *Apex Training System: Nutritional Guidelines for Altering Body Composition*.

26. U.S. Department of Health and Human Services. *Physical Activity and Health: A Report of the Surgeon General*. Atlanta, GA: Centers for Disease Control and Prevention; 1996.

27. Vereeke West R. The female athlete. The triad of disordered eating, amenorrhea and osteoporosis. *Sports Med*. 1998;26(2):63-71.

28. Verkhoshansky YV, Siff MC. *Supertraining*. 6th ed. Denver, CO: Supertraining International; 2003.

29. Volek JS, Houseknecht K, Kraemer WJ. Nutritional strategies to enhance performance of high-intensity exercise. *Strength Cond*. 1997;19:11-17.

30. Walberg JL, Leidy MK, Sturgill DJ, Hinkle DE, Ritchey SJ, Sebolt DR. Macronutrient needs in weight lifters during caloric restriction. *Med Sci Sports Exerc.* 1987;19:S70.

31. Wang Z, et al. Resting energy expenditure-fat-free mass relationship: New insights provided by body composition modeling, *Am J Physiol Endocrinol Metab.* 2000;279(3):E539-E545.

32. Zatsiorsky VM. *Science and Practice of Strength Training.* Champaign, IL: Human Kinetics; 1995.

Chapter 17

1. American College of Sports Medicine. *ACSM's Guidelines for Exercise Testing and Prescription.* 5th ed. Philadelphia: Lippincott Williams & Wilkins; 1995.

2. Arnold MD, Mayhew JL, LeSuer D, McCormick J. Accuracy of predicting bench press and squat performance from repetition: at low and high intensity. *J Strength Cond Res.* 1995;9:205-206. [Abstract].

3. Baechle TR, Earle RW. *Fitness Weight Training.* Champaign, IL: Human Kinetics; 1995.

4. Baechle TR, Earle RW, eds. *NSCA's Essentials of Strength Training and Conditioning.* 3rd ed. Champaign, IL: Human Kinetics; 2008.

5. Baechle TR, Earle RW. *Weight Training: Steps to Success.* 3rd ed. Champaign, IL: Human Kinetics; 2006.

6. Berger RA. Strength improvement. *Strength Health.* 1972, August.

7. Bompa TO. *Periodization of Strength: The New Wave in Strength Training.* Toronto: Verita; 1993.

8. Bompa TO. *Theory and Methodology of Training.* Dubuque, IA: Kendall/Hunt; 1983.

9. Brzycki M. Accent on intensity. *Scholastic Coach.* 1988;97:82-83.

10. Chu DA. Plyometrics: The link between strength and speed. *Nat Strength Cond Assoc J.* 1983;5(2):20-21.

11. DeLorme TL. Restoration of muscle power by heavy resistance exercises. *J Bone Joint Surg.* 1945;27:645.

12. Earle RW. Weight training exercise prescription. In: *Essentials of Personal Training Symposium Workbook.* Lincoln, NE: NSCA Certification Commission; 2006.

13. Enoka RM. Muscle strength and its development. New perspectives. *Sports Med.* 1988;6:146-168.

14. Fleck SJ, Kraemer WJ. *Designing Resistance Training Programs.* 2nd ed. Champaign, IL: Human Kinetics; 1997.

15. Fleck SJ. Periodized strength training: A critical review. *J Strength Cond Res.* 1999;13(1):82-89.

16. Garhammer J. A review of power output studies of Olympic and powerlifting: Methodology, performance prediction and evaluation tests. *J Strength Cond Res.* 1993;7(2):76-89.

17. Garhammer J. Weight lifting and training. In: Vaughan CL, ed. *Biomechanics of Sport,* Boca Raton, FL: CRC Press; 1989:169-211.

18. Häkkinen K, Pakarinen A, Alen M, et al. Relationships between training volume, physical performance capacity, and serum hormone concentrations during prolonged training in elite weight lifters. *Int J Sports Med.* 1987;8(Suppl):61-65.

19. Hedrick A. Training for hypertrophy. *Strength Cond J.* 1995;17(3):22-29.

20. Henneman E. Relation between size of motor neurons and their susceptibility to discharge. *Science.* 1957;126:1345-1347.

21. Hoeger W, Barette SL, Hale DF, Hopkins DR. Relationship between repetitions and selected percentages of one repetition maximum. *J Appl Sport Sci Res.* 1987;1(1):11-13.

22. Jones A. *Nautilus Training Principles.* Bulletin No. 2. Deland, FL: Nautilus; 1971.

23. Kraemer WJ. A series of studies: The physiological basis for strength training in American football: Fact over philosophy. *J Strength Cond Res.* 1997;11(3):131-142.

24. Newton RU, Kraemer WJ. Developing explosive muscular power: Implications for a mixed methods training strategy. *Nat Strength Cond Assoc J.* 1994;16:(5):20-31.

25. O'Shea P. Throwing speed. *Sports Fitness.* 1985;August:66-67,89-90.

26. Pauletto B. Sets and repetitions. *Nat Strength Cond Assoc J.* 1985;7(6):67-69.

27. Poliquin C. Five steps to increasing the effectiveness of your strength training program. *Nat Strength Cond Assoc J.* 1998;10:34-39.

28. Rippetoe M, Kilgore L. *Starting Strength: A Simple and Practical Guide for Coaching Beginners.* Wichita Falls, TX: Aasgaard; 2005.

29. Rippetoe M, Kilgore L, Pendlay G. *Practical Programming for Strength Training.* Wichita Falls, TX: Aasgaard; 2006.

30. Santa Maria DL, Grzybinski P, Hatfield B. Power as a function of load for a supine bench press exercise. *Nat Strength Cond Assoc J.* 1984;6(6):58.

31. Siff MC, Verkhoshansky Y. *Supertraining.* Escondido, CA: Sports Training; 1994.

32. Simmons L. Training by percents. *Powerlifting USA.* 1988;12(2):21.

33. Starr B. *The Strongest Shall Survive: Strength Training for Football.* 1st ed. Washington, DC: Fitness Products; 1978.

34. Stone MH, Keith R, Kearney JT, Wilson GD, Fleck SJ. Overtraining: A review of the signs and symptoms of overtraining. *J Appl Sport Sci Res.* 1991;5:35-50.

35. Tesch PA. Training for bodybuilding. In: Komi PV, ed. *Strength and Power in Sport: The Encyclopedia of Sports Medicine.* London: Blackwell Scientific; 1993.

36. Verhoshansky Y. *Fundamentals of Special Strength Training in Sport.* Livonia, MI: Sportivny Press; 1976.

37. Verkhoshansky YV, Siff MC. *Supertraining.* 6th ed. Denver, CO: Supertraining International; 2003.

38. Zatsiorsky VM. *Science and Practice of Strength Training*. Champaign, IL: Human Kinetics; 1995.

Chapter 18

1. Baechle TR, Earle RW, eds. *NSCA's Essentials of Strength Training and Conditioning*. 3rd ed. Champaign, IL: Human Kinetics; 2008.
2. Bellew JW, Yates JW, Gater DR. The initial effects of low-volume strength training on balance in untrained older men and women. *J Strength Cond Res*. 2003;17(1):121-128.
3. Cullinen K, Caldwell M. Weight training increases fat-free mass and strength in untrained young women. *J Amer Diet Assoc*. 1998;98(4):414-418.
4. Delavier F. *Strength Training Anatomy*. 3rd ed. Champaign, IL: Human Kinetics; 2010.
5. Fenstermacher S. *ACSM's Resources for the Personal Trainer*. 3rd ed. Philadelphia: Lippincott Williams & Wilkins; 2010.
6. Hunter G, Wetzstein C, Fields D, Brown A, Bamman M. Resistance training increases total energy expenditure and free-living physical activity in older adults. *J Appl Physiol*. 2000;89:977-984.
7. Hurley B. Does strength training improve health status? *Strength Cond*. 1994;16:7-13.
8. Kinakin K. *Optimal Muscle Training*. Champaign, IL: Human Kinetics; 2009.
9. Potvin AN. *Dumbbell Handbook: The Quick Reference Guide to Dumbbell Exercises*. Jespersen M, ed. Blaine, WA: Productive Fitness; 2005.
10. Potvin AN. *The Great Body Ball Handbook*. Jespersen M, ed. Blaine, WA: Productive Fitness; 2007.
11. Potvin AN. *The Great Stretch Tubing Handbook*. Jespersen M, ed. Blaine, WA: Productive Fitness; 2007.
12. Rippetoe M, Kilgore L. *Starting Strength: A Simple and Practical Guide for Coaching Beginners*. Wichita Falls, TX: Aasgaard; 2005.
13. Stone M, Blessing D, Byrd R, Tew J, Boatwright D. Physiological effects of a short term resistance training program on middle-aged untrained men. *Nat Strength Cond Assoc J*. 1982;4:16-20.
14. Thompson WR, et al., eds. *ACSM's Guidelines for Exercise Testing and Prescription*. 8th ed. Philadelphia: Lippincott Williams & Wilkins; 2010.
15. Verkhoshansky YV, Siff MC. *Supertraining*. 6th ed. Denver, CO: Supertraining International; 2003.
16. Waterbury C. *Muscle Revolution: The High-Performance System for Building a Bigger, Stronger, Leaner Body*. Chad Waterbury; 2006.
17. Zatsiorsky VM. *Science and Practice of Strength Training*. Champaign, IL: Human Kinetics; 1995.

Chapter 19

1. Adams K, O'Shea JP, O'Shea KL, Climstein M. The effect of six weeks of squat, plyometric and squat-plyometric training power production. *J Appl Sports Sci Res*. 1992;6:36-41.
2. Baechle TR, Earle RW, eds. *NSCA's Essentials of Strength Training and Conditioning*. 3rd ed. Champaign, IL: Human Kinetics; 2008.
3. Baechle TR, Earle RW. *Weight Training: Steps to Success*. 3rd ed. Champaign, IL: Human Kinetics; 2006.
4. Bonato P, Cheng MS, Gonzalez-Cueto J, Leardini A, O'Connor J, Roy SH. EMG-based measures of fatigue during a repetitive squat exercise. *IEEE Eng Med Biol Mag*. 2001 Nov-Dec;20(6):133-43. PubMed PMID: 11838245.
5. Cressey E, Fitzgerald M. *Maximum Strength: Get Your Strongest Body in 16 Weeks With the Ultimate Weight-Training Program*. Philadelphia, PA: Da Capo Lifelong; 2008.
6. Delavier F. *Strength Training Anatomy*. 3rd ed. Champaign, IL: Human Kinetics; 2010.
7. Escamilla RF. Knee biomechanics of the dynamic squat exercise. *Med Sci Sports Exerc*. 2001 Jan;33(1):127-41. Review. PubMed PMID: 11194098.
8. Gallagher, M. *The Purposeful Primitive: Using the Primordial Laws of Fitness to Trigger Inevitable, Lasting and Dramatic Physical Change*. Dragon Door Publications; 2008.
9. Hamlyn N, Behm DG, Young WB. Trunk muscle activation during dynamic weight-training exercises and isometric instability activities. *J Strength Cond Res*. 2007 Nov;21(4):1108-12. PubMed PMID: 18076231.
10. Hansen, J. *Natural Bodybuilding*. Champaign, IL: Human Kinetics; 2005.
11. Hatfield FC. *Bodybuilding: A Scientific Approach*. Chicago: Contemporary Books; 1984.
12. Hatfield FC. *Power: A Scientific Approach*. Chicago: Contemporary Books; 1989.
13. Isear JA Jr, Erickson JC, Worrell TW. EMG analysis of lower extremity muscle recruitment patterns during an unloaded squat. *Med Sci Sports Exerc*. 1997 Apr;29(4):532-9. PubMed PMID: 9107637.
14. Kinakin K. *Optimal Muscle Training*. Champaign, IL: Human Kinetics; 2009.
15. Larson GD Jr, Potteiger JA. A comparison of three different rest intervals between multiple squat bouts. *J Strength Cond Res*. 1997;11(2):115-118.
16. Matuszak ME, Fry AC, Weiss LW, Ireland TR, McKnight MM. Effect of rest interval length on repeated 1 repetition maximum back squats. *J Strength Cond Res*. 2003 Nov;17(4):634-7. PubMed PMID: 14636099.
17. McKean MR, Dunn PK, Burkett BJ. The lumbar and sacrum movement pattern during the back squat exercise. *J Strength Cond Res*. 2010 Oct;24(10):2731-41. PubMed PMID: 20885195.
18. Poliquin C. *The Poliquin Principles*. Napa, CA: Dayton Publishers & Writers Group; 1997.
19. Rippetoe M, Kilgore L. *Starting Strength: A Simple and Practical Guide for Coaching Beginners*. Wichita Falls, TX: Aasgaard; 2005.
20. Rippetoe M, Kilgore L, Pendlay G. *Practical Programming for Strength Training*. Wichita Falls, TX: Aasgaard; 2006.

21. Starr B. *The Strongest Shall Survive: Strength Training for Football*. 1st ed. Washington, DC: Fitness Products; 1978.
22. Verkhoshansky YV, Siff MC. *Supertraining*. 6th ed. Denver, CO: Supertraining International; 2003.
23. Yates D, McGough P. *A Portrait of Dorian Yates: The Life and Training Philosophy of the World's Best Bodybuilder*. HNL Publishing; 2006.
24. Zatsiorsky VM. *Science and Practice of Strength Training*. Champaign, IL: Human Kinetics; 1995.

Chapter 20

1. Aarskog R, Wisnes A, Wilhelmsen K, Skogen A, Bjordal JM. Comparison of two resistance training protocols, 6RM versus 12RM, to increase the 1RM in healthy young adults. A single-blind, randomized controlled trial. *Physiother Res Int.* 2012 Sep;17(3):179-86. PubMed PMID: 22147680.
2. Baechle TR, Earle RW, eds. *NSCA's Essentials of Strength Training and Conditioning*. 3rd ed. Champaign, IL: Human Kinetics; 2008.
3. Barnett C, et al. Effects of variation on the bench press exercise on the EMG activity of five shoulder muscles. *J Strength Cond Res.* 1995;9:222-227.
4. Bellar DM, et al. The effects of combined elastic- and free-weight tension vs. free-weight tension on 1-RM strength in the bench press. *J Strength Cond Res.* 2011;25(2):459-463.
5. Brechue WF, Mayhew JL. Upper-body work capacity and 1RM prediction are unaltered by increasing muscular strength in college football players. *J Strength Cond Res.* 2009 Dec;23(9):2477-86. PubMed PMID: 19910827.
6. Clemons JM, Aaron C. Effect of grip width on the myoelectric activity of the prime movers in the bench press. *J Strength Cond Res.* 1997;11(2):82-87.
7. Contreras B, Leahey S. The best damn bench press article period. *T-Nation.* 2011,15 Dec. Web.
8. Cressey E, Fitzgerald M. *Maximum Strength: Get Your Strongest Body in 16 Weeks With the Ultimate Weight-Training Program*. Philadelphia: Da Capo Lifelong; 2008.
9. Delavier F. *Strength Training Anatomy*. 3rd ed. Champaign, IL: Human Kinetics; 2010.
10. Duffey MJ, Challis JH. Fatigue effects on bar kinematics during the bench press. *J Strength Cond Res.* 2007;21(2):556-560.
11. Elliott BC, Wilson GJ, Kerr G. A biomechanical analysis of the sticking region in the bench press. *Medicine and Science in Sports and Exercise* 1989;21(4):450-462.
12. Gallagher, M. *The Purposeful Primitive: Using the Primordial Laws of Fitness to Trigger Inevitable, Lasting and Dramatic Physical Change.* Dragon Door Publications; 2008.
13. Ghigiarelli JJ, et al. The effects of a 7-week heavy elastic band and weight chain program on upper-body strength and upper-body power in a sample of division 1-AA football players. *J Strength Cond Res.* 2009;23(3):756-64.

14. Glass SC, and Armstrong T. Electromyographical activity of the pectoralis muscle during incline and decline bench press. *J Strength Cond Res.* 1997;11:163-167.
15. Goodman P, et al. No difference in 1RM strength and muscle activation during the barbell chest press on a stable and unstable surface. *J Strength Cond Res.* 2008;22(1):88-94.
16. Hansen J. *Natural Bodybuilding*. Champaign, IL: Human Kinetics; 2005.
17. Hatfield FC. *Bodybuilding: A Scientific Approach*. Chicago: Contemporary Books; 1984.
18. Hatfield FC. *Power: A Scientific Approach*. Chicago: Contemporary Books; 1989.
19. Kinakin K. *Optimal Muscle Training*. Champaign, IL: Human Kinetics; 2009.
20. Król H, Golas A, Sobota G. Complex analysis of movement in evaluation of flat bench press performance. *Acta Bioeng Biomech.* 2010;12(2):93-8. PubMed PMID: 20882947.
21. Lovell D, Mason D, Delphinus E, Eagles A, Shewring S, McLellan C. Does upper body strength and power influence upper body Wingate performance in men and women? *Int J Sports Med.* 2011 Oct;32(10):771-5. Epub 2011 May 26. PubMed PMID: 21618156.
22. Massey, et al. An analysis of full range of motion vs. partial range of motion training in the development of strength in untrained men. *J Strength Cond Res.* 2004;18(3):518–521.
23. Pearson SN, Cronin JB, Hume PA, Slyfield D. Kinematics and kinetics of the bench-press and bench-pull exercises in a strength-trained sporting population. *Sports Biomech.* 2009 Sep;8(3):245-54. PubMed PMID: 19891202.
24. Poliquin C. *The Poliquin Principles*. Napa, CA: Dayton Publishers & Writers Group; 1997.
25. Rhea MR, et al. Single versus multiple sets for strength: A meta-analysis to address the controversy. *Res Q Exerc Sport.* 2002;73(4):485-492.
26. Rippetoe M, Kilgore L. *Starting Strength: A Simple and Practical Guide for Coaching Beginners*. Wichita Falls, TX: Aasgaard; 2005.
27. Sakamoto A, Sinclair PJ. Muscle activations under varying lifting speeds and intensities during bench press. *Eur J Appl Physiol.* 2012 Mar;112(3):1015-25. PubMed PMID: 21735215.
28. Siegel JA, Gilders RM, Staron RS, Hagerman FC. Human muscle power output during upper- and lower-body exercises. *J Strength Cond Res.* 2002 May;16(2):173-8.
29. Starr, B. *The Strongest Shall Survive: Strength Training for Football*. 1st ed. Washington, DC: Fitness Products; 1978.
30. Tod DA, et al. "Psyching up" enhances force production during the bench press exercise. *J Strength Cond Res.* 2005;19:599-603.
31. V de Araujo Rocha, et al. Comparison among the EMG activity of the pectoralis major, anterior deltoids and triceps brachii during the bench press and peck deck exercises. *Revista Brasileira de Medicina do Esporte;* 2007.

32. Verkhoshansky YV, Siff MC. *Supertraining*. 6th ed. Denver, CO: Supertraining International; 2003.

33. Wilson JM, Loenneke JP, Jo E, Wilson GJ, Zourdos MC, Kim JS. The effects of endurance, strength, and power training on muscle fiber type shifting. *J Strength Cond Res*. 2012 Jun;26(6):1724-9. PubMed PMID: 21912291.

34. Wilson G, Elliott B, Kerr G. Bar path and force profile characteristics for maximal and submaximal loads in the bench press. *Int J Sport Biomech*. 1989;5:390-402.

35. Yates D, McGough P. *A Portrait of Dorian Yates: The Life and Training Philosophy of the World's Best Bodybuilder*. HNL Publishing; 2006.

36. Zatsiorsky VM. *Science and Practice of Strength Training*. Champaign, IL: Human Kinetics; 1995.

Chapter 21

1. Almstedt HC, Canepa JA, Ramirez DA, Shoepe TC. Changes in bone mineral density in response to 24 weeks of resistance training in college-age men and women. *J Strength Cond Res*. 2011 Apr;25(4):1098-103. PubMed PMID: 20647940.

2. Baechle TR, Earle RW, eds. *NSCA's Essentials of Strength Training and Conditioning*. 3rd ed. Champaign, IL: Human Kinetics; 2008.

3. Brown SP, Clemons JM, He Q, Liu S. Prediction of the oxygen cost of the deadlift exercise. *J Sports Sci*. 1994 Aug;12(4):371-5. PubMed PMID: 7932947.

4. Cholewicki J, McGill SM. Lumbar posterior ligament involvement during extremely heavy lifts estimated from fluoroscopic measurements. *J Biomech*. 1992 Jan;25(1):17-28. PubMed PMID: 1733981.

5. Chulvi-Medrano I, García-Massó X, Colado JC, Pablos C, de Moraes JA, Fuster MA. Deadlift muscle force and activation under stable and unstable conditions. *J Strength Cond Res*. 2010 Oct;24(10):2723-30. PubMed PMID: 20885194.

6. Cressey E, Fitzgerald M. *Maximum Strength: Get Your Strongest Body in 16 Weeks With the Ultimate Weight-Training Program*. Philadelphia: Da Capo Lifelong; 2008.

7. Delavier F. *Strength Training Anatomy*. 3rd ed. Champaign, IL: Human Kinetics; 2010.

8. Ebben WP, Feldmann CR, Dayne A, Mitsche D, Alexander P, Knetzger KJ. Muscle activation during lower body resistance training. *Int J Sports Med*. 2009 Jan;30(1):1-8. Epub 2008 Oct 30. PubMed PMID: 18975260.

9. Escamilla RF, Francisco AC, Fleisig GS, Barrentine SW, Welch CM, Kayes AV, Speer KP, Andrews JR. A three-dimensional biomechanical analysis of sumo and conventional style deadlifts. *Med Sci Sports Exerc*. 2000 Jul;32(7):1265-75. PubMed PMID: 10912892.

10. Escamilla RF, Francisco AC, Kayes AV, Speer KP, Moorman CT 3rd. An electromyographic analysis of sumo and conventional style deadlifts. *Med Sci Sports Exerc*. 2002 Apr;34(4):682-8. PubMed PMID: 11932579.

11. Fry AC, Webber JM, Weiss LW, Harber MP, Vaczi M, Pattison NA. Muscle fiber characteristics of competitive power lifters. *J Strength Cond Res*. 2003 May;17(2):402-10. PubMed PMID: 12741885.

12. Gallagher, Marty. *The Purposeful Primitive: Using the Primordial Laws of Fitness to Trigger Inevitable, Lasting and Dramatic Physical Change*. Dragon Door Publications; 2008.

13. Hales ME, Johnson BF, Johnson JT. Kinematic analysis of the powerlifting style squat and the conventional deadlift during competition: Is there a cross-over effect between lifts? *J Strength Cond Res*. 2009 Dec;23(9):2574-80. PubMed PMID: 19910816.

14. Hamlyn N, Behm DG, Young WB. Trunk muscle activation during dynamic weight-training exercises and isometric instability activities. *J Strength Cond Res*. 2007 Nov;21(4):1108-12. PubMed PMID: 18076231.

15. Hansen J. *Natural Bodybuilding*. Champaign, IL: Human Kinetics; 2005.

16. Hatfield FC. *Bodybuilding: A Scientific Approach*. Chicago: Contemporary Books; 1984,

17. Kinakin K. *Optimal Muscle Training*. Champaign, IL: Human Kinetics; 2009.

18. Poliquin C. *The Poliquin Principles*. Napa, CA: Dayton Publishers & Writers Group; 1997.

19. Rippetoe M, Kilgore L. *Starting Strength: A Simple and Practical Guide for Coaching Beginners*. Wichita Falls, TX: Aasgaard; 2005.

20. Starr B. *The Strongest Shall Survive: Strength Training for Football*. 1st ed. Washington, DC: Fitness Products; 1978.

21. Swinton PA, Stewart A, Agouris I, Keogh JW, Lloyd R. A biomechanical analysis of straight and hexagonal barbell deadlifts using submaximal loads. *J Strength Cond Res*. 2011 Jul;25(7):2000-9. PubMed PMID: 21659894.

22. Verkhoshansky YV, Siff MC. *Supertraining*. 6th ed. Denver, CO: Supertraining International; 2003.

23. Yates D, McGough P. *A Portrait of Dorian Yates: The Life and Training Philosophy of the World's Best Bodybuilder*. HNL Publishing; 2006.

24. Zatsiorsky VM. *Science and Practice of Strength Training*. Champaign, IL: Human Kinetics; 1995.

Chapter 22

1. *ACSM's Resource Manual for Guidelines for Exercise Testing and Prescription*. 3rd ed. Baltimore: Lippincott Williams & Wilkins; 1998.

2. American College of Sports Medicine. Position stand: The recommended quantity and quality of exercise for developing and maintaining cardiorespiratory and muscular fitness, and flexibility in healthy adults. *Med Sci Sports Exerc*. 1998;30(6):975-991.

3. American College of Sports Medicine. Position stand: The recommended quantity and quality of exercise for developing and maintaining cardiorespiratory and muscular fitness in healthy adults. *Med Sci Sports Exerc.* 1990;22(2):265-274.

4. Baechle TR, Earle RW, eds. *NSCA's Essentials of Strength Training and Conditioning.* 3rd ed. Champaign, IL: Human Kinetics; 2008.

5. Blair SN, Kohl HW, Barlow CE, Paffenbarger RS Jr, Gibbons LW, Macera CA. Changes in physical fitness and all-cause mortality. A prospective study of healthy and unhealthy men. *J Amer Med Assoc.* 1995;273(14):1093-1098.

6. Brooks GA, Fahey TD, White TP. *Exercise Physiology: Human Bioenergetics and Its Application.* 2nd ed. Mountain View, CA: Mayfield; 1996.

7. Burleson MA, O'Bryant HS, Stone MH, Collins MA, Triplett-McBride T. Effect of weight training exercise and treadmill exercise on post-exercise oxygen consumption. *Med Sci Sports Exerc.* 1998;30(4):518-522.

8. Costill DL, Fink WJ, Pollock ML. Muscle fiber composition and enzyme activities of elite distance runners. *Med Sci Sports Exerc.* 1976;8:96-102.

9. Dudley GA, Djamil R. Incompatibility of endurance- and strength-training modes of exercise. *J Appl Physiol.* 1985;59:1446-1451.

10. Enoka RM. Muscle strength and its development. New perspectives. *Sports Med.* 1988;6:146-168.

11. Fitts RH. Cellular mechanisms of muscle fatigue. *Physiol Rev.* 1994;49-94.

12. Fleck SJ, Kraemer WJ. *Designing Resistance Training Programs.* Champaign, IL: Human Kinetics; 1987.

13. Fletcher GF, Balady G, Blair SN, Blumenthal J, Caspersen C, Chaitman B, Epstein S, Sivarajen Froelicher ES, Froelicher VF, Pina IL, Pollock ML. Benefits and recommendations for physical activity programs for all Americans. A statement for health professionals by the Committee on Exercise and Cardiac Rehabilitation of the Council on Clinical Cardiology, American Heart Association. *Circulation.* 1996;94:857-862.

14. Gettman LR, Ward P, Hagan RD. A comparison of combined running and weight training with circuit weight training. *Med Sci Sports Exerc.* 1982;14(3):229-234.

15. Gillette CA, Bullough RC, Melby CL. Postexercise energy expenditure in response to acute aerobic or resistive exercise. *Int J Sport Nutr.* 1994;4(4):347-360.

16. Gore C, Whithers R. Effect of exercise intensity and duration on post-exercise metabolism. *J Appl Physiol.* 1990;68:2362-2368.

17. Hagerman PS. Aerobic endurance training design. In: Baechle TR, Earle RW, eds. *NSCA's Essentials of Personal Training,* Champaign, IL: Human Kinetics; 2004.

18. Henritze J, Weltman A, Schurrer RL, Barlow K. Effects of training at and above the lactate thresh-old on the lactate threshold and maximal oxygen uptake. *Eur J Appl Physiol.* 1985;54:84-88.

19. Holloszy JO, Coyle EF. Adaptations of skeletal muscle to endurance exercise and their metabolic consequences. *J Appl Physiol.* 1984;56:831-838.

20. Holly RG, Shaffrath JD. Cardiorespiratory endurance. In: Johnson EP, ed. *ACSM's Resource Manual for Guidelines for Exercise Testing and Prescription.* 3rd ed. Baltimore: Lippincott Williams & Wilkins; 1998:437-447.

21. Karvonen J. Importance of warm-up and cool-down on exercise performance. *Med Sports Sci* 1992;35:182-214.

22. Lambert EV, Bohlmann I, Cowling K. Physical activity for health: Understanding the epidemiological evidence for risk benefits. *Int Sport Med J.* 2001;1(5):1-15.

23. McArdle WO, Katch FI, Katch VL. In: *Exercise Physiology: Energy, Nutrition, and Human Performance.* 3rd ed. Philadelphia: Lea & Febiger; 1991.

24. National Institutes of Health: Consensus Development Panel on Physical Activity and Cardiovascular Health. Physical activity and cardiovascular health. *J Amer Med Assoc.* 1996;276:214-246.

25. Nieman DC. *Exercise Testing and Prescription.* 5th ed. Boston: McGraw-Hill; 2003.

26. Pollock ML, Wilmore JH. *Exercise in Health and Disease: Evaluation and Prescription for Prevention and Rehabilitation.* 2nd ed. Philadelphia: Saunders; 1990.

27. Potteiger JA. Aerobic endurance exercise training. In: Baechle TR, Earle RW, eds. *NSCA's Essentials of Strength Training and Conditioning.* 2nd ed. Champaign, IL: Human Kinetics; 2000:495-509.

28. Powers SK, Howley ET. *Exercise Physiology: Theory and Application to Fitness and Performance.* 6th ed. New York: McGraw-Hill; 2006.

29. Saltin B, Henriksson J, Nygaard E, Andersen P. Fiber types and metabolic potentials of skeletal muscles in sedentary man and endurance runners. In: Milvy P, ed. *Marathon: Physiological, Medical, Epidemiological, and Psychological Studies.* New York: New York Academy of Sciences; 1977:3-29.

30. Sharkey BJ. Intensity and duration of training and the development of cardiorespiratory fitness. *Med Sci Sports Exerc.* 1970;2:197-202.

31. Swain DP, Abernathy KS, Smith CS, Lee SJ, Bunn SA. Target heart rates for the development of cardiorespiratory fitness. *Med Sci Sports Exerc.* 1994;26:112-116.

32. U.S. Department of Health and Human Services. *Physical Activity and Health: A Report of the Surgeon General.* Atlanta, GA: Centers for Disease Control and Prevention; 1996.

33. Velasquez KS, Wilmore JH. Changes in cardiorespiratory fitness and body composition after a 12-week bench step training program. *Med Sci Sports Exerc.* 1993;24(Suppl):S78.

34. Verkhoshansky YV, Siff MC. *Supertraining.* 6th ed. Denver, CO: Supertraining International; 2003.

35. Whaley MH, Kaminsky LA, Dwyer GB, Getchell LH, Norton LA. Predictors of over- and underachievement of age-predicted maximal heart rate. *Med Sci Sports Exerc.* 1992;24(10):1173-1179.
36. Wilmore JH, Costill DL. *Physiology of Sport and Exercise.* 3rd ed. Champaign, IL: Human Kinetics; 2005.

Chapter 23
1. Alter MJ. *Science of Flexibility.* 2nd ed. Champaign, IL: Human Kinetics; 1996.
2. Andersen JC. Stretching before and after exercise: Effect on muscle soreness and injury risk. *J Athl Train.* 2005;40(3):218-220.
3. Anthony CP, Koltboff NJ. *Textbook of Anatomy and Physiology.* 9th ed. St. Louis, MO: Mosby; 1975.
4. Baechle TR, Earle RW, eds. *NSCA's Essentials of Personal Training.* Champaign, IL: Human Kinetics; 2004.
5. Baechle TR, Earle RW, eds. *NSCA's Essentials of Strength Training and Conditioning.* 3rd ed. Champaign, IL: Human Kinetics; 2008.
6. Beaulieu JA. Developing a stretching program. *Physician Sports Med.* 1981;9:59-69.
7. Behm DG, Bambury A, Cahill F, Power K. Effect of acute static stretching on force, balance, reaction time, and movement time. *Med Sci Sports Exerc.* 2004;36(8):1397-1402.
8. Bourne G. The basic facts about flexibility in a nutshell. *Modern Athlete and Coach.* 1995;33(2):3-4,35.
9. Church JB, Wiggins MS, Moode FM, Crist R. Effect of warm-up and flexibility treatments on vertical jump performance. *J Strength Cond Res.* 2001;15(3):332-336.
10. Cornwell A, Nelson AG, Sideaway B. Acute effects of stretching on the neuromuscular properties of the triceps surae muscle complex. *Eur J Appl Physiol.* 2002;86(5):428-434.
11. Davis DS, Ashby PE, McCale KL, McQuain JA, Wine JM. The effectiveness of 3 stretching techniques on hamstring flexibility using consistent stretching parameters. *J Strength Cond Res.* 2005;19(1):27-32. PubMed PMID: 15705041.
12. DiNubile N, ed. Scientific, medical, and practical aspects of stretching. In: *Clinics in Sports Medicine.* Philadelphia: Saunders; 1991:63-86.
13. Enoka RM. *Neuromechanics of Human Movement.* 3rd ed. Champaign, IL: Human Kinetics; 2001.
14. Evjenth O, Hamburg J. *Muscle Stretching in Manual Therapy—A Clinical Manual.* Alfta, Sweden: Alfta Rehab; 1984.
15. Fleck SJ, Kraemer WJ. *Designing Resistance Training Programs.* 3rd ed. Champaign, IL: Human Kinetics; 2003.
16. Fradkin AJ, Gabbe BJ, Cameron PA. Does warming up prevent injury in sport: The evidence from randomized controlled trials. *J Sci Med Sport.* 2006;9(3):214-220.

17. Gambetta V. Stretching the truth: The fallacies of flexibility. *Sports Coach.* 1997;20(3):7-9.
18. Gleim GW, McHugh MP. Flexibility and its effects on sports injury and performance [review]. *Sports Med.* 1997;24(5):289-299.
19. Gremion G. Is stretching for sports performance still useful? A review of the literature. *Rev Med Suisse.* 2005;27(28):1830-1834.
20. Herbert RD, Gabriel M. Effects of stretching before and after exercise on muscle soreness and risk of injury: A systematic review. *Br Med J.* 2002;325:468-470.
21. Hoffman J. *Physiological Aspects of Sports Performance and Training.* Champaign, IL: Human Kinetics; 2002.
22. Holcomb WR. Improved stretching with proprioceptive neuromuscular facilitation. *Nat Strength Cond Assoc J.* 2000;22(1):59-61.
23. Johansson PH, Lindstrom L, Sundelin G, Lindstrom B. The effects of pre-exercise stretching on muscular soreness, tenderness and force loss following heavy eccentric exercise. *Scand J Med Sci Sports.* 1999;9(4):219-225.
24. Kurz T. *Stretching Scientifically: A Guide to Flexibility Training.* 4th ed. Island Pond, VT: Stadion; 2003.
25. Leighton JR. A study of the effect of progressive weight training on flexibility. *J Assoc Phys Ment Rehabil.* 1964;18:101.
26. Mann DP, Jones MT. Guidelines to the implementation of a dynamic stretching program. *Strength Cond J.* 1999;21(6):53-55.
27. McAtee RE, Charland J. *Facilitated Stretching.* 3rd ed. Champaign, IL: Human Kinetics; 2007.
28. Nino, J. When could stretching be harmful? *Strength Cond J.* 1999;21(5):57-58.
29. Poterfield J, DeRosa C. *Mechanical Low Back Pain: Perspectives in Functional Anatomy.* Philadelphia: Saunders; 1991.
30. Shrier I. Does stretching improve performance? A systematic and critical review of the literature (review). *Clin J Sport Med.* 2004;14(5):267-273.
31. Starr B. *The Strongest Shall Survive: Strength Training for Football.* 1st ed. Washington, DC: Fitness Products; 1978.
32. Thomas M. The functional warm-up. *Strength Cond J.* 2000;22(2):51-53.
33. Verkhoshansky YV, Siff MC. *Supertraining.* 6th ed. Denver, CO: Supertraining International; 2003.

Chapter 24
1. Allerheilegen B, Rogers R. Plyometrics program design. *Strength Cond.* 1995;17(4):26-31.
2. Baechle TR, Earle RW, eds. *NSCA's Essentials of Strength Training and Conditioning.* 3rd ed. Champaign, IL: Human Kinetics; 2008.
3. Banister EW. Modeling elite athletic performance. In: MacDougall JD, Wenger HA, Green HJ, eds. *Physiological Testing of the High-Performance Athlete.* Champaign, IL: Human Kinetics; 1991:403-424.

4. Blattner S, Noble L. Relative effects of isokinetic and plyometric training on vertical jumping performance. *Res Q.* 1979;50(4):583-88.

5. Bosco C, Vittori C. Biomechanical characteristics of sprint running during maximal and supramaximal speed. *New Stud Athlet.* 1986;1(1):39-45.

6. Brown LE, Ferrigno VA, Santana JC. *Training for Speed, Agility, and Quickness.* Champaign, IL: Human Kinetics; 2000.

7. Chu D. Plyometrics: The link between strength and speed. *Nat Strength Cond Assoc J.* 1983;5(2):20-21.

8. Chu D, Korchemny R. Sprinting stride actions: Analysis and evaluation. *Nat Strength Cond Assoc J.* 1989;(6):6-8,82-85.

9. Delecluse C. Influence of strength training on sprint running performance: Current findings and implications for training. *Sports Med.* 1997 Sep;24(3):147-156. Review. PubMed PMID: 9327528.

10. Dintiman GB, Ward RD, and Tellez T. *Sports Speed.* Champaign, IL: Human Kinetics; 1998.

11. Faccioni A. Assisted and resisted methods for speed development (part 1). *Mod Athlete Coach.* 1994;32(2):3-6.

12. Harland MJ, Steele JR. Biomechanics of the sprint start. *Sports Med.* 1997;23(1):11-20.

13. Harre D, ed. *Principles of Sports Training.* Berlin: Sportverlag; 1982.

14. Hochmuth G. *Biomechanics of Athletic Movement.* 4th ed. Berlin: Sportverlag; 1984.

15. Kawamori N, Haff GG. The optimal training load for the development of muscular power. *J Strength Cond Res.* 2004;18(3):675-684.

16. Kozlov I, Muravyev V. Muscles and the sprint. *Sov Sports Rev.* 1992:27(6):192-195.

17. Leierer S. A guide for sprint training. *Athlet J.* 1979;59(6):105-106.

18. National Strength and Conditioning Association. Position statement: Explosive/plyometric exercises. *Nat Strength Cond Assoc J.* 1993;15(3):16.

19. Newton RU, Kraemer WJ. Developing explosive muscular power: Implications for a mixed methods training strategy. *Strength Cond.* 1994;16(5):20-31.

20. Plisk SS. The angle on agility. *Training Cond.* 2000;10(6):37-43.

21. Romanova N. The sprint: Nontraditional means of training (a review of scientific studies). *Soviet Sports Review.* 1990;25(2):99-102.

22. Schmidt RA, Wrisberg CA. *Motor Learning and Performance.* 4th ed. Champaign, IL: Human Kinetics; 2007.

23. Siff MC. *Supertraining.* 6th ed. Denver: Supertraining Institute; 2003.

24. Thorstensson A. Speed and acceleration. In: Dirix A, Knuttgen HG, Tittel K, eds. *The Olympic Book of Sports Medicine.* Oxford: Blackwell Scientific; 1991:218-229.

25. Verkhoshansky Y, Tatyan V. Speed-strength preparation of future champions. *Soviet Sports Review* 1983;18(4):166-170.

26. Verkhoshansky YV. Principles for a rational organization of the training process aimed at speed development. *New Stud Athlet.* 1996;11(2-3):155-160.

27. Verkhoshansky YV. Quickness and velocity in sports movements. *New Stud Athlet.* 1996;11(2-3):29-37.

28. Verkhoshansky YV, Siff MC. *Supertraining.* 6th ed. Denver: Supertraining International; 2003.

29. Wilson GJ, Murphy AJ, Giorgi A. Weight and plyometric training: Effects on eccentric and concentric force production. *Can J Appl Physiol.* 1996;21:301-315.

30. Zatsiorsky VM, Kraemer WJ. *Science and Practice of Strength Training.* 2nd ed. Champaign, IL: Human Kinetics; 2006.

Chapter 25

1. American College of Sports Medicine. Position stand: The recommended quantity and quality of exercise for developing and maintaining cardiorespiratory and muscular fitness in healthy adults. *Med Sci Sports Exerc.* 1990;22:265-274.

2. Baechle TR, Earle RW, eds. *NSCA's Essentials of Strength Training and Conditioning.* 3rd ed. Champaign, IL: Human Kinetics; 2008.

3. Behm DG, Anderson K, Curnew RS. Muscle force and activation under stable and unstable conditions. *J Strength Cond Res.* 2002;16(3):416-22.

4. Bompa TO. *Theory and Methodology of Training.* Dubuque, IA: Kendall/Hunt; 1983.

5. Clark MA. *Integrated Training for the New Millennium.* Thousand Oaks, CA: National Academy of Sports Medicine; 2001.

6. Cressey EM, West CA, Tiberio DP, Kraemer WJ, Maresh CM. The effects of ten weeks of lower-body unstable surface training on markers of athletic performance. *J Strength Cond Res.* 2007 May;21(2):561-7. PubMed PMID: 17530966.

7. Duval J. Traditional and unique approaches to strength training programs. *Strength Cond.* 1998;20(5):28-29.

8. Enoka RM. *Neuromechanical Basis of Kinesiology.* 2nd ed. Champaign, IL: Human Kinetics; 1994.

9. Fleck SJ, Kraemer WJ. *Designing Resistance Training Programs.* 2nd ed. Champaign, IL: Human Kinetics; 1997.

10. Fleck SJ. Periodized strength training: A critical review. *J Strength Cond Res.* 1999;13(1):82-89.

11. Gillam GM. Effects of frequency of weight training on muscle strength enhancement. *J Sports Med Phys Fitness.* 1981;21:432-436.

12. Harman E, Johnson M, Frykman P. CSCS coaches' school: Program design: A movement-oriented approach to exercise prescription. *Nat Strength Cond Assoc J.* 1992;14(1):47-54.

13. Jones A. *Nautilus Training Principles*. Bulletin No. 2. Deland, FL: Nautilus; 1971.

14. Matveyev LP. *Periodization of Sports Training*. Moscow: Fizkultura i Sport; 1966.

15. Mentzer M, Little J. *High-Intensity Training the Mike Mentzer Way*. Chicago: Contemporary Books; 2003.

16. Pauletto B. Choice and order of exercise. *Nat Strength Cond Assoc J*. 1986;8(2):71-73.

17. Philbin J. *High-Intensity Training*. Champaign, IL: Human Kinetics; 2004.

18. Stone MH, Collins D, Plisk S, Haff G, Stone ME. Training principles: Evaluation of modes and methods of resistance training. *Strength Cond J*. 2000;22(3):65-76.

19. Verkhoshansky YV, Siff MC. *Supertraining*. 6th ed. Denver, CO: Supertraining International; 2003.

20. Yates D, McGough P. *A Portrait of Dorian Yates: The Life and Training Philosophy of the World's Best Bodybuilder*. HNL Publishing; 2006.

21. Zatsiorsky VM. *Science and Practice of Strength Training*. Champaign, IL: Human Kinetics; 1995.

Chapter 26

1. American Academy of Pediatrics. Strength training by children and adolescents. *Pediatr*. 2001;107:1470-1472.

2. *ACSM's Exercise Management for Persons With Chronic Diseases and Disabilities*. 2nd ed. Champaign, IL: Human Kinetics; 2003.

3. *ACSM's Guidelines for Graded Exercise and Prescription*. 6th ed. Philadelphia: Lippincott Williams & Wilkins; 2000.

4. American Academy of Pediatrics. Strength training by children and adolescents. *Pediatr*. 2001;107:1470-1472.

5. American College of Obstetricians and Gynecologists. Exercise during pregnancy and the postpartum period. *Int J Gynecol Obstet*. 2002;77:79-81.

6. American College of Sports Medicine. Exercise and physical activity for older adults. *Med Sci Sports Exerc*. 1998;30:992-1008.

7. Arendt E, Dick R. Knee injury patterns among men and women in collegiate basketball and soccer: NCAA data and review of literature. *Am J Sports Med*. 1995;23:694-701.

8. Baechle TR, Earle RW, eds. *NSCA's Essentials of Strength Training and Conditioning*. 3rd ed. Champaign, IL: Human Kinetics; 2008.

9. Blimkie C. Benefits and risks of resistance training in youth. In: Cahill B, Pearl A, eds. *Intensive Participation in Children's Sports*. Champaign, IL: Human Kinetics; 1993:133-167.

10. British Association of Exercise and Sport Sciences. BASES position statement on guidelines for resistance exercise in young people. *J Sport Sci*. 2004;22:383-390.

11. Campbell W, Crim M, Young V, Evans W. Increased energy requirements and changes in body composition with resistance training in older adults. *Am J Clin Nutr*. 1994;60:167-175.

12. Cheung L, Richmond J, eds. *Child Health, Nutrition and Physical Activity*. Champaign, IL: Human Kinetics; 1995.

13. Christmas C, Andersen R. Exercise and older patients. Guidelines for the clinician. *J Am Geriatr Soc*. 2000;48:318-324.

14. Conley M, Rozeneck R. Health aspects of resistance exercise and training: NSCA position statement. *Strength Cond J*. 2001;23(6):9-23.

15. Corbin C, Pangrazi R, Welk G. Toward an understanding of appropriate physical activity levels of youth. *Physical Activity and Fitness Research Digest*. 1994;1(8):1-8.

16. De Loes M, Dahlstedt L, Thomee R. A 7-year study on risks and costs of knee injuries in male and female youth participants in 12 sports. *Scand J Med Sci Sports*. 2000;10:90-97.

17. Drinkwater B. Weight-bearing exercise and bone mass. *Phys Med Rehabill Clin N Am*. 1995;6:567-578.

18. Evans W. Exercise training guidelines for the elderly. *Med Sci Sports Exerc*. 1999;31:12-17.

19. Faigenbaum A, Kraemer W, Cahill B, Chandler J, Dziados J, Elfrink L, Forman E, Gaudiose M, Micheli L, Nitka M, Roberts S. Youth resistance training: Position statement paper and literature review. *Strength Cond J*. 1996;18:62-75.

20. Faigenbaum A. Strength training for children and adolescents. *Clin Sports Med*. 2000;19:593-619.

21. Faigenbaum A, Westcott W. *Strength and Power for Young Athletes*. Champaign, IL: Human Kinetics; 2000.

22. Faigenbaum A, Kraemer W, Cahill B, Chandler J, Dziados J, Elfrink L, Forman E, Gaudiose M, Micheli L, Nitka M, Roberts S. Youth resistance training: Position statement paper and literature review. *Strength Cond J*. 1996;18:62-75.

23. Falk B, Eliakim A. Resistance training, skeletal muscle and growth. *Pediatr Endocrinol Rev*. 2003;1:120-127.

24. Frontera W, Meredith C, O'Reilly K, Knuttgen H, Evans W. Strength conditioning in older men: Skeletal muscle hypertrophy and improved function. *J App Physiol*. 1988;64:1038-1044.

25. George D, Stakiw K, Wright C. Fatal accident with weightlifting equipment: Implications for safety standards. *Can Med Assoc J*. 1989;140:925-926.

26. Haff GG. Roundtable discussion: Youth resistance training. *Strength Cond J*. 2003;25(1):49-64.

27. Henwood T, Taaffe D. Improved physical performance in older adults undertaking a short-term programme of high-velocity resistance training. *Gerontology*. 2005;51:108-115.

28. Hurley B, Hagberg J. Optimizing health in older persons: Aerobic or strength training? In: J. Holloszy, ed. *Exercise and Sport Sciences Reviews*. Philadelphia: Wilkins & Wilkins; 1998: 61-89.

29. Karlsson M, Vergnaud P, Delmas P, Obrant K. Indicators of bone formation in weight lifters. *Calc Tiss Int*. 1995;56:177-180.

30. Kraemer W, Mazzetti S, Nindl B, Gotshalk L, Bush J, Marx J, Dohi K, Gomez A, Miles M, Fleck S, Newton R, Häkkinen K. Effect of resistance training on women's strength/power and occupational performances. *Med Sci Sports Exerc*. 2001;33:1011-1025.

31. Lauback L. Comparative muscle strength of men and women: A review of the literature. *Aviat Space Environ Med*. 1976;47:534-542.

32. MacRae P, Feltner M, Reinsch S. A 1-year exercise program for women: Effect on falls, injury and physical performance. *J Aging Phys Act*. 1994;2:127-142.

33. Malina RM, Bouchard C, Bar-Or O. *Growth, Maturation, and Physical Activity*. 2nd ed. Champaign, IL: Human Kinetics; 2004.

34. McCartney N, Hicks A, Martin J, Webber C. A longitudinal trial of weight training in the elderly-continued improvements in year two. *J Gerontol A-Biol*. 1996;51:B425-B433.

35. Menkes A, Mazel S, Redmond R, Koffler K, Libanati C, Gunberg C, Zizic T, Hagberg J, Pratley R, Hurley B. Strength training increases regional bone mineral density and bone remodeling in middle-aged and older men. *J Appl Physiol*. 1993;74:2478-2484.

36. Micheli L. Strength training in the young athlete. In: Brown E, Branta C, eds. *Competitive Sports for Children and Youth*. Champaign, IL: Human Kinetics; 1988:99-105.

37. Miller A, MacDougall J, Tarnopolsky M, Sale D. Gender differences in strength and muscle fiber characteristics. *Eur J Appl Physiol*. 1992;66:254-262.

38. Myers A, Young Y, Langlois J. Prevention of falls in the elderly. *Bone*. 1996;18(Suppl):87S-101S.

39. National Association for Sport and Physical Education. *Physical Activity for Children: A Statement of Guidelines*. Reston, VA: NASPE; 1998.

40. National Strength and Conditioning Association. Strength training for female athletes. *Nat Strength Cond Assoc J*. 1989;11:43-55,29-36.

41. Orr R, de Vos N, Singh N, Ross D, Stavrinos T, Fiatarone Singh M. Power training improves balance in healthy older adults. *J Gerontal A Biol Sci Med Sci*. 2006;61:78-85.

42. Payne V, Morrow J, Johnson L. Resistance training in children and youth: A meta-analysis. *Res Q Exerc Sport*. 1997;68:80-89.

43. Rians C, Weltman A, Cahill B, Janney C, Tippitt S, Katch FI. Strength training for prepubescent males: Is it safe? *Am J Sports Med*. 1987;15:483-489.

44. Roos RJ. The Surgeon General's report: A prime source for exercise advocates. *Phys Sportsmed*. 1997;25(4):122-131.

45. Sallis JF, Patrick K, Long BJ. Overview of the International Consensus Conference on Physical Activity Guidelines for Adolescents. *Pediatr Exerc Sci*. 1994;6:299-301.

46. Snow-Harter C, Bouxsein M, Lewis B, Carter D, Marcus R. Effects of resistance and endurance exercise on bone mineral status of young women. A randomized exercise intervention trial. *J Bone Mineral Res*. 1992;7:761-769.

47. Taunton J, Martin A, Rhodes E, Wolski L, Donnelly M, Elliot J. Exercise for older women: Choosing the right prescription. *Br J Sports Med*. 1997;31:5-10.

48. United States Department of Health and Human Services. *Healthy People 2010: Understanding and Improving Health*. 2nd ed. Washington, DC: U.S. Government Printing Office; 2000.

49. Volek J, Forsythe C, Kraemer W. Nutritional aspects of women strength athletes. *Br J Sports Med*. 2006;40:742-748.

50. West R. The female athlete: The triad of disordered eating, amenorrhea and osteoporosis. *Sports Med*. 1998;26:63-71.

51. Westcott WL, Baechle TR. *Strength Training for Seniors*. Champaign, IL: Human Kinetics; 1999:1-2.

52. Wikkinen K, Häkkinen A. Muscle cross-sectional area, force production and relaxation characteristics in women at different ages. *Eur J Appl Physiol*. 1991.62:410-414.

Chapter 27

1. Anderson MK, Hall SJ, eds. *Fundamentals of Sports Injury Management*. Baltimore: Lippincott Williams & Wilkins; 1997.

2. Arrington ED, Miller MD. Skeletal muscle injuries. *Orthop Clin North Am*. 1995;26(3):411-422.

3. Baechle TR, Earle RW, eds. *NSCA's Essentials of Strength Training and Conditioning*. 3rd ed. Champaign, IL: Human Kinetics; 2008.

4. Barrett GR, Noojin FK, Hartzog CW, Nash CR. Reconstruction of the anterior cruciate ligament in females: A comparison of hamstring versus patellar tendon autograft. *Arthroscopy*. 2002;18(1):46-54.

5. Chaitow L. *Cranial Manipulation Theory and Practice: Osseous and Soft Tissue Approaches*. London: Churchill Livingstone; 1999.

6. De Lorme TL. Restoration of muscle power by heavy resistance exercise. *J Bone Joint Surg*. 1945;27:645-667.

7. Ellenbecker TS, Davies GJ. *Closed Kinetic Chain Rehabilitation*. Champaign, IL: Human Kinetics; 2001.

8. Fleck SJ, Kraemer WJ. *Designing Resistance Training Programs*. 3rd ed. Champaign, IL: Human Kinetics; 2003.

9. Gross ML, Brenner SL, Esformes I, Sonzogni JJ. Anterior shoulder instability in weight lifters. *Am J Sport Med*. 1993;21(4):599-603.

10. Gross MT. Chronic tendinitis: Pathomechanics of injury, factors affecting the healing response, and treatment. *J Orthop Sport Phys*. 1992;16(6):248-261.

11. Häkkinen A, Sokka T, Kotaniemi A, Hannonen P. A randomized two-year study of the effects of dynamic strength training on muscle strength, disease activity, functional capacity, and bone mineral density in early rheumatoid arthritis. *Arthritis Rheum.* 2001;44(3):515-522.

12. Kibler WB. The role of the scapula in athletic shoulder function. *Am J Sport Med.* 1998;26:325-337.

13. Kovaleski JE, Gurchiek LR, Spriggs DH. Musculoskeletal injuries: Risks, prevention and care. In: American College of Sports Medicine, ed. *ACSM's Resource Manual for Guidelines for Exercise Testing and Prescription.* 3rd ed. Baltimore: Lippincott Williams & Wilkins; 1998.

14. Leadbetter WB. Cell-matrix response in tendon injury. *Clin Sport Med.* 1992;11:533-578.

15. Liebenson C. Active rehabilitation protocols. In: Liebenson C, ed. *Rehabilitation of the Spine.* Baltimore: Lippincott Williams & Wilkins; 1996.

16. Mense S, Simons DG. *Muscle Pain. Understanding its Nature, Diagnosis, and Treatment.* Philadelphia: Lippincott Williams & Wilkins; 2001.

17. Parsons IM, Apreleva M, Fu FH, Woo SL. The effect of rotator cuff tears on reaction forces at the glenohumeral joint. *J Orthopaed Res.* 2002;20(3, May):439-446.

18. Potach DH, Borden R. Rehabilitation and reconditioning. In: Baechle TR, Earle RW, eds. *NSCA's Essentials of Strength Training and Conditioning.* 2nd ed. Champaign, IL: Human Kinetics; 2000.

19. Tippett SR. *Coaches Guide to Sport Rehabilitation.* Champaign, IL: Leisure Press; 1990.

20. Verkhoshansky YV, Siff MC. *Supertraining.* 6th ed. Denver, CO: Supertraining International; 2003.

21. Zatsiorsky VM. *Science and Practice of Strength Training.* Champaign, IL: Human Kinetics; 1995.

Index

Note: The italicized *f* and *t* following page numbers refer to figures and tables, respectively.

About the Author

Tim Henriques has been with the National Personal Training Institute (NPTI) since its inception and serves as the director of NPTI Virginia, Maryland, and DC. Before working with NPTI he was a full-time personal trainer, working with the companies One to One Fitness and Fitness Image and Results before running his own business. He continues to train clients and work with athletes outside of NPTI as well as write and lecture on health and fitness.

Henriques has been competing in powerlifting for two decades and has made several notable accomplishments in that sport. He was a collegiate All-American powerlifter and set many state and national records. He set the Virginia state record for the deadlift by lifting 700 pounds at a body weight of 198 pounds. He set the national record for the strict curl in 2013. He currently coaches a powerlifting team called Team Force, who won the Federation Championships in 2011 and 2013. He has also competed in arm wrestling and strongman competitions. He is lifetime drug free.

Henriques earned his degree in kinesiology, along with minors in coaching and psychology, from James Madison University. He was born and raised in Fairfax County, Virginia, where he resides with his wife, Christina; their boys Nathan, Ryan, and Collin; and their dog, Pongo.

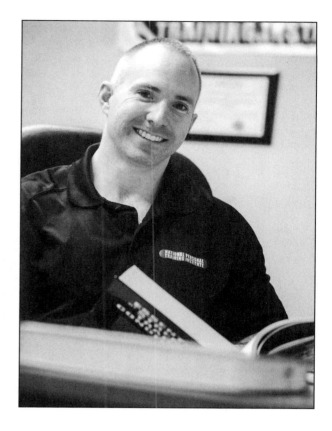

About NPTI

NPTI MISSION STATEMENT

As the nation's largest system of schools devoted to personal training, The National Personal Training Institute's (NPTI) mission is to prepare its students to become personal trainers and fitness professionals. NPTI strongly believes that self-study and online courses are not sufficient to become a qualified personal trainer and instead advocates that personal trainers need to partake in a formal education program that is approved by the Department of Education. Our graduates are ready to enter the work force and benefit the community as they are well versed in the scope of practice for personal trainers and knowledgeable on the subjects of health and fitness related to personal training. We strive to provide a high quality and worthwhile education experience that each student values and would recommend to their peers.

WHO WE ARE

The **National Personal Training Institute** (NPTI), founded in 2000, was created to raise the standard in personal training education. Acknowledging that the current state of online personal training courses were wanted, NPTI developed a comprehensive system to provide the necessary education to ensure that personal trainers were not only certified but also qualified. NPTI is an actual school for personal trainers—students attend classes, listen to lectures, complete homework, take tests, and participate in extensive practical-based, hands-on workshops. Students are taught both the art and science of personal training. NPTI currently has over 30 campuses throughout the United States and Canada. Businesses appreciate the in-depth education and practical experience that our graduates have, and they appreciate those students that choose to go above and beyond with their fitness education by attending NPTI. Thousands of students graduate from NPTI every year and go on to work in commercial fitness settings, rehab centers, weight loss clinics, personal training studios, and collegiate athletic centers; many graduates go on to operate their own personal training-based businesses as well.

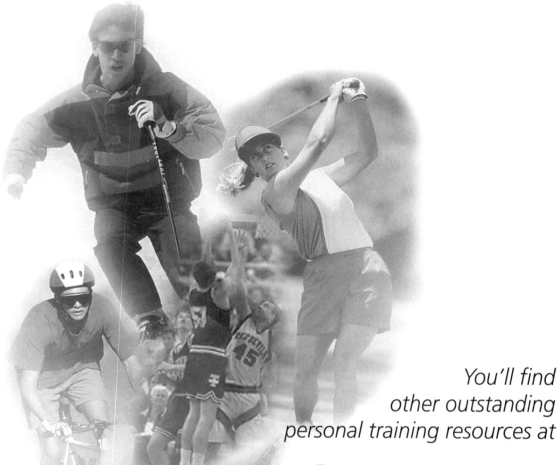